THIRD EDITION

Chemotherapy and Biotherapy Guidelines and Recommendations for Practice

EDITED BY
MARTHA POLOVICH, MN, RN, AOCN®
JULIE M. WHITFORD, RN, BSN, OCN®
MIKAELA OLSEN, RN, MS, OCN®

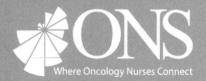

ONS
Where Oncology Nurses Connect

ONCOLOGY NURSING SOCIETY
PITTSBURGH, PA

ONS Publishing Division

Publisher: Leonard Mafrica, MBA, CAE
Director, Commercial Publishing: Barbara Sigler, RN, MNEd
Managing Editor: Lisa M. George, BA
Technical Content Editor: Angela D. Klimaszewski, RN, MN
Staff Editor: Amy Nicoletti, BA
Copy Editor: Laura Pinchot, BA
Graphic Designer: Dany Sjoen

Chemotherapy and Biotherapy Guidelines and Recommendations for Practice (Third Edition)

Library of Congress Control Number: 2009921267

ISBN: 978-1-890504-81-6

Publisher's Note

This book is published by the Oncology Nursing Society (ONS). ONS neither represents nor guarantees that the practices described herein will, if followed, ensure safe and effective patient care. The recommendations contained in this book reflect ONS's judgment regarding the state of general knowledge and practice in the field as of the date of publication. The recommendations may not be appropriate for use in all circumstances. Those who use this book should make their own determinations regarding specific safe and appropriate patient-care practices, taking into account the personnel, equipment, and practices available at the hospital or other facility at which they are located. The editors and publisher cannot be held responsible for any liability incurred as a consequence from the use or application of any of the contents of this book. Figures and tables are used as examples only. They are not meant to be all-inclusive, nor do they represent endorsement of any particular institution by ONS. Web sites mentioned are provided for information only; the hosts are responsible for their own content and availability. Unless otherwise indicated, dollar amounts reflect U.S. dollars.

Mention of specific products and opinions related to those products do not indicate or imply endorsement by ONS.

ONS publications are originally published in English. Publishers wishing to translate ONS publications must contact the ONS Publishing Division about licensing arrangements. ONS publications cannot be translated without obtaining written permission from ONS. (Individual tables and figures that are reprinted or adapted require additional permission from the original source.) Because translations from English may not always be accurate or precise, ONS disclaims any responsibility for inaccuracies in words or meaning that may occur as a result of the translation. Readers relying on precise information should check the original English version.

Printed in the United States of America

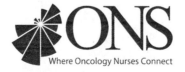

Oncology Nursing Society
Integrity • Innovation • Stewardship • Advocacy • Excellence • Inclusiveness

Contributors

Editors

Martha Polovich, MN, RN, AOCN®
Associate Director, Clinical Practice
Duke Oncology Network
Durham, North Carolina
Safe Handling; Flare Reaction; Irritation; Acute Infusion Reactions

Julie M. Whitford, RN, BSN, OCN®
Clinical Nurse Liaison
Amgen Inc.
Tulsa, Oklahoma
Myelosuppression: Anemia and Thrombocytopenia; Fatigue

MiKaela Olsen, RN, MS, OCN®
Oncology and Bone Marrow Transplant Clinical Nurse Specialist
The Sidney Kimmel Comprehensive Cancer Center at Johns Hopkins Hospital
Baltimore, Maryland
Gastrointestinal and Mucosal Side Effects; Alopecia

Authors

Cheryl D. Bednar-Gilbert, RN, OCN®, BS
Nurse Educator
Cancer Care Associates
Oklahoma City, Oklahoma
Cutaneous Toxicity

Carol Stein Blecher, RN, MS, AOCN®, APNC
Advanced Practice Nurse/Clinical Educator
Trinitas Comprehensive Cancer Center
Elizabeth, New Jersey
Care of the Patient Receiving Cancer Therapy

Paul F. Davis, MSN, RN-C, AOCNS®
Oncology Clinical Nurse Specialist
Duke Raleigh Hospital
Raleigh, North Carolina
Ocular Toxicity

Seth Eisenberg, RN, ADN, OCN®
Professional Practice Coordinator, Infusion Services
Seattle Cancer Care Alliance
Seattle, Washington
Cancer Therapy Goals and Response

Joanne P. Finley, RN, MS
Patient Education Coordinator
The Sidney Kimmel Comprehensive Cancer Center at Johns Hopkins Hospital
Baltimore, Maryland
Anorexia

Cindy Jo Horrell, MS, AOCN®
Oncology Nurse Practitioner
Lakeland Regional Cancer Center
Lakeland, Florida
Hepatotoxicity; Pancreatitis

Catherine Jansen, RN, PhD, OCN®
Oncology Clinical Nurse Specialist
Kaiser Permanente Medical Center
San Francisco, California
Cancer Treatment–Related Cognitive Changes

Anne Katz, RN, PhD
Clinical Nurse Specialist
CancerCare Manitoba
Winnipeg, Manitoba
Canada
Alterations in Sexuality; Reproductive Alterations

Alice S. Kerber, MN, RN, AOCN®
Clinical Nurse Specialist, Cancer Screening and Genetics
Saint Joseph's Hospital
Atlanta, Georgia
Ethical Issues Related to Cancer Therapy; Legal Issues Related to Cancer Therapy

Kristine B. LeFebvre, MSN, RN, AOCN®
Project Manager, Education Team
Oncology Nursing Society
Pittsburgh, Pennsylvania
Nursing Education and Management

Pamela J. Malloy, MN, RN, OCN®
End-of-Life Nursing Education Consortium (ELNEC)
    Project Director
American Association of Colleges of Nursing
Washington, District of Columbia
*Definition of Cancer; Treatment Modalities; The Drug
Development Process*

Paula M. Muehlbauer, RN, MSN, OCN®
(at the time of this writing)
Clinical Nurse Specialist
National Institutes of Health
Bethesda, Maryland
(at the time of publication)
Clinical Nurse Specialist, VA Nursing Academy
VA San Diego Healthcare System
San Diego, California
Principles of Antineoplastic Therapy

Lisa Schulmeister, RN, MN, APRN-BC, OCN®, FAAN
Oncology Nursing Consultant
River Ridge, Louisiana
Extravasation

Nonniekaye Shelburne, RN, MS, AOCN®, CRNP
Clinical Nurse Specialist
National Institutes of Health
Bethesda, Maryland
Principles of Antineoplastic Therapy

Brenda K. Shelton, MS, RN, CCRN, AOCN®
Clinical Nurse Specialist
The Sidney Kimmel Comprehensive Cancer Center at
    Johns Hopkins Hospital
Baltimore, Maryland
Cardiovascular Toxicity; Pulmonary Toxicity

Stephanie Shields, PharmD
Pharmacy Manager
Peachtree Hematology and Oncology Consultants
Atlanta, Georgia
Table 5. Characteristics of Cytotoxic Agents

Janice L. Skinner, CRNP
Nurse Practitioner, Program Coordinator
Bone Marrow Transplant
The Sidney Kimmel Comprehensive Cancer Center at
    Johns Hopkins Hospital
Baltimore, Maryland
Neurotoxicity

Tracy Skripac, RN, MSN, AOCN®, CHPN
Project Manager, Education Team
Oncology Nursing Society
Pittsburgh, Pennsylvania
Hemorrhagic Cystitis; Nephrotoxicity

Michael Smart, RN, BSN, OCN®
Staff Nurse, Oncology
Huntsville Hospital
Huntsville, Alabama
Verification and Maintenance of Treatment as Planned

Michael Steinberg, PharmD, BCOP
Associate Professor of Pharmacy Practice
Massachusetts College of Pharmacy and Health Sciences
Worcester, Massachusetts
*Table 7. Characteristics of Biologic Agents; Table 8.
Characteristics of Targeted Therapies*

Wendy Stiver, RN-BC, BSN, MA
Complex Care Coordinator
Alere
South Pasadena, California
Pretreatment; Treatment

Barbara J. Wilson, MS, RN, OCN®, AOCN®, ACNS-BC
Clinical Faculty
University of Mary
Bismarck, North Dakota
Myelosuppression: Introduction and Neutropenia

Laura Zitella, RN, MS, NP, AOCN®
Nurse Practitioner
Stanford Hospital and Clinics
Stanford, California
Post-Treatment Care

*The editors acknowledge the authors involved in the previous editions of this work
for their contributions that remain unchanged in this edition.*

Field Reviewers

Janet Cogswell, MS, RN, ACNS-BC, AOCN®
Lead Coordinator, Outpatient Hematology-Oncology
VA New Jersey Healthcare System
East Orange, New Jersey

Eileen M. Glynn-Tucker, RN, MS
Nurse Educator and Consultant
Green Oaks, Illinois

Jean M. Rosiak, RN, MSN, ANP-BC, AOCNP®
Nurse Practitioner
Aurora Medical Group
Milwaukee, Wisconsin

Gail M. Sulski, RN, MS, FNP, AOCNP®
Bone Marrow Transplant Nurse Practitioner
City of Hope/Banner BMT Program
Phoenix, Arizona

Disclosure

Editors and authors of guidelines provided by the Oncology Nursing Society are expected to disclose to the participants any significant financial interest or other relationships with the manufacturer(s) of any commercial products.

A vested interest may be considered to exist if a faculty member is affiliated with or has a financial interest in commercial organizations that may have a direct or indirect interest in the subject matter. A "financial interest" may include, but is not limited to, being a shareholder in the organization; being an employee of the commercial organization; serving on an organization's speakers bureau; or receiving research from the organization. An "affiliation" may be holding a position on an advisory board or some other role of benefit to the commercial organization. Vested interest statements appear in the front matter for each offering.

Contributors are expected to disclose any unlabeled or investigational use of products discussed in their content.

This information is acknowledged solely for the information of the readers.

The contributors provided the following disclosure and vested interest information:

Janet Cogswell, MS, RN, ACNS-BC, AOCN®, EPIC speakers bureau (Millennium), faculty; Educational Concepts Group (Bayer and Onyx), faculty

Paul F. Davis, MSN, RN-C, AOCNS®, Amgen Inc., speaker

Anne Katz, RN, PhD, Pfizer Inc., honorarium

Kristine B. LeFebvre, MSN, RN, AOCN®, Oncology Nursing Society, employee

MiKaela Olsen, RN, MS, OCN®, Amgen Inc., speaker, honoraria

Martha Polovich, MN RN AOCN®, Carmel Pharma, honoraria and travel expenses

Lisa Schulmeister, RN, MN, APRN-BC, OCN®, FAAN, TopoTarget USA, paid consultant; Advogent, speaker (supported through an educational grant from Baxter); Infusion Nurses Society, honoraria

Brenda K. Shelton, MS, RN, CCRN, AOCN®, Amgen Inc., speakers bureau; Bristol-Myers Squibb, speaker bureaus and advisory board

Tracy Skripac, RN, MSN, AOCN®, CHPN, Oncology Nursing Society, contractual employee at the time of authorship, salaried employee at the time of publishing

Michael Steinberg, PharmD, BCOP, Pfizer Inc., speaker

Gail M. Sulski, RN, MS, FNP, AOCN®, Millennium Pharmaceuticals, speaker, honoraria; Amgen Inc., speaker, honoraria

Julie M. Whitford, RN BSN, OCN®, Amgen Inc., employee

Barbara J. Wilson, MS, RN, OCN®, AOCN®, ACNS-BC, Sanofi-Aventis, speakers bureau

Table of Contents

Preface

The Oncology Nursing Society (ONS) *Chemotherapy and Biotherapy Guidelines and Recommendations for Practice* is now in its third edition. Since its first chemotherapy-related publication in 1984, ONS has provided leadership in this important area of oncology nursing practice. The goal of the publication has always been competent oncology nursing practice, which promotes patient safety. After 25 years, these guidelines have formed the foundation for the delivery of quality cancer care. While ONS is not a regulatory agency and, therefore, does not decide what treatments may be considered "standard of care," ONS provides the information contained in these guidelines based on evidence and research. Each institution or practice needs to make its own decision on whether to add a medication to its formulary based on the information that is available.

Because cancer treatment has changed since publication of the 2005 edition, the authors and editors have provided new and updated information to reflect those advances. The content related to targeted therapies and oral therapies has been expanded. Information on the management of skin, pulmonary, and cardiac toxicity has been updated accordingly. A chapter on treatment-related cognitive changes has been added. New tables and figures are included, and previous tables have been updated to provide information on newly approved drugs and care of the patients who receive them.

ONS gratefully acknowledges the authors and editors who have contributed to previous editions of this manual as well as the editors and authors of the material presented in this edition. The content has undergone an extensive peer review by both external reviewers and trainers for the ONS Chemotherapy and Biotherapy Course. Thanks to all who have participated in the preparation of this publication.

Abbreviations Used in This Manual

ACE—angiotensin-converting enzyme

ADL—activity of daily living

AHRQ—Agency for Healthcare Research and Quality

AIDS—acquired immunodeficiency syndrome

AJCC—American Joint Committee on Cancer

AML—acute myeloid leukemia

ANC—absolute neutrophil count

APHON—Association of Pediatric Hematology/Oncology Nurses

APOE—apolipoprotein E

ARB—angiotensin-receptor blocker

ASCO—American Society of Clinical Oncology

ASHP—American Society of Health-System Pharmacists

AUC—area under the plasma concentration versus time curve

BCG—bacillus Calmette-Guérin

BID—twice daily

BMT—bone marrow transplant

BRAT—bananas, rice, apples or applesauce, toast

BRCA1—breast cancer 1 gene

BRCA2—breast cancer 2 gene

BSA—body surface area

BSC—biologic safety cabinet

BUN—blood urea nitrogen

C—Celsius

CBC—complete blood count

cc—cubic centimeter

CFR—Code of Federal Regulations

cGy—centigray; unit of absorbed radiation dos equal to one hundredth of a gray

CHF—congestive heart failure

CHOP—cyclophosphamide, doxorubicin, vincristine, prednisone

CIN—chemotherapy-induced neutropenia

CINV—chemotherapy-induced nausea and vomiting

CN—cranial nerve

CNS—central nervous system

COG—Children's Oncology Group

CR—complete response

CrCl—creatinine clearance

CSF—colony-stimulating factor

CT—computed tomography

CTCAE—Common Terminology Criteria for Adverse Events

CTEP—Cancer Therapy Evaluation Program

CTZ—chemoreceptor trigger zone

CVAD—central vascular access device

CVC—central venous catheter

CXR—chest x-ray

D5W—5% dextrose in water

DHHS—U.S. Department of Health and Human Services

dl—deciliter

DNA—deoxyribonucleic acid

EAB—ethics advisory board

ECG—electrocardiogram

ECOG—Eastern Cooperative Oncology Group

EGF—epidermal growth factor

EGFR—epidermal growth factor receptor

EGFRI—epidermal growth factor receptor inhibitor

EORTC—European Organisation for Research and Treatment of Cancer

EPO—erythropoietin

ER/PR—estrogen receptor/progesterone receptor

ESA—erythropoiesis-stimulating agent

5-FU—5-fluorouracil

5HT$_3$—5-hydroxytryptamine-3 (serotonin)

FACT—Functional Assessment of Cancer Therapy evaluation tool

FDA—U.S. Food and Drug Administration

fL—femtoliter

g—gram

G-CSF—granulocyte–colony-stimulating factor

GFR—glomerular filtration rate

GI—gastrointestinal

GM-CSF—granulocyte macrophage–colony-stimulating factor

GVHD—graft-versus-host disease

Gy—gray; universal unit of absorbed radiation dose

Hct—hematocrit

HD—hazardous drug

HEPA—high-efficiency particulate air

HER—human epidermal growth factor receptor

Hg—mercury

Hgb—hemoglobin

HIV—human immunodeficiency virus

HPV—human papillomavirus

hr—hour

HSC—hematopoietic stem cell

HSCT—hematopoietic stem cell transplant

IARC—International Agency for Research on Cancer

IC—informed consent

IFN—interferon

Ig—immunoglobulin

IL—interleukin

ILD—interstitial lung disease

IM—intramuscular

INS—Infusion Nurses Society

IP—intraperitoneal

IRB—institutional review board

IT—intrathecal

ITP—immune thrombocytopenic purpura

IU—international units

IV—intravenous

IVF—in vitro fertilization

JCAHO—Joint Commission on Accreditation of Healthcare Organizations

KPS—Karnofsky Performance Status

L—liter

LAR—legally authorized representative

LFT—liver function test

LVEF—left ventricular ejection fraction

m—meter

MASCC—Multinational Association of Supportive Care in Cancer

mcg—microgram

MCV—mean corpuscular volume

MD—medical doctor

MDR—multidrug resistance

MDS—myelodysplastic syndrome

mEq—milliequivalent

mg—milligram

MHC—major histocompatibility complex

μ—micro

min—minute

ml—milliliter

mmol—millimole

MoAb—monoclonal antibody

MOPP—mechlorethamine, vincristine, procarbazine, prednisone

MSDS—material safety data sheet

msec—millisecond

mTOR—mammalian target of rapamycin

MUGA—multigated acquisition scan

NCCN—National Comprehensive Cancer Network

NCI—National Cancer Institute

NF-κB—nuclear factor-κB

NHL—non-Hodgkin lymphoma

NIH—National Institutes of Health

NIOSH—National Institute for Occupational Safety and Health

NK—natural killer

NKT—cells that have markers of both NK cells and T cells

NO—nitric oxide

NP—nurse practitioner

NPO—nothing by mouth

NRC—U.S. Nuclear Regulatory Commission

NS—normal saline

Abbreviations *(Continued)*

NSAID—nonsteroidal anti-inflammatory drug

NSCLC—non-small cell lung cancer

OHRP—Office for Human Research Protections

ONS—Oncology Nursing Society

OSHA—Occupational Safety and Health Administration

OTC—over the counter

P&P—policy and procedure

PBPC—peripheral blood progenitor cell

PD—progressive disease

PDE5—phosphodiesterase-5

PEC—primary engineering control

P-gp—p-glycoprotein

PICC—peripherally inserted central catheter

PO—oral

PPE—personal protective equipment

PR—partial response

PT—prothrombin time

PTT—partial thromboplastin time

QID—four times daily

QOL—quality of life

RBC—red blood cell

RCCT—randomized controlled clinical trial

RDI—relative dose intensity

RECIST—Response Evaluation Criteria in Solid Tumors

RiT—radioimmunotherapy

RNA—ribonucleic acid

RSO—radiation safety officer

RTK—receptor tyrosine kinases

SC—subcutaneous

SCr—serum creatinine

SD—stable disease

SIADH—syndrome of inappropriate antidiuretic hormone

SSRI—selective serotonin reuptake inhibitor

TB—tuberculosis

TBI—total body irradiation

T_c—cytotoxic T cells

T_H—helper T cells

TID—three times daily

TLS—tumor lysis syndrome

T_M—memory T cells

TNF—tumor necrosis factor

TNM—tumor, node, metastasis staging classification for solid tumors

T_{reg}—T regulatory cells

T_s—suppressor T cells

USP—United States Pharmacopeia

VA—vestibular apparatus

VAD—vascular access device

VC—vomiting center

VEGF—vascular endothelial growth factor

VEGFR—vascular endothelial growth factor receptor

VOD—veno-occlusive disease

VTE—venous thromboembolism

WBC—white blood cell

WHO—World Health Organization

Generic Medications and Brand-Name Equivalents

This list is not comprehensive; more than one company may manufacture or market a product by the same name. Although every effort was made to ensure the accuracy of this information at press time, product and company information change frequently; therefore, the publishers and contributors disclaim responsibility for the accuracy of this list. Before using this information, verify it to ensure that it is up-to-date. Cited trademark status pertains to the United States only. Not all products listed are available in the United States. This list is not an assertion of trademark ownership or an endorsement of any product.

Aldesleukin (IL-2, Chiron Corporation; Proleukin®, Novartis Oncology)

Alemtuzumab (anti-CD52, Campath®, Bayer HealthCare Pharmaceuticals Inc.)

Altretamine (Hexalen®, MGI Pharma Inc.)

Amphadase™ [bovine] (hyaluronidase injection, Amphastar Pharmaceuticals)

Arsenic trioxide (Trisenox®, Cephalon)

Asparaginase (Elspar®, Merck)

Azacitidine (Vidaza®, Celgene Corporation)

Bendamustine (Treanda®, Cephalon)

Bevacizumab (anti-VEGF, Avastin®, Genentech)

Bexarotene (Targretin®, Eisai Inc.)

Bismuth subsalicylate (Pepto-Bismol®, Procter & Gamble)

Bleomycin (Blenoxane®, Bristol-Myers Squibb)

Bortezomib (Velcade®, Millennium Pharmaceuticals)

Bupropion (Wellbutrin®, GlaxoSmithKline)

Busulfan (Oral: Myleran®, GlaxoSmithKline; IV: Busulfex®, Otsuka Pharmaceuticals)

Calcium polycarbophil (Equalactin®, Numark Laboratories; FiberCon®, Wyeth Consumer Healthcare)

Capecitabine (Xeloda®, Hoffmann-La Roche, Inc.)

Carboplatin (Paraplatin®, Bristol-Myers Squibb)

Carmustine (BiCNU®, Bristol-Myers Squibb; Gliadel®, MGI Pharma Inc.)

Cetuximab (Erbitux®, ImClone Systems)

Chlorambucil (Leukeran®, GlaxoSmithKline)

Cisplatin (Platinol®, Bristol-Myers Squibb)

Cladribine (Leustatin®, Ortho Biotech)

Clindamycin (Cleocin®, Pharmacia & Upjohn; Clindaderm®, Paddock Laboratories Inc.)

Clofarabine (Clolar™, Genzyme)

Cyclophosphamide (Cytoxan®, Bristol-Myers Squibb)

Cytarabine (cytosine arabinoside, ARA-C, Cytosar-U®, Teva Parenteral Medicines)

Cytarabine liposomal (DepoCyt®, Pacira Pharms, Inc.)

Dacarbazine (DTIC®, Bayer HealthCare Pharmaceuticals Inc.)

Dactinomycin (actinomycin D, Cosmegen®, Ovation Pharmaceuticals, Inc.)

Darbepoetin (Aranesp®, Amgen Inc.)

Dasatinib (Sprycel®, Bristol-Myers Squibb)

Daunorubicin (daunomycin, Cerubidine®, Bedford Laboratories, Sanofi-Aventis, and Wyeth Ayerst)

Daunorubicin citrate liposomal (DaunoXome®, Diatos, S.A.)

Decitabine (Dacogen®, MGI Pharma Inc.)

Denileukin diftitox (Ontak®, Ligand Pharmaceuticals Inc., Seragen)

Dexrazoxane for injection (Totect®, TopoTarget; Zinecard®, Pfizer Inc.)

Diphenoxylate HCl (Lomotil®, Pfizer Inc.)

Docetaxel (Taxotere®, Sanofi-Aventis)

Doxorubicin (Adriamycin®, Pharmacia & Upjohn; Rubex® [DSC], Bristol-Myers Squibb)

Doxorubicin liposomal (Doxil®, Ortho Biotech)

Eculizumab (Soliris®, Alexion Pharmaceuticals, Inc.)

Epinephrine (EpiPen® Auto-Injector, Dey, L.P.)

Epirubicin (Ellence®, Pfizer Inc.)

Epoetin alfa (Epogen®, Procrit®, Amgen Inc.)

Erlotinib (Tarceva®, OSI Pharmaceuticals, Inc.)

Etoposide (VP-16, VePesid®, Etopophos®, Bristol-Myers Squibb)

Filgrastim (G-CSF, Neupogen®, Amgen Inc.)

Floxuridine (FUDR®, Hospira)

Fludarabine (Fludara®, Bayer HealthCare Pharmaceuticals Inc.)

Fluorouracil (5-fluorouracil, 5-FU, Adrucil®, Pharmacia & Upjohn, and Teva Parenteral Medicines)

Gefitinib (Iressa®, AstraZeneca)

Gemcitabine (Gemzar®, Eli Lilly and Co.)

Gemtuzumab ozogamicin (anti-CD33, Mylotarg®, Wyeth Pharmaceuticals)

Granisetron transdermal (Sancuso®, ProStrakan)

Human papillomavirus quadrivalent (types 6, 11, 16, and 18) vaccine, recombinant (Gardasil®, Merck)

Hyaluronidase human injection, (recombinant) (Hylenex®, Baxter Healthcare Corporation)

Hyaluronidase injection (Hydase™, Akorn Inc.)

Hydroxyurea (Hydrea®, Bristol-Myers Squibb; Mylocel®, Barr Laboratories Inc.)

Ibritumomab tiuxetan (anti-CD20 antibody, Zevalin®, IDEC Pharmaceuticals Corporation)

Idarubicin (Idamycin®, Pharmacia & Upjohn)

Ifosfamide (Ifex®, Bristol-Myers Squibb)

Imatinib mesylate (Gleevec®, Novartis Oncology)

Interferon alfa-2a (Roferon-A®, Hoffmann-La Roche, Inc.)

Interferon alfa-2b (Intron A®, Schering-Plough)

Interferon gamma (Actimmune®, Intermune)

Interleukin-2 (Aldesleukin, Proleukin®, Novartis Oncology)

Intracorporeal injections (Caverject®, Pfizer Inc.; Trimix)

Intraurethral pellets (MUSE®, Vivus Pharmaceuticals)

Irinotecan (Camptosar®, Pfizer Inc.)

Ixabepilone (Ixempra®, Bristol-Myers Squibb)

Lapatinib (Tykerb®, GlaxoSmithKline)

Lenalidomide (Revlimid®, Celgene Corporation)

Levamisole (Eramisol®, Janssen Pharmaceuticals)

Lomustine (CeeNu®, Bristol-Myers Squibb)

Generic Medications and Brand-Name Equivalents *(Continued)*

Loperamide (Imodium® A-D, McNeil-PPC, Inc.)

Mechlorethamine (nitrogen mustard, Mustargen®, Ovation Pharmaceuticals, Inc.)

Megestrol acetate (Megace®, Bristol-Myers Squibb)

Melphalan (Alkeran®, GlaxoSmithKline)

Mercaptopurine (6-MP, Purinethol®, Teva Pharmaceuticals)

Methotrexate (MTX, Rheumatrex®; STADA Pharmaceuticals, Inc.; Trexall™, Duramed Pharmaceuticals, Inc.)

Methylphenidate (Ritalin®, Novartis Pharmaceuticals Corp.)

Minocycline (Minocin®, Triax Pharmaceuticals, and Lederle Laboratories)

Mitomycin (Mutamycin®, Bristol-Myers Squibb)

Mitotane (Lysodren®, Bristol-Myers Squibb)

Mitoxantrone (Novantrone®, EMD Serono, Inc.)

Modafinil (Provigil®, Cephalon)

Mupirocin (Bactroban®, GlaxoSmithKline)

Nelarabine (Arranon®, GlaxoSmithKline)

Nilotinib (Tasigna®, Novartis Oncology)

Octreotide (Sandostatin®, Novartis Oncology)

OncoVAX® (Vaccinogen, Inc.)

Oprelvekin (IL-11, Neumega®, Wyeth Pharmaceuticals)

Oxaliplatin for injection (Eloxatin®, Sanofi-Aventis)

Paclitaxel (Taxol®, Bristol-Myers Squibb)

Paclitaxel protein-bound particles; albumin-bound (Abraxane™, Abraxis BioSciences, with AstraZeneca)

Palifermin (rHuKGF, Kepivance®, Amgen Inc.)

Panitumumab (Vectibix®, Amgen Inc.)

Paroxetine (Paxil®, GlaxoSmithKline)

Pegaspargase (Oncaspar®, Enzon Pharmaceuticals)

Pegfilgrastim (Neulasta®, Amgen Inc.)

Pemetrexed (Alimta®, Eli Lilly and Co.)

Pentostatin (Nipent®, Hospira)

Pertuzumab (Omnitarg™, Genentech)

Procarbazine (Matulane®, Sigma Tau Pharmaceuticals)

Rituximab (anti-CD20 antibody, Rituxan®, Genentech, and IDEC Pharmaceuticals Corporation)

Romiplostim (Nplate™, Amgen Inc.)

Sargramostim (GM-CSF, Leukine®, Bayer HealthCare Pharmaceuticals Inc.)

6-mercaptopurine (Purinethol®, Teva Pharmaceuticals)

Sorafenib (Nexavar®, Bayer HealthCare Pharmaceuticals Inc.)

Streptozocin (Zanosar®, Teva Pharmaceuticals)

Sunitinib (Sutent®, Pfizer Inc.)

Temozolomide (Temodar®, Schering-Plough)

Temsirolimus (Torisel®, Wyeth Pharmaceuticals)

Teniposide (VM-26, Vumon®, Bristol-Myers Squibb)

Thalidomide (Thalomid®, Celgene Corporation)

Thioguanine (6-thioguanine, 6-TG, GlaxoSmithKline)

Thiotepa (Thioplex®, Amgen Inc.)

Topotecan (Hycamtin®, GlaxoSmithKline)

Tositumomab I-131 (Bexxar®, GlaxoSmithKline)

Trastuzumab (anti-HER2 antibody, Herceptin®, Genentech)

Trimetrexate (Neutrexin®, MedImmune)

Uracil and tegafur (UFT®, Bristol-Myers Squibb)

Valrubicin (Valstar®, Indevus Pharmaceuticals, Inc.)

Vinblastine (Velban®, Eli Lilly and Co.)

Vincristine (Oncovin®, Eli Lilly and Co.; Vincasar PFS®, Teva Parenteral Medicines)

Vinorelbine (Navelbine®, Pierre Fabre)

Vitrase® [ovine] (hyaluronidase injection, ISTA Pharmaceuticals)

Vorinostat (Zolinza®, Merck)

Warfarin (Coumadin®, Bristol-Myers Squibb)

Other brand-name products mentioned:

Alpha-Keri®, Novartis Consumer Health

Ambu® bag, Ambu Inc.

Anthelios®, La Roche-Posay

Aquaphor®, Beiersdorf, Inc.

Aveeno® oatmeal bath, Johnson & Johnson Consumer Companies, Inc.

Basis® soap, Beiersdorf, Inc.

Cetaphil®, Galderma Laboratories, Inc.

Cremophor®, BASF Corp.

Dermablend®, Recovery Elements

Dove®, Unilever

Ensure®, Ross Products

Gelclair®, EKR Therapeutics, Inc.

Ivory®, Procter & Gamble

Lubriderm®, Johnson & Johnson

Mylanta®, Johnson & Johnson and Merck Consumer Pharmaceuticals Co.

Neutrogena®, Neutrogena

Neutrogena Norwegian Formula® hand cream, Neutrogena

Nivea®, Beiersdorf, Inc.

PhaSeal®, Carmel Pharma, Inc.

Replens®, Lil' Drug Store Products, Inc.

Vacutainer®, Beckton Dickinson & Co.

Vaseline Intensive Care® Advanced Healing Lotion, Unilever

I. Introduction

A. Definition of cancer
1. Historically, cancer was described as a large group of malignant diseases with some or all of the following characteristics (Merkle & Loescher, 2005; Volker, 2005).
   a) Abnormal cell proliferation caused by a series of cellular and/or genetic alterations or translocations.
   b) Lack of controlled growth and cell division that leads to the formation of tumors and to invasion of tissues that are proximate to tumor cells.
   c) Ability to spread (metastasize) to distant site(s) and establish secondary tumors.
   d) Involves any tissue of the body.
   e) Evades natural cell death (apoptosis).
2. Currently, with the discovery of new information about molecular and cellular activity, cancer is believed to be only a few diseases (Loescher & Whitesell, 2003) that result from faulty or abnormal genetic expression caused by changes in deoxyribonucleic acid (DNA).
   a) The transcription of DNA into a single strand of messenger ribonucleic acid (RNA) may be changed.
   b) When abnormal messenger RNA exists, the synthesis of amino acids is changed, and the protein structure is abnormal as well.
3. Normal cells may undergo the changes as outlined by Loescher and Whitesell (2003) because of
   a) Spontaneous transformation: No causative agent is identified, but cellular characteristics are typical of cancer cells.
   b) Exposure to chemical or physical carcinogens: Environmental factors are continuously being studied. Chronic or occupational exposure to substances such as asbestos, benzene, radiation, tobacco, arsenic, nickel, and some chemotherapeutic agents is implicated in the development of cancers. The National Institute for Occupational Safety and Health (NIOSH) identified 135 substances as carcinogens in 2005 (NIOSH, 2005; Olsen, 2005; U.S. Department of Health and Human Services [DHHS], 2005a, 2005b; World Health Organization [WHO], 2008).
   c) Genetic alterations: Mutations are permanent changes in DNA sequencing of the base pairs, resulting in a cell with malignant properties. Some mutations are of no concern, but those that give rise to a clone of malignant cells form tumors. *TP53* is an example of a tumor suppressing gene that

is altered in many cancers (Giarelli, Jacobs, & Jenkins, 2002; Loescher & Whitesell, 2003; National Cancer Institute [NCI], n.d.; Volker, 2005).
   d) Exposure to viruses: Genetic changes can occur to cells through viruses. The human papillomavirus (HPV) is an example of a virus that is a primary cause of cervical cancer (NCI, 2006b).
4. Figure 1 provides a summary of genetic changes that may result in tumor formation. The properties of transformed cells are changes in the cytology, cell membrane, and growth and development.
5. Grading and differentiation: Differentiation is based on how closely tumor cells resemble normal cells in their structure and maturity. It is the process of cells developing and becoming fully mature and fully functional. Cells are obtained by biopsy or surgical removal for examination by a cytopathologist. Cancer cells appear different from those of the surrounding normal tissue. A tumor's level of differentiation can vary over time, and cells with several grades of differentiation may exist within a single tumor. The higher the grade, the more aggressive the tumor (Greene et al., 2002; Omerod, 2005).
   a) GX—grade cannot be assessed
   b) G1—well differentiated (resembles the parent cell)
   c) G2—moderately differentiated
   d) G3—poorly differentiated (bears little resemblance to the parent cell)
   e) G4—undifferentiated (impossible to tell which cell is the parent)
6. Staging: The purpose of staging is to verify the extent of the disease by assessing the location and size of the primary tumor, determining lymph node involvement, and confirming if there are additional tumors. This enables the doctor to determine prognosis, plan the best treatment, and identify clinical trials that may

Figure 1. Clonal Evolution in Cancer

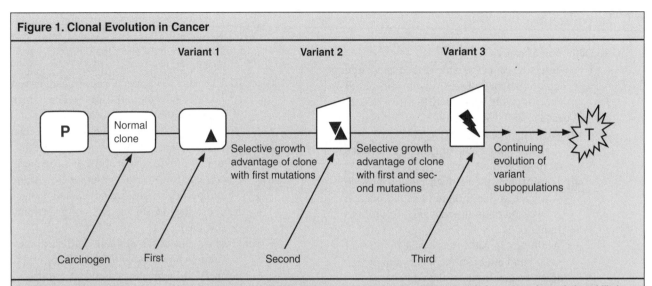

Specific genetic alterations in evolving tumors may range from gene mutations to major chromosomal aberrations (genetic instability). This figure illustrates a carcinogen-induced genetic change in a progenitor normal cell P, which produces a cell with selective growth advantage allowing clonal expansion to begin. In this case, gene mutations produce variant cells. Because they are at a disadvantage metabolically or immunologically, most variant cells are nonviable. If one variant has a selective advantage, its progeny becomes the predominant subpopulation until another variant appears. The sequential selection of variant subpopulations in each tumor (T) differs because of genetic instability, which positively or negatively affects cell proliferation.

Note. From "Biology of Cancer" (p. 6), by C.J. Merkle and L.J. Loescher in C.H. Yarbro, M.H. Frogge, and M. Goodman (Eds.), *Cancer Nursing: Principles and Practice* (6th ed.), 2005, Sudbury, MA: Jones and Bartlett. Copyright 2005 by Jones and Bartlett. Reprinted with permission.

be suitable for a patient. Staging provides a common language with which doctors can communicate about a patient's case. Staging criteria are unique for each type of cancer (American Joint Committee on Cancer [AJCC], 2008).

a) In general, evaluating the stage for solid tumors includes assessing the involvement of three factors originally developed by AJCC. Additional information about cancer staging is available online at www.cancerstaging.org.

(1) T—tumor (local involvement, invasion): The primary tumor is measured to document its size and to determine the depth of invasion of the tumor.

(2) N—nodes (nodal involvement): Lymph nodes in the area of the primary tumor are examined for the evidence of disease spread. Their size, number, and location are documented.

(3) M—metastasis (metastatic involvement): Studies are done to determine if the primary tumor has metastasized to distant location(s) (AJCC, 2008; Greene et al., 2002).

b) Lymphomas, leukemias, and multiple myeloma are hematologic malignancies that are staged according to other systems. For example, non-Hodgkin lymphoma is evaluated with a combination of staging systems including the WHO's classification of lymphoid neoplasms, the Ann Arbor staging system, and the International Prognostic Index (Armitage, 2005).

c) Most pediatric cancers are staged according to the TNM system; however, Hodgkin lymphoma, non-Hodgkin lymphoma, rhabdomyosarcoma, neuroblastoma, retinoblastoma, liver cancer, and Wilms tumor have separate staging systems (Guarino, 2007; NCI, 2007; Roebuck et al., 2007).

7. Depending upon the clinical presentation, laboratory values, and suspected malignancy, specimens obtained should be submitted for cytogenetics, assays for cell surface markers, flow cytometry, or other studies.

B. Treatment modalities: Table 1 summarizes the history of cancer therapy. A variety of modalities are used to treat cancer. Treatment may include one or more of the following interventions.

1. Surgery (Gillespie, 2005; Szopa, 2005)

a) Is a precise local treatment

b) May remove all of the primary tumor or a portion of it

c) May be the method of obtaining specimens for cytopathology

Table 1. History of Cancer Therapy

Period	Events
Pre 20th century	• 1500s: Heavy metals are used systemically to treat cancers; however, their effectiveness is limited and their toxicity is great (Burchenal, 1977). • 1890s: William Coley, MD, develops and explores the use of Coley's toxins, the first nonspecific immunostimulants used to treat cancer.
World War I	• Sulfur-mustard gas is used for chemical warfare; servicemen who are exposed to nitrogen mustard experience bone marrow and lymphoid suppression (Gilman, 1963; Gilman & Philips, 1946).
World War II	• Congress passes National Cancer Institute (NCI) Act in 1937. • Alkylating agents are recognized for their antineoplastic effect (Gilman & Philips). • Thioguanine and mercaptopurine are developed (Guy & Ingram, 1996). • 1946: NCI-identified cancer research areas include biology, chemotherapy, epidemiology, and pathology. • 1948: Divisions within NCI and external institutions are identified to conduct research (Zubrod, 1984). • Folic acid antagonists are found to be effective against childhood acute leukemia (Farber et al., 1948). • Antitumor antibiotics are discovered.
1950s	• 1955: National Chemotherapy Program, developed with congressional funding, is founded to develop and test new chemotherapy drugs. • 1957: Interferon is discovered. • The Children's Cancer Group, the first cooperative group dedicated to finding effective treatments for pediatric cancer, is formed.
1960s–1970s	• Development of platinum compounds begins. • Multidrug therapy improves remission rate without severe toxicity; mechlorethamine, vincristine, procarbazine, and prednisone (MOPP), the first combination chemotherapy, is used and found to be curative against Hodgkin disease (Noonan, 2007). • Clinical trials of bacillus Calmette-Guérin and *Corynebacterium parvum,* nonspecific immunostimulants, begin. • Chemotherapy is used with surgery and radiation as cancer treatment. • Development of hybridoma technology begins. • NCI starts its Biological Response Modifier Program. • Tamoxifen is synthesized in 1962; first used in 1969.
1970s	• The National Cancer Act of 1971 provides funding for cancer research; director is appointed by and reports to the President of the United States. • Doxorubicin phase I trials begin. • Adjuvant chemotherapy begins to be a common cancer treatment (Bonadonna et al., 1985; Fisher et al., 1986).
1980s	• Community Clinical Oncology Programs are developed in 1983 to contribute to NCI chemotherapy clinical trials. • Use of multimodal therapies increases (Eilber et al., 1984; Marcial et al., 1988). • Focus turns to symptom management to alleviate dose-limiting toxicities related to neutropenia, nausea and vomiting, and cardiotoxicity. • Clinical trials for dexrazoxane (ICRF-187) as a cardioprotectant begin (Speyer et al., 1988). • New chemotherapeutic agents are available. • Scientists begin to investigate recombinant DNA technology. • Trials of monoclonal antibodies and cytokines begin. • Effector cells (lymphokine-activated killer cells and tumor-infiltrating lymphocytes) are grown ex vivo. • 1986: U.S. Food and Drug Administration (FDA) approves interferon alfa. • 1989: FDA approves erythropoietin.
1990s	• New classifications of drugs (e.g., taxanes) are developed. • In clinical trials, paclitaxel is found to be effective against ovarian and breast cancers (Rowinsky et al., 1992). • FDA approves granulocyte–colony-stimulating factor and granulocyte macrophage–colony-stimulating factor, interleukin-2, interleukin-11, rituximab, trastuzumab, and denileukin diftitox. • Clinical trials of gene therapy and antiangiogenic agents begin. • FDA approves filgrastim for use in bone marrow transplantation and chemotherapy-induced neutropenia, severe chronic neutropenia, and peripheral blood stem cell transplantation. • FDA approves ondansetron for prevention of chemotherapy-induced nausea and vomiting; other 5-hydroxytryptamine-3 ($5HT_3$) receptor antagonists are in clinical trials (Perez, 1995). • As a result of improved symptom management, dose intensity becomes a focus. • FDA approves new analogs (e.g., vinorelbine) (Abeloff, 1995).

(Continued on next page)

Table 1. History of Cancer Therapy *(Continued)*	
Period	**Events**
1990s *(cont.)*	• Scientists focus on the sequencing of agents (Bonadonna et al., 1995). • The genetic basis of cancers becomes an important factor in cancer risk research (e.g., *BRCA1* for breast cancer, renal cell cancer) (Gnarra et al., 1995; Hoskins et al., 1995; Miki et al., 1994). • Aromatase inhibitors are approved for breast cancer treatment. This approval marks a step forward for hormonal therapy.
2000s	• The Children's Oncology Group, a cooperative group combining the efforts of several groups, is formed to further the advancement of cancer treatment for children. • Scientists complete a working draft of the human genome. • Theory of immune surveillance continues, and biotherapy is used to target and mount defense against certain antigens on malignant cells (e.g., gemtuzumab ozogamicin binds to CD33 on leukemic cells, rituximab binds to CD20-positive non-Hodgkin lymphoma cells). • Radioimmunotherapy (RIT) is used to deliver radioactivity directly to select tumor cells, avoiding damage to healthy tissue (e.g., ibritumomab tiuxetan, tositumomab I-131). • FDA approves antiangiogenic agents (bevacizumab was the first). • Neurokinin-1 antagonist (aprepitant) is used, in combination with other antiemetic drugs, to prevent chemotherapy-induced nausea and vomiting. • Therapeutic vaccine trials for existing cancers (e.g., OncoVAX®, an autologous tumor cell vaccine, is in phase III studies for stage II colon cancer), and FDA approves a prophylactic vaccine (Gardasil®) for the prevention of human papillomavirus infections that cause cervical cancer.

d) May be the only treatment a patient requires

e) May be preceded or followed by other modalities

f) May be used in the palliative setting to alleviate or lessen intolerable symptoms

2. Radiation therapy (Gosselin-Acomb, 2005; Witt, 2005)

 a) Like surgery, is a local treatment in that a beam is precisely directed at a specific target

 b) May follow surgery to prevent recurrence of the primary tumor

 c) Is more effective for some diseases than others

 d) Is sometimes used after chemotherapy because radiation can permanently damage bone marrow, making it impossible to give chemotherapy in the doses needed for curative therapy

 e) Often is given in combination with chemotherapy (chemoradiation)

3. Chemotherapy/hormonal therapies (Temple & Poniatowski, 2005; Tortorice, 2005)

 a) Are systemic therapies, rather than local treatments, as drugs are distributed throughout the body by the bloodstream

 b) May be used as single agents or more commonly in combination with other drugs

 c) Are limited by toxic effects on normal tissues

 d) May have a tumoricidal effect in hormone-sensitive tumors because of reduction or blockage of the source of the hormone or receptor site where hormone is active

4. Biotherapy/targeted agents (Gale, 2005)

 a) Are systemic treatments

 b) May modify the patient's own immune defenses

 c) May be so specific as to target a single receptor on the surface of tumor cells

 d) May cause side effects and toxicities that differ from those of other antineoplastic agents

 e) May be combined with other treatment modalities

 f) May promote tumor regression

 g) May stimulate hematopoiesis

C. The drug development process: Although there is a sense of urgency to develop new and better therapies, protection of the public is of paramount importance. Steps to develop new anticancer agents are complex as well as time- and resource-consuming. NCI, a division of the National Institutes of Health (NIH), examines thousands of agents yearly to discover new ones for testing. Only a small percentage are selected for preclinical testing, and even fewer are tested in phase I (see Table 2) clinical trials.

1. Development of new cytotoxic and other therapeutic agents

 a) Preclinical studies: Laboratory research using animal models often is conducted collaboratively by NCI and pharmaceutical companies. The NCI Cancer Therapy Evaluation Program (CTEP) will seek pharmaceutical sponsorship early once an agent is discovered because NCI does not market new agents. Pharmaceutical companies may seek CTEP codevelopment (Berg, 2008).

b) Preclinical studies involve lab analysis and animal subjects; they do not involve human subjects (Wong & Westendorp, 2008).

(1) Scientists undertake empirical or rational research to develop a new agent or a derivative of an existing agent that is more effective, has fewer side effects, or is less toxic than existing agents.

(2) The new agent is tested in vitro in various tumor cell lines. If the agent is effective, scientists undertake in vivo testing using mice or other research animals.

(3) The agent is tested for stability, solubility, and dose.

(4) Scientists perform studies involving animals to predict the initial dose that will be used in human studies.

2. Clinical trials involving humans: The purpose of a clinical trial is to study a new agent or device or combinations of agents by involving human volunteers in a scientific experiment. Scientists seek to evaluate the safety, effectiveness, and toxicities of a new drug or drug combinations

in humans. Clinical trials are vital to improve patient care. They play an important role in the reduction of cancer morbidity and mortality (Kosta & Gullatte, 2007). However, only 5% of adults with cancer enroll in clinical trials because some oncologists either do not have access to clinical trials or do not encourage participation, or because clinical trial databases can be unclear (Okie, 2006).

a) Regulating entities relevant to the protection of human research subjects: In addition to strict federal regulation, multiple regulatory groups oversee the participation of individuals in research (Brown & Markus, 2008).

(1) DHHS

(2) Office for Human Research Protections (OHRP), which regulates clinical trials sponsored or conducted by DHHS, enacted regulations in the Code of Federal Regulations (CFR) Title 45: Public Welfare and Human Services, *Protection of Human Subjects,* 45 CFR 46

(3) The U.S. Food and Drug Adminstration (FDA), which regulates clinical trials that involve the licensing of a drug or

Table 2. Phases of Cancer Clinical Trials

Phase and Number of Participants	Primary Goals	Characteristics
Phase 0 10–12 people	• Study pharmacodynamic and pharmacokinetic properties of a drug. • Identify drugs that do not produce desired effect, and avoid moving them into phase I trials. • Determine a dosing regimen for testing in standard clinical trials.	• Limited number of doses • Lower doses administered • Less risk to participant • Useful for molecularly targeted drugs with wide therapeutic indexes • Also useful for drugs that require development of biomarkers for future studies
Phase I 20–25 people	• Establish maximum tolerated dose and dosing schedule. • Evaluate toxicity. • Determine pharmacokinetics.	• Relapsed/refractory disease • Small number of patients • Dose-escalating cohorts • Variety of tumor types • Pharmacokinetic studies
Phase II < 100 people	• Determine antitumor activity in specific tumor types. • Evaluate toxicity.	• Groups of patients with same tumors • Measurable disease to assess response rates
Phase III 100–thousands	• Establish efficacy by assessing survival and time to progression. • Compare with current standard.	• Randomization between experimental treatment and standard treatment and/or control group • Large numbers of patients
Phase IV Hundreds to thousands	• Expand "off-label" use. • Further assess toxicity data and long-term safety. • Assess long-term effectiveness.	• Postmarketing trials and commercially available drugs

Note. From "History and Background of Clinical Trials" (p. 8), by S. Breslin in A.D. Klimaszewski, M.A. Bacon, H.E. Deininger, B.A. Ford, and J.G. Westendorp (Eds.), *Manual for Clinical Trials Nursing* (2nd ed.), 2008, Pittsburgh, PA: Oncology Nursing Society. Copyright 2008 by Oncology Nursing Society. Reprinted with permission.

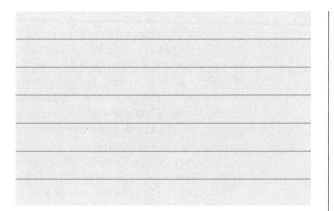

product, enacted regulations in the CFR Title 21: Food and Drugs, *Protection of Human Subjects*, 21 CFR 50

    (4) Institutional review boards (IRBs)

    (5) Ethics advisory boards

    (6) Data safety monitoring boards

b) Drug approval process

    (1) Research protocols are designed within an academic environment, through NCI, by pharmaceutical companies, or by cooperative research groups.

    (2) If the trial involves a new agent, the FDA reviews and approves the agent as an investigational new drug.

    (3) Table 2 presents an overview of the phases of clinical trials (Breslin, 2008). Funding may originate from public or private sources.

    (4) The FDA approves the new drug for commercial use when studies document its efficacy and safety.

    (5) The drug is marketed commercially.

    (6) Postmarketing studies are conducted to define new uses for approved drugs, as well as to monitor for toxicities, long-term safety, and long-term effectiveness (Breslin).

c) Pediatric involvement in clinical trials

    (1) More than 90% of pediatric patients with cancer receive treatment at centers affiliated with a multi-institution collaborative research group, such as the Children's Oncology Group (COG). Approximately 70% of children with cancer are treated in an NCI-sponsored clinical trial at some point during their illness (NCI, 2005).

    (2) In general, new drugs are tested in adults before researchers undertake studies involving children. In clinical trials with children, the first dose of the agent being studied is usually 80% of the maximum tolerated adult dose.

    (3) Because a child's size and metabolism differ significantly from those of an adult, drug data derived from adults may not apply to children.

    (4) In phase IV studies, dosages may be changed or combinations of approved agents altered in an attempt to maintain or improve cure rate while increasing quality of life (QOL) and decreasing the late effects of treatment. Incorporating phase IV trials into studies involving children is less common (Gattuso, 2004).

    (5) The Association of Pediatric Hematology/Oncology Nurses (APHON) has developed and provides the APHON Pediatric Chemotherapy and Biotherapy Provider Program, which standardizes nurses' education regarding the administration of chemotherapy and biotherapy to the pediatric population. For more information, visit APHON's Web site at www.aphon.org.

d) Nurses' roles regarding clinical trials: Nurses may

    (1) Help patients find clinical trials. Helpful resources include (Trocky & Brandt, 2008)

        (a) NIH's Clinical Trials Web site (http://clinicaltrials.gov), which lists clinical trials and provides education about clinical trials for the consumer

        (b) NCI's Cancer Trials Support Unit (www.ctsu.org), which focuses on phase III clinical trials

        (c) Coalition of National Cancer Cooperative Groups' TrialCheck® (www.trialcheck.org/services), which focuses on cooperative group oncology trials

        (d) Pharmaceutical company registry Web sites, such as GlaxoSmithKline (www.gsk-clinicalstudyregister .com) and Eli Lilly (www.lillytrials .com/initiated/initiated.html)

        (e) Internationally, nationally, and locally developed and maintained registries

    (2) Support prospective participants as they decide whether to enroll. When a patient is considering participation in a clinical trial, he or she may be facing stressors in addition to the enrollment decision, including a new diagnosis of cancer, disease progres-

sion, financial concerns, psychosocial distress, disruption with career, and role changes at home. Nurses can help by screening for psychological distress at every visit and referring the patient to social work services, pastoral services, or mental health services as appropriate (Klimaszewski, 2008b).

(3) Ensure informed consent (IC) if the patient decides to participate.

(a) IC is a heavily regulated *process* to protect human rights, of which the IC document is only a part (Klimaszewski, 2008a). Steps in the IC process are delineated in

Table 3. Nurses can help in the IC process by

i) Ensuring that the patient and/or family understand the purpose of participation in the clinical trial and allowing adequate time for them to receive answers to all of their questions. This will involve arranging for time with the clinical investigator and/or clinical trial nurse.

ii) Providing educational materials as required. All materials presented to patients and families must be language-specific,

Table 3. Steps in the Informed Consent Process	
Step	**Key Elements**
Initial meeting	Provide subject and family with the informed consent (IC) document. Discuss the IC document logically with subject and one or more members of the research team. Encourage subject and family to take notes. Provide adequate time for subject and family members to consider participation and have all questions answered. Provide subject with a video, audiotape, or interactive computer program to help him or her to understand the information in the IC document. Parents will represent subjects under age 18. If subject is between ages 6 and 18, ask for assent to participate, and provide an assent document for signature.
Time to read and consider participation	Subject is afforded adequate time to review the IC document at his or her leisure. Subject discusses the IC document with family, friends, social workers, clergy, a subject representative, or other trusted advisers. Subject records questions and concerns for discussion at next meeting.
Assessment of understanding	Discuss subject's questions and concerns that were recorded at home. Assess subject's understanding with interactive questioning, a written questionnaire, or by having the patient explain specific parts of the IC document in his or her own words. Document assessment of subject's understanding. Answer subject's questions until the patient states that he or she has enough information to make a decision. Document subject's statement regarding his or her decision.
Questions	Encourage subject to ask questions until the participant is satisfied with his or her understanding of the IC document. Encourage subject to record questions while away from the clinic and either bring them to the next meeting or schedule a visit to have the questions discussed.
New information	Assure subject that any new information available will be shared. Follow-up on assurance. Provide subject with an updated IC document for signature (as required). Document subject's understanding of new information in the presence of family. Document subject's signing of the new IC, review of IC, and that all subject's questions were answered. Provide copy of the IC form to subject.
Communication techniques	Videotapes, audiotapes, interactive computer programs, discussions with qualified professional and lay individuals
Supplemental materials	Videotapes, audiotapes, written materials, interactive computer programs

Note. Based on information from National Cancer Institute, 2006a, 2006c.
From "Informed Consent" (p. 101), by A.D. Klimaszewski in A.D. Klimaszewski, M.A. Bacon, H.E. Deininger, B.A. Ford, and J.G. Westendorp (Eds.), *Manual for Clinical Trials Nursing* (2nd ed.), 2008, Pittsburgh, PA: Oncology Nursing Society. Copyright 2008 by Oncology Nursing Society. Reprinted with permission.

developmentally appropriate, and accurate.

   iii) Documenting the patient's understanding of the clinical trial, follow-up and test schedules, and his or her right to withdraw at any time (Klimaszewski, 2008a).

(b) The institution's IRB will review/ revise the IC document for format and appropriateness of reading level for the patient and family. OHRP and FDA regulations about the IC document are found in the CFR and may be viewed at www.cancer.gov/clinicaltrials/ understanding/simplification-of-informed-consent-docs/page4#. A basic consent document must (DHHS, 2005c)

   i) State that the study involves research, provide an explanation of the purpose of the research, identify the possible duration of the subject's participation, and describe the procedure(s).

   ii) Describe foreseeable risks or discomforts that the subject might encounter.

   iii) Describe benefits to the subject or to any others.

   iv) Disclose appropriate alternative treatments that may be advantageous to the subject, if applicable.

   v) Describe how confidentiality of records that identify the subject will be managed.

   vi) Explain whether any compensation or other medical treatments will be made available if injury occurs. If injury does occur, explain what medical treatments will be available and where subjects can obtain further information.

   vii) Clearly document for the subject a contact who will answer questions about the research and whom to contact if the subject sustains a research-related illness or injury.

   viii) Describe that the subject may discontinue participation in the clinical trial at any time without penalty or loss of further treatment(s) and that participation in the clinical trial is voluntary.

(c) A nurse should ensure that the parents or legally authorized representative (LAR) of pediatric patients understand the concepts of consent, assent, and dissent as they relate to a child's participation in research. While the parents/LAR must provide consent, assent is a minor's affirmative agreement to participate in research. Allowing the right to assent honors a minor's autonomy to the extent that he or she has developed the capacity to make informed choices. If a minor does not object to participation, assent cannot be presumed (Baylis, Downie, & Kenny, 1999; Klimaszewski, 2008a). Dissent is a child's active refusal to participate in research. A sample assent form may be accessed at www.cancer .gov/clinicaltrials/conducting/ informed-consent-guide/page5.

(4) Work with clinical trial participants as appropriate. Make certain that all participation by nursing is within the scope of practice guidelines for the state where the patient is receiving care (Krumm & Garrett, 2007). Clinical investigators are responsible for ensuring that all staff involved in the conduct of the clinical trial

(a) Have a general familiarity with the study and protocol

(b) Have a clear understanding of the protocol and investigational product relevant to the tasks they will be performing

(c) Are aware of regulatory requirements and standards pertaining to the conduct of clinical trials and human subject protection

(d) Are competent to perform the tasks that they are delegated

(e) Are given additional training as necessary (FDA, 2007).

(5) Have additional responsibilities depending upon the phase of the clinical trial.

(a) Verify that the patient, parent, or LAR has given IC, that the original document is in the patient's medical record, and that the patient has received a copy before any study tests are performed or any study treatments are administered.

(b) Clarify technical explanations of procedures and treatments. Document.

(c) Document pretreatment assessment data.

(d) Measure height and weight; check dose calculations with a physician, pharmacist, or another qualified (i.e., chemotherapy-biotherapy trained) nurse.

(e) Have emergency medications and equipment available as appropriate. Document.

(f) Instruct the patient to report changes or symptoms experienced during and after drug administration. Document.

(g) Assess the patient's desire to continue by verbally affirming consent prior to beginning drug infusion. Patients have the right to withdraw at any time. Document.

(h) Administer the drug(s) according to the protocol. Document.

(i) Assess and evaluate drug reactions. Use the NCI Common Terminology Criteria for Adverse Events (CTCAE), available online at http://ctep.info.nih.gov/reporting/ctc.html, to document individual toxicities and help to identify trends in the study population.

(j) Follow up with telephone calls to assess the patient for delayed or chronic side effects as appropriate. Document (Bales & Dearing, 2008; Klimaszewski, 2008a; Wood, 2008).

3. "Fast-track" designation of drugs: Several chemotherapy and biotherapy drugs are given the designation of "fast-track" because of the need to accelerate the development of the drug and to enhance communication and cooperation between the FDA and pharmaceutical companies (Roberts & Chabner, 2004). Examples of just a few of the chemotherapy and biotherapy drugs that have been fast-tracked include docetaxel, irinotecan, tositumomab I-131, and cetuximab. There are many benefits of fast-track designation. These include (McBride, 2007)

a) Opportunities to promote early communication between the company submitting the drug and the FDA, thereby improving the efficiency of the development of the drug.

b) Sections of the new drug application can be submitted instead of all components.

c) Evaluations of various studies can be requested, using surrogate end points.

d) Priority reviews and accelerated approval expedites the study and approval of drugs that are promising.

References

Abeloff, M. (1995). Vinorelbine (Navelbine) in the treatment of breast cancer: A summary. *Seminars in Oncology, 22*(2, Suppl. 5), 1–4.

American Joint Committee on Cancer. (2008, July). *What is cancer staging?* Retrieved August 14, 2008, from http://www.cancerstaging.org/mission/whatis.html

Armitage, J.O. (2005). Staging non-Hodgkin lymphoma. *CA: A Cancer Journal for Clinicians, 55*(6), 368–376.

Bales, C.A., & Dearing, D. (2008). Administration of protocol agents. In A.D. Klimaszewski, M. Bacon, H.E. Deininger, B.A. Ford, & J.G. Westendorp (Eds.), *Manual for clinical trials nursing* (2nd ed., pp. 189–192). Pittsburgh, PA: Oncology Nursing Society.

Baylis, F., Downie, J., & Kenny, N. (1999). Children and decision making in health research. *IRB: A Review of Human Subjects Research, 21*(4), 5–10.

Berg, D.T. (2008). Sponsoring agencies: Industry. In A.D. Klimaszewski, M. Bacon, H.E. Deininger, B.A. Ford, & J.G. Westendorp (Eds.), *Manual for clinical trials nursing* (2nd ed., pp. 55–58). Pittsburgh, PA: Oncology Nursing Society.

Bonadonna, G., Valgussa, P., Rossi, A., Brambilla, C., Zambetti, M. & Veronesi, U. (1985). Ten-year experience with CMF-based adjuvant chemotherapy in resectable breast cancer. *Breast Cancer Research and Treatment, 5*, 95–115.

Bonadonna, G., Zambetti, M., & Valgussa, P. (1995). Sequential or alternating doxorubicin and CMF regimens in breast cancer with more than three positive nodes: Ten-year results. *JAMA, 273*(7), 542–547.

Breslin, S. (2008). History and background of clinical trials. In A.D. Klimaszewski, M. Bacon, H.E. Deininger, B.A. Ford, & J.G. Westendorp (Eds.), *Manual for clinical trials nursing* (2nd ed., pp. 3–9). Pittsburgh, PA: Oncology Nursing Society.

Brown, S.D., & Markus, S. (2008). Introduction to legal and regulatory issues. In A.D. Klimaszewski, M. Bacon, H.E. Deininger, B.A. Ford, & J.G. Westendorp (Eds.), *Manual for clinical trials nursing* (2nd ed., pp. 79–89). Pittsburgh, PA: Oncology Nursing Society.

Burchenal, J.H. (1977). The historical development of cancer chemotherapy. *Seminars in Oncology, 4*(2), 135–148.

Eilber, F.R., Morton, D.L., Eckhardt, J., Grant, T., & Weisenburger, T. (1984). Limb salvage for skeletal and soft tissue sarcomas. *Cancer, 53*(12), 2579–2584.

Farber, S., Diamond, L.K., Mercer, R.D., Sylvester, R.F., & Wolff, J.A. (1948). Temporary remissions in acute leukemia in children produced by folic acid antagonist, 4-aminopteroly-glutamic acid (aminopterin). *New England Journal of Medicine, 238*(23), 787–793.

Fisher, B., Fisher, E., & Redmond, C. (1986). Ten-year results from the NSABP clinical trial evaluating the use of L-phenylalanine mustard (L-PAM) in the management of primary breast cancer. *Journal of Clinical Oncology, 4*(6), 929–941.

Gale, D.M. (2005). Nursing implications of biotherapy and molecular targeted therapy. In J.K. Itano & K.N. Taoka (Eds.), *Core cur-*

riculum for oncology nursing (4th ed., pp. 763–784). St. Louis, MO: Elsevier Saunders.

Gattuso, J.S. (2004). Clinical trials. In N.E. Kline (Ed.), *Essentials of pediatric oncology nursing: A core curriculum* (2nd ed., pp. 80–81). Glenview, IL: Association of Pediatric Oncology Nurses.

Giarelli, E., Jacobs, L.A., & Jenkins, J. (2002). Cancer prevention, screening, and early detection: Human genetics. In K. Jennings-Dozier & S. Mahon (Eds.), *Cancer prevention, detection, and control: A nursing perspective* (pp. 99–141). Pittsburgh, PA: Oncology Nursing Society.

Gillespie, T.W. (2005). Surgical therapy. In C.H. Yarbro, M.H. Frogge, & M. Goodman (Eds.), *Cancer nursing: Principles and practice* (6th ed., pp. 212–228). Sudbury, MA: Jones and Bartlett.

Gilman, A. (1963). The initial clinical trial of nitrogen mustard. *American Journal of Surgery, 105,* 574–578.

Gilman, A., & Philips, F.J. (1946). The biological actions of therapeutic applications of the b-chloroethyl amines and sulfides. *Science, 103*(2675), 409–415.

Gnarra, J., Lerman, M., Zbar, B., & Linehan, W.M. (1995). Genetics of renal-cell carcinoma and evidence for a critical role for von Hippel-Lindau in renal tumorigenesis. *Seminars in Oncology, 22*(1), 3–8.

Gosselin-Acomb, T.K. (2005). Principles of radiation therapy. In C.H. Yarbro, M.H. Frogge, & M. Goodman (Eds.), *Cancer nursing: Principles and practice* (6th ed., pp. 229–249). Sudbury, MA: Jones and Bartlett.

Greene, F.L., Page, D.L., Fleming, I.D., Fritz, A., Balch, C.M., Haller, D.G., et al. (Eds.). (2002). *AJCC cancer staging manual* (6th ed.). New York: Springer.

Guarino, J. (2007). Diagnosis, cytogenetics, and staging. In N.E. Kline (Ed.), *The pediatric chemotherapy and biotherapy curriculum* (2nd ed., pp. 10–15). Glenview, IL: Association of Pediatric Hematology/Oncology Nurses.

Guy, J.L., & Ingram, B.A. (1996). Medical oncology—The agents. In R. McCorkle, M. Grant, M. Frank-Stromborg, & S.B. Baird (Eds.), *Cancer nursing: A comprehensive textbook* (2nd ed., pp. 359–394). Philadelphia: Saunders.

Hoskins, K., Stopfer, J., Calzone, K., Merajver, S., Febbeck, T., Garber, J., et al. (1995). Assessment and counseling for women with a family history of breast cancer. *JAMA, 273*(7), 577–585.

Klimaszewski, A.D. (2008a). Informed consent. In A.D. Klimaszewski, M. Bacon, H.E. Deininger, B.A. Ford, & J.G. Westendorp (Eds.), *Manual for clinical trials nursing* (2nd ed., pp. 97–105). Pittsburgh, PA: Oncology Nursing Society.

Klimaszewski, A.D. (2008b). Psychosocial considerations. In A.D. Klimaszewski, M. Bacon, H.E. Deininger, B.A. Ford, & J.G. Westendorp (Eds.), *Manual for clinical trials nursing* (2nd ed., pp. 133–140). Pittsburgh, PA: Oncology Nursing Society.

Kosta, J.A., & Gullatte, M.M. (2007). Clinical trials. In M.M. Gullatte (Ed.), *Clinical guide to antineoplastic therapy: A chemotherapy handbook* (2nd ed., pp. 481–489). Pittsburgh, PA: Oncology Nursing Society.

Krumm, S., & Garrett, M.R. (2007). Legal issues in chemotherapy administration. In M.M. Gullatte (Ed.), *Clinical guide to antineoplastic therapy: A chemotherapy handbook* (2nd ed., pp. 513–526). Pittsburgh, PA: Oncology Nursing Society.

Loescher, L.J., & Whitesell, L. (2003). The biology of cancer. In A.S. Tranin, A. Masny, & J. Jenkins (Eds.), *Genetics in oncology practice: Cancer risk assessment* (pp. 23–56). Pittsburgh, PA: Oncology Nursing Society.

Marcial, V.A., Pajak, T.F., Kramer, S., Davis, L.W., Steta, J., Laramore, G.E., et al. (1988). Radiation Therapy Oncology Group (RTOG) studies in head and neck cancer. *Seminars in Oncology, 15*(1), 39–60.

McBride, D. (2007). Talactoferrin alpha receives fast-track designation for the treatment of non-small cell lung cancer. *ONS Connect, 22*(1), 6.

Merkle, C.J., & Loescher, L.J. (2005). Cancer biology. In C.H. Yarbro, M.H. Frogge, & M. Goodman (Eds.), *Cancer nursing: Principles and practice* (6th ed., pp. 3–25). Sudbury, MA: Jones and Bartlett.

Miki, Y., Swensen, J., Shattuck-Eidens, D., Futreal, P.A., Harshman, K., Tavtigian, S., et al. (1994). A strong candidate for the breast and ovarian cancer susceptibility gene BRCA1. *Science, 266*(5182), 66–71.

National Cancer Institute. (2005, November). *Care for children and adolescents with cancer: Questions and answers.* Retrieved November 15, 2007, from http://www.cancer.gov/cancertopics/factsheet/NCI/children-adolescents

National Cancer Institute. (2006a, March 24). *A guide to understanding informed consent: What to expect.* Retrieved July 5, 2006, from http://www.cancer.gov/clinicaltrials/conducting/informed-consent-guide/page5

National Cancer Institute. (2006b, June). *Human papillomaviruses and cancer: Questions and answers.* Retrieved November 15, 2007, from http://www.cancer.gov/cancertopics/factsheet/Risk/HPV

National Cancer Institute. (2006c, May 23). *Simplification of informed consent documents: Appendix 2: Code of federal regulations for the protection of human subjects in research.* Retrieved July 5, 2006, from http://www.cancer.gov/clinicaltrials/understanding/simplification-of-informedconsent-docs/page4#appendix2

National Cancer Institute. (2007, October). *Childhood liver cancer treatment (PDQ®): Health professional version: Stage information.* Retrieved August 18, 2008, from http://www.cancer.gov/cancertopics/pdq/treatment/childliver/HealthProfessional/page3

National Cancer Institute. (n.d.). *NCI dictionary of cancer terms: p53.* Retrieved August 20, 2008, from http://www.cancer.gov/templates/db_alpha.aspx?CdrID=45813

National Institute for Occupational Safety and Health. (2005, September). *Pocket guide to chemical hazards.* Retrieved August 20, 2008, from http://www.cdc.gov/niosh/npg/

Noonan, K. (2007). Introduction to B-cell disorders. *Clinical Journal of Oncology Nursing, 11*(1), 3–11.

Okie, S. (2006). Access before approval—A right to take experimental drugs? *New England Journal of Medicine, 355*(5), 437–440.

Olsen, S.J. (2005). Epidemiology and prevention of cancer. In J.K. Itano & K.N. Taoka (Eds.), *Core curriculum for oncology nursing* (4th ed., pp. 839–860). St. Louis, MO: Elsevier Saunders.

Omerod, K.F. (2005). Diagnostic evaluation, classification, and staging. In C.H. Yarbro, M.H. Frogge, & M. Goodman (Eds.), *Cancer nursing: Principles and practice* (6th ed., pp. 153–180). Sudbury, MA: Jones and Bartlett.

Perez, E. (1995). Review of the preclinical pharmacology and comparative efficacy of 5-hydroxytryptamine-3 receptor antagonists for chemotherapy-induced emesis. *Journal of Clinical Oncology, 13*(4), 1036–1043.

Roberts, T.G., & Chabner, B.A. (2004). Beyond fast-track for drug approvals. *New England Journal of Medicine, 351*(5), 501–505.

Roebuck, D.J., Aronson, D., Clatput, P., Czauderna, P., de Ville de Goyet, J., Gauthier, F., et al. (2007). 2005 PRETEXT: A revised staging system for primary malignant liver tumours of childhood developed by the SIOPEL group. *Pediatric Radiology, 37*(2),123–132.

Rowinsky, E., Onetto, N., Canetta, R., & Arbuck, S. (1992). Taxol: The first of the taxanes, an important new class of antitumor agents. *Seminars in Oncology, 19*(6), 646–662.

Speyer, J., Green, M., Dramer, E., Rey, M., Sanger, J., Ward, C., et al. (1988). Protective effect of the bispiperazinedione ICRF-187 against doxorubicin-induced cardiac toxicity in women with advanced breast cancer. *New England Journal of Medicine, 319*(12), 745–752.

Szopa, T.J. (2005). Nursing implications of surgical treatment. In J.K. Itano & K.N. Taoka (Eds.), *Core curriculum for oncology nursing* (4th ed., pp. 736–747). St. Louis, MO: Elsevier Saunders.

Temple, S.V., & Poniatowski, B.C. (2005). Nursing implications of antineoplastic therapy. In J.K. Itano & K.N. Taoka (Eds.), *Core curriculum for oncology nursing* (4th ed., pp. 785–801). St. Louis, MO: Elsevier Saunders.

Tortorice, P.V. (2005). Chemotherapy: Principles of therapy. In C.H. Yarbro, M.H. Frogge, & M. Goodman (Eds.), *Cancer nursing: Principles and practice* (6th ed., pp. 315–350). Sudbury, MA: Jones and Bartlett.

Trocky, N.M., & Brandt, C. (2008). Clinical trial registries. In A.D. Klimaszewski, M. Bacon, H.E. Deininger, B.A. Ford, & J.G. Westendorp (Eds.), *Manual for clinical trials nursing* (2nd ed., pp. 305–311). Pittsburgh, PA: Oncology Nursing Society.

U.S. Department of Health and Human Services. (2005a). *Carcinogens listed in the Eleventh Report: Part A. Known to be human carcinogens. Report on carcinogens, Eleventh edition; U.S. Department of Health and Human Services, Public Health Service, National Toxicology Program.* Retrieved August 20, 2008, from http://ntp.niehs.nih.gov/ntp/roc/eleventh/known.pdf

U.S. Department of Health and Human Services. (2005b). *Carcinogens listed in the Eleventh Report: Part B. Reasonably anticipated to be a human carcinogen. Report on carcinogens, Eleventh edition; U.S. Department of Health and Human Services, Public Health Service, National Toxicology Program.* Retrieved August 20, 2008, from http://ntp.niehs.nih.gov/ntp/roc/eleventh/reason.pdf

U.S. Department of Health and Human Services. (2005c, June). *Code of federal regulations, Title 45: Public Welfare, Part 46: Protection of Human Subjects.* Retrieved December 3, 2007, from http://www.hhs.gov/ohrp/humansubjects/guidance/45cfr46.htm

U.S. Food and Drug Administration. (2007, May). *Guidance for industry. Protecting the rights, safety, and welfare of study subjects—supervisory responsibilities of investigators.* Retrieved August 20, 2008, from http://www.fda.gov/cber/gdlns/studysub.pdf

Volker, D.L. (2005). Biology of cancer and carcinogenesis. In J.K. Itano & K.N. Taoka (Eds.), *Core curriculum for oncology nursing* (4th ed., pp. 443–464). St. Louis, MO: Elsevier Saunders.

Witt, M.E. (2005). Nursing implications of radiation therapy. In J.K. Itano & K.N. Taoka (Eds.), *Core curriculum for oncology nursing* (4th ed., pp. 748–762). St. Louis, MO: Elsevier Saunders.

Wong, S.F., & Westendorp, J. (2008). Investigational agents and procurement of research study drugs. In A.D. Klimaszewski, M. Bacon, H.E. Deininger, B.A. Ford, & J.G. Westendorp (Eds.), *Manual for clinical trials nursing* (2nd ed., pp. 179–188). Pittsburgh, PA: Oncology Nursing Society.

Wood, L.S. (2008). Adverse events. In A.D. Klimaszewski, M. Bacon, H.E. Deininger, B.A. Ford, & J.G. Westendorp (Eds.), *Manual for clinical trials nursing* (2nd ed., pp. 197–214). Pittsburgh, PA: Oncology Nursing Society.

World Health Organization. (2008, July). *What causes cancer? Fact sheet No. 297: Cancer.* Retrieved August 19, 2008, from http://www.who.int/mediacentre/factsheets/fs297/en/print.html

Zubrod, C.G. (1984). Origins and development of chemotherapy research at the National Cancer Institute. *Cancer Treatment Reports, 68*(1), 9–19.

D. Ethical issues related to cancer therapy
  1. Healthcare realities that present potential ethical issues
    a) Medical advances: Advances in technology allow healthcare professionals to sustain life longer than ever before. However, this ability may not always be employed for the right reasons. Life-sustaining measures may be employed because the healthcare professional (Kerber, 2006; Pence, 2004; Pendry, 2007)
      (1) Did not discuss the patient's wishes before a crisis developed
      (2) Was reluctant to or did not communicate medical treatment options with a grief-stricken family
      (3) Feared legal liability
      (4) Followed the traditional treatment protocol, which emphasizes treatment rather than supportive care measures
      (5) Was experiencing moral distress related to personal values or biases.
    b) Changing healthcare environment: Staffing shortages, reallocation of resources, consolidation, and corporatization have resulted in growing administrative dominance over clinical practice (Agency for Healthcare Research and Quality [AHRQ], 2000; Institute of Medicine, 2004; Pendry, 2007).
    c) Increasing numbers of uninsured and insufficiently insured individuals: Even with insurance, copayments can lead to debt. Children and the working poor are most affected by lack of coverage, and some people with insurance are unable to obtain reimbursement for certain treatments, such as bone marrow transplant (BMT) or off-label use of medications (Hoffman, Schoen, Rowland, & Davis, 2001; O'Donnell, 2004).
    d) Increases in a culturally diverse populace: Cultural and communication differences

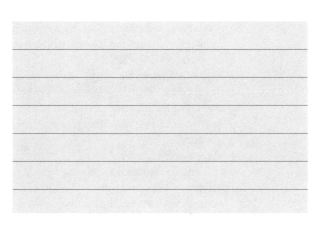

present a range of challenges, from discussion of diagnosis and prognosis to decisions about who will provide long-term care (Balsa, Seiler, McGuire, & Bloche, 2003; O'Donnell, 2004; Searight & Gafford, 2005).

    e) Use of unproven cancer treatments: Increasing use of unproven treatments, either in conjunction with or as a substitute for conventional treatment, is the result of many factors, including the unpredictable nature of individual response to cancer and its treatment, the need for control, belief in individual rights and determination, and cultural and spiritual beliefs (O'Donnell, 2004; Sheridan-Leos, Schulmeister, & Hartranft, 2006).

2. Ethical issues that oncology nurses face in daily practice (Cassells, Jenkins, Lea, Calzone, & Johnson, 2003; Kerber, 2006; Pendry, 2007) relate to
    a) End-of-life decisions
    b) IC
    c) Patient autonomy and decision-making capacity
    d) The right to refuse treatment
    e) Undertreatment of pain
    f) The healthcare environment and reform
    g) Access to care
    h) Confidentiality
    i) Scientific integrity
    j) Nurse-family conflicts
    k) Nurse-physician conflicts
    l) Physician-family conflicts
    m) Participation in clinical research.

3. The Joint Commission on Accreditation of Healthcare Organizations (JCAHO, 2005) requires that a nurse be able to request an ethics consultation within the clinical institution to assist in evaluating the decision-making capacity of an individual as well as to assist with problem resolution.

4. The characteristics of ethical decisions: Ethical decisions maximize the following (Beauchamp & Childress, 2001; Cassells et al., 2003; Kerber, 2006).
    a) Autonomy: Independent decision making by an individual in accordance with his or her own best interest
    b) Nonmaleficence: The duty to do no harm
    c) Beneficence: The duty to act in the best interest of the involved person
    d) Justice: Equitable distribution of available resources
    e) Veracity: Truth-telling
    f) Fidelity: Faithfulness to promises made
    g) Advocacy: Support given to others to assist in their decision-making ability

E. Legal issues related to cancer therapy: Adhering to national, state, and institutional standards is a fundamental responsibility of all nurses (Birke, 2004; Dearing, 2008).
1. The acts and standards guiding nursing practice
    a) Nurse practice acts: State laws that define nursing performance in fundamental terms for each state
    b) Oncology Nursing Society *Statement on the Scope and Standards of Oncology Nursing Practice* (Brant & Wickham, 2004) describes the minimum standard of care to which a patient with cancer is entitled.
    c) *Infusion Nursing Standards of Practice* (Infusion Nurses Society, 2006) describes the current standard of nursing practice for IV therapy.
    d) Institution-specific standards may be set forth in
        (1) Standards of practice
        (2) Nursing policy and procedure manuals
        (3) Job descriptions
        (4) IRB decisions.
2. Common legal issues
    a) Medication errors: A nurse is the final checkpoint in the medication administration process; therefore, legal issues regarding medication errors frequently affect nurses.
        (1) Prevalence
            (a) As reported by the Institute of Medicine (2004), 3.7% of inpatients experienced an adverse event related to a medication error.
            (b) Preventable adverse drug events caused one out of five injuries or deaths to patients in hospitals (AHRQ, 2000).
            (c) Sixty-three percent of the oncology nurses that participated in a 1999 study by Schulmeister reported chemotherapy errors in their institutions (Schulmeister, 1999; Sheridan-Leos et al., 2006).
        (2) Risks associated with the administration of cytotoxic agents (Birner, 2003; Schulmeister, 2006; Sheridan-Leos et al., 2006)
            (a) Toxicity
            (b) Low margin for dosing error (Use of high-dose ablative therapy leaves essentially no margin for error.)
            (c) Widely varying dosages and administration schedules (Doses

and schedules may be patient-specific.)

   (d) Doses often are modified based on patients' clinical status and response.

   (e) Complicated and varying medications, schedules, and regimens

(3) Types of chemotherapy medication errors (Clancy, Farquhar, & Sharp, 2005; Sheridan-Leos, 2007)

   (a) Administration of the wrong dose (under- or overdosing)

   (b) Schedule and timing errors

   (c) Use of the wrong drug

   (d) Infusion rate errors

   (e) Omission of drugs or hydration

   (f) Improper drug preparation

   (g) Route errors (e.g., intrathecal [IT] versus IV)

   (h) Administration to the wrong patient

   (i) Administration when lab values not appropriate

(4) Factors contributing to medication errors in chemotherapy: Most medication errors are system-related and not attributable to individual negligence or misconduct (AHRQ, 2000; Sheridan-Leos, 2007).

   (a) Stress

   (b) Understaffing

   (c) Lack of experience administering chemotherapy

   (d) Unclear or ambiguous chemotherapy orders

   (e) Lack of experience administering the specific chemotherapy drug with which the error occurred

   (f) Fatigue

   (g) Illegible handwriting

   (h) Inaccessibility of information about chemotherapy drugs

   (i) Chemotherapy drug packaging or vial difficult to read or understand

   (j) Increasing number of complicated schedules and new drug combinations

(5) Strategies for preventing medication errors have been described by the American Society of Health-System Pharmacists (ASHP, 2002; see also Santell, Protzel, & Cousins, 2004) and include the following.

   (a) Verify all pertinent clinical patient information, including patient's measured height and weight, labo-

ratory results, and body surface area (BSA).

   (b) Ensure that up-to-date drug information and other resources are readily available to clinicians.

   (c) Support institutional policy that prohibits verbal orders for chemotherapy.

   (d) Use preprinted, standardized forms or computer-generated forms to order cytotoxic drugs when possible.

   (e) Avoid the use of abbreviations, acronyms, coined names, and other ambiguous methods of communicating drug information.

   (f) Provide ongoing education to patients about their medications, and encourage them to ask questions and seek clarification before their drugs are administered.

   (g) Ensure adherence to institutional policies and procedures.

   (h) Verify all chemotherapy doses, scheduling, and dosing calculation (see section IV.B: Verification and Maintenance of Treatment as Planned). Support institutional policy for a systematic method of dose verification.

   (i) Review orders in an environment with minimal distractions.

   (j) Ensure that only experienced oncology nurses who are competent in administering cytotoxic therapy administer cytotoxic therapy.

b) Documentation issues (ASHP, 2002; Gialanella, 2004; Sheridan-Leos et al., 2006): The duty to keep accurate records is a fundamental legal nursing responsibility. The medical record is scrutinized in the event of litigious action and is believed to reflect the care rendered (i.e., "If it wasn't charted, it wasn't done").

(1) Common documentation errors include

   (a) Omitting observations of significance

   (b) Failing to document the patient's response to an intervention

   (c) Failing to document patient teaching and understanding

   (d) Failing to document what was taught and to whom.

(2) Documentation should include the following direct and indirect nursing actions.

    (a) Telephone conversations, particularly those in which the nurse gives the patient instructions or advice

    (b) Pertinent conversations with the patient, family, or other caregivers

    (c) Interagency referrals

    (d) Cytotoxic drug administration: See Appendices 1 and 2.

    (e) The record should include

      i) Patient's name

      ii) Date and time of therapy

      iii) Drug name, dose, route of administration, and infusion duration

      iv) Volume and type of fluids administered

      v) Assessment of the site before, during, and after infusion

      vi) Information about infusion device (e.g., vein selection, needle size, type of device, infusion pump)

      vii) Verification of blood return before, during, and after IV therapy.

    (f) Patient assessment and evaluation of the patient response to and tolerance of treatment

    (g) Patient and family education related to drugs received, toxicities, toxicity management, and follow-up care

    (h) Post-treatment or discharge instructions

  c) Issues related to IC process: The patient must give IC for treatment, enrollment in a clinical trial, or participation in nursing research (Birke, 2004; Klimaszewski, 2008; White, Keller, & Horrigan, 2003).

    (1) The IC document must state the right of the patient to refuse or discontinue treatment at any time.

    (2) The IC document and, subsequently, physicians and nurses, must guarantee patients that ongoing support and care will be provided if they decline or discontinue treatment connected with the trial or research.

    (3) Nurses and physicians have different but complementary roles in the IC process.

    (4) See Section I.C for additional information on the IC process and the nurse's role.

References

Agency for Healthcare Research and Quality. (2000). *Translating research into practice: Reducing errors in health care* (AHRQ Publication No. 00-PO58). Rockville, MD: Author. Retrieved November 13, 2007, from http://www.ahrq.gov/research/errors.htm

American Society of Health-System Pharmacists. (2002). ASHP guidelines on preventing medication errors with antineoplastic agents. *American Journal of Health-System Pharmacists, 59*(17), 1648–1668.

Balsa, A., Seiler, N., McGuire, T., & Bloche, M. (2003). Clinical uncertainty and healthcare disparities. *American Journal of Law and Medicine, 29*(2–3), 203–219.

Beauchamp, T.L., & Childress, J.F. (2001). *Principles of biomedical ethics* (5th ed.). New York: Oxford University Press.

Birke, M. (2004). Elder law, Medicare, and legal issues in older patients. *Seminars in Oncology, 31*(2), 282–292.

Birner, A. (2003). Safe administration of oral chemotherapy. *Clinical Journal of Oncology Nursing, 7*(2), 158–162.

Brant, J.M., & Wickham, R.S. (Eds.). (2004). *Statement on the scope and standards of oncology nursing practice.* Pittsburgh, PA: Oncology Nursing Society.

Cassells, J.M., Jenkins, J., Lea, D.H., Calzone, K., & Johnson, E. (2003). An ethical assessment framework for addressing global genetic issues in clinical practice. *Oncology Nursing Forum, 30*(3), 383–390.

Clancy, C., Farquhar, M.B., & Sharp, B. (2005). Focus on patient safety. Patient safety in nursing practice. *Journal of Nursing Care Quality, 20*(3), 193–197.

Dearing, D. (2008). Legislative issues. In A.D. Klimaszewski, M. Bacon, H.E. Deininger, B.A. Ford, & J.G. Westendorp (Eds.), *Manual for clinical trials nursing* (2nd ed., pp. 115–122). Pittsburgh, PA: Oncology Nursing Society.

Gialanella, K. (2004). Documentation. *Advance for Nurses, 6*(14), 17–19.

Hoffman, C., Schoen, C., Rowland, D., & Davis, L. (2001). Gaps in health care coverage in working age Americans and the consequences. *Journal of Health Care for the Poor and Underserved, 12*(3), 272–289.

Infusion Nurses Society. (2006). Infusion nursing standards of practice. *Journal of Infusion Nursing, 29*(Suppl. 1), S1–S92.

Institute of Medicine. (2004). *Keeping patients safe: Transforming the work environment of nurses.* Washington, DC: National Academies Press.

Joint Commission on Accreditation of Healthcare Organizations. (2005). *Comprehensive accreditation manual for hospitals.* Oakbrook Terrace, IL: Author.

Kerber, A.S. (2006). Legal and ethical issues concerning the older adult with cancer. In A. Reb & D. Cope (Eds.), *An evidence-based ap-*

proach to the treatment and care of the older adult with cancer (pp. 561–578). Pittsburgh, PA: Oncology Nursing Society.

Klimaszewski, A.D. (2008). Informed consent. In A.D. Klimaszewski, M. Bacon, H.E. Deininger, B.A. Ford, & J.G. Westendorp (Eds.), *Manual for clinical trials nursing* (2nd ed., pp. 97–105). Pittsburgh, PA: Oncology Nursing Society.

O'Donnell, P. (2004). Ethical issues in end-of-life care: Social work facilitation and proactive interventions. In J. Berzoff & P.R. Silverman (Eds.), *Living with dying: A handbook for end-of-life healthcare practitioners* (pp. 171–187). New York: Columbia University Press.

Pence, G.E. (2004). *Classic cases in medical ethics* (4th ed.). New York: McGraw-Hill Higher Education.

Pendry, P. (2007). Moral distress: Recognizing it to retain nurses. *Nursing Economics, 25*(4), 217–221.

Santell, J.P., Protzel, M.M., & Cousins, D. (2004). Medication errors in oncology practice. *U.S. Pharmacist, 29*(4). Retrieved September 28, 2008, from http://www.uspharmacist.com/index.asp?show=article&page=8_1259.htm

Schulmeister, L. (1999). Chemotherapy medication errors: Description, severity, and contributing factors. *Oncology Nursing Forum, 26*(6), 1033–1042.

Schulmeister, L. (2006). Preventing chemotherapy errors. *Oncologist, 11*(5), 463–468.

Searight, H.R., & Gafford, J. (2005). Cultural diversity at the end of life: Issues and guidelines for family physicians. *American Family Physician, 71*(3). Retrieved September 28, 2008, from http://www.aafp.org/afp/20050201/515.html

Sheridan-Leos, N. (2007). A model of chemotherapy education for novice oncology nurses that supports a culture of safety. *Clinical Journal of Oncology Nursing, 11*(4), 545–551.

Sheridan-Leos, N., Schulmeister, L., & Hartranft, S. (2006). Failure mode and effect analysis: A technique to prevent chemotherapy errors. *Clinical Journal of Oncology Nursing, 10*(3), 393–398.

White, M.K., Keller, V., & Horrigan, L.A. (2003). Beyond informed consent: The shared decision making process. *Journal of Clinical Outcomes Management, 10*(6), 323–328.

II. Cancer Therapy Goals and Response

A. Goals of cancer therapy (Otto, 2007)
1. Prevention (Brown & Humble, 2007)
2. Cure
   a) The prolonged absence of detectable disease
   b) The desired outcome for all patients, but one that is not always achievable
3. Control
   a) An extension of life when cure is unrealistic
   b) Preventing the growth of cancer cells without complete elimination of the disease (Gosselin-Acomb, 2005)
   c) Reducing existing disease without preventing the development of new disease
4. Palliation
   a) Comfort when supposed cure or control of the disease is impossible
   b) Reduction of side effects and symptoms, including pain (Brown & Humble, 2007; Ellison & Chevlen, 2002; Gaddis & Gullatte, 2007)
   c) May include surgery, radiation therapy, or chemotherapy-biotherapy, individually or in combination (Ferrans, 2005; Otto, 2007)
5. Adjuvant therapy: Therapy following the primary treatment modality, such as surgery or radiation. The goal of adjuvant therapy is to target minimal disease or micrometastases for patients at high risk for recurrence (Otto, 2007).
6. Neoadjuvant therapy: The use of one or more treatment modalities prior to the primary therapy (e.g., chemotherapy before surgery). Goal is to shrink the primary tumor to improve the effectiveness of surgery and/or decrease the likelihood of micrometastases (Otto, 2007).
7. Chemoprevention: The use of selected pharmaceutical agents to prevent cancer in high-risk individuals (e.g., administration of tamoxifen to women whose personal health history indicates they are at a statistically increased risk for developing breast cancer) (Brown & Humble, 2007; Sporn & Lippman, 2003).
8. Myeloablation: Obliteration of bone marrow in preparation for peripheral blood stem cell or bone marrow transplantation.
9. Immunosuppression: Blunting the patient's immunogenic response in preparation for a stem cell transplant. The conditioning regimen involves the administration of chemotherapy, often with radiation. Myeloablative regimens require lethal doses; nonmyeloablative (sometimes referred to as "mini-transplants") use nonlethal doses (Poliquin, 2007).

B. Factors affecting response to treatment
1. Tumor burden: The inverse relationship between the number of tumor cells and response implies that the smaller the tumor, the higher the rate of response (Evans & Bitran, 2001; Tortorice, 2005). This is because as the tumor mass increases in size, the growth rate begins to slow, thus decreasing the effectiveness of antineoplastic therapy.
2. Rate of tumor growth: Tumor doubling time (time for the tumor to double in mass) and growth fraction (proportion of proliferating cells in relation to the total number of tumor cells) are important factors affecting response. Chemotherapeutic agents are most active against rapidly growing tumors (Evans & Bitran, 2001; Otto, 2007).
3. Drug resistance
   a) Newer theories explaining the various pathways of drug resistance have recently emerged based on a better understanding of how cytotoxic drugs affect malignant cell apoptosis. These theories help to explain why chemosensitive tumors may not be completely eliminated (Tortorice, 2005).
   b) A complex biochemical pathway involving a multitude of receptors and enzymes is implicated and is dependent upon the type of cell and chemotherapeutic agent (Tortorice, 2005).
   c) Research (Tortorice, 2005) points to a complex interaction among cytotoxic agents, chemical messengers (transporters that affect drug delivery to the tumor) (Gaddis & Gullatte, 2007), and the genetic ability of malignant cells to avoid chemotherapy-induced apoptosis because of their high rate of genetic instability.
   d) Tumor cells may be inherently resistant to antineoplastic agents or develop resistance after drug exposure due to the emergence of resistant clones. Single-agent or multidrug

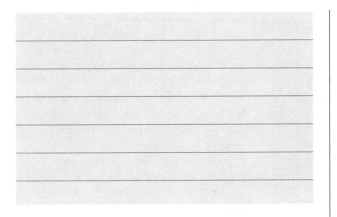

resistance (MDR) may occur and may be caused by a number of factors.

(1) Insufficient dosing may lead to the development of resistant cell clones arising from random mutations in cellular DNA (Barton-Burke & Wilkes, 2006; Chu & DeVita, 2005).

(2) Chemotherapy may kill sensitive cells while leaving behind cells resistant to treatment administered (Tortorice, 2005).

(3) MDR occurs when malignant cells are exposed to cytotoxic agents possessing dissimilar mechanisms of action and appears to be caused by mutations in the malignant cells' regulatory system (Chu & DeVita, 2005; Tortorice, 2005). Several pathways are thought to be responsible for MDR and include alterations in the metabolism of chemotherapy within the tumor, the ability of tumor cells to repair damaged DNA (thus bypassing apoptosis), and decreased uptake by formerly susceptible cells (Tortorice). MDR pathways include the following.

(a) Overexpression of the MDR-1 gene, which encodes for the cell membrane efflux pump P-glycoprotein (P-gp), is believed to be responsible for resistance by its ability to remove toxic molecules (i.e., chemotherapy) from inside the cell before the drug can reach the DNA. The presence of P-gp is a poor prognostic indicator (Barton-Burke & Wilkes, 2006; Tortorice 2005).

(b) Resistance to topoisomerase drugs (e.g., doxorubicin) can occur when the tumor develops the ability to change the binding properties of topoisomerase enzymes (Tortorice, 2005).

(c) MDR also can occur from increased levels of normally protective enzymes (e.g., glutathione S-transferase), which facilitate the elimination of platinum compounds and alkylating agents from malignant cells (Tortorice, 2005).

(4) Impaired metabolism may result in reduced drug activation or increased drug deactivation.

(5) Other types of resistance include the following.

(a) Acquired resistance is the result of further mutations after exposure to additional drugs (Chu & DeVita, 2005).

(b) Emergent resistance occurs after the affected cells survive an exposure to an environmental carcinogen (e.g., tobacco).

(c) Cells may temporarily be less responsive because of changes in environment or stimuli or have permanent resistance (Goldie, 2008).

(d) Temporary resistance may be caused by poor blood supply to tumor, which prevents a therapeutic dose of drug from being delivered (Tortorice, 2005).

(6) Overcoming drug resistance remains a high priority. Researchers continue to look for ways to deactivate the P-gp in malignant cells and to identify new agents that alter the apoptotic pathways, increase the effectiveness of current chemotherapy, and interact with specific characteristics associated with the DNA in malignant cells (Barton-Burke & Wilkes, 2006).

C. Treatment strategies
1. Combination versus single-agent therapy (Burris, 2001; Haskell, 2001; Langhorne & Barton-Burke, 2001; Tortorice, 2005)

a) Tumor cell populations are heterogeneous; therefore, a combination of agents with different mechanisms of action is able to increase the proportion of cells killed at any one time.

b) Combination chemotherapy reduces the possibility of drug resistance by using drugs that have different mechanisms of action.

c) Agents selected for use in combination chemotherapy have proven efficacy as single agents.

d) Combination chemotherapy may use the principle of drug synergy to maximize the effects of another drug. Synergy is affected by the rate of tumor cell proliferation, as well as by whether the drugs are administered sequentially or simultaneously (e.g., leucovorin potentiates the cytotoxicity of 5-fluorouracil [5-FU]) (Brown & Humble, 2007).

e) Drugs with similar toxicities generally are avoided, although this is not always possible. For example, both paclitaxel and cisplatin can cause peripheral neuropathy as single agents but often are used together (Argyriou et al., 2007).

2. Dose or dose intensity (dose over total time of delivery) of chemotherapy
   a) Cycles are designed to permit organ recovery from the damage to normal tissues. Because the average time for white blood cell (WBC) nadir is 10–14 days, many regimens are based upon this repeating cycle.
   b) Administering a drug like 5-FU at a steady concentration over a period of time increases cell kill (Howland & Mycek, 2006). Current research efforts are directed toward reducing the amount of time between standard doses of chemotherapy to increase dose density (Citron et al., 2003; Pfreundschuh et al., 2004; Tortorice, 2005). By reducing the time between chemotherapy cycles, tumor regrowth may be diminished. This strategy has resulted in longer survival for patients with breast, ovarian, and colon cancers and lymphoma (Tortorice). The prophylactic use of the colony-stimulating factor pegfilgrastim has allowed for dose-dense chemotherapy regimens that would otherwise result in unacceptable neutropenia (Burdette-Radoux et al., 2007; von Minckwitz et al., 2007).
   c) Nurses should be aware that dose reduction or delay resulting from chemotherapy side effects, scheduling conflicts, or any other reason may have a negative impact on patient survival (Tortorice, 2005). Optimal cell kill is achieved by delivering sufficient doses of chemotherapy at intervals corresponding with the phase of tumor cells. Proactive management of symptoms and educating patients on the importance of maintaining the prescribed dosing schedule are paramount.

3. Hormone receptor status
   a) Tumors that grow more rapidly in the presence of a specific hormone may be suppressed with the administration of an antihormonal agent. The presence of estrogen and/or progesterone receptors is prognostic for breast cancer. Patients who are positive (ER/PR) demonstrate better overall survival rates (Yackzan, 2007).
   b) This factor has become increasingly important in cancer therapy.

D. Measuring response
   1. Measuring tumor response
      a) Objective tumor response is assessed through a quantitative measurement such as surgical examination, imaging studies, and/or serum tumor markers. Measurements recorded at the time of diagnosis are compared to those recorded after completing a course of treatment.
      b) Tumor response has historically been classified according to the following categories (Perry, Anderson, & Donehower, 2000).
         (1) Complete response (CR): Absence of all signs and symptoms of cancer for at least one month using objective criteria (e.g., quantitative bidimensional tumor measurement)
         (2) Partial response (PR): At least a 50% reduction of measurable tumor mass for one month without development of new tumors
         (3) Stable disease (SD): A reduction in tumor mass of less than 50% or less than a 25% increase in tumor growth
         (4) Progressive disease (PD): Growth of 25% or more or development of new tumors
         (5) Relapse
            (a) After CR, a new tumor appears or the original tumor reappears.

(b) With PR, a new tumor appears or the original tumor increases in size.

c) Response Evaluation Criteria in Solid Tumors (RECIST) guidelines were developed in 1999 by an international task force including the European Organisation for Research and Treatment of Cancer (EORTC), NCI of the United States, and the National Cancer Institute of Canada Clinical Trials Group.

   (1) Guidelines are intended to facilitate communication between researchers and clinicians (Therasse, Eisenhauer, & Buyse, 2006).

   (2) Considerable variation exists between the RECIST and WHO criteria for evaluating response (Mazumdar, Smith, & Schwartz, 2004; Schwartz et al., 2006). These variations create a challenge for evaluating the effectiveness of therapies being studied in clinical trials.

2. The WHO (Therasse et al., 2000) recognizes that diagnostic technologies (e.g., computed tomography [CT] scans, magnetic resonance imaging) have led to confusion regarding three-dimensional measurement of disease. As a result, the reported response criteria vary among research groups.

3. RECIST guidelines include the following (Therasse et al., 2000).

a) Response to a clinical trial is used to decide whether an agent or regimen demonstrated results that are promising enough to warrant further testing (prospective end point).

b) At baseline, tumors must be measurable in at least one dimension (using metrics) by calipers or a ruler. Baseline measurements must be obtained within four weeks of initiating therapy. (Nonmeasurable lesions include bone lesions, ascites, pleural or pericardial effusions, leptomeningeal disease, and inflammatory breast cancer.)

c) The same method and technique used at baseline must be used to evaluate response for reporting and follow-up.

d) If the primary end point is response to treatment, the patient must have at least one measurable lesion at baseline. If only one measurable lesion is present, it must be confirmed by cytology or histology.

e) Measurable lesions, up to 5 per organ or 10 in total, are identified as "target" lesions.

   (1) Lesions selected are the longest in diameter; suitable for follow-up measurement.

   (2) The sum of the longest diameter for each lesion is calculated and reported as the *baseline sum longest diameter*. This sum is used as the reference to compare response.

   (3) All other non–target lesions are measured and recorded if possible. Their presence or absence can be noted for follow-up but is not included in the response evaluation.

f) Using RECIST criteria

   (1) CR is the disappearance of all target lesions.

   (2) PR is a 30% reduction in the sum of the longest diameter of target lesions as compared to the baseline.

   (3) PD is a 20% increase in the longest diameter compared to the smallest sum recorded since treatment was initiated.

   (4) Follow-up should be protocol-specific.

     (a) Every other cycle (6–8 weeks) is reasonable for follow-up.

     (b) Patients who discontinue therapy because of deterioration of their health condition without evidence of PD are identified as "symptomatically deteriorated" and not included in the PR, SD, or PD groups.

     (c) At the conclusion of treatment, follow-up tests and schedules will be based upon the goal of the study. If time to a specific event, such as recurrence or death, is the primary end point of the study, measurements must be compared to the baseline.

     (d) The duration of overall response is measured from when the measurement criteria were met for CR or PR until the first date a recurrence or PD was measured.

     (e) The duration of SD is the time from initiation of therapy until the criteria are met for PD.

g) Reporting using RECIST results: All patients in the study must be assessed at the end of the study. Patients are assigned to one of the following categories.

   (1) CR
   (2) PR
   (3) SD
   (4) PD
   (5) Early death from disease
   (6) Early death from toxicity

4. Measuring patient response

a) Response according to performance status scales

   (1) After tumor type, patient activity level or performance status is the most impor-

tant factor to consider when determining appropriate treatment (Ellison & Chevlen, 2002). Several performance scales are currently in use. Of these, the Karnofsky, Eastern Cooperative Oncology Group (ECOG), and WHO scales are the most common for adults. Patients who have lower performance scores (e.g., bedridden) may not be able to withstand the rigors of an aggressive treatment regimen and may experience a decrease in QOL. Performance scales also are used as part of inclusion/exclusion criteria for clinical trials (Omerod, 2005). A Web page for converting between scales is available through the FDA at www.fda.gov/cder/cancer/perstat .htm.

(2) See Table 4, which compares four different performance status scales.

Table 4. Performance Status Scales/Scores[a]

Karnofsky		WHO		ECOG (Zubrod)		Lansky[b]	
% Score	Functional Status	Score	Functional Status	Score	Functional Status	Score	
100	Normal, no complaints or evidence of disease	0	Fully active and able to carry out all pre-disease activities without restriction	0	Asymptomatic	100	Fully active, normal
90	Able to carry out normal activity; minor signs or symptoms of disease	1	Restricted in strenuous activity but ambulatory and able to carry out light work	1	Symptomatic; fully ambulatory	90	Minor restrictions in physically strenuous activity
80	Normal activity with effort; some signs or symptoms of disease					80	Active, but tires more quickly
70	Cares for self; unable to carry out normal activity or do active work	2	Ambulatory and capable of all self-care but unable to do any light work; up and about more than 50% of waking hours	2	Symptomatic; in bed less than 50% of day	70	Both greater restriction of and less time spent in play activity
60	Requires occasional assistance but able to care for most needs					60	Up and around, but minimal active play; keeps busy with quieter activities
50	Requires considerable assistance and frequent medical care	3	Capable of only limited self-care; confined to bed or chair more than 50% of waking hours	3	Symptomatic; in bed more than 50% of day but not bedridden	50	Gets dressed but lies around much of the day; no active play but able to participate in all quiet play and activities
40	Disabled; requires special care and assistance					40	Mostly in bed; participates in quiet activities
30	Severely disabled; hospitalization indicated although death not imminent	4	Completely disabled; unable to carry out any self-care and confined totally to bed or chair	4	Bedridden	30	In bed; needs assistance even for quiet play
20	Very sick; hospitalization necessary; active supportive treatment necessary					20	Often sleeping; play entirely limited to very passive activities

(Continued on next page)

Table 4. Performance Status Scales/Scores[a] *(Continued)*

Karnofsky		WHO		ECOG (Zubrod)		Lansky[b]	
% Score	Functional Status	Score	Functional Status	Score	Functional Status	Score	
10	Moribund; fatal processes progressing rapidly					10	No play; does not get out of bed
0	Dead					0	Unresponsive

[a] Karnofsky and Lansky performance scores are intended to be multiples of 10.
[b] The conversion of the Lansky to ECOG scales is intended for NCI reporting purposes only.

ECOG—Eastern Cooperative Oncology Group; NCI—National Cancer Institute; WHO—World Health Organization

Note. From "Diagnostic Evaluation, Classification, and Staging" (p. 177), by K. Omerod in C.H. Yarbro, M.H. Frogge, and M. Goodman (Eds.), *Cancer Nursing: Principles and Practice* (6th ed.), 2005, Sudbury, MA: Jones and Bartlett. Copyright 2005 by Jones and Bartlett, www.jbpub.com. Adapted wtih permission.

(a) Karnofsky Performance Status (KPS) scale: Evaluates adult performance in terms of percentage; a lower score indicates poorer performance (Karnofsky & Burchenal, 1949).

(b) ECOG and Zubrod scales: Evaluate adult performance on a 0–5 scale; a higher score indicates poorer performance (Oken et al., 1982).

(c) WHO scale: Scales developed by the United Nations and include performance and toxicity grading.

(d) The Lansky Performance scale was developed specifically for children, as the KPS scale is often not applicable in pediatric populations (Lansky, List, Lansky, Ritter-Sterr, & Miller, 1987).

References

Argyriou, A.A., Polychronopoulos, P., Koutras, A., Xiros, N., Petsas, T., Argyriou, K., et al. (2007). Clinical and electrophysiological features of peripheral neuropathy induced by administration of cisplatin plus paclitaxel-based chemotherapy. *European Journal of Cancer Care, 16*(3), 231–237.

Barton-Burke, M., & Wilkes, G. (2006). Cancer chemotherapy and cell cycle kinetics. In M. Barton-Burke & G.M. Wilkes (Eds.), *Cancer therapies* (pp. 21–28). Sudbury, MA: Jones and Bartlett.

Brown, D., & Humble, A. (2007). Cellular mechanisms of chemotherapy. In M.M. Gullatte (Ed.), *Clinical guide to antineoplastic therapy: A chemotherapy handbook* (2nd ed., pp. 1–15). Pittsburgh, PA: Oncology Nursing Society.

Burdette-Radoux, S., Wood, M.E., Olin, J.J., Laughlin, R.S., Crocker, A.M., Ashikaga, T., et al. (2007). Phase I/II trial of adjuvant dose-dense docetaxel/epirubicin/cyclophosphamide (TEC) in stage II and III breast cancer. *Breast Journal, 13*(3), 274–280.

Burris, H.A. (2001). Combination chemotherapy. In M.C. Perry (Ed.), *The chemotherapy source book* (3rd ed., pp. 69–73). Philadelphia: Lippincott Williams & Wilkins.

Chu, E., & DeVita, E., Jr. (2005). *Physicians' cancer chemotherapy drug manual*. Sudbury, MA: Jones and Bartlett.

Citron, M.L., Berry, D.A., Cirrincione, C., Hudis, C., Winer, E.P., Gradishar, W.J., et al. (2003). Randomized trial of dose-dense versus conventionally scheduled and sequential versus concurrent combination chemotherapy as postoperative adjuvant treatment of node-positive primary breast cancer: First report of Intergroup Trial C9741/Cancer and Leukemia Group B Trial 9741. *Journal of Clinical Oncology, 21*(8), 1431–1439.

Ellison, N.M., & Chevlen, E.M. (2002). Palliative chemotherapy. In A. Berger, R. Portenoy, & D. Weissman (Eds.), *Principles and practice of palliative care and supportive oncology* (2nd ed., pp. 698–709). Philadelphia: Lippincott Williams & Wilkins.

Evans, A.M., & Bitran, J.D. (2001). Adjuvant chemotherapy. In M.C. Perry (Ed.), *The chemotherapy source book* (3rd ed., pp. 48–69). Philadelphia: Lippincott Williams & Wilkins.

Ferrans, C. (2005). Quality of life as an outcome of cancer care. In C.H. Yarbro, M.H. Frogge, & M. Goodman (Eds.), *Cancer nursing: Principles and practice* (6th ed., pp. 183–200). Sudbury, MA: Jones and Bartlett.

Gaddis, J.S., & Gullatte, M.M. (2007). Pharmacologic principles of chemotherapy. In M.M. Gullatte (Ed.), *Clinical guide to antineoplastic therapy: A chemotherapy handbook* (2nd ed., pp. 19–37). Pittsburgh, PA: Oncology Nursing Society.

Goldie, J.H. (2008). Drug resistance. In M.C. Perry (Ed.), *The chemotherapy source book* (4th ed., pp. 37–48). Philadelphia: Lippincott Williams & Wilkins.

Gosselin-Acomb, T.K. (2005). Principles of radiation therapy. In C.H. Yarbro, M.H. Frogge, & M. Goodman (Eds.), *Cancer nursing: Principles and practice* (6th ed., pp. 229–249). Sudbury, MA: Jones and Bartlett.

Haskell, C.M. (2001). Principles of cancer chemotherapy. In C. Haskell (Ed.), *Cancer treatment* (5th ed., pp. 62–86). Philadelphia: Saunders.

Howland, R.D., & Mycek, M.J. (2006). Anticancer drugs. In R.A. Harvey & P.C. Champe (Eds.), *Lippincott's illustrated reviews: Pharmacology* (3rd ed., pp. 453–484). Philadelphia: Lippincott Williams & Wilkins.

Karnofsky, D.A., & Burchenal, J.H. (1949). The clinical evaluation of chemotherapeutic agents in cancer. In C. MacLeod (Ed.), *Evaluation of chemotherapeutic agents* (pp. 191–205). New York: Columbia University Press.

Langhorne, M., & Barton-Burke, M. (2001). Chemotherapy administration: General principles for nursing practice. In M. Barton-Burke, G. Wilkes, & K. Ingwersen (Eds.), *Cancer chemotherapy: A nursing process approach* (3rd ed., pp. 608–643). Sudbury, MA: Jones and Bartlett.

Lansky, S., List, M., Lansky, L., Ritter-Sterr, C., & Miller, D. (1987). The measurement of performance in childhood cancer patients. *Cancer, 60*(7), 1651–1656.

Mazumdar, M., Smith, A., & Schwartz, L.H. (2004). A statistical simulation study finds discordance between WHO criteria and RECIST guideline. *Journal of Clinical Epidemiology, 57*(4), 358–365.

Oken, M.M., Creech, R.H., Tormey, D.C., Horton, J., Davis, T.E., McFadden, E.T., et al. (1982). Toxicity and response criteria of the Eastern Cooperative Oncology Group. *American Journal of Clinical Oncology, 5*(6), 649–655.

Omerod, K. (2005). Diagnostic evaluation, classification, and staging. In C.H. Yarbro, M.H. Frogge, & M. Goodman (Eds.), *Cancer nursing: Principles and practice* (6th ed., pp. 153–180). Sudbury, MA: Jones and Bartlett.

Otto, S.E. (2007). Chemotherapy. In M. Langhorne, J. Fulton, & S.E. Otto (Eds.), *Oncology nursing* (5th ed., pp. 362–376). St. Louis, MO: Elsevier Mosby.

Perry, M.C., Anderson, S.M., & Donehower, R.C. (2000). Chemotherapy. In M. Abeloff, J. Armitage, A. Lichter, & J. Niederhuber (Eds.), *Clinical oncology* (2nd ed., pp. 378–422). Philadelphia: Churchill Livingstone.

Pfreundschuh, M., Truemper, L., Kloess, M., Schmits, R., Feller, A.C., Ruebe, C., et al. (2004). 2-weekly or 3-weekly CHOP chemotherapy with or without etoposide for the treatment of elderly patients with aggressive lymphomas: Results of the NHL-B2 trial of the DSHNHL. *Blood, 104*(3), 634–641.

Poliquin, C. (2007). Conditioning regimens in hematopoietic stem cell transplantation. In S. Ezzone & K. Schmit-Pokorny (Eds.), *Blood and marrow stem cell transplantation: Principles, practice and nursing insights* (3rd ed., pp. 109–143). Sudbury, MA: Jones and Bartlett.

Schwartz, L.H., Colville, J.A., Ginsberg, M.S., Wang, L., Mazumdar, M., Kalaigian, J., et al. (2006). Measuring tumor response and shape change on CT: Esophageal cancer as a paradigm. *Annals of Oncology, 17*(6), 1018–1023.

Sporn, M.B., & Lippman, S.M. (2003). Chemoprevention of cancer. In D. Kufe, R. Pollack, R. Weichselbaum, R. Bast, T. Ganster, J. Holland, et al. (Eds.), *Cancer medicine* (6th ed., pp. 413–422). Hamilton, Ontario, Canada: BC Decker.

Therasse, P., Arbuck, S.G., Eisenhauer, E.A., Wanders, J., Kaplan, R.S., Rubenstein, L., et al. (2000). New guidelines to evaluate the response to treatment in solid tumors. *Journal of the National Cancer Institute, 92*(3), 205–214.

Therasse, P., Eisenhauer, E.A., & Buyse, M. (2006). Update in methodology and conduct of cancer clinical trials. *European Journal of Cancer, 42*(10), 1322–1330.

Tortorice, P.V. (2005). Chemotherapy: Principles of therapy. In C.H. Yarbro, M.H. Frogge, & M. Goodman (Eds.), *Cancer nursing: Principles and practice* (6th ed., pp. 315–350). Sudbury, MA: Jones and Bartlett.

von Minckwitz, G., Kummel, S., du Bois, A., Eiermann, W., Eidtmann, H., Gerber, B., et al. (2007). Pegfilgrastim +/– ciprofloxacin for primary prophylaxis with TAC (docetaxel/doxorubicin/cyclophosphamide) chemotherapy for breast cancer. Results from the GEPARTRIO study. *Annals of Oncology, 19*(2), 292–298.

Yackzan, S.G. (2007). Pathophysiology and staging of breast cancer. In S.M. Mahon (Ed.), *Site-specific cancer series: Breast cancer* (pp. 51–62). Pittsburgh, PA: Oncology Nursing Society.

III. Principles of Antineoplastic Therapy

A. Life cycle of cells (Brown & Humble, 2007; Otto, 2007; Vermeulen, Van Bockstaele, & Berneman, 2003): The cell life cycle is a five-stage reproductive process occurring in both normal and malignant cells (see Figure 2).

1. **Gap 0 (G0)**
   a) Resting phase
   b) Cells are temporarily out of the cycle and not actively proliferating, while all other cellular activities are occurring.
   c) Cells continue in this phase until there is a stimulus to enter the active cell cycle, leading to cell division.
   d) Because they are not dividing, cells in G0 phase are considered protected from exposure to many chemotherapeutic agents.

2. **Gap 1 (G1)**
   a) Postmitotic phase
   b) Cells begin the first phase of reproduction by synthesizing proteins and RNA necessary for cell division.

3. **Synthesis (S):** DNA is synthesized.

4. **Gap 2 (G2)**
   a) Premitotic (or postsynthetic) phase
   b) The second phase of protein and RNA synthesis occurs.
   c) Preparation for mitotic spindle formation occurs.
   d) The cell is now prepared to actively divide.

5. **Mitosis (M)**
   a) Cell division occurs.
   b) Shortest phase of the cell life cycle.
   c) At the conclusion of mitosis, two daughter cells have been formed. They either reenter

Figure 2. Cell Life Cycle

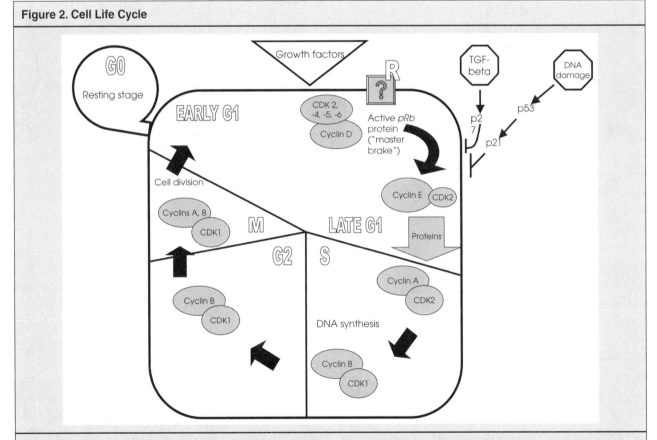

The cell cycle consists of four active stages (G1, S, G2, M) that are controlled by proteins called cyclins. The cyclins (D, E, A, B) activate upon forming complexes with enzymes called cyclin-dependent kinases (CDKs). Upon activation, the cyclin-CDK complexes allow the cell to progress through each specific cell-cycle stage. Present throughout the cell cycle, the cyclin-CDK complexes serve as checkpoints, or monitors, of the cell cycle. Inhibitory proteins—such as p21, p27, and p53—prevent progression through the cell cycle if DNA damage is present or if the nutrients or oxygen necessary to support cellular proliferation is in short supply. Inhibitory proteins, in turn, are regulated by inhibitory growth factors and TGFB. Cyclin-CDK complexes and pRb ("the master brake") tightly regulate the R (restriction) point. Once past R, the cell cycle "turns on," and progression through the cell cycle is inevitable. The stability of the inhibitory proteins and cyclin-CDK complexes are altered in cancer. Normal cell-cycle controls are absent and uncontrolled cellular proliferation prevails.

Note. From "Biology of Cancer" (p.15), by J. Gibbon and L. Loescher in C.H. Yarbro, M.H. Frogge, & M. Goodman (Eds.), *Cancer Nursing: Principles and Practice* (6th ed.), 2005, Sudbury, MA: Jones and Bartlett. Copyright 2005 by Jones and Bartlett, www.jbpub.com. Reprinted with permission.

the cell cycle to again reproduce or begin to perform the specific functions of the tissue for which they are programmed.

B. Chemotherapeutic agents: Drugs are classified according to pharmacologic action or their effect on cell reproduction (i.e., the cell life cycle as described previously). See Table 5.
  1. Cell-cycle– or phase-specific drugs exert effect within a specific phase of the cell cycle (Brown & Humble, 2007; Hande, 2004).
    a) These drugs have the greatest tumor cell kill when given in divided but frequent doses, or as a continuous infusion with a short cycle time. This will allow the maximum number of cells to be exposed to the drug at the specific time in their life cycle when they are vulnerable to the drug.
    b) Classifications include antimetabolites, plant alkaloids (camptothecins, epipodo-phyllotoxins, taxanes, and vinca alkaloids), and miscellaneous agents.
  2. Cell-cycle– or phase-nonspecific drugs exert effect in all phases of the cell cycle, including the G0 resting phase (Brown & Humble, 2007; Hande, 2004).
    a) Cell-cycle–nonspecific drugs are effective in treating tumors with more slowly dividing cells.
    b) If the cancer is sensitive to the agent used, the drug is incorporated into the cell. The cell kill may not be instantaneous but may occur when the cell attempts to divide.
      1) The destruction of tumor cells will be directly proportional to the amount of the drug administered.
      2) These drugs are given intermittently, allowing the individual to recover from dose-limiting toxicities before the drug is repeated.
      3) The most frequent dose-limiting toxicity is suppression of the bone marrow.
    c) Classifications include alkylating agents, antitumor antibiotics, hormonal therapies, and nitrosoureas.

C. Actions of the immune system
  1. It is essential to understand the immune system in order to understand how biotherapy works.
  2. The immune system (see Figure 3) is a highly specialized and adaptive system that protects an individual by providing
    a) Defense against foreign organisms.
    b) Homeostasis: Destruction of aging or damaged cells.

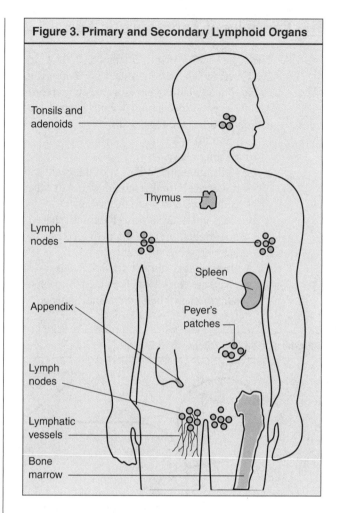

Figure 3. Primary and Secondary Lymphoid Organs

    c) Surveillance: Identification of foreign, or nonself, substances (Hyde, 2000; Janeway, Travers, Walport, & Shlomchik, 2005).

D. Types of immune response
  1. An immune response is the reaction of the immune system against a foreign substance.
  2. Any substance capable of producing such a response is called an antigen.
  3. There are two types of immune response (see Table 6).
    a) Innate, or nonspecific, immunity (see Figure 4) is essential for inducing the proper adaptive immune response (Janeway et al., 2005). Innate immunity does not generate immunologic memory and involves the following (Hyde, 2000; Janeway et al.).
      (1) Physical barriers (skin and mucous membranes)
      (2) Mechanical barriers (coughing, sneezing, and blinking)
      (3) Chemical barriers (tears and sweat)
      (4) Inflammatory responses (production of monocytes, macrophages, and polymorphonuclear cells)

Table 6. Innate and Adaptive Immune Responses

Immune Response	Mechanism of Action	Cells Primarily Involved
Innate	• Primary line of defense • Nonspecific • No memory	• Neutrophils • Monocytes, macrophages • Large granular lymphocytes (natural killer cells)
Adaptive	• Secondary line of defense • Specific memory	• Lymphocytes • T cells (in cell-mediated immunity) • B cells (in humoral immunity)

(5) Complement activation

(6) Acute-phase protein production (e.g., interleukin [IL]-2)

(7) Production of large granular lymphocytes (natural killer [NK] or NK and NKT cells)

b) Adaptive, or specific, immunity is the secondary line of defense and involves the following (Hyde, 2000; Janeway et al., 2005).

(1) Immunologic memory and specificity

(2) Collaboration of B cells and T cells

(3) Three types of adaptive immunity are the following.

(a) Humoral immunity (see Figure 5): B lymphocytes, memory B cells, and plasma cells mediate humoral immunity. The result is the production of immunoglobulins (Igs).

(b) Cell-mediated immunity (see Figure 6): Cell-mediated immunity is mediated by T cells and their cytokine products. This type of immunity does not involve an antibody; it does involve the following (Janeway et al., 2005).

　i) Cytotoxic T cells (T_C), usually CD8 positive

　ii) Helper T cells (T_H1 or T_H2), usually CD4 positive

(c) T regulatory cells, also known as suppressor T cells (T_S)

　i) T regulatory cells: These cells display the markers CD4 and CD25 and act to limit the activity of other immune effector cells.

　ii) Their major role is thought to be to prevent the onset of immunity to normal tissues of the body and to limit the inflammatory response that can occur with infections.

Figure 4. Innate (Nonspecific) Immune Response

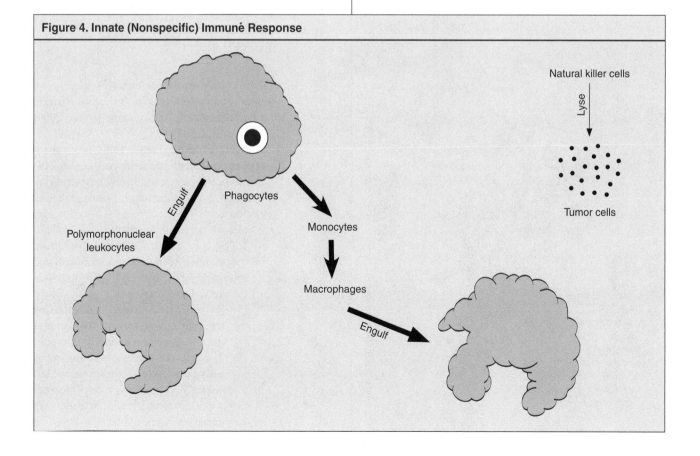

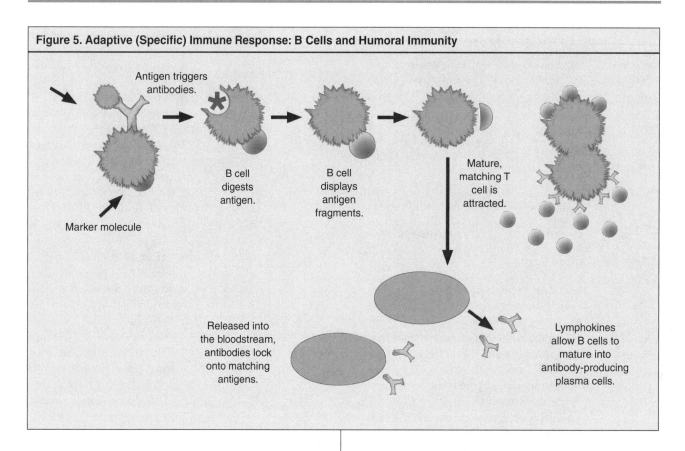

Figure 5. Adaptive (Specific) Immune Response: B Cells and Humoral Immunity

Antigen triggers antibodies.

Marker molecule

B cell digests antigen.

B cell displays antigen fragments.

Mature, matching T cell is attracted.

Released into the bloodstream, antibodies lock onto matching antigens.

Lymphokines allow B cells to mature into antibody-producing plasma cells.

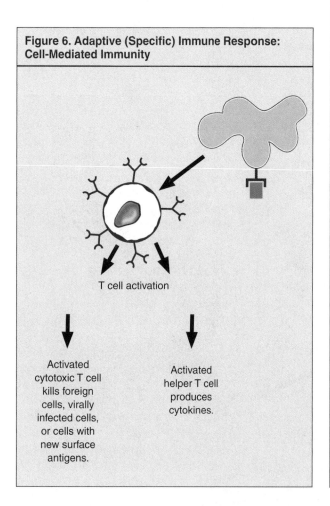

Figure 6. Adaptive (Specific) Immune Response: Cell-Mediated Immunity

T cell activation

Activated cytotoxic T cell kills foreign cells, virally infected cells, or cells with new surface antigens.

Activated helper T cell produces cytokines.

iii) Animals and people without T regulatory cells develop a variety of inflammatory disorders primarily involving the bowel, skin, and liver.

E. Cells of the immune system (see Figure 7): The immune response involves the intricate interaction of a number of cells and proteins (Hyde, 2000; Janeway et al., 2005).
   1. Antigen-presenting cells: Cells (e.g., macrophages, B cells, dendritic cells) that efficiently present antigen to T cells; only dendritic cells are capable of initiating a primary immune response.
   2. T cells (Hyde, 2000; Janeway et al., 2005)
      a) Helper (T_H cells): Cells that coordinate the immune response and cell-mediated immunity; they are required to maintain cytotoxic T cell responses.
         (1) T_H1 cells are necessary for activating macrophages and are involved in production of certain antibody isotypes.
         (2) T_H2 cells are effective activators of B cells particularly in primary responses.
      b) Cytotoxic (T_C cells): Cells that kill foreign cells, virally infected cells, or cells with new surface antigens

Figure 7. Cells of the Immune System

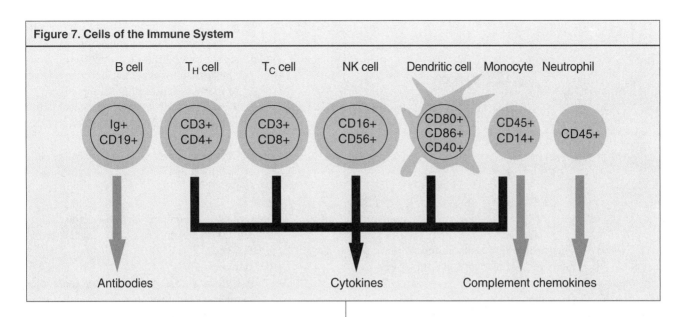

c) T regulatory cells/suppressor (T_{reg} cells/T_S cells): Cells that interfere with development of immune reaction when recognizing antigen; their primary role is to modulate the severity of inflammation produced by infection but also play an important role to prevent autoimmunity and may be involved in malignancy.

d) Memory T cells (T_M cells): Cells that recognize specific antigens and induce recall responses

3. NK cells: Cells that are cytotoxic to tumor cells and virally infected autologous cells by producing substances that can bind to and destroy foreign invaders, without having to identify a specific antigen; NK cells identify foreign substances by their lack of identifying surface molecules.

4. NKT cells: Cells that have markers both of NK cells and T cells

5. B lymphocytes: Plasma cell precursors; plasma cells manufacture Ig (an antibody) specific to an initiating antigen.

6. Antibodies: Protein products of plasma cells; also known as immunoglobulins, they enhance effector-cell functions.

a) The majority of peripheral blood antibody is IgG.

b) IgM is the first antibody produced in response to antigen and is followed by antibody switching to the other types.

c) IgA is present in bodily secretions and helps to prevent infections at sites where the environment interacts with the body, such as the nose and lungs.

d) IgD is present in slight amounts in normal serum. There is some controversy over the exact biologic function; however, IgD may have some antibody function for penicillin, diphtheria, and insulin.

e) IgE exists in trace amounts in normal serum and is associated with immediate hypersensitivity reactions. IgE antibodies are generated when combined with certain antigens, thus activating the release of histamine from mast cells.

7. Cytokines: Glycoprotein products of immune cells such as lymphocytes and macrophages. Cytokines mediate effector defense functions. Cytokines themselves usually are not cytotoxic.

F. Tumor escape mechanisms: When immune surveillance fails, tumor formation occurs. The theories set forth to explain this process include the following (Janeway et al., 2005; Muehlbauer & Schwartzentruber, 2003; Sondel, Rakhmilevich, de Jong, & Hank, 2001).

1. Altered immunogenicity

a) Tumors can be targeted by the immune system either through cell surface molecules that function as targets for antibody responses or intracellular molecules that are presented within the context of the major histocompatibility complex (MHC) molecules.

b) Antigen expression on the tumor-cell surface is altered, allowing the antigen to go unrecognized by the humoral immune system.

c) Alternatively, cell-mediated immune response can be blunted through loss or alteration of the MHC molecules or loss or mutation of the peptide epitope that binds to the MHC molecule and is recognized by the T cells.

2. Antigen modulation

a) Antibodies produced as part of the immune response cause antigens to enter the tumor cell or leave it completely.

b) This further limits the ability of the immune cells to recognize the tumor cell as nonself.
3. Immune suppression
    a) The tumor itself produces substances that alter or inhibit the body's immune response.
    b) One example of such a factor is transforming growth factor beta, which inhibits the activity of T cells.
4. Acquired deficiencies to immune sensitivity: This includes age- and disease-associated alterations such as decreased or increased apoptosis and signaling defects of T cells.
5. Immunologic aging: Alterations in T-cell functions cause declines in T-cell proliferation, generation of T killer cells, production of IL-2, and signal transduction of lymphocytes.
6. Tumors do not give off inflammatory warning signals to simulate an immune response.

G. Principles of biotherapy
1. Biotherapy: The use of agents derived from biologic sources or agents that affect biologic responses (Rieger, 2001)
2. Theory of immune surveillance
    a) The transformation of a cell from normal to malignant involves a number of genetic mutations over a span of years.
    b) As cells differentiate, they produce proteins (antigens) on their surface that the immune system recognizes as nonself; an immune response can be mounted in defense (Rieger, 2001).
3. Methods of biotherapeutic action: Experts propose that biotherapeutic agents work by doing one or more of the following (Rieger, 2001).
    a) Enhancing the patient's own immune response
    b) Altering the milieu in which cancer cells grow by modifying the actions of the normal cells in the area of the tumor

c) Increasing the vulnerability of cancer cells to the body's own immune system
d) Altering the pathway by which normal cells transform into malignant cells, which may be more preventive than therapeutic
e) Preventing the metastasis of cancer cells
f) Enhancing the repair of normal cells damaged by treatment
g) Changing cancer cells so they behave like healthy cells

H. Categories of biotherapy (Janeway et al., 2005; Rieger, 2001; Rosenberg, 2000; Sondel et al., 2001)
1. Cytokines
    a) Cytokines are small protein molecules released by diverse cells throughout the body providing communication between the cells of the immune system.
    b) Cytokines generally are activated by a stimulus and induce responses by binding to specific receptors. Cells expressing receptors for specific cytokines can either be activated or inhibited, which alters the immune effector function.
    c) Cytokines affect the growth and differentiation of white blood cells and regulate immune and inflammatory responses.
    d) Cytokines may enhance cytotoxic activity and secrete additional cytokines, resulting in an amplification of the immune response. This enhanced immune activation stimulates proliferation or activation and recruitment of additional immune effector cells.
    e) Cytokines are multifunctional substances having proinflammatory, anti-inflammatory, and regulatory functions in the immune system.
    f) The cytokines include a variety of ILs, interferons (IFNs), tumor necrosis factors (TNFs), and transforming growth factor. Examples include IL-1, -2, -3, -4, -6, -8, 10, and -15 and IFN-α and IFN-ß.
    g) These cytokines regulate antibody production and the functions of B and T cells, as well as interact with antigen-presenting cells and NK cells.
    h) Examples of cytokines used for therapeutic purposes include
        (1) IFNs
        (2) ILs
        (3) Hematopoietic growth factors.
2. Monoclonal antibodies (MoAbs) (for nomenclature, see Figure 8) (Battiato, 2005; Muehlbauer, Cusack, & Morris, 2006; Rieger, Green, & Murray, 2001; Schmidt & Wood, 2003)
    a) General

(1) Derived from human or mouse or combinations thereof
  (a) Murine: Derived from mouse antibody; less effective because they lack the ability to bind to the Fc receptor
  (b) Chimeric: Combination of mouse and human antibodies
  (c) Humanized: Small part mouse fused with human
  (d) Human: Only human antibodies
(2) Cell surface proteins can function as targets for binding MoAbs.
(3) MoAbs have been used to target host tissues or proteins that support tumor growth, such as growth factors and growth factor receptors, or they may merely identify targets that are relatively unique to the tumor cell population.
(4) MoAbs also may inhibit the binding of growth factors to their respective receptors on the cell surface and shut off downstream signaling that stimulates tumor cell growth.
(5) Antibodies recognize and bind to specific antigens.
  (a) Depending on the particular class and subtype, an antibody can interact with other serum proteins, such as the complement system, or Fc-receptors on cells to activate normal immune functions that selectively eliminate the antigen or totally eliminate the target cell expressing that antigen.

  (b) Antibody-dependent cellular cytotoxicity is thought to be the major mechanism for response to most MoAbs: This type of response is believed to involve a three-step process.
    i) The antibody binds to the antigen of the tumor cell.
    ii) NK cells recognize the antibody-covered tumor cells.
    iii) Cytotoxic proteins are released to destroy tumor cells.
  (c) Alternatively, MoAbs can act directly on the tumor cell to induce cell death.
b) Unconjugated antibodies (Groch, 2002; Muehlbauer et al., 2006; Schmidt & Wood, 2003)
  (1) Unconjugated MoAbs are unmodified and do not have cytotoxic agents or radioisotopes attached to them. Their antitumor activity solely results from the actions of the MoAb on its targets.
  (2) Examples
    (a) Rituximab
    (b) Trastuzumab
    (c) Cetuximab
    (d) Bevacizumab
    (e) Pantitumumab
c) Conjugated antibodies
  (1) Physically attached to antitumor agents such as radioisotopes, chemotherapy drugs, toxins, or other biologic agents.
  (2) After targeting specific antigens, conjugated MoAbs attack tumors by releasing the attached antitumor agents into the cells or by concentrating high

Figure 8. Types of Monoclonal Antibodies

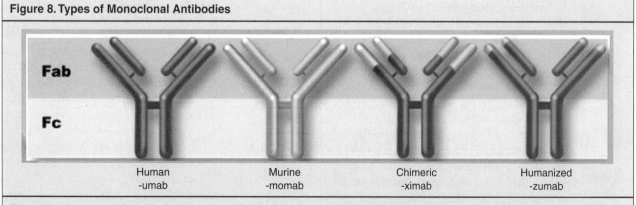

| Human | Murine | Chimeric | Humanized |
| -umab | -momab | -ximab | -zumab |

Fab—variable portion; this portion is the antigen-binding site that recognizes and binds to a specific antigen; Fc—this portion is at the end, or stem, of the antibody. It signals the cells of the immune system to destroy the target, or cell, it is bound onto.

Note. From *Biomolecular Targeted Therapies in Cancer Treatment* [Slide kit], by Oncology Education Services, Inc., 2003, Pittsburgh, PA: Author. Copyright 2003 by Oncology Education Services, Inc. Reprinted with permission.

levels of local radioactive emissions to the site.

(3) An advantage of radioimmunotherapy is its ability to kill cells at a distance; no need to bind to the tumor cells directly to have beneficial effects.

(4) Examples of conjugated MoAbs

    (a) Gemtuzumab ozogamicin (Mylotarg®) conjugated with calicheamicin, an antitumor antibiotic

    (b) Radioisotope conjugates (antibodies labeled with a radioisotope): Ibritumomab tiuxetan (Zevalin®) (Biogen Idec Inc. & Genentech, Inc., 2008), and iodine-131 tositumomab (Bexxar®) (Corixa Corp. & GlaxoSmithKline, 2003)

I. Principles of radioimmunotherapy (RIT) (Bruner, Gosselin-Acomb, & Haas, 2005)

  1. RIT is a radiopharmaceutical cancer treatment that employs radionuclide-labeled, or radiolabeled, MoAbs.

    a) These antibodies, which are administered systemically by IV injection, recognize tumor-associated antigens to deliver radioactivity to tumor cells selectively (Kaminski et al., 1996).

    b) Radiolabeled MoAbs have an important and growing role in cancer therapy (Groch, 2002; Hainsworth, 2003; Larson, Divgi, Sgouros, Cheung, & Scheinberg, 2000; Wahl et al., 1998).

  2. The goal of RIT is to destroy or inactivate cancer cells while preserving the integrity of normal tissues (Dunne-Daly, 1999).

  3. Each radionuclide emits radiation particles and/or rays with energies that are characteristic of that specific radionuclide. Depending on its type, a radionuclide can emit one, two, or three types of emissions (Bruner et al., 2005).

    a) Alpha particles

      (1) Consist of two protons and two neutrons (the nucleus of a helium atom)

      (2) These particles have poor penetrating ability. Alpha particles cannot penetrate the outermost layers of skin, and they travel a maximum distance of 5 cm.

      (3) A sheet of paper is sufficient to block the radiation source, or a distance of 5 cm between the radiation source and the point will shield the radiation.

      (4) The skin of an alpha-irradiated patient is adequate to protect others from radiation exposure; in other words, alpha particles are not external hazards, but ingestion or inhalation can be lethal or produce secondary malignancies.

      (5) However, contact with an irradiated patient's excreted body fluids may be hazardous. The use of universal precautions is sufficient.

    b) Beta particles

      (1) Are electrons.

      (2) Have greater penetration abilities than do alpha particles.

      (3) Like alpha particles, beta particles are not external hazards. The patient's skin or thick plastic shielding is usually adequate protection from beta particles.

      (4) Yttrium-90 (such as Zevalin) (Biogen Idec Inc. & Genentech, Inc., 2008) emits beta particles.

      (5) After RIT, the following apply.

        (a) The patient's body fluids are temporarily radioactive.

        (b) The patient should receive specific discharge instructions to limit family exposure.

    c) Gamma rays

      (1) Are high-energy gamma-emitting radionuclides.

      (2) Protection from these rays is achieved by maintaining a specific distance from the radioactive source and the point (the distance is specific to the radioisotope used), and using appropriate shielding.

      (3) Patients receiving this type of radionuclide may have to be in radiation isolation and behind lead shields (Bruner et al., 2005).

      (4) Iodine-131 emits high-energy beta particles and gamma rays. The thyroid gland concentrates iodine and is at risk of damage if radioactive iodine is ingested.

4. Care should include the following (Bruner et al., 2005).

   a) Restrict people from entering the room during infusion.

   b) Observe time and distance limitations based on recommendations of the Radiation Safety Officer or nuclear pharmacist.

   c) Release patient after administration based on specific guidelines that vary by state.

   d) Pregnant women and children should avoid contact with the patients.

   e) Body fluids are radioactive for a period of time depending on the half-life and elimination of the isotope.

   f) Provide patient-specific discharge instructions to limit family exposure.

   g) Low-energy, or weak, gamma-emitting radionuclides: Special precautions usually are not necessary (Bruner et al., 2005).

5. Immunoconjugated radioactive biologic agents should be handled according to guidelines for the specific isotope used (see Bruner et al., 2005, for specifics).

6. Radioactive isotopes must be administered by licensed professionals.

J. Toxin-conjugated molecules

1. Toxins such as diphtheria or *Pseudomonas* exotoxin are potent inhibitors of cell viability. One molecule of diphtheria toxin delivered intracellularly is capable of inhibiting protein synthesis that results in the death of the cells.

2. Antibodies and cytokines can be used to target these toxic molecules to cancer cells and depend upon the uptake of these toxins by the cells to cause their death.

3. The strategy of delivering toxins intracellularly has resulted in FDA approval of two agents for the treatment of malignancy.

   a) Gemtuzumab ozogamicin for the treatment of leukemia

   b) Denileukin diftitox for the treatment of mycosis fungoides

K. Therapeutic uses for biotherapeutic agents (see Table 7): Biotherapeutic agents have been shown to

1. Cure, when used as a primary or adjuvant therapy.

2. Improve overall response or increase disease-free survival when used in conjunction with conventional therapies (Rieger, 2001; Rosenberg, 2000).

3. Control or stabilize disease.

4. Maintain or enhance QOL.

L. Supportive uses for biotherapeutic agents

1. Biotherapeutic agents can decrease the severity of toxicities associated with other therapeutic modalities (e.g., hematopoietic growth factors can lessen the side effects of chemotherapy).

2. Uses for biotherapeutic agents in research: Numerous biotherapy agents are in clinical trials, including cancer vaccines, dendritic cells, tumor-infiltrating lymphocytes, other interleukins, antiangiogenic agents, and gene therapy (NIH, n.d.; Rosenberg, 2000).

M. Biotherapeutic strategies: Advances in the knowledge of molecular biology have led to the development of a number of agents referred to as targeted therapies. These agents may be further divided into those that target the antigenic properties of the tumor cell itself (e.g., MoAbs) and those that target intracellular processes. A growing number of unique molecular targets have been identified within cancer cells resulting in the discovery of novel new agents, many of which are oral. See Table 8 for a list of targeted therapies.

1. Signal transduction and targeted therapies (Gale, 2003; Kimmelman, Bafico, & Aaronson, 2001; Mendelsohn, Baird, Fan, & Markowitz, 2001; Schwartz & Shah, 2005; Wilkes, 2006; Wilkes, Esper, & Muehlbauer, 2006) (See Table 8, and refer to Figure 9 for common terminology.)

   a) Cellular growth, function, and apoptosis are regulated by a complex network of biochemical and molecular messengers. This is referred to as cell signaling.

   b) Signal transduction is the generation of a signal from either outside the cell (growth

---

Figure 9. Common Terminology in Cell Signaling

- Ligands: Molecules, such as growth factors, that activate receptors, such as growth factor receptors, on the surface of the cell
- Ligand binding: The process by which the ligand attaches to a specific receptor site and activates the receptor, thereby activating the signaling pathway. This is similar to antigen-antibody binding.
- Monomer: Single receptor, inactivated state
- Dimerization: Activation of receptor through monomer pairing. Dimerization occurs between two adjacent receptors that have bound ligand. That is, two monomers that are side by side on the surface of the cell are paired and activated by the ligand. The joining activates a series of signals.
- Phosphorylation: Activation of a chemical process to initiate signaling such as with tyrosine kinase
- Heterodimerization: The pairing of two different ligand-bound receptors together, such as Erb1 and Erb2
- Homodimerization: The joining of two receptors of the same subtype, such as two Erb1 (HER1) receptors or two Erb2 (HER2), Erb3 (HER3), or Erb4 (HER4) receptors

factors and growth factor receptors) or inside the cell (tyrosine kinase receptors) that produces a signaling cascade that travels down a pathway to the cell nucleus and delivers a signal for the cell to divide.

(1) The nucleus then directs the cell activities. This could include cell proliferation, induction of angiogenesis, increased growth factor production, or inhibition of apoptosis.

(2) Receptor tyrosine kinases (RTK) contain several domains, including an extracellular ligand-binding domain, transmembrane domain, and an intracellular domain containing protein tyrosine kinase.

(3) Activation of RTK triggers a biochemical cascade of cell signaling events. This signal transduction can initiate on the ligands on the extracellular domain, sending a signal across the transmembrane to intracellular tyrosine kinase and on to the nucleus of the cell.

(4) Tyrosine kinases modify themselves as well as other cellular proteins by putting phosphate molecules on the amino acid tyrosine.
   (a) This activity is necessary for receptor signaling.
   (b) Targeted therapies are directed toward specific molecules (targets) along a cellular signaling pathway that is involved in tumor growth, proliferation, and/or invasion.

(5) Targeted therapies moderate, control, and/or kill cancer cells and work differently than either chemotherapy or radiation therapy (see Figure 10).

(6) Therapies targeting intracellular pathways, or tyrosine kinase receptors, are small molecules and to date are mostly oral therapies. Because of the need for long-term inhibition of signaling, chronic oral therapy represents the most rational approach to dosing.
   (a) Erlotinib
   (b) Sorafenib
   (c) Sunitinab
   (d) Imitanib

(7) Therapies targeting growth factor receptors in the extracellular pathways are generally MoAbs (see previous section).

(8) Mammalian target of rapamycin (mTor) kinase inhibition: Temsirolimus

2. Growth factors
   a) Growth factors are produced by cells in all body tissues.
   b) Growth factors are primarily responsible for initiating the complex cell signaling that is required to maintain cell viability and cell division.
   c) These factors can influence cells in either a positive or negative way, including affecting cell survival, apoptosis, and differentiation.
   d) Growth factors bind with their specific receptors and initiate a cascade of intracellular signaling.
   e) Examples of growth factors
      (1) Epidermal growth factor (EGF), which binds to the epidermal growth factor receptor (EGFR)
      (2) Vascular endothelial growth factor (VEGF), which binds to the vascular endothelial growth factor receptor (VEGFR)
   f) Redundancies exist in cell signaling. Several extracellular signals may lead to the activation of the same pathway.
      (1) The final response of the cell may differ depending on the response from the nucleus.
      (2) Additionally, despite this redundancy with stimuli, the kinetics and extent of activation may vary, leading to vastly different outcomes.

N. Angiogenesis and antiangiogenic agents (Carmeliet & Jain, 2000; Ellis & Fidler, 2001; Gasparini, 1999; Libutti & Pluda, 2000; Muehlbauer, 2003; Papetti & Herman, 2002; Risau, 1995; Viale, 2007; Wilkes, 2007; Yancopoulos et al., 2000)
   1. Angiogenesis is the development of new blood vessels. It is a complex, multistep process that is required for a host of normal functions, including wound healing, tissue repair, reproduction, growth, and development.
   2. Under normal circumstances, angiogenesis is tightly controlled by a balance of stimulators and inhibitors.

Figure 10. Cancer Treatments: Mechanisms of Action

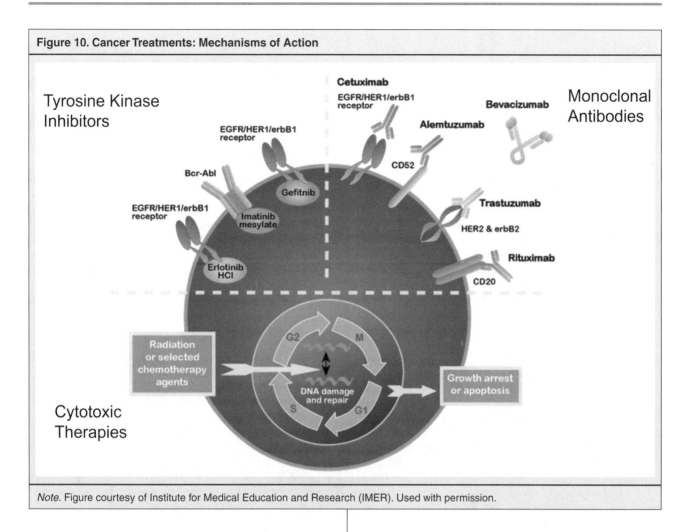

Note. Figure courtesy of Institute for Medical Education and Research (IMER). Used with permission.

3. In malignant angiogenesis, that balance is upset, leading to a cascade of irregular molecular and cellular events that contribute to tumor neovascularization.

4. In the context of tumor growth, angiogenesis refers to the growth of new vessels within a tumor. The new vessels develop from the existing vascular network and provide a blood supply for the tumor.

   a) VEGF and basic fibroblast growth factor (bFGF) are circulating growth factors known to induce angiogenesis. Their presence has been reported to correlate with extent of disease, clinical status, and survival.

   b) Endothelial cells line the vasculature of normal tissues. In a resting state, they provide a homeostatic barrier that prevents the uncontrolled extravasation of intravascular components and inhibits coagulation.

   c) When a tumor begins to grow in normal tissue, tumor cells release factors that elicit responses from the surrounding endothelium. The result is vascular growth from normal tissue into the tumor.

   d) Neovascularization contributes to tumor invasion and metastasis.

      (1) Tumor vasculature is permeable and disorganized with a weak basement membrane. These conditions facilitate the migration of endothelial cells.

      (2) VEGF can cause accumulation of endothelial cells and stimulate further tumor angiogenesis.

      (3) Blood flow in tumors is sluggish, thus inducing hypoxia and acidosis. Tumor hypoxia further induces tumor angiogenesis.

      (4) Hypoxia and acidosis may contribute to chemotherapy and radiotherapy resistance because of lack of oxygen.

5. Antiangiogenic agents

   a) Mechanism of action: Antiangiogenic agents target the neovasculature of tumors to halt their growth, prevent tumor invasion, and preclude metastatic diffusion. Potentially, antiangiogenic agents are ideal for use with other cancer therapy modalities because antiangiogenic agents maximize the efficacy of the other therapies.

b) Side effects: Table 7 presents a list of some of the side effects of antiangiogenic agents.

6. Administration: Always review the clinical research protocol or the updated Micromedex information (www.micromedex.com) before administering an antiangiogenic agent as well as all other chemotherapeutic agents. Know the side effects, interventions, drug interactions, and diagnostic studies that apply to the agent that will be used.

References

Aronoff, G.R., Bennett, W.M., Berns, J.S., Brier, M.E., Kasbekar, N., Mueller, B.A., et al. (Eds.). (2007). *Drug prescribing in renal failure: Dosing guidelines for adults and children* (5th ed.). Philadelphia: American College of Physicians.

Ascherman, J.A., Knowles, S.L., & Attkiss, K. (2000). Docetaxel (Taxotere) extravasation: A report of five cases with treatment recommendations. *Annals of Plastic Surgery, 45*(4), 438–441.

Battiato, L. (2005). Biologic and targeted therapy. In C.H. Yarbro, M.H. Frogge, & M. Goodman (Eds.), *Cancer nursing: Principles and practice* (6th ed., pp. 510–558). Sudbury, MA: Jones and Bartlett.

Biogen Idec Inc. & Genentech, Inc. (2008). Zevalin [Package insert]. South San Francisco, CA: Author.

Brown, D., & Humble, A. (2007). Cellular mechanisms of chemotherapy. In M.M. Gullatte (Ed.), *Clinical guide to antineoplastic therapy: A chemotherapy handbook* (2nd ed., pp. 1–17). Pittsburgh, PA: Oncology Nursing Society.

Bruner, D.W., Gosselin-Acomb, T., & Haas, M. (Eds.). (2005). *Manual for radiation oncology nursing practice and education* (3rd ed.). Pittsburgh, PA: Oncology Nursing Society.

Camp, M.J., Gilmore, J.W., Gullatte, M.M., & Hutcherson, D.A. (2007). Antineoplastic agents. In M.M. Gullatte (Ed.), *Clinical guide to antineoplastic therapy: A chemotherapy handbook* (2nd ed., pp. 81–356). Pittsburgh, PA: Oncology Nursing Society.

Carmeliet, P., & Jain, R.K. (2000). Angiogenesis in cancer and other diseases. *Nature, 407*(6801), 249–257.

Chu, E., & DeVita, V.T., Jr. (2006). *Physicians' cancer chemotherapy drug manual.* Sudbury, MA: Jones and Bartlett.

Corixa Corp. & GlaxoSmithKline. (2003). Bexxar [Package insert]. Seattle, WA, & Philadelphia: Author.

Dunne-Daly, C.F. (1999). Principles of radiotherapy and radiobiology. *Seminars in Oncology Nursing, 15*(4), 250–259.

Ellis, L.M., & Fidler, I.J. (2001). Tumor angiogenesis. In J. Mendelsohn, P.M. Howley, M.A. Israel, & L.A. Liotta (Eds.), *The molecular basis of cancer* (2nd ed., pp. 173–185). Philadelphia: Saunders.

Gale, D.M. (2003). Molecular targets in cancer therapy. *Seminars in Oncology Nursing, 19*(3), 193–205.

Gasparini, G. (1999). The rationale and future potential of angiogenesis inhibitors in neoplasia. *Drugs, 58*(1), 17–38.

GlaxoSmithKline. (2008). Alkeran [Package insert]. Retrieved December 11, 2008, from http://us.gsk.com/products/assets/us_alkeran-injection.pdf

Groch, M.W. (2002, February 9–10). *New perspectives on PET.* Paper presented at the Mid-Winter Educational Symposium, Society of Nuclear Medicine, Scottsdale, AZ. Retrieved December 7, 2004, from http://www.mcdscapc.com/viewarticle/440520

Hainsworth, J.D. (2003, May 31–June 3). *Non-Hodgkin lymphoma: Where do we stand today?* Paper presented at the 39th Annual Meeting of the American Society of Clinical Oncology, Chicago, IL. Retrieved December 7, 2004, from http://www.medscape.com/viewarticle/457534

Hande, K. (2004). Principles and pharmacology of chemotherapy. In J.P. Greer, J. Foerster, J. Lukens, G.M. Rodgers, F. Paraskevas, & B. Glader (Eds.), *Wintrobe's clinical hematology* (11th ed., pp. 1945–1947). Philadelphia: Lippincott Williams & Wilkins.

Hyde, R.M. (Ed.). (2000). *Immunology* (4th ed.). Philadelphia: Lippincott Williams & Wilkins.

Janeway, C.A., Travers, P., Walport, M., & Shlomchik, M.J. (2005). *Immunobiology: The immune system in health and disease* (6th ed.). New York: Garland Science.

Kaminski, M.S., Zasakny, K.R., Francis, I.R., Fenner, M.C., Ross, C.W., Milik, A.W., et al. (1996). Iodine-131-anti-B1 radioimmunotherapy for B-cell lymphoma. *Journal of Clinical Oncology, 14*(7), 1974–1981.

Keefe, D.M., Schubert, M.M., Elting, L.S., Sonis, S.T., Epstein, J.B., Raber-Durlacher, J.E., et al.; Mucositis Study Section of the Multinational Association of Supportive Care in Cancer and the International Society for Oral Oncology. (2007). Updated clinical practice guidelines for the prevention and treatment of mucositis. *Cancer, 109*(5), 820–831.

Kimmelman, A., Bafico, A., & Aaronson, S.A. (2001). Oncogenes and signal transduction. In J. Mendelsohn, P.M. Howley, M.A. Israel, & L.A. Liotta (Eds.), *The molecular basis of cancer* (2nd ed., pp. 115–133). Philadelphia: Saunders.

Larson, S.M., Divgi, C., Sgouros, G., Cheung, N.K.V., & Scheinberg, D.A. (2000). Monoclonal antibodies: Basic principles: Radioisotope conjugates. In S.A. Rosenberg (Ed.), *Principles and practice of the biologic therapy of cancer* (2nd ed., pp. 396–412). Philadelphia: Lippincott Williams & Wilkins.

Libutti, S.K., & Pluda, J.M. (2000). Antiangiogenesis: Clinical applications. In S.A. Rosenberg (Ed.), *Principles and practice of the biologic therapy of cancer* (2nd ed., pp. 844–861). Philadelphia: Lippincott Williams & Wilkins.

Mendelsohn, J., Baird, A., Fan, Z., & Markowitz, S.D. (2001). In J. Mendelsohn, P.M. Howley, M.A. Israel, & L.A. Liotta (Eds.), *The molecular basis of cancer* (2nd ed., pp. 137–161). Philadelphia: Saunders.

Muehlbauer, P.M. (2003). Anti-angiogenesis in cancer therapy. *Seminars in Oncology Nursing, 19*(3), 180–192.

Muehlbauer, P.M., Cusack, G., & Morris, J.C. (2006). Monoclonal antibodies and side effect management. *Oncology, 20*(10, Suppl., Nurse Ed.), 11–21.

Muehlbauer, P.M., & Schwartzentruber, D.J. (2003). Cancer vaccines. *Seminars in Oncology Nursing, 19*(3), 206–216.

National Institutes of Health. (n.d.). *ClinicalTrials.gov.* Retrieved January 18, 2008, from http://www.clinicaltrials.gov

Otto, S.E. (2007). Chemotherapy. In M.E. Langhorne & S.E. Otto (Eds.), *Oncology nursing* (5th ed., pp. 362–376). St. Louis, MO: Elsevier Mosby.

Papetti, M., & Herman, I.M. (2002). Mechanisms of normal and tumor derived angiogenesis. *American Journal of Cell Physiology, 282*(5), C947–C970.

Patel, P.N. (2006). Methylene blue for management of ifosfamide-induced encephalopathy. *Annals of Pharmacotherapy, 40*(2), 299–303.

Rieger, P.T. (2001). Biotherapy. In P.T. Rieger (Ed.), *Biotherapy: A comprehensive overview* (pp. 3–37). Sudbury, MA: Jones and Bartlett.

Rieger, P.T., Green M., & Murray J.L. (2001). Monoclonal antibodies: Applications in solid tumors and other diseases. In P.T. Rieger (Ed.), *Biotherapy: A comprehensive overview* (pp. 317–355). Sudbury, MA: Jones and Bartlett.

Risau, W. (1995). Differentiation of endothelium. *Federation of American Societies for Experimental Biology Journal, 9*(10), 926–933.

Rosenberg, S.A. (Ed.). (2000). *Principles and practice of the biologic therapy of cancer*. Philadelphia: Lippincott Williams & Wilkins.

Schmidt, K.C., & Wood, B.A. (2003). Trends in cancer therapy: Role of monoclonal antibodies. *Seminars in Oncology Nursing, 19*(3), 169–179.

Schwartz, G.K., & Shah, M.A. (2005). Targeting the cell cycle: A new approach to cancer therapy. *Journal of Clinical Oncology, 23*(36), 9408–9421.

Solimando, D.A., Jr. (2008). *Drug information handbook for oncology* (7th ed.). Hudson, OH: Lexi-Comp.

Sondel, P.M., Rakhmilevich, A.L., de Jong, J.L.O., & Hank, J.A. (2001). Cellular immunity and cytokines. In J. Mendelsohn, P.M. Howley, M.A. Israel, & L.A. Liotta (Eds.), *The molecular basis of cancer* (2nd ed., pp. 535–571). Philadelphia: Saunders.

Spratto, G.R., & Woods, A.L. (2007). *PDR nurses drug handbook*. Montvale, NJ: Thomson Healthcare.

Vermeulen, K., Van Bockstaele, D.R., & Berneman, Z.N. (2003). The cell cycle: A review of regulation, deregulation, and therapeutic targets in cancer. *Cell Proliferation, 36*(3), 131–149.

Viale, P.H. (2007). The biology of angiogenesis. *Supplement to Oncology* (Nurse Edition), *21*(14), 5–11.

Wahl, R.L., Zasadny, K.R., MacFarlane, D., Francis, I.R., Ross, C.W., Estes, J., et al. (1998). Iodine-131 anti-B1 antibody for B-cell lymphoma: An update on the Michigan phase I experience. *Journal of Nuclear Medicine, 39*(Suppl. 8), 21S–27S.

Wilkes, G. (2006). Molecular targeted therapy. In M. Barton-Burke & G.M. Wilkes (Eds.), *Cancer therapies* (pp. 181–214). Sudbury, MA: Jones and Bartlett.

Wilkes, G. (2007). Clinical use of antiangiogenic agents: Dosing, side effects, and management. *Oncology Nurse Edition, 21*(14), 16–23.

Wilkes, G., Esper, P., & Muehlbauer, P. (2006). *Cancer biology webcourse*. Pittsburgh, PA: Oncology Nursing Society.

Wilkes, G.M., & Barton-Burke, M. (2008). *Oncology nursing drug handbook*. Sudbury, MA: Jones and Bartlett.

Yancopoulos, G.D., Davis, S., Gale, N.W., Rudge, J.S., Wiegand, S.J., & Holash, J. (2000). Vascular-specific growth factors and blood vessel formation. *Nature, 407*(6801), 242–248.

Table 5. Characteristics of Cytotoxic Agents

Classification	Mechanism of Action	Medication Name(s)	Route of Administration	Indications	Side Effects	Nursing Considerations
Alkylating agent	Breaks DNA helix strand, thereby interfering with DNA replication	Altretamine (Hexalen®)	PO	Ovarian cancer	Neurotoxicity, peripheral neuropathy, nausea, vomiting, skin rash, hypersensitivity, elevation of LFTs, abdominal cramps, diarrhea, myelosuppression	Monitor for progressive neurologic toxicity. Instruct patients to take after meals and at bedtime.
		Bendamustine (Treanda®)	IV	CLL, B-cell NHL	Neutropenia, pyrexia, thrombocytopenia, nausea, vomiting, leukopenia	Infuse over 30–60 min. Take precautions for TLS in high-risk patients. Monitor closely for infusion reactions.
		Busulfan (Oral: Myleran®) (IV: Busulfex®)	IV, PO	CML, BMT preparation	Profound tachycardia, hypertension, chest pain, myelosuppression, hyperpigmentation, alopecia, sperm or ovarian suppression, confusion, seizures, mucositis, pulmonary fibrosis, nausea, vomiting, insomnia, hyperglycemia, blurred vision. Venous occlusive disease has been reported in patients receiving doses >16 mg/kg in conjunction with alkylating agents for stem cell transplant (Solimando, 2008).	Monitor blood counts closely. If the leukocyte count is < 20,000/mm³, discontinue drug. Administer seizure prophylaxis. Instruct patients to take on an empty stomach to decrease risk of nausea and vomiting.
		Carboplatin (Paraplatin®)	IV	Ovarian cancer	Thrombocytopenia, neutropenia (myelosuppression is more pronounced with renal impairment), nausea, vomiting, hypersensitivity reaction, mild alopecia, skin rash	Drug is an irritant. Drug is light sensitive. Carboplatin exhibits much less renal toxicity than does cisplatin, so rigorous hydration is unnecessary unless renal dysfunction exists. Monitor blood counts closely, and reduce the dose per protocol. Specific dosing guidelines are recommended for carboplatin. See Figures 14, 15, and 16. Give after taxanes in sequential regimens to limit myelosuppression and enhance efficacy. Premedicate with a 5HT₃ antagonist and dexamethasone for nausea and vomiting. Check creatinine level prior to each dose (AUC dosing). Have emergency medications available for hypersensitivity reaction, which usually occurs after the seventh dose. Perform hypersensitivity skin test.

(Continued on next page)

Table 5. Characteristics of Cytotoxic Agents (Continued)

Classification	Mechanism of Action	Medication Name(s)	Route of Administration	Indications	Side Effects	Nursing Considerations
Alkylating agent (cont.)		Chlorambucil (Leukeran®)	PO	CLL, HD, NHL	Myelosuppression, ovarian or sperm suppression, nausea, vomiting, secondary malignancy, hyperuricemia, pulmonary fibrosis, seizure (increased risk in children with nephrotic syndrome)	Toxicity may increase if the patient has used barbiturates. Contraindicated in patients with seizure history and within one month of radiation and/or cytotoxic therapy.
		Cisplatin (Platinol®)	IV	Ovarian, testicular, bladder, cervical, breast, prostate, and head and neck cancers, leukemia, Wilms tumor; brain tumors	Severe nephrotoxicity, severe acute and delayed nausea, vomiting, dose-limiting myelosuppression, ototoxicity, neurotoxicity, hyperuricemia, hypersensitivity reaction, hypomagnesemia, peripheral neuropathy	Cisplatin is an irritant with vesicant potential if > 20 ml of concentrated solutions 0.5 mg/ml is extravasated. Hold the drug if the patient's SCr is > 1.5 mg/dl; otherwise, irreversible renal tubular damage may occur (Aronoff et al., 2007). Amifostine may be used as a renal protectant. Rigorous hydration is necessary to prevent nephrotoxicity. Use mannitol to achieve osmotic diuresis. Premedicate for nausea and vomiting. Consider obtaining a baseline audiogram.
		Cyclophosphamide (Cytoxan®)	Intrapleural, IV, PO	Breast and ovarian cancers, MM, leukemias, lymphomas, neuroblastoma, retinoblastoma, mycosis fungoides	Hemorrhagic cystitis, vomiting, dose-limiting myelosuppression, nausea, alopecia, secondary malignancy, testicular or ovarian failure High-dose: acute cardiomyopathy, syndrome of inappropriate antidiuretic hormone	Give the dose, whether IV or PO, early in the day. Ensure adequate hydration. If given PO, have patients drink plenty of fluids (2–3 L/day) (Solimando, 2008). Have patients empty their bladder frequently and before bed to prevent hemorrhagic cystitis. Mesna may be considered in conjunction with IV fluids for prevention of hemorrhagic cystitis. Pelvic irradiation potentiates hemorrhagic cystitis. When used with radiation therapy, potential for radiation recall exists with subsequent doses of cyclophosphamide.

(Continued on next page)

Table 5. Characteristics of Cytotoxic Agents *(Continued)*

Classification	Medication Name(s)	Mechanism of Action	Route of Administration	Indications	Side Effects	Nursing Considerations
Alkylating agent *(cont.)*	Dacarbazine (DTIC®)		IV	Malignant melanoma, HD, soft-tissue sarcoma, fibrosarcoma, neuroblastoma	Severe neutropenia and thrombocytopenia (with nadir at 2–3 weeks or more), severe nausea and vomiting for up to 12 hrs, anorexia, alopecia, rash, flu-like syndrome, hypotension, hypersensitivity reaction (uncommon), photosensitivity, hepatic dysfunction	Dacarbazine is an irritant that may cause tissue necrosis if extravasated. Administer by infusion over 30–60 min. May cause severe pain and burning at the injection site and along the course of the vein. To reduce these effects, increase the diluent, reduce the infusion rate, and apply cold compresses to the needle insertion site and along the vein. Protect solution from light (pink solution indicates decomposition). Flu-like syndrome may occur up to seven days after drug administration; treat symptoms. Reduce doses for patients with poor renal function.
	Ifosfamide (Ifex®)		IV	Testicular cancer, head and neck cancers, NHL, sarcomas, breast cancer, pancreatic cancer	Hemorrhagic cystitis, nausea, alopecia, vomiting, myelosuppression, neurotoxicity (somnolence, confusion, hallucinations, depressive psychoses, and encephalopathy). Methylene blue has been used to treat ifosfamide-induced encephalopathy; reports have also shown that the encephalopathy may spontaneously resolve (Patel, 2006).	Premedicate for nausea and vomiting with a serotonin antagonist and dexamethasone. Administer the drug over 30 min or more. To prevent hemorrhagic cystitis, **always administer with mesna.** Mesna may be given PO, as a bolus dose, or continuous infusion or mixed in the bag with the ifosfamide. Mesna dose should be 60%–100% of the ifosfamide dose (based on weight). Refer to package insert for specific dosing recommendations.
	Mechlorethamine (nitrogen mustard, Mustargen®)		IV	HD, NHL, CLL, CML, mycosis fungoides	Severe nausea, vomiting, alopecia, myelosuppression, pain or phlebitis at IV site, chills, fever, testicular or ovarian failure	Drug is a vesicant. Administer the agent over several minutes, through the side arm of a free-flowing IV. Flush with 125–150 ml NS postinfusion. If extravasation occurs, the antidote is sodium thiosulfate. Use mechlorethamine as soon after preparation as possible (15–30 min); it is extremely unstable. Do not mix mechlorethamine with any other drug. Premedicate with aprepitant. Administer 5HT$_3$ antagonist and dexamethasone for nausea and vomiting.

(Continued on next page)

Table 5. Characteristics of Cytotoxic Agents (Continued)

Classification	Mechanism of Action	Medication Name(s)	Route of Administration	Indications	Side Effects	Nursing Considerations
Alkylating agent (cont.)		Melphalan (Alkeran®)	IV, PO	MM; ovarian, testicular, and breast cancers; melanoma; sarcoma	Myelosuppression, nausea, vomiting, mucositis, hypersensitivity reaction	Avoid extravasation. Administer via central line if poor peripheral venow access (GlaxoSmithKline, 2008). Myelosuppression may be delayed and last four to six weeks, so monitor blood counts carefully. Hold or reduce dose per institutional protocol. Instruct patients to take on an empty stomach. Ice chips applied to oral cavity are recommended during high-dose melphalan administration to prevent oral mucositis (Keefe et al., 2007).
		Oxaliplatin (Eloxatin®)	IV	Colorectal cancer	Anaphylactic reaction, neurotoxicity (fatigue, fever, pain, headache, insomnia) that is aggravated by cold temperatures; peripheral neuropathy (it is not recommended to administer magnesium and calcium intravenously for prophylaxis, as doing so may affect tumor response rates), nausea, vomiting, diarrhea, myelosuppression, pulmonary fibrosis	Consider a dose reduction in patients with renal dysfunction. Monitor for acute, reversible effects and persistent neurotoxicity. For 3–4 days after therapy, patients should avoid consuming cold drinks and foods and breathing cold air (cover mouth with scarf). Do not prepare or infuse in sodium chloride or other chloride-containing solutions. D5W solution is recommended. Premedicate with a 5HT₃ antagonist and dexamethasone for nausea and vomiting.
		Temozolomide (Temodar®)	PO	Treatment of adult patients with refractory anaplastic astrocytoma who have experienced disease progression on nitrosoureas and procarbazine; or with newly diagnosed glioblastoma multiforme	Dose-limiting myelosuppression, nausea, vomiting, headache, fatigue, photosensitivity, liver toxicity, rash	Warn patients to avoid sun exposure for several days after therapy. Do not open capsules. Instruct patients to take on an empty stomach to decrease risk of nausea and vomiting. Do not administer if patients have had an allergic reaction to dacarbazine. Administer PCP prophylaxis with trimethoprim-sulfamethoxazole in patients receiving with radiation therapy for 42-day regimen. Bedtime administration may be advised (Solimando, 2008).
		Thiotepa (Thioplex®)	IV, SC, IM, IT, intravesical, ophthalmic, intratumoral	Bladder, breast, and ovarian cancers; HD, NHL, lymphoma, sarcoma	Hypersensitivity reaction, myelosuppression, ovarian or sperm suppression, nausea, vomiting, pain at infusion site, rash, fever, skin burn, mucositis, hemorrhagic cystitis	Thiotepa is primarily excreted in the urine; monitor renal function carefully. Myelosuppression may be delayed (14–28 days). Use skin care measures when using high-dose therapy.

(Continued on next page)

Table 5. Characteristics of Cytotoxic Agents *(Continued)*

Classification	Medication Name(s)	Mechanism of Action	Route of Administration	Indications	Side Effects	Nursing Considerations
Antimetabolite	Azacitidine (Vidaza®)	Azacitidine is believed to cause hypomethylation of DNA and direct cytotoxicity on abnormal hematopoietic cells in the bone marrow. Abnormal cells, including cancer cells, no longer respond to normal growth control mechanisms. The cytotoxic effects of azacitidine cause the death of these cells, whereas nonproliferating cells are relatively insensitive to the medication.	SC, IV	Patients with specific subtypes of MDS	Bone marrow suppression (including neutropenia, thrombocytopenia, and anemia), nausea, vomiting, diarrhea, fatigue, fever, erythema at injection site, elevated SCr, renal failure, hypokalemia, renal tubular acidosis, hepatic coma	IV: Mix in NS or LR only. Infuse over 10–40 min. Administration should be completed within 1 hr of reconstitution. SC: Gently roll syringe between palms to mix medication immediately prior to administration. Divide doses > 4 ml into two syringes and inject into two separate sites. Invert the syringe 2–3 times and roll vigorously between palms prior to administration. Draw 0.2 ml of air into syringe prior to administration to prevent contamination of skin layers and decreasing irritation. Do not use ice on injection site, as it may decrease drug absorption. Rotate sites for administration among thigh, abdomen, and upper arm. Administer new injections at least one inch from old site. Avoid sites that are tender, bruised, red, or hard. Monitor CBC and liver and renal function during therapy. Drug is contraindicated in patients with hypersensitivity to azacitidine or mannitol and those with advanced malignant hepatic tumors. Medication has been shown to have teratogenic effects. Female patients should avoid becoming pregnant while taking this medication. Male patients should be advised not to father a child while receiving therapy.
	Capecitabine (Xeloda®)	Acts in S phase; inhibits enzyme production for DNA synthesis, leading to strand breaks or premature chain termination	PO	Breast and metastatic colon cancers	Diarrhea, palmar-plantar erythrodysesthesia, mucositis, nausea, vomiting, anemia, increased bilirubin, fatigue	Patient education regarding importance of reporting toxicity and dose reduction is critical. Drug is contraindicated in patients with known hypersensitivity to 5-fluorouracil. Monitor PT and INR closely, as capecitabine increases effect of warfarin. Administer with food and water.
	Cladribine (Leustatin®)		IV	Hairy cell leukemia, NHL	Myelosuppression, fever, nausea, vomiting, neurotoxicity, hypersensitivity reaction, TLS	Allopurinol and IV hydration are recommended for patients with high tumor burden to prevent TLS. Use with caution in patients with liver and renal dysfunction.

(Continued on next page)

Table 5. Characteristics of Cytotoxic Agents *(Continued)*

Classification	Mechanism of Action	Medication Name(s)	Route of Administration	Indications	Side Effects	Nursing Considerations
Antimetabolite *(cont.)*	A purine nucleoside antimetabolite that incorporates into the DNA chain inhibiting DNA repair.	Clofarabine (Clolar™)	IV	Patients 1–21 years old with relapsed or refractory ALL after at least two prior regimens	Nausea, vomiting, diarrhea, bone marrow suppression (including anemia, leukopenia, thrombocytopenia, neutropenia, and febrile neutropenia), infection, hepatobiliary toxicity, renal toxicity; rare cases of systemic inflammatory response syndrome/capillary leak syndrome and cardiac toxicity, including tachycardia, pericardial effusion, and left ventricular systolic dysfunction	Continuous IV fluid administration during the five days of chemotherapy administration is encouraged to reduce the risk of TLS and other adverse effects. Use prophylactic steroids to help to prevent systemic inflammatory response syndrome and capillary leak syndrome. Allopurinol should be given if hyperuricemia is expected. Monitor respiratory status and blood pressure during infusion. Monitor renal and hepatic function during the days of administration. Monitor hematologic status closely following treatment.
		Cytarabine (cytosine arabinoside, ARA-C, Cytosar-U®)	IV, SC, IT, IM	ALL, AML, CML, HD, NHL, CNS leukemia	Myelosuppression, nausea, vomiting, anorexia, fever, mucositis, diarrhea, hepatic dysfunction, pruritus, localized pain and/or thrombophlebitis at IV site; photophobia High-dose: cerebellar toxicity, keratitis (treat with dexamethasone ophthalmic drops), dermatologic toxicities	Determine if the ordered dose is a standard dose or a high dose; administer the agent according to institutional guidelines. Note: Toxicities vary depending upon rate of high-dose cytarabine administration. Continuous-infusion cytarabine is associated with pulmonary toxicity (fluid overload), and bolus dose administration is associated with cerebellar toxicities. Specific nursing interventions are warranted for each. For IT administration: Use preservative-free saline. Allopurinol and IV hydration are recommended for newly diagnosed patients with AML or patients with high tumor burden to prevent TLS.
		Cytarabine liposomal (DepoCyt®)	IT only	Lymphomatous meningitis	High-dose: mucositis, diarrhea	Do not use in pediatric patients. Administer IT only. Patients should lie flat for one hour after lumbar puncture. Monitor closely for immediate toxic reactions.
		Decitabine (Dacogen®)	IV	MDS	Myelosuppression, fatigue, nausea, cough, constipation, diarrhea, hyperglycemia, petechiae	Delay treatment if SCr ≥ 2 or total bilirubin ≥ 2 times upper limit of normal, until resolved. Use within 15 min of reconstitution. If this is not possible, return to pharmacy so solution can be prepared in cold infusion fluid.

(Continued on next page)

Table 5. Characteristics of Cytotoxic Agents (Continued)

Classification	Medication Name(s)	Mechanism of Action	Route of Administration	Indications	Side Effects	Nursing Considerations
Antimetabolite (cont.)	Floxuridine (FUDR®)		Intra-arterial, IV	Adenocarcinoma of GI tract with metastasis to liver, gallbladder, or bile duct	Myelosuppression, nausea, vomiting, diarrhea, mucositis, alopecia, photosensitivity, darkening of the veins, abdominal pain, gastritis, enteritis, hepatotoxicity, palmar-plantar erythrodysesthesia	Do not use in pediatric patients. Recommendations about dose reduction apply to patients with compromised liver function. Adjust dose per institutional protocol and monitor patients' hepatic function carefully.
	Fludarabine (Fludara®)		IV	CLL, low-grade lymphoma	Myelosuppression, nausea, vomiting, diarrhea, rash, neurotoxicity, interstitial pneumonitis	Administer as a 30-min infusion. Monitor PFTs. Allopurinol and IV hydration are recommended for newly diagnosed patients with CLL or patients with high tumor burden to prevent TLS.
	Fluorouracil (5-fluorouracil, 5-FU, Adrucil®)		IV, topical	Colorectal, breast, pancreatic, stomach, esophageal, and head and neck cancers	Myelosuppression, nausea, anorexia, vomiting, diarrhea, mucositis, alopecia, ocular toxicities (e.g., increased lacrimation, photosensitivity), darkening of the veins, dry skin; cardiac toxicity (rare)	Ensure that patients take year-round photosensitivity precautions; encourage sunscreen use if patients must be exposed. Leucovorin often is given concurrently to enhance 5-FU activity. Apply ice chips to the oral cavity 10–15 min pre- and post-IV bolus dose 5-FU to reduce mucositis in patients with GI malignancies.
	Gemcitabine (Gemzar®)		IV	Pancreatic, breast, and ovarian cancers; NSCLC	Myelosuppression (especially anemia), nausea, vomiting, fever, flu-like symptoms, rash, pulmonary toxicity with increased infusion time	Do not use in pediatric patients. Infuse over 30 min; infusion longer than 60 min or more than weekly can increase pulmonary toxicity. Myelosuppression is a dose-limiting toxicity.
	Mercaptopurine (6-MP, Purinethol®)		PO, IV (not available in the United States)	ALL, AML, CML, NHL	Myelosuppression, mucositis, nausea, hyperuricemia	Reduce oral dose by 75% when used concurrently with allopurinol. Patients should take drug on an empty stomach, one hour before meals or two hours after meals.

(Continued on next page)

Table 5. Characteristics of Cytotoxic Agents *(Continued)*

Classification	Mechanism of Action	Medication Name(s)	Route of Administration	Indications	Side Effects	Nursing Considerations
Antimetabolite *(cont.)*		Methotrexate (MTX)	IM, IV, IT, PO	HD, NHL, leukemia; CNS metastasis; lung, breast, and head and neck cancers; gestational trophoblastic tumor; osteogenic sarcoma; rheumatoid arthritis	Mucositis, nausea, myelosuppression, oral or GI ulceration, renal toxicity, photosensitivity, liver toxicity, neurotoxicity associated with high-dose therapy	Drug is yellow in color. **High doses must be followed by leucovorin and vigorous hydration.** Follow dosing schedule carefully. Monitor serum methotrexate levels until ≤ 0.1 mmol. Monitor urine pH and maintain ≥ 7 before treatment and until methotrexate levels ≤ 0.1 mmol. Instruct patients on strict mouth care. Patients must take photosensitivity precautions. Ensure that patients avoid taking multivitamins with folic acid. Multiple drug interactions (e.g., NSAIDs, alcohol, aspirin, warfarin, aminoglycosides) are possible (Camp et al., 2007). Methotrexate is contraindicated in patients with pleural or pericardial effusions and ascites because of severe toxicity from methotrexate accumulation.
		Nelarabine (Arranon®)	IV	Relapsed or nonrespondent T-cell acute lymphoblastic leukemia and T-cell lymphoblastic lymphoma to two cycles of chemotherapy	Myelosuppression, headache, nausea, vomiting, diarrhea, constipation, cough, dyspnea, neurologic toxicities (somnolence, seizures, ataxia)	Given as undiluted IV infusion over 2 hours for adults and 1 hour for pediatrics. Administer with appropriate supportive care medications to prevent hyperuricemia and TLS. Discontinue for $\geq$ grade 2 neurologic events.

(Continued on next page)

Table 5. Characteristics of Cytotoxic Agents (Continued)

Classification	Medication Name(s)	Mechanism of Action	Route of Administration	Indications	Side Effects	Nursing Considerations
Antimetabolite (cont.)	Pemetrexed (Alimta®)	Disrupts folate-dependent metabolic processes essential for cell replication	IV	Given in combination with cisplatin for the treatment of malignant pleural mesothelioma; nonsquamous NSCLC initial treatment in combination with cisplatin or as a single-agent after prior chemotherapy	Side effects with pemetrexed plus cisplatin regimen include myelosuppression, fatigue, nausea, vomiting, chest pain, and dyspnea. Side effects are reduced with vitamin supplementation. Renal and liver toxicity.	To reduce treatment-related hematologic and GI toxicity, administer folic acid, 350–1,000 mcg PO, daily starting 1 week prior to the first cycle and daily for three weeks after final cycle. Give vitamin B_{12} injection, 1,000 mcg IM, 1 week before first cycle and repeat every nine weeks until treatment is completed. Dexamethasone 4 mg BID for 3 days starting the day before treatment decreases incidence of skin rash. Monitor CBC on days 8 and 15. Hold treatment if absolute neutrophil count < 1,500 cells/mm³, platelet count < 100,000 cells/mm³, or creatinine clearance < 45 ml/min. Monitor renal and hepatic function. The concurrent use of ibuprofen may increase the risk of renal damage.
	Pentostatin (Nipent®)		IV	Hairy cell leukemia, CLL, lymphoma	Myelosuppression, fever, chills, nausea, vomiting, rash, renal failure, confusion, hepatic enzyme elevation, lymphocytopenia, heightened infection risk	Administer with 500–1,000 ml 5% dextrose in ½ NS solution prior to the infusion and an additional 500 ml after infusion.
	Thioguanine (6-thioguanine, 6-TG)		PO	ALL, AML, CML	Myelosuppression, hyperuricemia, nausea, hepatotoxicity, diarrhea	No dose reduction is necessary when this drug is used concurrently with allopurinol. Administer on an empty stomach.
	Trimetrexate (Neutrexin®)		IV	Colorectal and head and neck cancers, non-small cell lung cancer, PCP, toxoplasmosis	Myelosuppression, mucositis, nausea, vomiting, alopecia, headache, rash	Monitor renal and hepatic function. Use with caution in patients with abnormal renal and hepatic function.
	Uracil and tegafur (UFT®)		PO	Breast, colorectal, gastric, and pancreatic cancers	Diarrhea, nausea, vomiting, fatigue, rash, neurotoxicity, myelosuppression	Instruct patients to take with a large glass of water on an empty stomach.

(Continued on next page)

Table 5. Characteristics of Cytotoxic Agents (Continued)

Classification	Mechanism of Action	Medication Name(s)	Route of Administration	Indications	Side Effects	Nursing Considerations
Antitumor antibiotic	Binds with DNA, thereby inhibiting DNA and RNA synthesis	Bleomycin (Blenoxane®)	IV, SC, IM, intracavitary	Malignant pleural effusion; squamous cell cancer of head and neck; cervical, vulvar, penile, and testicular cancers; melanoma; HD; NHL	Hypersensitivity or anaphylactic reaction (rare), hyperpigmentation, alopecia, photosensitivity, renal toxicity, hepatotoxicity, pulmonary fibrosis, fever, chills	Patients with lymphoma have a higher incidence of anaphylaxis after receiving bleomycin than do other patients who receive the drug. Therefore (per institutional protocol), a test dose of 1–2 units IV, IM, or SC may be administered before the first dose of bleomycin in patients with lymphoma. Patients who have received prior bleomycin are at risk for pulmonary toxicity when exposed to oxygen during surgery. Ensure that patients and family members understand the lifelong necessity of disclosing previous use of bleomycin when future needs for anesthesia occur to prevent a fatal episode of pulmonary failure. Because of the dose-related incidence of pulmonary fibrosis, the cumulative lifetime dose should not exceed 400 units. PFTs are recommended at initiation of bleomycin and every 1–2 months thereafter. Consider stopping drug if a 30%–35% decrease from pretreatment values occurs. Acetaminophen and an antihistamine may decrease fever and chills in first 24 hrs after administration.
		Dactinomycin (actinomycin D, Cosmegen®)	IV	Ewing sarcoma, Wilms tumor, testicular cancer, gestational trophoblastic disease, rhabdomyosarcoma	Myelosuppression, nausea, vomiting, alopecia, mucositis, diarrhea, ovarian or sperm suppression, radiation recall (hyperpigmentation of previously irradiated areas)	Dactinomycin is a vesicant. This drug may be ordered in micrograms, so check the dose carefully.
		Mitomycin (Mutamycin®)	IV	Pancreatic, stomach, colon, breast, lung, bladder, head and neck, and esophageal cancers	Myelosuppression, nausea, vomiting, anorexia, alopecia, mucositis, renal toxicity, pulmonary toxicity, fatigue	Drug is purple in color. Mitomycin is a vesicant. Nadir occurs 4–8 weeks after treatment begins. Acute shortness of breath and bronchospasm can occur very suddenly when this drug is given with a vinca alkaloid.

(Continued on next page)

Table 5. Characteristics of Cytotoxic Agents (Continued)

Classification	Mechanism of Action	Medication Name(s)	Route of Administration	Indications	Side Effects	Nursing Considerations
Antitumor antibiotic (cont.)		Mitoxantrone (Novantrone®)	IV	Breast and prostate cancers, lymphoma, ANLL	Myelosuppression, arrhythmia (if patient was treated with doxorubicin), nausea, vomiting, mucositis, alopecia; drug may turn the urine blue-green and can cause sclera to turn bluish.	Mitoxantrone is an irritant with vesicant potential. Drug is blue in color. The risk of cardiotoxicity with mitoxantrone is less than that with doxorubicin, but prior anthracycline use, chest irradiation, or cardiac disease can increase the patient's risk.
Antitumor antibiotic (anthracycline)	Binds with DNA, thereby inhibiting DNA and RNA synthesis	Daunorubicin (Cerubidine®, Daunomycin®)	IV	ALL in children, ANLL	Myelosuppression, nausea, vomiting, alopecia, cardiotoxicity, hyperuricemia, radiation recall, ovarian or sperm suppression; drug may turn the urine red.	Drug is red in color. Daunorubicin is a vesicant. Test patients' cardiac ejection fraction scan before starting therapy.
		Daunorubicin citrate liposomal (DaunoXome®)	IV	AIDS-related Kaposi sarcoma	Myelosuppression, nausea, vomiting, alopecia, cardiotoxicity, hyperuricemia, radiation recall, ovarian or sperm suppression; drug may turn the urine red.	Drug is red in color. Daunorubicin citrate liposomal is not a vesicant but should be considered an irritant, and caution should be taken to avoid extravasation. Consider a dose reduction in patients with liver dysfunction. Test patients' cardiac ejection fraction before starting daunorubicin liposomal therapy. This drug must be mixed in D5W only. Do not use in-line filters.
		Doxorubicin (Adriamycin®)	IV	Breast, ovarian, prostate, stomach, thyroid, small cell lung, and liver cancers; squamous cell cancer of the head and neck; MM, HD, NHL, ALL, AML; Wilms tumor	Myelosuppression, nausea, vomiting, alopecia, mucositis, dose-limiting cardiotoxicity, radiation recall, arrhythmia, hyperuricemia, photosensitivity; drug may turn the urine red.	Drug is red in color. Doxorubicin is a vesicant. Doxorubicin may cause a flare reaction. Test patients' cardiac ejection fraction before starting therapy. Do not exceed a lifetime cumulative dose of 550 mg/m² (450 mg/m² if the patient has had prior or chest irradiation or concomitant cyclophosphamide treatment). Consider initiating dexrazoxane for patients who have received a cumulative dose of 300 mg/m² and are continuing doxorubicin treatment. In pediatrics, dexrazoxane may be used concurrently.

(Continued on next page)

Table 5. Characteristics of Cytotoxic Agents *(Continued)*

Classification	Mechanism of Action	Medication Name(s)	Route of Administration	Indications	Side Effects	Nursing Considerations
Antitumor antibiotic (anthracycline) *(cont.)*		Doxorubicin liposomal (Doxil®)	IV	AIDS-related Kaposi sarcoma, ovarian cancer, MM in combination with bortezomib	Myelosuppression, nausea, vomiting, alopecia, mucositis, dose-limiting cardiotoxicity, arrhythmia, hyperuricemia, radiation recall; palmar-plantar erythrodysesthesia, photosensitivity; drug may turn the urine red.	Drug is red in color. Doxorubicin liposomal is not a vesicant but should be considered an irritant, and caution should be taken to avoid extravasation. The same warnings as with conventional doxorubicin apply regarding cardiovascular complications. Use only with D5W. Do not substitute for Adriamycin. Start infusion at 1 mg/min over at least 30 min to minimize infusion-related reactions.
		Epirubicin (Ellence®)	IV	Breast cancer	Myelosuppression, nausea, vomiting, mucositis, diarrhea, cardiotoxicity, alopecia, radiation recall; drug may turn the urine red as drug concentrates in and is metabolized by RBCs.	Drug is red in color. Epirubicin is a vesicant. Consider a dose reduction in patients with liver dysfunction. Reduce dose by 50% in patients with SCr > 5 mg/dl. Test patients' cardiac ejection fraction before starting epirubicin therapy. Cimetidine increases the AUC of epirubicin by 50% (Camp et al., 2007).
		Idarubicin (Idamycin®)	IV	ANLL	Myelosuppression, nausea, vomiting, alopecia, vein itching, cardiomyopathy, radiation recall, rash, mucositis, diarrhea; drug may turn the urine red.	Drug is red-orange in color. Idarubicin is a vesicant. Infuse slowly over 10–15 min into free-flowing side arm infusion. The cardiotoxicity of idarubicin is less than that of daunorubicin. Cumulative doses > 150 mg/m² idarubicin are associated with decreased ejection fraction. Local reactions (hives at injection site) may occur.
		Valrubicin (Valstar®)	Intravesical	Intravesical therapy of BCG-refractory in situ bladder cancer	Dysuria, bladder spasm, urinary incontinence, leukopenia, neutropenia, hyperglycemia; drug may turn the urine red.	Do not use in pediatrics. Valrubicin is administered as an intravesicular bladder lavage.

(Continued on next page)

Table 5. Characteristics of Cytotoxic Agents (Continued)

Classification	Mechanism of Action	Medication Name(s)	Route of Administration	Indications	Side Effects	Nursing Considerations
Miscellaneous	Degrades the chimeric PML/RAR alpha protein; degrades the NB4 human promyelocytic leukemia cells to cause partial maturation and trigger apoptosis; causes the release of toxic free radicals inside the cell that triggers apoptosis of the APL cell	Arsenic trioxide (Trisenox®)	IV	APL	Fatigue, prolonged QT interval, APL differentiation syndrome, leukocytosis, headache, nausea, vomiting, diarrhea, musculoskeletal pain, peripheral neuropathy	Use with caution with other agents that prolong QT/QTc interval. Obtain baseline ECG prior to therapy. Ensure QTc interval < 500 msec prior to infusion. Periodic QTc intervals should be measured during therapy (e.g., weekly) per institutional guidelines. Use with caution in patients with renal impairment. Monitor electrolytes during therapy. Maintain serum potassium > 4 mEq/L and magnesium > 1.8 mg/dl.
	Inhibits protein synthesis	Asparaginase (Elspar®)	IV, SC, IM	ALL	Nausea, vomiting, hepatotoxicity, fever, hyperglycemia, anaphylaxis, pancreatitis, coagulopathy, hypoalbuminemia, hypersensitivity reaction, renal toxicity	Giving the drug IM greatly reduces the incidence of anaphylaxis. Keep medications to treat anaphylaxis at bedside.
		Pegaspargase (Oncaspar®)	IM, IV	ALL (may be used upfront or for those who have developed hypersensitivity to asparaginase)	Hepatotoxicity, coagulopathy, anaphylaxis	Test dose is not needed. Longer half-life (5–6 days) than asparaginase (1–2 days), therefore dosed every 14 days versus daily or every 3 days. Risk of anaphylaxis is less than that of asparaginase.
	Acts in S phase as antimetabolite	Hydroxyurea (Hydrea®, Mylocel®)	PO	CML, malignant melanoma, squamous cell cancer of the head and neck, metastatic ovarian cancer, sickle cell anemia	Myelosuppression (especially severe anemia), nausea, vomiting, diarrhea, renal failure, mucositis, hyperuricemia, fever, rash	Adjust the dose according to WBC counts; monitor WBCs at least every 2 weeks, and stop treatment until counts recover. Do not change the dose too frequently in older patients because they may be more sensitive to the medication. Instruct patients on strict mouth care. Doses may be divided within the 24-hr period to decrease nausea and vomiting.
	Inhibits adrenal steroid production	Mitotane (Lysodren®)	PO	Adrenocortical cancer	Nausea, vomiting, mucositis, adrenal insufficiency	Monitor patients on warfarin therapy closely with PT/INR. Adrenal steroid replacement is indicated.

(Continued on next page)

Table 5. Characteristics of Cytotoxic Agents *(Continued)*

Classification	Mechanism of Action	Medication Name(s)	Route of Administration	Indications	Side Effects	Nursing Considerations
Miscellaneous *(cont.)*	May inhibit protein, RNA, and DNA synthesis	Procarbazine (Matulane®)	PO	HD, brain tumors	Myelosuppression, nausea, vomiting	Patients should avoid foods high in tyramine, such as aged cheeses, air-dried or cured meats, fava or broad bean pods, tap/draft beer, wine (over 120 ml), vermouth, marmite concentrate, sauerkraut, and other soybean condiments because procarbazine inhibits monoamine oxidase. Patients also should avoid alcohol for possible Antabuse®-like reaction.
	Inhibits the enzymatic activity of HDAC, which allows for the accumulation of acetyl groups on the histone lysine residue, which results in cell cycle arrest and/or apoptosis of some transformed cells	Vorinostat (Zolinza®)	PO	Cutaneous T-cell lymphoma	Diarrhea, fatigue, nausea, thrombocytopenia, thromboembolism, anorexia, dysgeusia	Instruct patients to take once daily with food. Monitor CBC, electrolytes, glucose, and SCr every 2 weeks during first 2 months and monthly afterward because of possible hyperglycemia and QT prolongation. Capsules should not be opened or crushed. Drug may interact with Coumadin® (increasing PT/INR) and other HDAC inhibitors (valproic acid) (severe thrombocytopenia and GI bleeding).
	Semi-synthetic analog of epothilone B; binds to beta-tubulin on microtubles, leading to cell death by blocking cells in mitotic phase of cell division cycle	Ixabepilone (Ixempra®)	IV	Metastatic or locally advanced breast cancer in combination with capecitabine in patients after failure of an anthracycline or taxane	Peripheral sensory neuropathy, myelosuppression, fatigue, myalgia, alopecia, nausea, vomiting, mucositis, diarrhea, musculoskeletal pain	CYP3A4 inhibitors may increase ixabepilone concentration, and CYP3A4 inducers may decrease ixabepilone concentration. Avoid St. John's wort. Premedicate with diphenhydramine and famotidine or ranitidine 1 hr prior to dose to decrease chance of hypersensitivity reaction. Mix only in LR in non-PVC bag. Administer through 0.2–1.2 micron in-line filter.

(Continued on next page)

Table 5. Characteristics of Cytotoxic Agents (Continued)

Classification	Mechanism of Action	Medication Name(s)	Route of Administration	Indications	Side Effects	Nursing Considerations
Nitrosourea	Breaks DNA helix, interfering with DNA replication; crosses the blood-brain barrier	Carmustine (BiCNU®)	IV, implantation (Gliadel® wafer)	HD, NHL, CNS tumors, MM, BMT, malignant melanoma	Nausea, vomiting, myelosuppression, renal toxicity, hepatic toxicity, pulmonary fibrosis, ovarian or sperm suppression	Carmustine crosses the blood-brain barrier. Nadir occurs 4–6 weeks after therapy starts. Because of delayed toxicity, successive treatments usually are given no more frequently than once every 6–8 weeks. Rapid infusion may cause burning along the vein and flushing of the skin. Long-term therapy can result in irreversible pulmonary fibrosis, which may present as an insidious cough and dyspnea or sudden respiratory failure.
		Lomustine (CeeNu®)	PO	Pancreatic, liver, gastric, and colorectal cancers; CNS and brain tumors; MM, HD, NHL	Myelosuppression (severe), nausea, vomiting, alopecia, renal toxicity, hepatic toxicity, mucositis, anorexia, pulmonary fibrosis	Lomustine crosses the blood-brain barrier. Because of delayed myelosuppression, do not repeat the dose more than once every 6 weeks. Administer on an empty stomach. Monitor PFTs, LFTs, and renal function.
		Streptozocin (Zanosar®)	IV	Metastatic islet-cell pancreatic carcinoma, carcinoid tumor	Renal toxicity, myelosuppression, nausea, vomiting, hyperglycemia, proteinuria	Nephrotoxicity may be dose limiting. This drug may alter glucose metabolism in some patients. Rapid infusion may cause burning along the vein.
Plant alkaloid (camptothecin)	Acts in S phase; topoisomerase I inhibitors; causes double-strand DNA changes	Irinotecan (Camptosar®)	IV	Metastatic colorectal cancer	Diarrhea, myelosuppression, alopecia	Do not use in pediatrics. This drug can cause early and late diarrhea, which can be dose limiting. Early diarrhea can occur within 24 hrs of administration and generally is cholinergic. Many institutions use atropine to treat this early diarrhea. Refer to institutional protocol regarding the dosing and administration of atropine and other antidiarrheals.
		Topotecan (Hycamtin®)	IV	Metastatic ovarian cancer, cervical cancer, SCLC	Myelosuppression, diarrhea, alopecia, nausea, vomiting, headache	Prior to administration, dilute the appropriate volume of reconstituted solution with either NS IV solution or D5W IV solution.

(Continued on next page)

Table 5. Characteristics of Cytotoxic Agents (Continued)

Classification	Mechanism of Action	Medication Name(s)	Route of Administration	Indications	Side Effects	Nursing Considerations
Plant alkaloid (epipodophyllotoxin)	Induces irreversible blockade of cells in premitotic phases of cell cycle (late G2 and S phases); interferes with topoisomerase II enzyme reaction	Etoposide (VP-16, VePesid®, Etopophos®)	IV, PO	Breast and testicular cancers, SCLC, MM, BMT	Myelosuppression, nausea, vomiting, alopecia, anorexia, orthostatic hypotension, hyperuricemia, hypersensitivity reaction, anaphylaxis High-dose: mucositis, diarrhea	Do not administer this drug by means of rapid IV infusion or IV push. Infuse it over 30–60 min to avoid hypotension. Monitor patients' blood pressure during infusion. Prior to use, dilute the drug to a final concentration of 0.2–0.4 mg/ml to prevent precipitation. Monitor for crystallization during infusion. If a patient has an allergic reaction to etoposide, premedicate with diphenhydramine. Do not administer to patients with bilirubin > 5 mg/dl.
		Teniposide (VM-26, Vumon®)	IV	Childhood ALL	Myelosuppression, hypotension, pulmonary toxicity, anaphylaxis, nausea, vomiting	Do not administer via rapid infusion; infuse over 30–60 min. To avoid hypotension, monitor patients' blood pressure during the infusion. Drug may cause an allergic reaction. Administer through non-PVC tubing.
Plant alkaloid (taxane)	Stabilizes microtubules, inhibiting cell division; effective in G2 and M phases	Docetaxel (Taxotere®)	IV	NSCLC; breast, head and neck, prostate, and gastric cancers	Myelosuppression, hypersensitivity reaction, fluid retention, alopecia, skin and nail changes, mucositis, nausea, vomiting, paresthesia, neurotoxicity	Do not use in pediatrics. Docetaxel is an irritant. Extravasation may lead to edema, erythema, and occasional pain and blister formation. Premedicate as follows to reduce the severity of hypersensitivity reaction and fluid retention: dexamethasone 8 mg PO BID, beginning 1 day prior to docetaxel treatment and continuing for the day of treatment and 1 day after. Refer to institutional guidelines for additional pretreatment requirements. Do not use PVC tubing or bags to administer docetaxel.

(Continued on next page)

Table 5. Characteristics of Cytotoxic Agents *(Continued)*

Classification	Mechanism of Action	Medication Name(s)	Route of Administration	Indications	Side Effects	Nursing Considerations
Plant alkaloid (taxane) *(cont.)*		Paclitaxel (Taxol®)	IV	Metastatic breast, ovarian, head and neck cancers; NSCLC; AIDS-related Kaposi sarcoma	Myelosuppression, alopecia, peripheral neurotoxicity, hypersensitivity reaction, facial flushing, myalgia, fatigue, cardiac arrhythmias, mucositis, diarrhea	Do not use in pediatrics. Paclitaxel is an irritant and potential vesicant. Extravasation may lead to local pain, edema, and erythema at the infusion site. There are reports of necrosis. Pretreat as follows to help to prevent hypersensitivity reaction, including anaphylaxis, 30–60 min before treatment: cimetidine 300 mg or famotidine 20 mg IV, diphenhydramine 50 mg IV, and (unless contraindicated) dexamethasone 20 mg IV (Solimando, 2008). Filter paclitaxel with a 0.2 micron in-line filter. Use glass bottles or non-PVC (polyolefin or polypropylene) bags to administer paclitaxel; do not use PVC tubing or bags.
		Paclitaxel protein-bound particles; albumin-bound (Abraxane™)	IV	Treatment of metastatic breast cancer after failure of combination chemotherapy or relapse within six months of adjuvant therapy	Myelosuppression, sensory neuropathy, myalgia, arthralgia, nausea, vomiting, diarrhea, mucositis, alopecia	Drug is free of solvents; therefore, no premedication is required to prevent hypersensitivity reactions. Consider dose reduction by about 20% for severe sensory neuropathy; resume treatment with reduced dose when neuropathy improves to grade 1 or 2 (Solimando, 2008). Do not use in patients with baseline neutrophil counts < 1,500 cells/mm^3.
Plant alkaloid (vinca alkaloid)	Acts in late G2 phase, blocking DNA production, and in M phase, preventing cell division	Vinblastine (Velban®)	IV	Testicular cancer, squamous cell cancer of the head and neck, HD, Kaposi sarcoma, histiocytosis	Myelosuppression, alopecia, anorexia, jaw pain, peripheral neuropathy, constipation, paralytic ileus	Vinblastine is a vesicant. Generally, neurotoxicity occurs less frequently with vinblastine than with vincristine; however, it can occur with high doses. **Drug is fatal if given intrathecally.**

(Continued on next page)

Table 5. Characteristics of Cytotoxic Agents (Continued)

Classification	Medication Name(s)	Mechanism of Action	Route of Administration	Indications	Side Effects	Nursing Considerations
Plant alkaloid (vinca alkaloid) (cont.)	Vincristine (Oncovin®)		IV	ALL, HD, NHL, CML, sarcoma, breast cancer, SCLC, neuroblastoma, Wilms tumor	Peripheral neuropathy, alopecia, constipation, paralytic ileus, jaw pain, foot drop	Vincristine is a vesicant. Neurotoxicity is cumulative but often reversible; conduct a neurologic evaluation before each dose. Withhold dose if severe paresthesia, motor weakness, or other abnormality develops. Reduce dose in the presence of significant liver disease. Stool softeners and/or a stimulant laxative may help to prevent severe constipation. **Drug is fatal if given intrathecally.**
	Vinorelbine (Navelbine®)		IV	NSCLC, breast and ovarian cancers, HD	Myelosuppression, nausea, vomiting, neurotoxicity, peripheral neuropathy, alopecia	Do not use in pediatrics. Vinorelbine is a vesicant. Administer via IV push over 6–10 min through the side port of a free-flowing IV, then flush with 75–125 ml solution. **Drug is fatal if given intrathecally.**

AIDS—acquired immunodeficiency syndrome; ALL—acute lymphocytic leukemia; AML—acute myeloid leukemia; ANLL—acute nonlymphocytic leukemia; APL—acute promyelocytic leukemia; AUC—area under the plasma concentration versus time curve; BCG—bacillus Calmette-Guérin; BID—twice daily; BMT—bone marrow transplant; CBC—complete blood count; CLL—chronic lymphocytic leukemia; CML—chronic myeloid leukemia; CNS—central nervous system; D5W—5% dextrose in water; dl—deciliter; DNA—deoxyribonucleic acid; ECG—electrocardiogram; 5HT$_3$—5-hydroxytryptamine-3; GI—gastrointestinal; HD—Hodgkin disease; HDAC—histone deacetylases; hr—hour; IM—intramuscular; INR—international normalized ratio; IT—intrathecal; IV—intravenous; kg—kilogram; LFT—liver function test; LR—lactated Ringer's solution; MDS—myelodysplastic syndrome; mcg—microgram; mEq—milliequivalent; mg—milligram; ml—milliliter; mmol—millimole; min—minute; MM—multiple myeloma; msec—millisecond; NHL—non-Hodgkin lymphoma; NS—normal saline; NSAID—nonsteroidal anti-inflammatory drug; NSCLC—non-small cell lung cancer; PCP—Pneumocystis carinii pneumonia; PFT—pulmonary function test; PO—oral; PT—prothrombin time; PVC—polyvinyl chloride; QTc—QT interval corrected; RBC—red blood cell; RNA—ribonucleic acid; SC—subcutaneous; SCLC—small cell lung cancer; SCr—serum creatinine; TLS—tumor lysis syndrome; WBC—white blood cell

Note. Based on information from Aronoff et al., 2007; Ascherman et al., 2000; Camp et al., 2007; Chu & DeVita, 2006; Solimando, 2008; and manufacturers' prescribing information.

Table 7. Characteristics of Biologic Agents

Classification	Medication Name(s)	Mechanism of Action	Route of Administration	Indications	Side Effects	Nursing Considerations
Colony-stimulating factor (CSF)	Darbepoetin (Aranesp®)	Stimulates erythropoiesis via the same mechanism as endogenous erythropoietin	SC	Treatment of anemia associated with chronic renal failure whether or not the patient is receiving dialysis Treatment of anemia in patients with nonmyeloid malignancies where anemia is caused by concomitantly administered chemotherapy	Hypertension, skin rash, urticaria, pure red cell aplasia, myalgia, infection, fatigue, edema, diarrhea, thrombotic events	Risk of death and serious cardiovascular events is increased if Hgb > 12 g/dl when administered. Ensure adequate iron stores in patients prior to and during use. Drug may be administered every 1, 2, or 3 weeks, but maintain consistent dosing schedule. Use lowest effective dose. Do not shake vials or syringes containing drug. Store in refrigerator. Do not freeze.
	Epoetin alfa (Procrit®)	Stimulates erythropoiesis via the same mechanism as endogenous erythropoietin	SC	Treatment of anemia associated with chronic renal failure whether or not the patient is receiving dialysis; anemia associated with treatment using zidovudine in HIV-infected patients; anemia in patients with nonmyeloid malignancies where anemia is caused by concomitant use of chemotherapy; and in patients scheduled to undergo elective noncardiac, nonvascular surgery to reduce the need for allogeneic red blood cell transfusions	Hypertension, skin rash, urticaria, pure red cell aplasia, myalgia, infection, fatigue, edema, diarrhea, thrombotic events	Risk of death and serious cardiovascular events is increased if Hgb > 12 g/dl when administered. Ensure adequate iron stores in patients prior to and during use. May be given 3 times weekly or as a single weekly dose. Use lowest effective dose. Do not shake vials or syringes containing drug. Store in refrigerator. Do not freeze.

(Continued on next page)

Table 7. Characteristics of Biologic Agents *(Continued)*

Classification	Mechanism of Action	Medication Name(s)	Route of Administration	Indications	Side Effects	Nursing Considerations
Colony-stimulating factor (CSF) *(cont.)*	Regulates the production of neutrophils within the bone marrow	Filgrastim (G-CSF, Neupogen®)	SC, IV	Used to decrease the incidence of infection in patients with neutropenic fever associated with myelosuppressive anticancer treatments for nonmyeloid malignancies Used to reduce the time to neutrophil recovery and duration of fever following induction or consolidation chemotherapy in patients with AML Used to reduce the duration of neutropenia and associated sequelae in patients receiving myeloablative chemotherapy prior to BMT Used to mobilize hematopoietic progenitor cells into peripheral blood for collection via leukapheresis Used for chronic administration to reduce the incidence and duration of sequelae of neutropenia in patients with congenital, cyclic, or idiopathic neutropenia	Allergic reactions including urticaria, rash, and facial edema; rare risk of splenic rupture; ARDS, nausea, vomiting, bone pain, fever	Store in refrigerator. Do not freeze. Drug may be diluted with D5W solution. Do not dilute with saline solutions. Do not shake vials or syringes containing drug.
	Stimulates keratinocyte GFR to result in proliferation, differentiation, and migration of epithelial cells	Palifermin (rHuKGF, Kepivance®)	IV	Used to decrease the incidence and duration of severe oral mucositis in patients with hematologic malignancies receiving myelosuppressive chemotherapy prior to BMT	Skin rash, skin erythema, pruritus, fever, dysesthesia, tongue discoloration, tongue thickening, taste alterations, pain, arthralgias, elevated serum amylase, elevated serum lipase	Do not use within 24 hours before, during, or after administration of myelosuppressive chemotherapy. Administer for 3 days before and then 3 days after myelosuppressive chemotherapy. Do not shake reconstituted solution. Reconstituted product should not be used if stored at room temperature for longer than 1 hour. Do not filter reconstituted solution.

(Continued on next page)

Table 7. Characteristics of Biologic Agents *(Continued)*

Classification	Mechanism of Action	Medication Name(s)	Route of Administration	Indications	Side Effects	Nursing Considerations
Colony-stimulating factor *(cont.)*	Regulates the production of neutrophils within the bone marrow	Pegfilgrastim (Neulasta®)	SC	Used to decrease the incidence of infection related to neutropenia in patients with nonmyeloid malignancies receiving myelosuppressive chemotherapy	Allergic reactions including urticaria, rash, facial edema; rare risk of splenic rupture; ARDS, nausea, vomiting, bone pain, fever	Pegfilgrastim reduces renal clearance and prolongs persistence compared to filgrastim. Do not administer in the period beginning 14 days before until 24 hours after administration of myelosuppressive chemotherapy. Administer as a single 6 mg injection once per chemotherapy cycle. The 6 mg fixed dose should not be administered to children or adolescents weighing less than 45 kg. Store in refrigerator. Do not freeze. Do not shake vials or syringes containing drug.
	Induces committed progenitor cells to divide and differentiate in the GM pathways, including neutrophils, monocytes/macrophages, and myeloid-derived dendritic cells	Sargramostim (GM-CSF, Leukine®)	SC, IV	Used following induction chemotherapy in patients with AML to shorten neutrophil recovery and reduce incidence of infection. Used in patients for the mobilization of hematopoietic progenitor cells for collection via leukapheresis and to speed engraftment following autologous transplantation of progenitor cells. Used to accelerate myeloid recovery following allogeneic BMT. Used in patients with failure of engraftment following BMT	Edema, capillary leak syndrome, pleural or pericardial effusions, dyspnea, fever, abdominal pain, headache, chills, diarrhea, bone pain	Dilution for IV use should be in NS solution. Store in refrigerator. Do not freeze. Do not shake vials or syringes containing drug. Do not administer through in-line filter.

(Continued on next page)

Table 7. Characteristics of Biologic Agents (Continued)

Classification	Mechanism of Action	Medication Name(s)	Route of Administration	Indications	Side Effects	Nursing Considerations
Immunomodulator	Restores depressed immune function; stimulates antibodies to various antigens; stimulates T-cell activation and proliferation; potentiates monocyte and macrophage functions; and increases neutrophil mobility, adherence, and chemotaxis	Levamisole (Eramisol®)	PO	In combination with 5-fluorouracil in the treatment of colorectal cancer	Nausea, diarrhea, vomiting, dermatitis, fatigue, taste alterations, arthralgia, agranulocytosis	Perform routine hematologic monitoring. Flu-like syndrome often accompanies agranulocytosis; instruct patients to report symptoms. An Antabuse®-like effect may occur when taken concomitantly with alcohol. Monitor INR in patients taking warfarin, and adjust accordingly.
Interferon (IFN)	Mechanisms of activity are not clearly understood but include inhibition of viral replication, direct antiproliferation of tumor cells, and modulation of host immune response.	IFN alfa-2a (Roferon-A®)	SC, IM	Treatment of hairy cell leukemia, chronic hepatitis C, chronic-phase Philadelphia chromosome–positive CML	Fever, chills, hypersensitivity, malaise, headache, anorexia, fatigue, depression, suicidal ideation, nausea, vomiting, diarrhea, dizziness, impaired memory, agitation, alopecia, leukopenia, thrombocytopenia, anemia, injection site reactions	Store agent in refrigerator but do not freeze. Do not shake product. Protect from light. Product is stable for 30 days after reconstitution when stored in refrigerator. Advise patients to report feelings of depression or suicidal thoughts to a physician. Drug is contraindicated in patients with Child-Pugh class B or C hepatic insufficiency. Drug may aggravate hyperthyroidism or hypothyroidism in susceptible patients. Patients with diabetes may require adjustment of antidiabetic regimen.

(Continued on next page)

Table 7. Characteristics of Biologic Agents (Continued)

Classification	Mechanism of Action	Medication Name(s)	Route of Administration	Indications	Side Effects	Nursing Considerations
Interferon (IFN) (cont.)	Mechanisms of activity are not clearly understood but include inhibition of viral replication, direct antiproliferation of tumor cells, and modulation of host immune response.	IFN alfa-2B (Intron A®)	SC, IM, IV	Treatment of hairy cell leukemia, malignant melanoma, follicular lymphoma, condylomata acuminata, AIDS-related Kaposi sarcoma, chronic hepatitis B and C	Fever, chills, malaise, myalgia, headache, anorexia, fatigue, depression, suicidal ideation, nausea, vomiting, diarrhea, nephrotic syndrome, pancreatitis, psychosis, hallucinations, renal failure, renal insufficiency, leukopenia, anemia, thrombocytopenia	Store agent in refrigerator but do not freeze. Do not shake product. Protect from light. Product is stable for 30 days after reconstitution when stored in refrigerator. Drug is contraindicated in patients with liver impairment. Use with caution in patients with a history of cardiovascular disease. Preexisting ophthalmologic disorders, such as diabetic or hypertensive retinopathy, should be examined periodically during treatment. Drug may aggravate hyperthyroidism or hypothyroidism in susceptible patients.
		Interferon gamma, IFN-γ (Actimmune®)	SC	Reduces frequency and severity of infections related to chronic granulomatous disease. Also indicated for delaying progression of severe malignant osteopetrosis	Fever, headache, rash, chills, injection site tenderness, fatigue, diarrhea, vomiting, nausea, myalgia, arthralgia, myelosuppression, elevated hepatic transaminases	Hold therapy or reduce dose by 50% in cases of severe reactions. Flu-like syndrome may exacerbate preexisting cardiac conditions, such as CHF.

(Continued on next page)

Table 7. Characteristics of Biologic Agents *(Continued)*

Classification	Mechanism of Action	Medication Name(s)	Route of Administration	Indications	Side Effects	Nursing Considerations
Interleukin (IL)	Promotes proliferation, differentiation, and recruitment of T and B cells, NK cells, LAK cells, and tumor-infiltrating lymphocytes that enhance tumor-fighting capabilities; increases production of IFN gamma, IL-1, and TNF	Aldesleukin (IL-2, Proleukin®)	SC, IV	Treatment of renal cell carcinoma and metastatic melanoma	Fever, rigors, malaise, headache, myalgia, arthralgia, tachycardia, hypotension, cardiomyopathy, arrhythmias, capillary leak syndrome, dyspnea, nausea, vomiting, diarrhea, stomatitis, dizziness, anemia, thrombocytopenia, leukopenia, elevated transaminases, elevated serum creatinine, BUN, neurologic toxicities, skin rash, pruritus, hyperbilirubinemia	Do not use with an in-line filter. Do not mix with NS or bacteriostatic water. Store in refrigerator but do not freeze. Protect from light. Do not mix with other medications. Monitor fluid status, vital signs, mental status, and urine output. Hypotension is dose limiting and mimics septic shock; use IV boluses carefully; treatment may require vasopressor support. Drug is contraindicated in patients with cardiac disease, abnormal pulmonary function, or organ allografts. Assess fall risk during treatment.
	Stimulates megakaryocytopoiesis and thrombopoiesis	Oprelvekin (IL-11, Neumega®)	SC	Prevention of severe thrombocytopenia and reduced need for platelet transfusions in patients receiving chemotherapy	Anaphylaxis, dilutional anemia, diarrhea, dizziness, fever, fluid retention resulting in peripheral edema, pulmonary edema, dyspnea, capillary leak syndrome, atrial arrhythmias and exacerbation of preexisting pulmonary effusions, headache, nausea, vomiting, insomnia, rhinitis	Store in refrigerator but do not freeze. Reconstitute with sterile water and use within 3 hours of reconstitution. Do not shake or freeze following reconstitution. Protect from light.

AIDS—acquired immunodeficiency syndrome; AML—acute myeloid leukemia; ARDS—adult respiratory distress syndrome; BMT—bone marrow transplant; BUN—blood urea nitrogen; CHF—congestive heart failure; CML—chronic myeloid leukemia; D5W—5% dextrose in water; GFR—glomerular filtration rate; GM—granulocyte macrophage; GM-CSF—granulocyte macrophage-colony-stimulating factor; Hgb—hemoglobin; HIV—human immunodeficiency virus; IM—intramuscular; INR—international normalized ratio; IV—intravenous; LAK—lymphokine-activated killer; NK—natural killer; NS—normal saline; PO—oral; SC—subcutaneous; TNF—tumor necrosis factor

Note. Based on information from Camp et al., 2007; Spratto & Woods, 2007; Wilkes & Barton-Burke, 2008; and manufacturers' prescribing information.

Table 8. Characteristics of Targeted Therapies

Classification	Mechanism of Action	Medication Name(s)	Route of Administration	Indications	Side Effects	Nursing Considerations
Immunotoxin	Directs cytotoxic action of diphtheria toxin to cells that express the IL-2 receptor, resulting in inhibition of cellular protein synthesis leading to cell death	Denileukin diftitox (Ontak®)	IV	Treatment of patients with persistent or recurrent cutaneous T-cell lymphoma whose malignant cells express the CD25 component of the IL-2 receptor	Hypersensitivity, vascular leak syndrome, hypotension, edema, hypoalbuminemia, fever, chills, headache, rash, anorexia, reduced lymphocytes, increased transaminases, asthenia, infection, pain, nausea, vomiting, dyspnea, cough	The incidence of adverse effects diminishes after the first two treatment courses. Store at or below –10°C. Agent cannot be refrozen after thawing and must be brought to room temperature before preparing dose. Vials should not be heated. Avoid vigorous agitation. Use prepared solution within 6 hr. Do not infuse through a filter. Protect from light.
Miscellaneous biologic response modifiers (BRMs)	Exact antineoplastic mechanism is unclear but may be related to antiangiogenetic or anti-inflammatory properties.	Lenalidomide (Revlimid®)	PO	Treatment of patients with transfusion-dependent anemia secondary to low- or intermediate-risk MDS associated with the 5q chromosomal deletion; in combination with dexamethasone in patients with multiple myeloma who have received at least one prior therapy	Risk of fetal harm, neutropenia, thrombocytopenia, deep vein thrombosis, pulmonary embolism, pruritus, rash, dry skin, diarrhea, constipation, nausea, nasopharyngitis, cough, dyspnea, pharyngitis, fatigue, pyrexia, peripheral edema, asthenia, arthralgia, dizziness, headache, muscle cramps, upper respiratory tract infections	Females should avoid becoming pregnant during treatment and within 4 weeks of discontinuing treatment because of risk of fetal harm. A pregnancy test should be performed prior to initiating therapy. RevImlid is only available under the RevAssist® program to ensure patients are properly informed of fetal risks. Capsules should be taken with water. Capsules should be swallowed whole and not chewed, crushed, or broken.
	Exact antineoplastic mechanism is unclear but may be related to antiangiogenetic or anti-inflammatory properties.	Thalidomide (Thalomid®)	PO	Used in combination with dexamethasone for treatment in patients with newly diagnosed multiple myeloma; also indicated for treatment of erythema nodosum leprosum	Deep vein thrombosis, pulmonary embolism, drowsiness, somnolence, peripheral neuropathy, dizziness, orthostatic hypotension, neutropenia, confusion, anxiety, tremor, insomnia, depression, fatigue, fever, anemia, thrombocytopenia, constipation, anorexia, nausea, edema, bone pain, dyspnea, rash, dry skin, increased hepatic enzymes, increased SCr, muscle weakness	Females should avoid becoming pregnant beginning 4 weeks before treatment, during treatment, and within 4 weeks of discontinuing treatment because of risk of fetal harm. Perform a pregnancy test prior to initiating therapy. Thalomid must be dispensed and administered in compliance with the STEPS® program. Instruct male patients to never have unprotected sex with a woman who may become pregnant because of the same risk of fetal harm. Because of the potential for significant drowsiness, instruct patients to avoid situations where impaired mental and/or physical functioning could put themselves or others at risk of harm.

(Continued on next page)

Table 8. Characteristics of Targeted Therapies *(Continued)*

Classification	Medication Name(s)	Mechanism of Action	Route of Administration	Indications	Side Effects	Nursing Considerations
Monoclonal antibody (MoAb)	Alemtuzumab (anti-CD52, Campath®)	Binds to CD52 present on the surface of B and T cells, monocytes, macrophages, NK cells, and some granulocytes resulting in antibody-dependent lysis	IV	B-cell CLL	Anemia, thrombocytopenia, neutropenia, hypersensitivity, hypotension, fever, chills, rigors, fatigue, malaise, rash, urticaria, nausea, vomiting, diarrhea, dyspnea, increased risk of opportunistic infections	Premedicate with diphenhydramine and acetaminophen. Anti-infective prophylaxis for *Pneumocystis jeroveci* pneumonia and herpes virus is recommended. Dose modifications are recommended for neutropenia and thrombocytopenia. Do not shake. Drug must be used within 8 hr of dilution with dextrose or saline solutions.
	Bevacizumab (anti-VEGF, Avastin®)	Binds to and inhibits the activity of human VEGF to its receptors (FLT and KDR) blocking proliferation and formation of new blood vessels	IV	In combination with 5-fluorouracil-containing regimens as first- or second-line treatment for patients with metastatic carcinoma of the colon or rectum; may also be used in combination with carboplatin and paclitaxel for first-line treatment of patients with unresectable, locally advanced, recurrent, or metastatic nonsquamous NSCLC	Hemorrhage, hypertension, proteinuria, CHF, asthenia, diarrhea, abdominal pain, headache, neutropenia, hyponatremia, proteinuria, arterial thromboembolic events, GI perforation, wound healing complications, fistula formation in the GI tract, and/or intra-abdominal abscesses	Avoid use for at least 28 days after major surgery; surgical incision should be fully healed. Suspend treatment with bevacizumab several weeks before surgery. Store agent in refrigerator. Do not freeze. Do not shake. Protect from light. Diluted solution may be stored for up to 8 hr under refrigeration. Do not mix or administer with dextrose-containing solutions. Monitor blood pressure during treatment. Permanently discontinue medication if patients develop GI perforation, wound dehiscence requiring medical intervention, serious bleeding, nephrotic syndrome, or hypertensive crisis. Temporarily suspend if evidence of moderate to severe proteinuria and severe hypertension until evaluation and treatment are provided. Risk of CHF exists in patients who previously received anthracyclines.

(Continued on next page)

Table 8. Characteristics of Targeted Therapies *(Continued)*

Classification	Mechanism of Action	Medication Name(s)	Route of Administration	Indications	Side Effects	Nursing Considerations
Monoclonal antibody (MoAb) *(cont.)*	Binds to extracellular domain of the EGFR, resulting in inhibition of cell growth and induction of apoptosis, and decreased matrix metalloproteinase and VEGF production	Cetuximab (Erbitux®)	IV	Used in patients with EGFR-expressing metastatic colorectal cancer after failure of irinotecan- or oxaliplatin-based regimens Used with irinotecan or in patients with metastatic colorectal cancer who are intolerant of irinotecan Used in combination with radiation therapy to treat local or regionally advanced squamous cell carcinoma of the head and neck Used in recurrent or metastatic squamous cell carcinoma of the head and neck progressing after platinum-based therapy	Infusion-related reactions may include bronchospasm, fever, chills, rigors, angioedema, urticaria, hypotension, stridor, pulmonary toxicity, acneiform rash, dry skin and fissuring, malaise, asthenia, fever, diarrhea, fatigue, nausea, vomiting, anorexia, leukopenia, acneiform rash, hypomagnesemia, weight loss, pharyngitis	Serious, potentially fatal infusion reactions may occur. Cardiopulmonary arrest has occurred in patients when used in combination with radiation therapy. Dose modification is recommended following development of acneiform rash. Instruct patients to wear sunscreen and hats and limit sun exposure. Premedicate with an H1 antagonist. Administer through 0.22-micron in-line filter. Flush line with NS after infusion. Store agent in refrigerator. Do not freeze. Do not shake. Protect from light. Do not dilute. Discard unused portion after 8 hr at room temperature or 12 hr under refrigeration.
	Binds to the complement protein C5, which inhibits its cleavage to C5a and C5b; this inhibits formation of the terminal components C5b-9, thus mediating intravascular hemolysis.	Eculizumab (Soliris®)	IV	Treatment of patients with paroxysmal nocturnal hemoglobinuria to reduce hemolysis	Headache, nasopharyngitis, back pain, nausea; increases the risk of meningococcal infections	Do not administer as an IV push or bolus. Dilute to a final concentration of 5 mg/ml prior to administration. Administer by IV infusion over 35 min. Do not use in patients with unresolved serious *Neisseria meningitides* infection or those who are not currently vaccinated against *Neisseria meningitides*. Vaccinate patients at least 2 weeks prior to receiving the first dose of eculizumab. Revaccinate according to medical guidelines for vaccine use.

(Continued on next page)

Table 8. Characteristics of Targeted Therapies *(Continued)*

Classification	Mechanism of Action	Medication Name(s)	Route of Administration	Indications	Side Effects	Nursing Considerations
Monoclonal antibody (MoAb) *(cont.)*	Binds to CD33 expressed on AML cells resulting in internalization of antibody-antigen complex and subsequent release of calicheamicin toxin that binds to DNA resulting in double strand breaks and cell death	Gemtuzumab ozogamicin (anti-CD33, Mylotarg®)	IV	Treatment of CD33-positive AML in patients age 60 years or older in first relapse who are not considered candidates for standard chemotherapy	Severe neutropenia, anemia, thrombocytopenia, hypersensitivity, chills, fever, hypotension, dyspnea, pulmonary infiltrates, pulmonary edema, pleural effusions, severe veno-occlusive disease, peripheral edema, headache, rash, nausea, vomiting, diarrhea, anorexia, weakness, hyperbilirubinemia	Administer only by IV infusion. Store agent in refrigerator. Do not freeze. Protect from light during reconstitution and until completion of infusion. Premedicate with diphenhydramine, acetaminophen, and methylprednisolone. Neutropenia and thrombocytopenia are severe and prolonged. May result in TLS, and appropriate measures should be taken to prevent adverse sequelae.
	Binds to CD20 on B cells resulting in direct delivery of the radioactive isotope indium-111 or yttrium-90 that induces cell damage through the formation of free radicals	Ibritumomab tiuxetan (anti-CD20 antibody, Zevalin®)	IV	Treatment of relapsed or refractory low-grade, follicular, or transformed B-cell NHL	Severe and potentially life-threatening allergic reactions during infusion; fever, chills, rigors, headache, nausea, bronchospasm, dyspnea, myalgia, arthralgia, asthenia, prolonged B-cell lymphocytopenia, leukopenia, thrombocytopenia, neutropenia, anemia, severe cutaneous and mucocutaneous reactions, secondary leukemia, MDS	Drug is combined with rituximab. Administered dose cannot exceed 32 mCi regardless of patient's weight. Drug is not transported with radioisotope; radiolabeling must be done by appropriate personnel in a specialized facility. Drug is intended as single-course treatment. Monitor closely for extravasation. Store in refrigerator. Do not freeze.
	Binds to EGFR and competitively inhibits binding of ligands to this receptor; this prevents receptor autophosphorylation and activation of receptor-associated kinases that results in inhibition of cell growth, induction of apoptosis, decreased production of proinflammatory cytokines and VGFs, and internalization of EGFR	Panitumumab (Vectibix®)	IV	Single-agent treatment for EGFR-expressing metastatic colorectal carcinoma with disease progression on or following fluoropyrimidine-, oxaliplatin-, or irinotecan-containing regimens	Dermatologic toxicity including dermatitis acneform, pruritus, erythema, rash, skin exfoliation, paronychia, dry skin, and skin fissures, which may be complicated by abscesses and sepsis; fatigue, abdominal pain, hypomagnesemia, infusion reactions	Advise patients to wear sunscreen and hats to limit sun exposure. Dose modification is recommended following infusion-related reactions or dermatologic toxicity. Drug must be given by IV infusion pump via in-line filter. Dilute dose with NS. Do not shake diluted product. Store in refrigerator. Do not freeze. Protect from light. Use diluted solution within 6 hr at room temperature or within 24 hr if under refrigeration.

(Continued on next page)

Table 8. Characteristics of Targeted Therapies (Continued)

Classification	Mechanism of Action	Medication Name(s)	Route of Administration	Indications	Side Effects	Nursing Considerations
Monoclonal antibody (MoAb) (cont.)	Binds to CD20 on B cells resulting in activation of complement-dependent cytotoxicity as well as ADCC	Rituximab (anti-CD20 antibody, Rituxan®)	IV	Treatment of relapsed or refractory low-grade follicular CD20-positive B-cell NHL; first-line treatment of follicular CD20-positive B-cell NHL in combination with CVP chemotherapy regimen; treatment of low-grade, CD20-positive B-cell NHL in patients with stable disease or who achieve a partial or complete response with CVP chemotherapy; first-line treatment of diffuse large B-cell, CD20-positive NHL in combination with CHOP or other anthracycline-based chemotherapy regimen; in combination with methotrexate to reduce signs and symptoms of moderate to severe rheumatoid arthritis	Severe infusion-related reactions including urticaria, hypotension, angioedema, hypoxia, or bronchospasm; fever, chills, rigors, headache, dyspnea, myalgia, arthralgia, prolonged B-cell lymphopenia, leukopenia, infection, asthenia, nausea, rash, hepatitis B reactivation	Administer only by IV infusion. Store agent in refrigerator. Do not freeze. Do not shake product. Agent is stable for 24 hr under refrigeration. Consider premedication with acetaminophen and diphenhydramine. Infusion-related side effects may resolve with slowing or suspending infusion. The incidence of infusion-related side effects is reduced with subsequent infusions. Potential exists for development of TLS within 12–24 hr after infusion.
	Binds to CD20 on pre-B and mature lymphocytes resulting in apoptosis and ADCC; ionizing radiation caused by iodine-131 (I-131) results in additional cell death	Tositumomab I-131 (Bexxar®)	IV	Treatment of patients with CD20-positive relapsed or refractory, low-grade, follicular or transformed NHL including patients refractory to rituximab	Anaphylaxis, hypothyroidism, severe and prolonged thrombocytopenia, anemia, neutropenia, allergic reactions, asthenia, fever, infection, chills, rigors, sweating, nausea, vomiting, abdominal pain, rash, secondary leukemia/MDS	Agent is not indicated for initial treatment of CD20-positive NHL. Thyroid-blocking agents should be given 24 hr prior to tositumomab I-131 therapy and continued for 14 days after. The same IV tubing set must be used throughout the entire dosimetric or therapeutics step to prevent loss of drug. Instruct patients how to minimize exposure of other people to radioactivity that will remain in their system for several days. Only personnel trained in handling radioactive agents should prepare and administer this agent. Store in refrigerator. Do not freeze.

(Continued on next page)

Table 8. Characteristics of Targeted Therapies *(Continued)*

Classification	Mechanism of Action	Medication Name(s)	Route of Administration	Indications	Side Effects	Nursing Considerations
Monoclonal antibody (MoAb) *(cont.)*	Binds to the extracellular domain of HER2, resulting in mediation of ADCC against cells that overproduce HER2	Trastuzumab (anti-HER2 antibody, Herceptin®)	IV	In combination with treatment regimens of doxorubicin, cyclophosphamide, and paclitaxel for adjuvant treatment of patients with HER2-overexpressing node-positive breast cancer; as single-agent therapy for treatment of patients with metastatic breast cancer whose tumors overexpress the HER2 protein and have received one or more chemotherapy regimens for their disease; in combination with paclitaxel for treatment of patients with metastatic breast cancer whose tumors overexpress HER2 protein and who have not previously received chemotherapy for their disease	Infusion reactions of chills, fever, headache, dizziness, dyspnea, hypotension, rash and asthenia; pulmonary toxicity related to infusion; left ventricular cardiac dysfunction, hypersensitivity reactions, diarrhea, leukopenia, anemia, neutropenia, infection	Administer only by IV infusion. Store agent in refrigerator. Do not freeze. Solution reconstituted with bacteriostatic water is stable for 28 days under refrigeration. Solution reconstituted with sterile water must be used immediately and not saved. Do not shake product. HER2 protein overexpression is seen in 25%–30% of primary breast cancers. Do not administer concurrently with doxorubicin and cyclophosphamide; intended to be administered following completion of doxorubicin and cyclophosphamide. LVEF must be determined prior to initiation and during treatment.
Small molecule inhibitor	Inhibits chymotrypsin-like activity of 26S proteosome resulting in disruption of cellular hemostatic mechanisms that can lead to cell death	Bortezomib (Velcade®)	IV	Treatment of patients with multiple myeloma or mantle cell lymphoma who have received at least one prior therapy	Peripheral neuropathy, hypotension, nausea, vomiting, diarrhea, blurred vision, fatigue, myelosuppression	Do not use in pediatrics. Use with caution in patients with severe renal or hepatic disease. Monitor hydration status and treat as necessary.

(Continued on next page)

Table 8. Characteristics of Targeted Therapies *(Continued)*

Classification	Mechanism of Action	Medication Name(s)	Route of Administration	Indications	Side Effects	Nursing Considerations
Small molecule inhibitor *(cont.)*	Inhibits multiple tyrosine kinases, including BCR-ABL, SRC family, c-KIT, EPHA2, and PDGFRβ. Predicted to bind to multiple conformations of the *ABL* kinase	Dasatinib (Sprycel®)	PO	Treatment of adults with chronic, accelerated, or myeloid or lymphoid blast-phase CML with resistance or intolerance to prior therapy including imatinib; treatment of Ph+ ALL	Myelosuppression, fluid retention, including pleural and pericardial effusion; prolonged QT interval by ECG; diarrhea, nausea, abdominal pain, vomiting	Do not crush or cut tablets. Use with caution if patients are taking anticoagulants. Drug interactions can occur with CYP3A4 inducers (e.g., dexamethasone, phenytoin, carbamazepine) and substrates (e.g., cyclosporine, fentanyl, St. John's wort, antacids, H2 blockers, proton pump inhibitors). Elevation of transaminases or bilirubin, hypocalcemia, and hypophosphatemia may occur. Hypocalcemia may require oral calcium supplements.
	Inhibits the intracellular phosphorylation of tyrosine kinase associated with EGFR, expressed on the surfaces of normal and cancer cells	Erlotinib (Tarceva®)	PO	Treatment of locally advanced or metastatic NSCLC after failure of at least one prior chemotherapy regimen; also approved for use in combination with gemcitabine for the treatment of locally advanced, unresectable, or metastatic pancreatic carcinoma	Rash and diarrhea (may be severe [grades 3–4]); anorexia, fatigue, dyspnea; abnormal LFTs may be transient or associated with liver metastases; GI bleeding, conjunctivitis, and keratitis have occurred. There have been rare reports of serious ILD (acute onset of new or progressive pulmonary symptoms [e.g., dyspnea, cough, fever]); therapy should be interrupted for evaluation if these symptoms develop.	Cotreatment with ketoconazole or other potent CYP3A4 inhibitors may increase erlotinib levels, requiring a lower dose. Pretreatment with rifampicin and other CYP3A4 inducers (includes phenytoin, phenobarbital, and St. John's wort) may decrease erlotinib activity, requiring an increased dose. Monitor LFTs and consider dose reductions. Monitor INR in patients receiving warfarin. Monitor for GI bleeding and elevated INR. Diarrhea can be managed with loperamide. Both diarrhea and skin reactions may require dose reduction or temporary interruption of therapy.
	Although the exact antitumor action is unclear, gefitinib inhibits several tyrosine kinases present on cell surface receptors.	Gefitinib (Iressa®)	PO	For use as monotherapy in the treatment of locally advanced or metastatic NSCLC in patients who have failed to respond to either a platinum-based regimen or docetaxel	Diarrhea, rash, acne, dry skin, nausea, vomiting, pruritus, anorexia, asthenia, weight loss, increase in hepatic transaminases, ILD	Drug administration may be held for up to 14 days to help to manage poorly tolerated diarrhea. Evaluate for new onset or worsening of pulmonary symptoms.

(Continued on next page)

Table 8. Characteristics of Targeted Therapies (Continued)

Classification	Mechanism of Action	Medication Name(s)	Route of Administration	Indications	Side Effects	Nursing Considerations
Small molecule inhibitor (cont.)	Inhibits BCR-ABL tyrosine kinase created by the Ph+ genetic abnormality, inhibiting proliferation, and induces apoptosis in BCR-ABL–positive cell lines	Imatinib mesylate (Gleevec®)	PO	Treatment of patients with newly diagnosed Ph+ CML in chronic phase; treatment of patients with Ph+ CML in blast crisis, accelerated phase, or chronic phase after failure of IFN alfa therapy; treatment of patients with relapsed or refractory Ph+ ALL; treatment of patients with myelodysplastic/myeloproliferative disorders associated with PDGFR gene rearrangements; treatment of patients with systemic mastocytosis without certain c-Kit mutations; treatment of patients with hypereosinophilic syndrome and/or chronic eosinophilic leukemia in the presence of certain mutations; treatment of patients with unresectable, recurrent, and/or metastatic dermatofibrosarcoma protuberans; treatment of patients with unresectable and/or metastatic GIST; adjuvant treatment of resected GIST	Edema and fluid retention, GI irritation, nausea, vomiting, neutropenia, thrombocytopenia, hepatotoxicity	Weigh patients frequently, and monitor them for signs and symptoms of fluid retention. Ensure that patients take imatinib with food and a large glass of water. Monitor CBC, differential, and LFTs. Drugs that may increase plasma concentration include ketoconazole, itraconazole, erythromycin, and clarithromycin. Drugs that may decrease plasma concentration include dexamethasone, phenytoin, carbamazepine, rifampicin, phenobarbital, and St. John's wort. Interaction is possible in patients receiving warfarin. Advise women of childbearing age not to become pregnant while taking imatinib. Researchers have not conducted studies of the drug in pregnant women.

(Continued on next page)

Table 8. Characteristics of Targeted Therapies *(Continued)*

Classification	Mechanism of Action	Medication Name(s)	Route of Administration	Indications	Side Effects	Nursing Considerations
Small molecule inhibitor *(cont.)*	4-anilinoquinazoline kinase inhibitor of the intracellular tyrosine kinase domains of both EGFR and of HER2 receptors	Lapatinib (Tykerb®)	PO	Used in combination with capecitabine for the treatment of patients with advanced or metastatic breast cancer whose tumors overexpress HER2 and who have received prior therapy including an anthracycline, a taxane, and trastuzumab	Diarrhea, palmar-plantar erythrodysesthesia, nausea, rash, vomiting, fatigue; decreased LVEF	Instruct patients to take lapatinib at least 1 hr before or 1 hr after a meal. However, capecitabine should be taken with food or within 30 min of food. Dose should be taken once daily; do not divide the daily dose. Modify the dose for cardiac and other toxicities, severe hepatic impairment, and CYP3A4 drug interactions. Confirm normal ejection fraction before beginning drug. Severe diarrhea may be managed with antidiarrheal agents, and replace fluids and electrolytes if severe. Lapatinib may cause fetal harm when administered to pregnant women.
	Binds to and stabilizes the inactive conformation of BCR-ABL, the kinase produced by the Ph+	Nilotinib (Tasigna®)	PO	Treatment of chronic-phase and accelerated-phase Ph+ CML in adult patients resistant or intolerant to prior therapy including imatinib	Rash, pruritus, nausea, fatigue, headache, constipation, diarrhea, vomiting Serious reactions include thrombocytopenia, neutropenia, elevated lipase, hepatic and electrolyte abnormalities, prolonged QT interval. Sudden deaths have been reported.	Instruct patients to swallow capsules whole with water. No food should be consumed for at least 2 hr before the dose and 1 hr after. Do not use in patients with hypokalemia, hypomagnesemia, or long QT syndrome. CBC should be checked every 2 weeks for the first 2 months then monthly. Correct electrolyte abnormalities prior to treatment. ECG should be obtained at baseline, 7 days after initiation, and periodically to monitor QTc. Avoid concomitant use of strong inhibitors or inducers of CYP3A4. Dose reduction may be necessary if inhibitors must be given, and the QTc should be monitored closely. Do not use in patients who are pregnant or breastfeeding. Sexually active female patients should use effective contraception during treatment.

(Continued on next page)

Table 8. Characteristics of Targeted Therapies *(Continued)*

Classification	Mechanism of Action	Medication Name(s)	Route of Administration	Indications	Side Effects	Nursing Considerations
Small molecule inhibitor *(cont.)*	Multikinase inhibitor that is believed to decrease tumor cell signaling, angiogenesis, and apoptosis	Sorafenib (Nexavar®)	PO	Treatment of unresectable hepatocellular carcinoma and treatment of advanced renal cancer	Palmar-plantar erythrodysesthesia, rash, hypertension, myocardial infarction, mucositis, dyspepsia, increased lipase, increased amylase, diarrhea, nausea, vomiting, decreased appetite, increased risk of bleeding, peripheral neuropathy	Treatment continues until patients no longer benefit from therapy or until unacceptable toxicity occurs. Patients should be cautioned to prevent becoming pregnant during treatment and for 2 weeks after treatment has stopped. Sorafenib has been shown to cause birth defects or fetal loss.
	Decreases tumor cell proliferation and reduces tumor angiogenesis	Sunitinib (Sutent®)	PO	Treatment of GIST after disease progression while on imatinib or intolerance to imatinib; treatment of advanced renal cell carcinoma	Myelosuppression, left ventricular dysfunction, hypothyroidism, diarrhea, nausea, vomiting, stomatitis, dyspepsia, skin discoloration, depigmentation of hair, palmar-plantar erythrodysesthesia, fatigue, hypertension, bleeding, edema	Medication may be taken with or without food. Baseline ejection fraction should be obtained prior to initiation of sunitinib. Coadministration with ketoconazole, itraconazole, clarithromycin, atazanavir, indinavir, nefazodone, nelfinavir, ritonavir, saquinavir, telithromycin, or voriconazole may increase sunitinib concentrations. Grapefruit also may increase concentrations. Coadministration with dexamethasone, phenytoin, carbamazepine, rifampin, rifabutin, rifapentin, phenobarbital, or St. John's wort may decrease sunitinib concentrations.

(Continued on next page)

Table 8. Characteristics of Targeted Therapies *(Continued)*

Classification	Mechanism of Action	Medication Name(s)	Route of Administration	Indications	Side Effects	Nursing Considerations
Small molecule inhibitor *(cont.)*	Binds to the intracellular protein FKBP-12 resulting in inhibition of mTOR, causing an interruption of cell division	Temsirolimus (Torisel®)	IV	Treatment of advanced renal cell carcinoma	Rash, asthenia, mucositis, nausea, edema, hypersensitivity reactions, anorexia, myelosuppression, hyperglycemia, hyperlipemia, hypertriglyceridemia, elevated alkaline phosphatase, elevated SCr, lymphopenia, hypophosphatemia, elevated AST, ILD	Pretreat with prophylactic IV diphenhydramine 25–50 mg (or similar antihistamine) approximately 30 min before the start of each dose. Hyperglycemia and hyperlipemia are likely and may require treatment. Monitor lipid profiles. Monitor for symptoms of radiographic changes of ILD. Because of abnormal wound healing, use caution in the perioperative period. Patients should avoid receiving live vaccines and having close contact with those who have received live vaccines. Bowel perforations may occur; evaluate for fever, abdominal pain, bloody stools, and acute abdomen promptly. Women of childbearing potential should be advised of the potential hazard to the fetus and to avoid becoming pregnant. Monitor renal function at baseline and throughout treatment.

ADCC—antibody-dependent cellular cytotoxicity; ALL—acute lymphoblastic leukemia; AML—acute myeloid leukemia; AST—aspartate aminotransferase; CBC—complete blood count; CHF—congestive heart failure; CHOP—cyclophosphamide, doxorubicin, vincristine, prednisone; CLL—chronic lymphocytic leukemia; CML—chronic myeloid leukemia; CVP—cyclophosphamide, vincristine, prednisone; DNA—deoxyribonucleic acid; ECG—electrocardiogram; EGFR—epidermal growth factor receptor; GI—gastrointestinal; GIST—gastrointestinal stromal tumor; hr—hour; HER2—human epidermal growth factor receptor 2; IFN—interferon; IL—interleukin; ILD—interstitial lung disease; INR—international normalized ratio; IV—intravenous; LFT—liver function test; LVEF—left ventricular ejection fraction; mCi—millicurie; MDS—myelodysplastic syndrome; mg—milligram; min—minute; mTOR—mammalian target of rapamycin; NHL—non-Hodgkin lymphoma; NK—natural killer; NS—normal saline; NSCLC—non-small cell lung cancer; PDGFR—platelet-derived growth factor receptor; Ph+—Philadelphia chromosome-positive; PO—oral; QTc—QT interval corrected; SCr—serum creatinine; TLS—tumor lysis syndrome; VEGF—vascular endothelial growth factor; VGF—*Vaccinia* virus growth factor

Note. Based on information from manufacturers' prescribing information.

IV. Fundamentals of Administration

A. Safe handling: Many drugs used in the treatment of cancer are considered hazardous to healthcare workers. The term *hazardous* describes drugs that require special handling because of health risks that may result from exposure. These risks are a result of the inherent toxicities of the drugs (ASHP, 2006; NIOSH, 2004). According to the Occupational Safety and Health Administration (OSHA, 1995), safe levels of occupational exposure to hazardous agents cannot be determined, and no reliable method of monitoring work-related exposure exists. Therefore, it is imperative that those who work with hazardous drugs (HDs) adhere to practices designed to minimize occupational exposure.

1. Definition of HDs: The American Society of Hospital Pharmacists (1990) (now ASHP) provided the first definition of HDs [*a)–e)*]; NIOSH (2004) refined the definition [*f)*]. Drugs are considered hazardous if they exhibit one or more of the following characteristics:

   a) Carcinogenicity

   b) Teratogenicity or developmental toxicity

   c) Reproductive toxicity

   d) Organ toxicity at low doses

   e) Genotoxicity

   f) Drugs similar in structure or toxicity to drugs classified as hazardous using these criteria

2. Potential health risks associated with occupational exposure to HDs

   a) An increased risk of cancer among occupationally exposed nurses and pharmacy workers (Hansen & Olsen, 1994; Martin, 2005; Skov et al., 1992): The International Agency for Research on Cancer (IARC) publishes independent assessments of the carcinogenic risks of chemicals and has identified 10 drugs used in the treatment of cancer and two combination regimens as known human carcinogens. Other antineoplastic agents are classified as probable or possible carcinogens (see Table 9) (IARC, 2007).

   b) Structural defects in a fetus as a result of occupational exposure during pregnancy (Hemminki, Kyyronen, & Lindbohm, 1985; Peelen, Roeleveld, Heederik, Kromhout, & de Kort, 1999)

   c) Adverse reproductive outcomes, including fetal loss, miscarriage, or spontaneous abortions (Selevan, Lindbohm, Hornung, & Hemminki, 1985; Stucker et al., 1990;

Table 9. Carcinogens	
Exposure Risk	**Antineoplastic Drugs**
Group 1: Carcinogenic to humans	• Arsenic trioxide • Azathioprine • Busulfan • Chlorambucil • Cyclophosphamide • ECB • Melphalan • MOPP • Semustine • Tamoxifen • Thiotepa • Treosulfan
Group 2A: Probably carcinogenic to humans	• Azacitadine • Carmustine • Cisplatin • Doxorubicin • Etoposide • Lomustine • Nitrogen mustard • Procarbazine • Teniposide
Group 2B: Possibly carcinogenic to humans	• Amsacrine • Bleomycin • Dacarbazine • Daunorubicin • Mitomycin • Mitoxantrone • Streptozocin

ECB—etoposide, cisplatin, and bleomycin; MOPP—mustargen, vincristine, procarbazine, and prednisone

Note. Based on information from International Agency for Research on Cancer, 2007.

Valanis, Vollmer, & Steele, 1999); infertility (Fransman et al., 2007; Martin, 2005; Valanis, Vollmer, Labuhn, & Glass, 1997); preterm births and learning disabilities in offspring of nurses exposed during pregnancy (Martin, 2005)

   d) Chromosomal damage in healthcare workers following exposure to cytotoxic agents (Fuchs et al., 1995; Harrison, 2001; Sessink et al., 1994; Ursini et al., 2006)

   e) Acute symptoms such as hair loss, abdominal pain, nasal sores, contact dermatitis, allergic reactions, skin injury, and eye injury (Harrison, 2001; Valanis, Vollmer, Labuhn, & Glass, 1993a, 1993b)

3. Potential health risks associated with occupational exposure to biotherapy agents

   a) Limited data are available regarding the effects of occupational exposure to biologic agents.

   b) Most biologic agents do not affect DNA and do not cause genetic changes.

c) Antiangiogenic agents may pose a risk to a fetus during pregnancy (e.g., thalidomide [Celgene Corporation, 2005]).

d) Several targeted agents meet one or more of the criteria in the NIOSH definition of HDs and should be handled as hazardous (e.g., handled with personal protective equipment [PPE] and not crushed). These include imatinib mesylate, sorafenib, dasatinib, sunitinib malate, erlotinib, and vorinostat.

e) IFN is hazardous because of its reproductive toxicity (OSHA, 1995).

f) Conjugated MoAbs are hazardous because of the radioactive isotopes or toxins.

g) A list of drugs that should be handled as hazardous can be found in the NIOSH Alert (2004) Appendix A.

4. Potential routes of exposure to HDs

a) Absorption through skin or mucous membranes after direct drug contact or indirect drug contact from surfaces or objects that are contaminated with HDs

(1) Several studies reported measurable levels of cytotoxic agents in the urine of healthcare workers (Labuhn, Valanis, Schoeny, Loveday, & Vollmer, 1998; Pethran et al., 2003; Wick, Slawson, Jorgenson, & Tyler, 2003), most likely from dermal absorption.

(2) Multiple studies have documented contamination of the environment with HDs in drug preparation areas, drug administration areas, and patient care areas (Connor, Anderson, Sessink, Broadfield, & Power, 1999; Fransman, Vermeulen, & Kromhout, 2005; McDevitt, Lees, & McDiarmid, 1993; Schmaus, Schierl, & Funck, 2002; Sessink, Anzion, van den Broek, & Bos, 1992; Sessink, Boer, Scheefhals, Anzion, & Bos, 1992; Wick et al., 2003).

(3) Several researchers have detected drug contamination on the outside of drug vials when delivered by the manufacturers (Connor et al., 2005; Nygren, Gustavsson, Strom, & Friberg, 2002; Sessink, Boer et al., 1992). Cyclophosphamide, 5-FU, ifosfamide, and platinum have all been detected on vial exteriors using various wipe sampling and washing techniques. These findings indicate that nurses are at risk for skin exposure if they do not wear PPE while handling unopened drug vials.

b) Injection by injury from needlesticks or contaminated sharps (Schreiber et al., 2003)

c) Inhalation of drug aerosols, dust, or droplets (Dorr & Alberts, 1992; Harrison & Schultz, 2000; Kiffmeyer et al., 2002; Kromhout et al., 2000; Mason et al., 2005)

d) Ingestion through contaminated food, beverage, tobacco products, or other hand-to-mouth behavior (NIOSH, 2004)

5. The U.S. Department of Labor (1998) has established a five-tier hierarchy of hazard controls.

a) The best way to protect workers from a hazardous exposure is to **eliminate the hazard**, but this is not feasible with drug therapy.

b) **Substitution** of the hazardous material for a less-toxic substance is the second best method of hazard control.

c) Next on the hierarchy of controls is the use of **engineering controls**—machines or equipment—to isolate or contain the hazard to reduce exposure.

d) The fourth level of protection is **administrative controls**, which includes education and training of those responsible for HD handling.

e) The final level of protection is **PPE**, which places responsibility for protection on the nurse.

6. Guidelines regarding PPE

a) Types of apparel

(1) Gloves: Wear disposable gloves that are powder-free and have been tested for use with HDs. Latex gloves provide protection but should be used with caution because of the risk of latex sensitivity. Gloves made of nitrile (Singleton & Connor, 1999), polyurethane, or neoprene may provide protection (Connor, 1999). The American Society for Testing and Materials (2005) developed a

standard for testing gloves to determine their resistance to permeation by chemotherapy. The FDA requires permeation testing before gloves are labeled as chemotherapy-designated gloves. Double gloves are recommended for all handling activities (drug preparation, administration, and handling of contaminated waste) (ASHP, 2006; NIOSH, 2004). Inspect gloves for physical defects before use. Remove and discard gloves immediately after use; if a tear, puncture, or drug spill occurs; or after 30 minutes of wear (ASHP; NIOSH, 2004). Do not reuse gloves.

(2) Gowns: Wear a disposable, lint-free gown made of a low-permeability fabric, such as polyethylene-coated materials (Connor, 1993; Harrison & Kloos, 1999). The gown should have a solid front, long sleeves, tight cuffs, and back closure. The inner glove cuff should be worn under the gown cuff; the outer glove cuff should extend over the gown cuff to fully protect the skin. Discard the gown if it is visibly contaminated, before leaving drug handling areas, and after handling HDs. Gowns are meant for single use and should not be reapplied after removal (NIOSH, 2004) to prevent potential transfer of drug contamination to clothing.

(3) Respirators: Wear a NIOSH-approved respirator mask (such as a nonpowered, air-purifying, particulate-filter respirator) when there is a risk of aerosol exposure such as when administering an aerosolized HD or cleaning an HD spill. Consult the material safety data sheet (MSDS) for the respirator appropriate to the situation (NIOSH, 1996). Surgical masks do not provide respiratory protection.

(4) Eye and face protection: Wear a face shield or a combination of mask and face shield that provides splash protection whenever there is a possibility of splashing.

b) Situations requiring PPE: Wear PPE to reduce exposure whenever there is a risk of HDs being released into the environment, such as in the following situations (NIOSH, 2004).

(1) Introducing or withdrawing needles from vials

(2) Transferring drugs from vials to other containers using needles or syringes

(3) Opening ampules

(4) Expelling air from a drug-filled syringe

(5) Administering HDs by any route

(6) Spiking IV bags containing HDs and changing IV tubing

(7) Priming IV tubing

(8) Handling leakage from tubing, syringe, and connection sites

(9) Disposing of HDs and items contaminated by HDs

(10) Handling the body fluids of a patient who received hazardous agents in the past 48 hours

(11) Cleaning HD spills

7. Storage and labeling of chemotherapeutic agents

a) On the clinical unit

(1) Store chemotherapy drug containers in a location that limits exposure of healthcare workers and provides appropriate storage conditions (e.g., temperature and light).

(2) Use a distinct label on all drug containers to indicate the hazardous nature of the contents (OSHA, 1995).

(3) Have access to instructions (e.g., MSDS) regarding what to do in the event of accidental exposure.

(4) Check HD containers before taking them from the storage area to ensure that the packaging is intact and to detect any leakage or breakage.

b) In the home (Polovich, 2003) (see Appendix 3)

(1) Keep all HDs out of the reach of children and pets.

(2) Store HDs in containers that provide adequate protection from puncture or breakage.

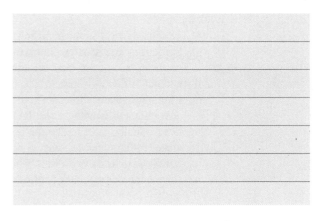

(3) Label containers to indicate the hazardous nature of their contents.

(4) Provide instructions listing the proper procedure for handling a damaged container.

(5) Store HDs in an area free of moisture and temperature extremes.

(6) Provide spill kits and instructions for their use.

(7) Give verbal and written instructions about handling and storing HDs and HD waste.

8. Safe handling while compounding HDs: Maintain sterile technique during the preparation of parenteral drugs. The U.S. Pharmacopeial Convention [USP] (2008) recently issued new standards for sterile products, including HDs. The environment in which HD preparation takes place must meet all standards for ventilation, including air exchanges per hour, particle counts, and negative pressure. For a full explanation of the standards, refer to the USP document.

   a) Chemotherapeutic drugs

   (1) Prepare cytotoxic drugs, including oral drugs that must be compounded or crushed, in a primary engineering control (PEC), such as a biologic safety cabinet (BSC) or a compounding aseptic containment isolator (ASHP, 2006; NIOSH, 2004; USP, 2008). The PEC should

   (a) Provide vertical laminar airflow. Vertical airflow carries contaminated air away from the operator and out of the environment.

   (b) Eliminate exhaust through a high-efficiency particulate air (HEPA) filter. Ideally, a PEC should be vented to the outside (ASHP, 2006; NIOSH, 2004; USP, 2008).

   (c) Have a fan that operates continuously (ASHP, 2006).

   (d) Be located in a buffer area with negative pressure.

   (e) Be used by individuals trained to employ techniques that reduce interference with airflow.

   (f) Be serviced according to the manufacturer's recommendations.

   (g) Be recertified after relocation, repair, filter replacement, and/or every six months (National Sanitation Foundation, 2007; OSHA, 1999).

(2) Wash hands before donning PPE.

(3) Wear chemotherapy-designated PPE.

(4) If desired, place a sterile, plastic-backed absorbent pad on the work surface. Such pads may interfere with airflow in a BSC (Minoia et al., 1998).

(5) Limit items placed in the PEC to avoid interfering with airflow (ASHP, 2006).

(6) Use safe technique when opening ampules (ASHP, 2006).

   (a) Clear fluid from the ampule neck.

   (b) Tilt the ampule away from yourself.

   (c) Wrap gauze or an alcohol pad around the neck of the ampule.

   (d) Break the ampule in the direction away from yourself.

   (e) Use a filtered needle to withdraw fluid.

(7) When reconstituting drugs provided in vials, avoid pressure buildup, which can result in the release of drug aerosols. Use a closed-system device (e.g., PhaSeal®) if available (NIOSH, 2004). According to NIOSH (2004, p. 44), "A closed-system device is a drug transfer device that mechanically prohibits the transfer of environmental contaminants into the system and the escape of hazardous drug or vapor concentrations outside the system."

(8) Use tubing and syringes with Luer lock fittings.

(9) Avoid overfilling syringes. A syringe that is too full may separate from the plunger end (OSHA, 1995).

(10) Spike IV bags and prime tubing with compatible fluid before adding cytotoxic drugs (ASHP, 2006; OSHA, 1995) or use a closed-system device to minimize the risk of exposure (Con-

nor, Anderson, Sessink, & Spivey, 2002; Wick et al., 2003).

(11) Place a label on each container that says "Cytotoxic Drug" or a similar, distinct warning.

(12) Wipe the outside of the container (e.g., syringe or IV bag) with moist gauze before placing it in a sealable bag for transport. Avoid contaminating the outside of the transport bag.

(13) Dispose of all material that has come into contact with a cytotoxic drug in a waste container designated for cytotoxic waste.

(14) Remove and discard outer gloves and gown. Then remove inner gloves.

(15) Wash hands with soap and water before leaving the work area.

b) Biotherapy drugs

(1) Use safe handling precautions for biotherapy agents that are considered hazardous (e.g., IFN) (NIOSH, 2004).

(2) Wear gloves when mixing biotherapy agents that are irritating to skin (e.g., rituximab [Genentech, Inc., 2000]).

(3) A nuclear pharmacist prepares radiolabeled MoAbs for infusion. Note: Federal and state laws require that radiation safety warning signs designate the areas in which radioisotopes are stored or used (Bruner, Haas, & Gosselin-Acomb, 2004).

9. Transporting chemotherapeutic drugs (OSHA, 1995)

a) Transport syringes containing HDs in a sealed container with the Luer lock end of the syringe capped. Do not transport syringes with attached needles.

b) Select a transport receptacle that can contain spillage if dropped (e.g., a leakproof, zipper-lock bag) and additional impervious packing material as necessary to avoid damage during transport.

c) Label the outermost receptacle with a distinct label to indicate that its contents are hazardous.

d) Ensure that whoever will be transporting the drugs has access to a spill kit and knows how to use it.

10. Safe handling considerations during administration of HDs (ASHP, 2006; OSHA, 1995)

a) Always wear PPE.

b) Work below eye level.

c) Ensure that a spill kit and hazardous waste container are available.

d) Use a closed-system device (NIOSH, 2004), or place a disposable, absorbent, plastic-backed pad underneath the work area to absorb droplets of the drug that may spill.

e) Use a closed-system device, or place a gauze pad under the syringe at injection ports to catch droplets during administration.

f) Use needles, syringes, and tubing with Luer lock connectors.

g) If priming occurs at the administration site, prime IV tubing with a fluid that does not contain the drug or by using the backflow method.

h) After drug administration, remove the IV container with the tubing attached (NIOSH, 2004; Polovich, 2003). Do not remove the spike from IV containers or reuse tubing.

i) Use detergent and water to wash surfaces that come into contact with HDs (Polovich, 2003).

j) Discard all contaminated material and PPE in a hazardous waste container.

11. Special precautions for radiation therapy: Special precautions are necessary to protect healthcare workers from exposure while caring for patients receiving some types of radiation therapy. Radiation protection standards and regulations are determined by the U.S. Nuclear Regulatory Commission (NRC), the FDA (radiopharmaceuticals), and state radiation regulatory agencies.

a) Occupational radiation exposure should be kept as low as reasonably achievable. This requires close collaboration between the healthcare team and the radiation safety officer (RSO). Three factors help to provide protection (McQuestion, 2007).

(1) Time: Limit the amount of time spent near the radioactive source. Radiation exposure is directly proportional to the amount of time spent near the source. (After a patient receives RIT,

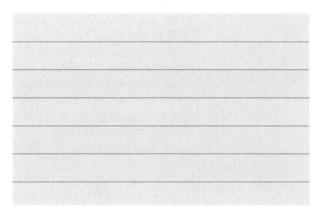

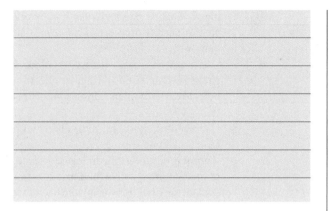

the patient is considered the radioactive source.)

(2) Distance: Maximize the amount of space between a point (what is to be protected) and the radioactive source. Radiation exposure decreases as the distance from the radioactive source increases.

(3) Shielding: Add a protective barrier placed between the radioactive source and the point. The type of shielding used depends on the type of radiation.

b) Radiation monitoring devices are used to measure occupational exposure.

(1) Monitoring of personnel: Personnel monitoring is required by law regardless of whether the patient is treated as an inpatient or outpatient. The film badge is the most widely used monitoring device. Each person caring for a patient receiving radiation therapy should be assigned a film badge that is only worn within the work environment, is changed according to institutional guidelines, and is not shared with anyone else (Bruner et al., 2004). A dosimeter is another kind of monitoring device. It can be a personal device or one that is shared after being reset.

(2) Monitoring of the environment: Environmental monitoring is done with a Geiger-Müller counter, which reacts to the presence of ionizing particles. After a course of inpatient RIT is completed and before the room is cleaned, the RSO surveys the room, linens, and garbage with the Geiger-Müller counter.

12. Handling a patient's body fluids

a) After chemotherapy

(1) Institute standard precautions (double gloves and disposable gown) when handling the blood, emesis, or excreta of a patient who has received chemotherapy within the previous 48 hours. Wear a face shield if splashing is possible (NIOSH, 2004).

(2) For an incontinent child or adult, clean the patient's skin well with each diaper change. Apply a protective barrier ointment to the skin of the patient's diaper area to decrease the chance of skin irritation from contact with urinary metabolites (Polovich, 2003).

(3) Flush the toilet with the lid down after disposing of excreta from a patient who has received cytotoxic agents within the past 48 hours. When a lid is not present, consider covering the open toilet with a plastic-backed pad to prevent splashing. Although there is no research to support the role of double-flushing in reducing exposure, it has been suggested in the past (Brown et al., 2001; Welch & Silveira, 1997) and may be helpful with low-volume-per-flush toilets (Polovich, 2003).

b) After RIT (Bruner et al., 2004)

(1) Institute standard precautions as previously noted when handling the patient's body fluids (e.g., sweat, saliva, urine, feces, blood, semen, vaginal fluid). The duration of precautions varies depending on the radionuclide's half-life.

(2) Consult the RSO or nuclear pharmacist.

13. Handling a patient's linens

a) After chemotherapy (Polovich, 2003)

(1) To the extent possible, preclude the need for laundering linens and clothing by using disposable linens or leakproof pads to contain HD-contaminated body fluids.

(2) If body fluids are present, use standard precautions when handling the linens of a patient who has received chemotherapy within 48 hours.

(3) Handle contaminated bed linens and clothing as follows.

(a) In the hospital setting

i) Handle linens with PPE and place into a leakproof bag.

ii) In most institutions, all linens are handled as contaminated by laundry personnel before washing.

(b) In the home setting (Polovich, 2003) (see Appendix 3)

i) Wearing gloves, place contaminated linens into a washable pillowcase, separate from other items.

ii) Machine wash linens and cloth diapers twice in hot water, with regular detergent, separately from other household items.

iii) Discard disposable diapers in plastic bags to prevent leakage.

iv) Discard used gloves and gowns in an appropriately labeled hazardous waste container.

b) After RIT (Bruner et al., 2004)

(1) If body fluids are present, use standard precautions when handling the linens of a patient who has received RIT.

(2) Keep linens in the hospital room until scanned and cleared by the RSO or nuclear pharmacist.

14. Disposal of HDs and materials contaminated with HDs

a) In the hospital setting (NIOSH, 2004)

(1) Place soft contaminated materials into a sealable, leakproof bag or a rigid cytotoxic waste container marked with a brightly colored label that cites the hazardous nature of the contents.

(2) Use puncture-proof containers for sharp or breakable items. Dispose of needles and syringes intact; do not break or recap needles or crush syringes.

(3) Seal containers when full.

(4) Do not dispose of drug-contaminated items in infectious waste (red) containers. Some facilities autoclave or microwave these materials (NIOSH, 2004; Smith, 2002), which does not deactivate HDs.

(5) Follow institutional policy regarding disposal of partial doses of chemotherapy when administration is interrupted.

(6) Only housekeeping personnel who have received instruction in safe-handling procedures should handle waste containers. These personnel should wear gowns with cuffs and a back closure and two pairs of disposable chemical-protective gloves.

b) In the home setting (Polovich, 2003) (see Appendix 3)

(1) Follow all the instructions applicable to the hospital setting except those

related to handling the filled waste container.

(2) Designate an area away from children and pets where filled containers await pickup.

(3) Follow county and state regulations regarding the disposal of hazardous wastes.

(4) Some agencies that provide HDs will arrange for proper disposal of contaminated equipment.

15. Procedures following acute accidental cytotoxic exposure: Improper technique, faulty equipment, or negligence in BSC operation can lead to exposure (OSHA, 1995).

a) Initial interventions

(1) In the event of skin exposure: Remove any contaminated garments and immediately wash contaminated skin with soap and water. Refer to the MSDS for agent-specific interventions.

(2) In case of eye exposure: Immediately flush the eye with saline solution or water for at least 15 minutes (OSHA, 1995), then seek emergency treatment. Ideally, each area designated for the handling of cytotoxic agents should contain an eyewash station. An acceptable alternative is a sterile saline IV container connected to IV tubing.

(3) In the event of inhalation exposure, move away from the area of exposure as quickly as possible. Depending on the severity of symptoms, seek emergency treatment from the employee health professional or emergency department. Refer to the MSDS for agent-specific interventions.

(4) For accidental ingestion, do not induce vomiting unless indicated in the

MSDS. Depending on the severity of symptoms, seek emergency treatment from the employee health professional or emergency department. Refer to the MSDS for agent-specific interventions.

b) Reporting (Polovich, 2003)
(1) In case of employee exposure: Report the exposure to the employee health department or as institutional policy requires.
(2) In case of patient exposure: Report the exposure as institutional policy requires. In addition, inform the patient's healthcare providers.

16. Spill management
a) Radioactive spills: In case of a spill of radiolabeled antibody or contamination with the radioactive body fluid of a patient recently treated with RIT (Bruner et al., 2004)
(1) Restrict access to the area and contact the RSO immediately. Never try to clean the area or touch the radioactive source. Adhere to the principles of time, distance, and shielding (see section IV.A.11, Special Precautions for Radiation Therapy).
(2) Follow other applicable NRC guidelines.

b) Cytotoxic spills: Spill kits should be available wherever HDs are stored, transported, prepared, or administered (see Figure 11). Everyone who works with HDs should be trained in spill cleanup. Individuals trained in handling hazardous materials (such as a Hazardous Materials Response Team) should clean up large spills whenever possible (OSHA, 2004b). In case of a spill involving a cytotoxic agent, follow these procedures.

(1) Immediately post a sign or signs that warn others of the presence of a hazardous spill. This will prevent others from being exposed.
(2) Don two pairs of gloves, a disposable gown, and a face shield.
(3) Wear a NIOSH-approved respirator (OSHA, 2004c).
(4) Use appropriate items in the spill-control kit to contain the spill.
(5) Clean up the spill according to its location and type. Do not use chemical inactivators, with the exception of sodium thiosulfate. (Sodium thiosulfate is used to inactivate mechlorethamine [nitrogen mustard]). Inactivators other than sodium thiosulfate may react with the spilled chemical to form potentially dangerous byproducts (Harrison, 2001).
(a) To clean up a spill on a hard surface (ASHP, 2006)
i) Wipe up liquids by using absorbent pads or spill-control pillows. Wipe up solids by using wet absorbent pads.
ii) Pick up glass fragments by using a small scoop or utility gloves worn over chemotherapy gloves. Place the glass in a puncture-proof container.
iii) Place puncture-proof container and contaminated materials into a leakproof waste bag. Seal the bag. Place the sealed bag inside another bag, appropriately labeled as hazardous waste. For the moment, leave the outer bag open.
iv) Clean the spill area thoroughly, from least contaminated to most contaminated areas, using a detergent solution followed by clean water. Repeat.
v) Use fresh detergent solution to wash any reusable items used to clean up the spill and items located in the spill area (e.g., an IV pump). Use water to rinse the washed items. Repeat the washing and rinsing.
vi) Remove PPE and place disposable items in the unsealed

Figure 11. Contents of an Antineoplastic Spill Kit

- Two pairs of disposable chemical-protective gloves (one should be a pair of utility gloves)
- Low permeability, disposable protective garments (coveralls or gown and shoe covers)
- Face shield
- Respirator
- Absorbent, plastic-backed sheets or spill pads
- Disposable toweling
- At least two sealable thick plastic hazardous waste disposal bags (prelabeled with an appropriate warning label)
- A disposable scoop for collecting glass fragments
- A puncture-resistant container for glass fragments

Note. Based on information from American Society of Health-System Pharmacists, 2006.

cytotoxic waste disposal bag.

vii) Seal the outer cytotoxic waste disposal bag and place it in a puncture-proof container.

viii) Follow institutional guidelines regarding cleaning or maintenance of equipment.

ix) Dispose of all material used in the cleanup process according to institutional policy and federal, state, and local laws (OSHA, 1995).

(b) To clean up a spill on a carpeted surface (note that carpet is not recommended in drug administration areas), ASHP (1990) recommends the following.

i) Don PPE, including a NIOSH-approved respirator.

ii) Use absorbent powder, not absorbent towels, to absorb the spill.

iii) Use a small vacuum, reserved for hazardous-drug cleanup only, to remove the powder. Dispose of the collection bag as hazardous waste; clean the outside of the vacuum before storing.

iv) Clean the carpet as usual.

v) Follow guidelines for a spill on a hard surface to clean and dispose of other contaminated items.

(c) To clean up a spill in a BSC (ASHP, 2006; OSHA, 1995)

i) If the volume of the spill is < 150 ml: Clean up the spill according to the guidelines for a spill on a hard surface.

ii) If the volume of the spill is > 150 ml: Clean up the spill as if it were a spill on a hard surface. Include the drain spillage trough in washing efforts. Then complete the following additional steps.

• If the spill was not contained in a small area or the drain spillage trough: Wash the affected areas with a cleaning agent designed to remove chemicals from stainless steel.

• If the spill contaminated the HEPA filter: Seal the BSC in plastic and label it as contaminated equipment. Schedule a BSC service technician to change the HEPA filter. Ensure that the BSC is not used before the filter is changed.

• Clean and/or dispose of contaminated items as described in the guidelines for spills on a hard surface.

(d) To clean up a spill in the home setting: See Figure 12.

(6) Report and document the spill according to institutional policy: For any spill greater than a few drops, complete a report about the spill and forward it to those specified by institutional policy (Harrison, 2001). Document the following.

(a) The name of the drug and the approximate volume spilled

(b) How the spill occurred

(c) Spill management procedures followed

(d) The names of personnel, patients, and others exposed to the spill

(e) A list of personnel notified of the spill

17. Requirements for policies regarding the handling of HDs: OSHA (2004a) requires that employers provide a safe or healthful workplace. Employers must implement policies and procedures related to the safe handling of HDs. Policies should address all aspects of handling these hazardous materials to protect employees, patients, customers, and the environment from exposure. Such policies must (NIOSH, 2004)

a) Outline procedures to ensure the safe storage, transport, administration, and disposal of hazardous agents.

b) Describe the procedure for identifying and updating the list of HDs used in the facility.

c) Require that all employees who handle HDs wear PPE.

d) Mandate that HDs be prepared in a BSC or containment isolator (USP, 2008).

e) Prohibit staff from eating, drinking, smoking, chewing gum, using tobacco, storing food, and applying cosmetics in areas where HDs are prepared or used.

f) Mandate training for all employees who prepare, transport, or administer HDs or

Figure 12. Spill Kit Procedure for Home Use

(Please review this procedure with your nurse.)

1. Do not touch the spill with unprotected hands.
2. Open the spill kit and put on both pairs of gloves. If the bag or syringe with chemotherapy drugs has been broken or is leaking and you have a catheter or implanted port in place, before cleaning the spill disconnect the catheter from the tubing and flush and cap it as usual.
3. Put on the gown (closes in back), face shield, and respirator.
4. Use spill pillows to contain spill—put around puddle to form a "V."
5. Use the absorbent sheets to blot up as much of the drug as possible.
6. Put contaminated clean-up materials directly into the plastic bag contained in the kit. Do not lay them on unprotected surfaces.
7. Use the scoop and brush to collect any broken glass, sweeping toward the V'd spill pillows, and dispose of the glass in the box of the kit.
8. While still wearing the protective gear, wash the area with dishwashing or laundry detergent and warm water, using disposable rags or paper towels, and put them in the plastic bag with other waste. Rinse the area with clean water and dispose of the towels in the same plastic bag.
9. Remove gloves, face shield, respirator, and gown and place them in the plastic bag. Put all contaminated materials, including the spill kit box, into the second large plastic bag, and seal and label the bag with the hazardous waste label in the kit.
10. Wash your hands with soap and water.
11. Call the home health nurse, clinic, or doctor's office promptly to report the spill. Plans need to be made to replace the spilled chemotherapy so the treatment can be completed. Arrangements will be made to have the waste material picked up or have you bring it to the hospital for proper disposal.
12. If the spill occurs on sheets or clothing, wash the items in hot water, separate from other wash. Wash clothing or bed linen contaminated with body wastes in the same manner.
13. Patients on 24-hour infusions should use a plastic-backed mattress pad to protect the mattress from contamination.

Following these procedures prevents undue exposure and ensures your safety. Call your nurse if you have any questions. Thank you.

Note. From "Home Chemotherapy Safety Procedures," by C. Blecke, 1989, *Oncology Nursing Forum, 16*(5), p. 721. Copyright 1989 by Oncology Nursing Society. Adapted with permission. Also based on information from National Institute for Occupational Safety and Health, 2004.

care for patients receiving these drugs. This training must include the risks of exposure, the appropriate procedures for minimizing exposure, and how training is documented (OSHA, 1994).

g) Require that documents such as MSDS are available to healthcare workers who handle HDs.

h) State that spills should be managed according to the institution's HD spill policy and procedure.

i) Set forth a plan for medical surveillance of personnel handling HDs.

j) Address HD handling around pregnancy. Even when all recommended precautions are used, the potential for exposure cannot be completely eliminated. Therefore, an additional level of protection is suggested for those most vulnerable to the reproductive and developmental effects of HDs. Employers should allow employees who are actively trying to conceive or are pregnant or breastfeeding to refrain from activities that may expose them and their infant to reproductive health hazards such as chemical, physical, or biologic agents. Alternate duty that does not include HD preparation or administration must be made available upon request to both men and women in the aforementioned situations or who have other medical reasons for not being exposed to HDs. The employee has the responsibility of notifying the employer of the specific situation (e.g., pregnancy, preconception, breastfeeding). The American College of Occupational and Environmental Medicine (1996) provides guidelines for managing reproductive hazard management.

k) Define quality improvement programs that monitor compliance with safe-handling policies and procedures.

References

American College of Occupational and Environmental Medicine. (1996). ACOEM reproductive hazard management guidelines (committee report). *Journal of Occupational Environmental Medicine, 38*(1), 83–90.

American Society for Testing and Materials. (2005). *D 6978-05 standard practice for assessment of resistance of medical gloves to permeation by chemotherapy drugs*. West Conshohocken, PA: Author.

American Society of Health-System Pharmacists. (2006). ASHP guidelines on handling hazardous drugs. *American Journal of Health-System Pharmacy, 63*(12), 1172–1193.

American Society of Hospital Pharmacists. (1990). ASHP technical assistance bulletin on handling cytotoxic and hazardous drugs. *American Journal of Hospital Pharmacy, 47*(5), 1033–1049.

Brown, K.A., Esper, P., Kelleher, L.O., O'Neil, J.E.B., Polovich, M., & White, J.M. (Eds.). (2001). *Chemotherapy and biotherapy guidelines and recommendations for practice*. Pittsburgh, PA: Oncology Nursing Society.

Bruner, D., Haas, M., & Gosselin-Acomb, T. (Eds.). (2004). *Manual for radiation oncology nursing practice and education* (3rd ed.). Pittsburgh, PA: Oncology Nursing Society.

Celgene Corporation. (2005). Thalomid [Package insert]. Summit, NJ: Author.

Connor, T.H. (1993). An evaluation of the permeability of disposable polypropylene-based protective gowns to a battery of cancer chemotherapy drugs. *Applied Occupational and Environmental Hygiene, 8*(9), 785–789.

Connor, T.H. (1999). Permeability of nitrile rubber, latex, polyurethane, and neoprene gloves to 18 antineoplastic drugs. *American Journal of Health-System Pharmacy, 56*(23), 2450–2453.

Connor, T.H., Anderson, R.W., Sessink, P.J., Broadfield, L., & Power, L.A. (1999). Surface contamination with antineoplastic agents in six cancer treatment centers in Canada and the United States. *American Journal of Health-System Pharmacy, 56*(14), 1427–1432.

Connor, T.H., Anderson, R.W., Sessink, P.J., & Spivey, S.M. (2002). Effectiveness of a closed-system device in containing surface contamination with cyclophosphamide and ifosfamide in an I.V. admixture area. *American Journal of Health-System Pharmacy, 59*(1), 68–72.

Connor, T.H., Sessink, P.J., Harrison, B.R., Pretty, J.R., Peters, B.G., Alfaro, R.M., et al. (2005). Surface contamination of chemotherapy drug vials and evaluation of new vial-cleaning techniques: Results of three studies. *American Journal of Health-System Pharmacy, 62*(5), 475–484.

Dorr, R.T., & Alberts, D.S. (1992). Topical absorption and inactivation of cytotoxic anticancer agents in vitro. *Cancer, 70*(Suppl. 4), 983–987.

Fransman, W., Roeleveld, N., Peelen, S., de Kort, W., Kromhout, H., & Heederik, D. (2007). Nurses with dermal exposure to antineoplastic drugs: Reproductive outcomes. *Epidemiology, 18*(1), 112–119.

Fransman, W., Vermeulen, R., & Kromhout, H. (2005). Dermal exposure to cyclophosphamide in hospitals during preparation, nursing and cleaning activities. *International Archives of Occupational and Environmental Health, 78*(5), 403–412.

Fuchs, J., Hengstler, J.G., Jung, D., Hiltl, G., Konetzko, J., & Oesch, F. (1995). DNA damage in nurses handling antineoplastic agents. *Mutational Research, 342*(1–2), 17–23.

Genentech, Inc. (2000). *Material safety data sheet—Rituximab.* South San Francisco, CA: Author.

Hansen, J., & Olsen, J.H. (1994). Cancer morbidity among Danish female pharmacy technicians. *Scandinavian Journal of Work and Environmental Health, 20*(1), 22–26.

Harrison, B.R. (2001). Risks of handling cytotoxic drugs. In M.C. Perry (Ed.), *The chemotherapy source book* (3rd ed., pp. 566–582). Philadelphia: Lippincott Williams & Wilkins.

Harrison, B.R., & Kloos, M.D. (1999). Penetration and splash protection of six disposable gown materials against fifteen antineoplastic drugs. *Journal of Oncology Pharmacy Practice, 5*(2), 61–66.

Harrison, B.R., & Schultz, C.D. (2000). Determination of tablet trituration dust in work zone air. *Journal of Oncology Pharmacy Practice, 6*(1), 23.

Hemminki, K., Kyyronen, P., & Lindbohm, M.L. (1985). Spontaneous abortions and malformations in the offspring of nurses exposed to anaesthetic gases, cytostatic drugs, and other potential hazards in hospitals, based on registered information of outcome. *Journal of Epidemiology and Community Health, 39*(2), 141–147.

International Agency for Research on Cancer. (2007). *Overall evaluations of carcinogenicity to humans. IARC Monographs,* Vols. 1–99 [Electronic version]. Retrieved November 8, 2007, from http://monographs.iarc.fr/ENG/Classification/crthall.php

Kiffmeyer, T.K., Kube, C., Opiolka, S., Schmidt, K.G., Schoppe, G., & Sessink, P.J.M. (2002). Vapour pressures, evaporation behaviour and airborne concentrations of hazardous drugs: Implications for occupational safety. *Pharmaceutical Journal, 268*(March 9), 321–337.

Kromhout, H., Hock, F., Uitterhoeve, R., Huijbers, R., Overmars, R.F., Anzion, R.B., et al. (2000). Postulating a dermal pathway for exposure to anti-neoplastic drugs among hospital workers: Applying a conceptual model to the results of three workplace surveys. *Annals of Occupational Hygiene, 44*(8), 551–560.

Labuhn, K., Valanis, B., Schoeny, R., Loveday, K., & Vollmer, W.M. (1998). Nurses' and pharmacists' exposure to antineoplastic drugs: Finds from industrial hygiene scans and urine mutagenicity tests. *Cancer Nursing, 21*(2), 79–89.

Martin, S. (2005). Chemotherapy handling and effects among nurses and their offspring [Abstract]. *Oncology Nursing Forum, 32*(2), 425.

Mason, H.J., Blair, S., Sams, C., Jones, K., Garfitt, S.J., Cuschieri, M.J., et al. (2005). Exposure to antineoplastic drugs in two UK hospital pharmacy units. *Annals of Occupational Hygiene, 49*(7), 603–610.

McDevitt, J.J., Lees, P.S., & McDiarmid, M.A. (1993). Exposure of hospital pharmacists and nurses to antineoplastic agents. *Journal of Occupational Medicine, 35*(11), 56–60.

McQuestion, M. (2007). Radiation protection and safety. In M.L. Haas, W.P. Hogle, G.J. Moore-Higgs & T.K. Gosselin-Acomb (Eds.), *Radiation therapy: A guide to patient care* (pp. 25–35). St. Louis, MO: Mosby.

Minoia, C., Turci, R., Sottani, C., Schiavi, A., Perbellini, L., Angeleri, S., et al. (1998). Application of high performance liquid chromatography/tandem mass spectrometry in the environmental and biological monitoring of health care personnel occupationally exposed to cyclophosphamide and ifosfamide. *Rapid Communications in Mass Spectrometry, 12*(20), 1485–1493.

National Institute for Occupational Safety and Health. (1996). *Summary for respirator users* [Electronic version]. Retrieved January 5, 2008, from http://www.cdc.gov/niosh/respsumm.html

National Institute for Occupational Safety and Health. (2004). *Preventing occupational exposure to antineoplastic and other hazardous drugs in health care settings.* Retrieved September 13, 2008, from http://www.cdc.gov/niosh/docs/2004-165

National Sanitation Foundation. (2007). *Standard NSF/ANSI standard 49-2007 for Class II (laminar flow) biohazard cabinetry.* Ann Arbor, MI: Author.

Nygren, O., Gustavsson, B., Strom, L., & Friberg, A. (2002). Cisplatin contamination observed on the outside of drug vials. *Annals of Occupational Hygiene, 46*(6), 555–557.

Occupational Safety and Health Administration. (1994). *Hazard communication standard 1910.1200.* Retrieved September 15, 2005, from http://www.osha.gov/pls/oshaweb/owadisp.show_document?p_table=STANDARDS&p_id=10099

Occupational Safety and Health Administration. (1995). *Controlling occupational exposure to hazardous drugs. OSHA technical manual* [Electronic version]. Retrieved August 31, 2005, from http://www.osha.gov/dts/osta/otm/otm_vi/otm_vi_2.html

Occupational Safety and Health Administration. (1999). *OSHA technical manual, TED 1-0.15A section VI, chapter II: Categorization of drugs as hazardous.* Retrieved January 5, 2008, from http://www.osha.gov/dts/osta/otm/otm_vi/otm_vi_2.html#2

Occupational Safety and Health Administration. (2004a). *Code of federal regulations. Title 29, Labor: Subpart: General: Definitions*

(Title 29, Part (29CFR 1910.2). Retrieved January 5, 2008, from http://www.access.gpo.gov/nara/cfr/waisidx_04/29cfr1910_04. html

Occupational Safety and Health Administration. (2004b). *Code of federal regulations. Title 29, Labor: Subpart: Hazardous waste operations and emergency response: Hazardous materials (29CFR1910.120)*. Retrieved January 5, 2008, from http://www.access.gpo.gov/nara/cfr/waisidx_04/29cfr1910_04 .html

Occupational Safety and Health Administration. (2004c). *Code of federal regulations. Title 29, Labor: Subpart: Personal protective equipment: Respiratory protection (29 CFR1910.134)*. Retrieved January 5, 2008, from http://www.access.gpo.gov/nara/cfr/ waisidx_04/29cfr1910_04.html

Peelen, S., Roeleveld, N., Heederik, D., Kromhout, H., & de Kort, W. (1999). [Toxic effects on reproduction in hospital personnel.] *Reproductie-toxische effecten bij ziekenhuispersoneel.* Amsterdam: Elsevier.

Pethran, A., Schierl, R., Hauff, K., Grimm, C.H., Boos, K.S., & Nowak, D. (2003). Uptake of antineoplastic agents in pharmacy and hospital personnel. Part I: Monitoring of urinary concentrations. *International Archives of Occupational and Environmental Health, 76*(1), 5–10.

Polovich, M. (Ed.). (2003). *Safe handling of hazardous drugs*. Pittsburgh, PA: Oncology Nursing Society.

Schmaus, G., Schierl, R., & Funck, S. (2002). Monitoring surface contamination by antineoplastic drugs using gas chromatography-mass spectrometry and voltammetry. *American Journal of Health-System Pharmacy, 59*(10), 956–961.

Schreiber, C., Radon, K., Pethran, A., Schierl, R., Hauff, K., Grimm, C.H., et al. (2003). Uptake of antineoplastic agents in pharmacy personnel. Part 2: Study of work-related factors. *International Archives of Occupational and Environmental Health, 76*(1), 11–16.

Selevan, S.G., Lindbohm, M.L., Hornung, R.W., & Hemminki, K. (1985). A study of occupational exposure to antineoplastic drugs and fetal loss in nurses. *New England Journal of Medicine, 313*(19), 1173–1178.

Sessink, P.J., Anzion, R.B., van den Broek, P.H., & Bos, R.P. (1992). Detection of contamination with antineoplastic agents in a hospital pharmacy department. *Pharmacy Weekly Science, 14*(1), 16–22.

Sessink, P.J., Boer, K.A., Scheefhals, A.P., Anzion, R.B., & Bos, R.P. (1992). Occupational exposure to antineoplastic agents at several departments in a hospital. Environmental contamination and excretion of cyclophosphamide and ifosfamide in urine of exposed workers. *International Archives of Occupational and Environmental Health, 64*(2), 105–112.

Sessink, P.J., Cerna, M., Rossner, P., Pastorkova, A., Bavarova, H., Frankova, K., et al. (1994). Urinary cyclophosphamide excretion and chromosomal aberrations in peripheral blood lymphocytes after occupational exposure to antineoplastic agents. *Mutational Research, 309*(2), 193–199.

Singleton, L.C., & Connor, T.H. (1999). An evaluation of the permeability of chemotherapy gloves to three cancer chemotherapy drugs. *Oncology Nursing Forum, 26*(9), 1491–1496.

Skov, T., Maarup, B., Olsen, J., Rorth, M., Winthereik, H., & Lynge, E. (1992). Leukaemia and reproductive outcome among nurses handling antineoplastic drugs. *British Journal of Industrial Medicine, 49*(12), 855–861.

Smith, C.A. (2002, Nov/Dec). Managing pharmaceutical waste—What pharmacists should know. *Journal of the Pharmacy Society of Wisconsin*, pp. 17–22.

Stucker, I., Caillard, J.F., Collin, R., Gout, M., Poyen, D., & Hemon, D. (1990). Risk of spontaneous abortion among nurses handling antineoplastic drugs. *Scandinavian Journal of Work and Environmental Health, 16*(2), 102–107.

Ursini, C.L., Cavallo, D., Colombi, A., Giglio, M., Marinaccio, A., & Iavicoli, S. (2006). Evaluation of early DNA damage in healthcare workers handling antineoplastic drug. *International Archives of Occupational and Environmental Health, 80*(2), 134–140.

U.S. Department of Labor. (1998). *Informational booklet on industrial hygiene*. Retrieved September 18, 2008, from http://www.osha .gov/Publications/OSHA3143/OSHA3143.htm

U.S. Pharmacopeial Convention. (2008, May 1). Pharmaceutical compounding sterile preparations. In U.S. Pharmacopeia (Ed.), *National formulary, 26th rev.* (31st ed.). Rockville, MD: Author.

Valanis, B., Vollmer, W.M., Labuhn, K., & Glass, A. (1993a). Acute symptoms associated with antineoplastic drug handling among nurses. *Cancer Nursing, 16*(4), 288–295.

Valanis, B., Vollmer, W.M., Labuhn, K., & Glass, A. (1993b). Association of antineoplastic drug handling with acute adverse effects in pharmacy personnel. *American Journal of Health-System Pharmacy, 50*(3), 455–462.

Valanis, B., Vollmer, W.M., Labuhn, K., & Glass, A. (1997). Occupational exposure to antineoplastic agents and self-reported infertility among nurses and pharmacists. *Journal of Occupational and Environmental Medicine, 39*(6), 574–580.

Valanis, B., Vollmer, W.M., & Steele, P. (1999). Occupational exposure to antineoplastic agents: Self-reported miscarriages and stillbirths among nurses and pharmacists. *Journal of Occupational and Environmental Medicine, 41*(8), 632–638.

Welch, J., & Silveira, J.M. (Eds.). (1997). *Safe handling of cytotoxic drugs: An independent study module* (2nd ed.). Pittsburgh, PA: Oncology Nursing Society.

Wick, C., Slawson, M.H., Jorgenson, J.A., & Tyler, L.S. (2003). Using a closed-system protective device to reduce personnel exposure to antineoplastic agents. *American Journal of Health-System Pharmacy, 60*(22), 2314–2320.

B. Verification and maintenance of treatment as planned
1. The treatment plan
   a) Maintaining the planned treatment schedule is important because systemic cancer treatments often have a narrow margin of therapeutic benefit.
      (1) With minor adjustments below therapeutic doses, tumor response and patient outcomes can be adversely affected (Schulmeister, 2006).
      (2) Conversely, minor adjustments above therapeutic doses may result in increased toxicity without increased benefit.
   b) Maintaining a treatment plan's dose intensity (doses as planned without dosage reductions or delays) is related to improved patient survival (Monk et al., 2006). Unfortunately, dose reductions or treatment delays often occur because of toxicities. In a study of patients with non-Hodgkin

lymphoma (NHL) (N = 4,522), only half received greater than 85% of the optimal dose intensity for their regimens (Lyman, Dale, Friedberg, Crawford, & Fisher, 2004).

c) As part of ensuring optimal patient outcomes, oncology nurses must evaluate the appropriateness of the treatment plan and perform several safety checks to ensure that the agents are given as intended with appropriate supportive care measures.

d) Verification of cancer treatment orders is not as simple as knowing a single recommended dose or maximum safe dose as is true of many non-oncology medications.

(1) Institutional policies and procedures (P&Ps) should detail the process for regimen and dose verification for cancer treatment orders. P&Ps should clearly define the steps to take when discrepancies, potentially inappropriate orders, or other concerns arise.

(2) The nurse evaluates the appropriateness of the treatment regimen considering the indication, route of administration, concomitant treatments, and other factors. For example, doses of methotrexate may range from 2.5 mg to 20,000 mg depending on the condition being treated.

(3) Dosage reductions and treatment delays with resulting reduction in dose intensity may occur when potential toxicities are not proactively addressed (Lenhart, 2005).

(a) The oncology nurse works with patients to ensure that treatments remain on schedule at planned doses. Assessment before, during, and after treatment with appropriate follow-up regarding identified needs is important.

(b) Providing appropriate support may reduce the severity of toxicities and help to maintain the planned treatment.

i) Growth factor support to prevent neutropenic complications was found to eliminate age as a predictive factor for dosage reductions and treatment delays in patients with NHL (Lyman et al., 2004).

ii) Teaching patients evidence-based infection prevention measures may reduce the risk of neutropenic fever (Zitella et al., 2006).

2. Concepts of dose density and dose intensity

a) Dose-dense therapy: A standard regimen that is given with less time between cycles is referred to as a *dose-dense* regimen.

(1) The rationale for dose-dense therapy is to minimize tumor regrowth between cycles.

(2) Hematopoietic growth factors reduce the severity and duration of neutropenia from myelosuppressive treatments, allowing the time between treatment cycles to be reduced.

b) Dose intensity: *Dose intensity* refers to the amount of drug given over a period of time (e.g., mg/m^2/week).

(1) Dose-dense regimens increase dose intensity.

(2) Maintaining dose intensity ensures optimal exposure of the tumor to chemotherapy agents.

(3) Treatment delays or dosage reductions decrease dose intensity.

(a) Decisions to delay treatments may occur because of lack of knowledge by both patients and nurses regarding the importance of dose intensity (Lenhart, 2005).

(b) Relative dose intensity (RDI) is expressed as a percentage derived by dividing the **actual dose** of chemotherapy given over a period of time by the **planned dose** of chemotherapy over the planned period of time (Lenhart, 2005).

i) Example: The plan calls for 100 mg/m^2 of an agent weekly for 4 weeks.

• The patient receives 100 mg/m^2 on weeks 1, 2, and 3, but only 75 mg/m^2 on week 4.

• The planned dose intensity was 100 mg/m^2/week or 400 mg/m^2/4 weeks.

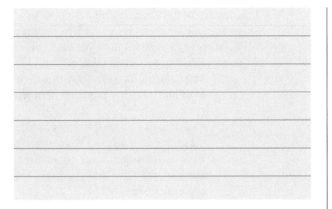

- The actual dose intensity was 375 mg/m²/4 weeks or 94 mg/m²/week.
- Therefore, the RDI was 94% (375 divided by 400).

    ii) Providing supportive care measures as needed to maintain dose intensity is extremely important to improving long-term survival.
- A study of patients with large cell lymphomas (N = 115) found that an RDI of 75% or greater was the single most important factor in predicting survival (Lenhart, 2005).
- A 20-year study of patients with breast cancer (N = 386) treated with adjuvant chemotherapy found that when RDI fell below 65%, survival rates were similar to not having received chemotherapy at all (Lenhart, 2005).

3. The role of the nurse in verifying the treatment plan and schedule
   a) Prior to initiating a cancer treatment regimen, oncology nurses should
    (1) Review the regimen and anticipated side effects.
    (2) Verify that the ordered regimen is appropriate for the indication.
    (3) If a nonstandard regimen or research protocol is used, ensure that a copy of the nonstandard regimen, protocol, or abstract is available to verify the ordered regimen.
    (4) Do not verify a dose with a previous treatment; always verify with a protocol.
   b) Verification includes
    (1) Checking that prescribed doses are within the normal range for the indication

    (2) Ensuring appropriate time intervals between scheduled treatments
    (3) Reviewing and documenting laboratory values and other factors that may require changes in treatment
    (4) Ensuring that all questions regarding orders are addressed prior to administration.
   c) Institutions must ensure that processes and tools are in place to enable appropriate verification of treatment regimens by the nurse.

4. Verification of patient understanding of the treatment plan
   a) See also Section VI.A. Patient Education.
   b) Verify that the patient and involved caregivers have received appropriate education. This should include
    (1) Verifying the patient's understanding of and IC for the therapy prior to initiating treatment
    (2) Providing written information regarding plan of care in language appropriate for the patient
    (3) Stressing the importance of maintaining the planned treatment schedule
    (4) Allowing opportunities for questions and assessment of understanding.
   c) Establish systems to monitor compliance with home regimens and return appointments.

5. Promoting continuity of care: Systems must be in place to ensure accurate/complete reporting of treatment plan/history when the patient moves from one healthcare setting to another. Incomplete or inaccurate communication between facilities can lead to treatment errors.
   a) A copy of the regimen should be provided to the new treating facility upon transfer.
   b) A summary of prior cancer treatments and current treatments should be communicated.
   c) Hospitalization or any change of healthcare setting is not in itself a reason to stop or delay treatments.

6. Verification of the chemotherapy and biotherapy orders: Nurses must familiarize themselves with the planned regimen and evaluate the need for clarification or additional information before providing treatment.
   a) The nurse is responsible for verifying that the planned regimen is appropriate and dosed within normal limits for the indication and schedule.
   b) Treating facilities must provide the resources to meet this responsibility.

(1) Drug and regimen references
(2) Internet availability (e.g., National Comprehensive Cancer Network [NCCN] guidelines, www.nccn.org)
(3) A copy of the protocol or reference for nonstandard regimens

7. Verification of dose modifications: If standard doses are modified, documentation describing the rationale should be provided. This allows the nurse to assess the appropriateness of dosing. Some reasons for dose modification include comorbid conditions, toxicities with previous treatment, or other factors, such as the following.

a) Obesity: Dose capping sometimes is used for obese patients. The intent is to prevent unnecessary toxicity with the higher doses called for with BSA and area under the plasma concentration versus time curve (AUC) calculations. Some evidence has shown that dose reductions related to obesity, while reducing toxicities, may result in decreased survival outcomes (Griggs, Sorbero, & Lyman, 2005).

b) Older age: Doses of chemotherapy sometimes are reduced in older adults because of their presumed inability to tolerate standard doses as renal function declines with age.

(1) Actual comorbid conditions and functional status may be better indicators to determine the need for dosage reductions. A growing body of evidence supports the use of standard doses in older adult patients with good performance status and without significant comorbidities. Dose reductions, while reducing toxicities, increase the risk for poor response to treatment (Burdette-Radoux & Muss, 2006).

(2) Appropriate growth factor support may improve the ability to maintain standard-dose regimens (Lenhart, 2005).

(3) One study found that standard-dose regimens of cisplatin and etoposide with granulocyte–colony-stimulating factor (G-CSF) support were well-tolerated in older adults. Compared to those with dose-reduced (or attenuated-dose) regimens (n = 28), those on standard regimens with G-CSF support (n = 67) demonstrated dramatically increased response rates and one-year survival (Ardizzoni et al., 2005).

c) Children: In pediatric oncology, agents typically dosed based on BSA are sometimes converted to mg/kg doses using the "rule of 30" (30 kg = 1 m^2). The rationale is that BSA dosing may not be accurate or optimal because of organ development in the very young (younger than three years) and small (less than 10 kg to less than 30 kg). However, no consensus exists regarding when and if these modifications should be used.

(1) Based on findings that several infants with Wilms tumors experienced toxicity-related deaths, recommendations were developed to calculate doses based on weight instead of BSA. Similar survival rates with less toxicity resulted.

(2) However, when using weight-based dosing of busulfan for allogeneic stem cell transplantation in young children, inadequate responses resulted from underdosing. The children's own immune systems recovered and rejected the transplants (Trigg, 2004).

d) Polypharmacy: Sometimes interactions between medications necessitate dosage adjustments. This can occur with primary treatment agents as well as supportive care medications.

(1) Aprepitant given to prevent chemotherapy-induced nausea and vomiting (CINV) increases the effect of dexamethasone. Except when dexamethasone is part of the cancer treatment itself, it is recommended that the dexamethasone dose be reduced when given concurrently with aprepitant (Flemm, 2004).

(2) Nurses need to be cognizant of the possibility of drug interactions that may enhance or diminish the efficacy of a specific drug. It is advisable to check with the oncology pharmacist if a patient is receiving multiple drugs for cancer therapy and multiple additional drugs for comorbid conditions such as diabetes, arthritis, and allergies.

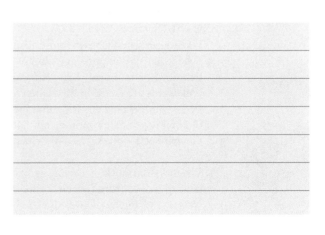

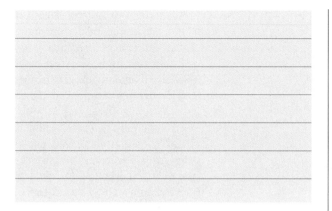

8. Evaluating the treatment orders
   a) Oncology nurses must evaluate treatment orders for clarity. The complexity of some treatment regimens increases the risk for ambiguity when orders are written.
   b) Use of preprinted orders and computer ordering systems has the potential to decrease the occurrences of ambiguous or incomplete orders.
9. Verification of dose calculations
   a) Errors in dose calculations may cause significant harm to patients. Therefore, two independent verifications of dosing calculations are required before initiating treatment.
   b) Two chemotherapy-competent individuals (e.g., nurses, pharmacists), in addition to the ordering prescriber, should perform a double-check of dosage calculations.
      (1) Independent calculations help to prevent bias errors. Each person performs calculations independently, and the results are compared.
      (2) Institutions must ensure that nurses administering cancer treatments are adequately trained in performing calculations. Processes should be developed to confirm that verifications are done and documented.
      (3) Weights and heights used for dose calculations must actually be measured.
   c) Several types of dosing (mg, mg/kg, mg/m^2, and AUC) may be used.
      (1) Fixed doses: This means the prescribed dose does not require calculations based on patient size. Many of the oral agents are dosed in this manner. Verification entails ensuring that the ordered dose is appropriate and that the patient receives the prescribed dose.
      (2) Weight-based dosing: Dosing is expressed as dose of drug per unit of body weight (e.g., mg/kg). Doses should be calculated using an accurately measured weight.
      (3) BSA-based dosing: Most cytotoxic chemotherapy drugs are dosed based on BSA, or the estimated total area of a person's skin expressed in square meters (m^2). BSA should be calculated using accurately measured current height and weight.
         (a) Advantages: The underlying assumption is that by incorporating both height and weight, BSA is a more reliable indicator than weight for predicting pharmacokinetics.
         (b) Disadvantages
            i) Increased complexity of calculations increases the chance for medication errors.
            ii) BSA dosing alone does not account for factors other than height and weight that could influence pharmacokinetics. For example, a male and female who both have a BSA of 2.0 may have vastly different renal and hepatic functions. Also, age and gender may play a role in pharmacokinetics.
            iii) For many chemotherapy agents, there is a lack of evidence supporting a correlation between BSA alone and drug clearance from the body (Gao, Klumpen, & Gurney, 2008). Evidence suggests that BSA is a poor predictor of drug action and clearance for topotecan, cisplatin, irinotecan, epirubicin, etoposide, and many other chemotherapy agents traditionally dosed based on BSA (Mathijssen et al., 2007).
            iv) A retrospective study of 33 investigational anticancer agents tested from 1991 through 2001 among 1,650 adult patients with cancer found that BSA was reliable in decreasing interpatient variability in five of the agents. These agents included paclitaxel and temozolomide (Baker et al., 2002). BSA has also proved to be a good tool in predicting drug clearance of docetaxel (de Jongh et al., 2001).

v) In addition to the current utilization of clinical factors in modifying BSA-based doses, future strategies may incorporate genotype and phenotype markers as well as therapeutic drug monitoring to achieve optimal doses (Gao et al., 2008).

vi) Despite the issues with BSA-based dosing, it remains the most common method for dosing many chemotherapy agents. Nurses should be aware of drug-specific recommendations for dosage adjustments that account for patient variability such as renal and liver function.

(c) At least seven different formulas are used for calculating BSA, each yielding slightly different results. For this reason, it should be clear which formula was used by the prescriber when calculating drug doses. In the United States, the most commonly used formulas are the Dubois and Dubois, Gehan and George, and Mosteller equations (see Figure 13) (Kouno, Katsumata, Mukai, Ando, & Watanabe, 2003).

i) The Mosteller equation (a simplified version of the more complex Gehan and George formula) is most commonly used (Kouno et al., 2003).

ii) An advantage of the Mosteller equation is that it can be car-

ried out with any calculator that has a square root function.

(d) Modifications made to the actual BSA to obtain adjusted doses should be clearly stated. If an ideal body weight is used instead of actual weight to calculate BSA, this should be indicated in the order.

(e) Although BSA calculators and slide rules are available, it is important to verify that the tools used are based on the same formula used in the treatment orders. Check the institution's policies and procedures regarding use of a specific formula versus BSA calculator or slide rule.

(f) In calculating dosages, the nurse should be aware of medication-specific circumstances that affect dosing. For example, vincristine is dosed based on BSA, but prescribers often cap the dose at a maximum of 2 mg regardless of the BSA to reduce toxicities (McEvoy, 2004). Not all physicians agree with this practice.

(4) Carboplatin and AUC-based dosing: AUC calculations are commonly used to determine carboplatin doses. AUC refers to the amount of drug exposure over time or the total drug concentration in plasma over a period of time (Solimando, 2007).

(a) The Calvert formula is used to determine the total dose of carboplatin in milligrams (see Figure 14). Target AUC is specified in the order.

(b) In practice, an estimated creatinine clearance (CrCl) is used more frequently than an actual glomerular filtration rate (GFR), as this would require a 24-hour urine collection.

(c) GFR = glomerular filtration rate = estimated creatinine clearance = CrCl

---

Figure 13. Formulas for Determining Body Surface Area (BSA)

Mosteller Equation (most commonly used in the United States):

$$\sqrt{\frac{\text{height in cm} \times \text{weight in kg}}{3{,}600}}$$

This formula is converted to inches and pounds as

$$\sqrt{\frac{\text{height in inches} \times \text{weight in pounds}}{3{,}131}}$$

Dubois and Dubois Equation:
BSA = 0.007184 × height in cm $^{0.725}$ × weight in kg $^{0.425}$

Gehan and George Equation:
BSA = 0.0235 × height in cm $^{0.42246}$ × weight in kg $^{0.51456}$

Note. Based on information from Kouno et al., 2003; Meyers, 2006.

Figure 14. Calvert Formula

Dose of carboplatin (mg) = (target AUC) × (GFR + 25)

Total dose calculated is in mg, not mg/m^2.

(d) Example: The order calls for "Carboplatin AUC 6."
  i) The calculated CrCl is 50 ml/min.
  ii) GFR + 25 (CrCl + 25) = 50 + 25 = 75
  iii) Target AUC × 75 = 6 × 75 = 450 mg
  iv) Carboplatin dose = 450 mg
(e) AUC dosing of carboplatin accounts for age, gender, weight, and renal function. Carboplatin drug clearance is strongly correlated with GFR, making carboplatin an ideal drug to be dosed based on AUC (de Jongh et al., 2001).
(f) Several formulas, each yielding significantly different results, exist for obtaining the value for GFR (estimated CrCl). Potential exists for errors in dosing when a different formula is used than that intended by the prescriber.
(g) Two common formulas used to obtain CrCl for carboplatin dosing are the Cockcroft-Gault and Jelliffe formulas (see Figures 15 and 16). The Cockcroft-Gault formula is the most commonly used in the United States. The Jelliffe method does not account for weight.
(h) Generally, the formulas for estimating CrCl are reliable. Exceptions include emaciated patients in whom actual CrCl is typically lower than estimated CrCl and patients with rapidly changing creatinine levels. With patients exhibiting a rise in CrCl of > 0.5–0.7 mg/dl/day, actual CrCl may be less than 10 ml/day (Solimando, 2007).

Figure 16. Calculation of Glomerular Filtration Rate: Jelliffe Method

Males:

$$CrCl\ (ml/min.) = \frac{\{98 - [0.8 \times (age - 20)]\}}{serum\ creatinine\ (mg/dl)}$$

Females:

$$CrCl\ (ml/min.) = \frac{\{98 - [0.8 \times (age - 20)]\}}{serum\ creatinine\ (mg/dl)} \times 0.9$$

Note. From "Carboplatin Dosing Accounting for the Renal and Hematologic Status of Patients," by T. Busse, 2003, *Clinical Journal of Oncology Nursing, 7*(1), p. 105. Copyright 2003 by Oncology Nursing Society. Reprinted with permission.

  (i) When creatinine levels are very low (< 0.6 mg/dl), many practitioners will adjust the creatinine value to 0.6 mg/dl when using the Jelliffe method for calculating GFR (Nagao et al., 2006).
  (j) Nurses practicing outside of the United States should be aware of adjustments required to GFR calculations based on differences in laboratories. A study in Japan found that GFR was significantly overestimated when using standard formulas. The causative factor had to do with laboratory differences in obtaining creatinine levels, and adjustments to the GFR formulas resolved overestimations (Ando et al., 2000).
10. When calculations do not agree
  a) Several factors can result in verification calculations yielding results that are different from the ordered doses.
    (1) A change in the patient's weight: Minor weight changes typically are not significant. However, patients should be weighed before each treatment cycle and the doses calculated based on the current weight.
    (2) Using different formulas for verifying calculations
    (3) An error in the calculations during the verification process: The first step when noting discrepancies in doses is to recheck the calculations.
    (4) An error in calculations during the ordering process: This is the primary purpose of the verification process.
  b) P&Ps should dictate the acceptable variance between the ordered dose and the recalculated dose. For example, a 5%

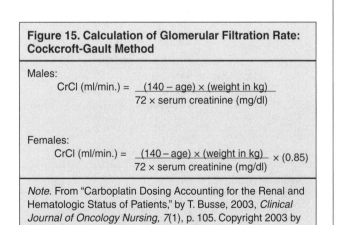

Figure 15. Calculation of Glomerular Filtration Rate: Cockcroft-Gault Method

Males:

$$CrCl\ (ml/min.) = \frac{(140 - age) \times (weight\ in\ kg)}{72 \times serum\ creatinine\ (mg/dl)}$$

Females:

$$CrCl\ (ml/min.) = \frac{(140 - age) \times (weight\ in\ kg)}{72 \times serum\ creatinine\ (mg/dl)} \times (0.85)$$

Note. From "Carboplatin Dosing Accounting for the Renal and Hematologic Status of Patients," by T. Busse, 2003, *Clinical Journal of Oncology Nursing, 7*(1), p. 105. Copyright 2003 by Oncology Nursing Society. Reprinted with permission.

variance rule is common practice. With this, as long as the recalculated dose is within 5% of the actual ordered dose, it is acceptable to proceed.

   (1) When the ordered dose is 100 mg, a 5% variance rule allows administration of the drug when recalculations fall between 95 mg and 105 mg.

   (2) Without a policy that states an acceptable variance, it is necessary for the nurse to clarify a dose discrepancy with the prescriber prior to administering treatment.

11. Rounding doses: Policy should indicate if rounding of doses is acceptable or expected.

12. Verification of oral agents

  a) See also Appendix 3.

  b) Oral formulations of chemotherapy and biologic agents require the same processes of verification as other types of systemic cancer treatments (Womer et al., 2002). Many oral agents are based on fixed dosing regimens, but some require BSA calculations. The orders and first dose should be verified by two chemotherapy-competent individuals when administered in a healthcare setting.

  c) Ensuring patient/caregiver understanding of the oral treatment regimen is critical when the agents are administered at home.

   (1) Some patients do not adhere to treatment regimens because of a lack of understanding related to inadequate preparation and/or assessment of abilities (Aisner, 2007).

   (2) Dispensing pharmacies are not always familiar with cancer medications and may not offer the necessary teaching required (Bartel, 2007).

   (3) Complex treatment schedules may make it difficult for some to maintain adherence. Providing patients with treatment calendars may be helpful.

   (4) Failure to adhere to the treatment regimen may result in poor outcomes. For example, tumor resistance can develop after only short periods of abstaining from imatinib. Patient education should include the importance of maintaining the regimen as ordered.

13. Verification of medication sequence

  a) The order in which chemotherapy and biotherapy agents are given may have an impact on the pharmacokinetics and pharmacodynamics of the agents. However, it is not always known if specific sequences of treatments result in better outcomes.

   (1) A review of 50 published studies evaluating 32 different chemotherapy regimens found only 11 regimens in which sequence did not seem to have an impact. For the others, improper sequencing of the chemotherapeutic agents had the potential for increasing toxicity and decreasing the effectiveness of the regimen (Stanford, Zondor, & Jumper, 2005).

   (2) Studies have demonstrated that hormonal agents in the treatment of ER/PR+ breast cancer should not be started until after completion of the chemotherapeutic regimens (Sertoli et al., 2002).

   (3) A study of patients with non-small cell lung cancer (NSCLC) (N = 80) demonstrated a more favorable tumor response rate (54%) when cisplatin preceded irinotecan versus the more traditional irinotecan-first approach (39%). This led to a recommendation for change in how this regimen is administered (Han et al., 2006).

  b) Some institutions develop algorithms to determine which agent is given first when no specific direction is given regarding sequence. In the absence of specific policy-driven direction, the nurse should seek clarification of sequence when the orders are not clear.

14. Standard therapy, research protocols, and tailored therapy

  a) Standard treatment regimens: These are treatment regimens determined to be most efficacious for a given cancer and patient conditions. Specific agents with specified doses, routes, rates, and sequence are identified within the regimen. All of the agents in a regimen constitute one cycle of treatment. The frequency of cycles is included within the standard treatment plan.

b) High-dose chemotherapy: Some chemotherapy regimens call for very high doses of the agents. With some types of cancer, the use of high-dose therapy is required to achieve potential cure.

(1) These regimens typically require much more supportive care (e.g., transfusions, growth factor support) because of severe myelosuppression and other toxicities.

(2) High-dose chemotherapy also sometimes is used with the goal of myeloablation before stem cell transplantation.

(3) Oncology nurses should be aware of toxicities that emerge when higher doses of agents are given. For example, high-dose cyclophosphamide carries the risk of cardiac toxicity that is not present in lower-dose regimens (Loerzel & Dow, 2003).

c) Research protocols: Researchers continue to investigate new agents and new ways of giving and combining older agents with the goal of improving tumor response to therapy and/or reducing the toxicity of therapy.

(1) When a research protocol is being used, it is imperative that the protocol is followed exactly as written.

(2) Failure to follow the protocol exactly can lead to difficulty in interpreting the research findings, thus rendering the data "unevaluable."

d) "Tailored" protocols: As the understanding of the interplay of tumor molecular biology, the role of genetics, and other factors continues to grow, it is speculated that a time will come when regimens will be individualized for patients. Predicting tumor response based on patient-specific data may result in the use of agents that are more likely to have a positive effect while eliminating toxic agents not likely to be of benefit. This is an area currently being investigated.

References

Aisner, J. (2007). Overview of the changing paradigm in cancer treatment: Oral chemotherapy. *American Journal of Health-System Pharmacy, 64*(Suppl. 5), S4–S7.

Ando, M., Minami, H., Ando, Y., Saka, H., Sakai, S., Yamamoto, M., et al. (2000). Multi-institutional validation study of carboplatin dosing formula using adjusted serum creatinine level. *Clinical Cancer Research, 6*(12), 4733–4738.

Ardizzoni, A., Favaretto, A., Boni, L., Baldini, E., Castiglioni, F., Antonelli, P., et al. (2005). Platinum-etoposide chemotherapy in elderly patients with small-cell lung cancer: Results of a randomized multicenter phase II study assessing attenuated-dose or full-dose with lenograstim prophylaxis. *Journal of Clinical Oncology, 23*(3), 569–575.

Baker, S.D., Verweij, J., Rowinski, E.K., Donehower, R.C., Schellens, J.H., Grochow, L.B., et al. (2002). Role of body surface area in dosing of investigational anticancer agents in adults, 1991-2001. *Journal of the National Cancer Institute, 94*(24), 1883–1888.

Bartel, S.B. (2007). Safe practices and financial considerations in using oral chemotherapeutic agents. *American Journal of Health-System Pharmacy, 64*(Suppl. 5), S8–S14.

Burdette-Radoux, S., & Muss, H.B. (2006). Adjuvant chemotherapy in the elderly: Whom to treat, what regimen? *Oncologist, 11*(3), 234–242.

de Jongh, F.E., Verweij, J., Loos, W., de Wit, R., de Jonge, M.J.A., & Planting, A.S.T. (2001). Body-surface area–based dosing does not increase accuracy of predicting cisplatin exposure. *Journal of Clinical Oncology, 19*(17), 3733–3739.

Flemm, L.A. (2004). Aprepitant for chemotherapy-induced nausea and vomiting. *Clinical Journal of Oncology Nursing, 8*(3), 303–306.

Gao, B., Klumpen, H.J., & Gurney, H. (2008). Dose calculation of anticancer drugs. *Expert Opinion on Drug Metabolism and Toxicology, 4*(10), 1307–1319.

Griggs, J.J., Sorbero, M.E.S., & Lyman, G.H. (2005). Undertreatment of obese women receiving breast cancer chemotherapy. *Archives of Internal Medicine, 165*(11), 1267–1273.

Han, J.Y., Lim, H.S., Lee, D.H., Ju, S.Y., Lee, S.Y., Kim, H.Y., et al. (2006). Randomized phase II study of two opposite administration sequences of irinotecan and cisplatin in patients with advanced nonsmall cell lung carcinoma. *Cancer, 106*(4), 873–880.

Kouno, T., Katsumata, N., Mukai, H., Ando, M., & Watanabe, T. (2003). Standardization of the body surface area (BSA) formula to calculate the dose of anticancer agents in Japan. *Japanese Journal of Clinical Oncology, 33*(6), 309–313.

Lenhart, C. (2005). Relative dose intensity: Improving cancer treatment and outcomes. *Oncology Nursing Forum, 32*(4), 757–764.

Loerzel, V.W., & Dow, K.H. (2003). Cardiac toxicity related to cancer treatment. *Clinical Journal of Oncology Nursing, 7*(5), 557–562.

Lyman, G.H., Dale, D.C., Friedberg, J., Crawford, J., & Fisher, R.I. (2004). Incidence and predictors of low chemotherapy dose-intensity in aggressive non-Hodgkin lymphoma: A nationwide study. *Journal of Clinical Oncology, 22*(21), 4302–4311.

Mathijssen, R.H., deJong, F.A., Loos, W.J., van der Bol, J.M., Verweij, J., & Sparreboom, A. (2007). Flat-fixed dosing versus body surface area based dosing of anticancer drugs in adults: Does it make a difference? *Oncologist, 12*(8), 924–926.

McEvoy, G.K. (2004). Vincristine sulfate. In G.K. McEvoy (Ed.), *AHFS drug information 2004* (pp. 1168–1171). Bethesda, MD: American Society of Health-System Pharmacists.

Meyers, E. (2006). *RNotes: Nurse's clinical pocket guide* (2nd ed.). Philadelphia: F.A. Davis.

Monk, J.P., Phillips, G., Waite, R., Kuhn, J., Schaaf, L.J., Otterson, G.A., et al. (2006). Assessment of tumor necrosis factor alpha blockade as an intervention to improve tolerability of dose-intensive chemotherapy in cancer patients. *Journal of Clinical Oncology, 24*(12), 1852–1859.

Nagao, S., Fujiwara, K., Kagawa, R., Kozuka, Y., Oda, T., Maehata, K., et al. (2006). Is the adjustment of serum creatinine level < 0.6 mg/dl to 0.6 mg/dl justified in estimates of carboplatin clearance calculated by the Jelliffe formula? *Journal of Clinical Oncology, 2006 ASCO Annual Meeting Proceedings Part I, 24*(18S), 5072.

Schulmeister, L. (2006). Preventing chemotherapy errors. *Oncologist, 11*(5), 463–468.

Sertoli, M.R., Pronzato, P., Venturini, M., Del Mastro, L., Querirolo, P., Vecchio, S., et al. (2002). A randomized study of concurrent versus sequential adjuvant chemotherapy and tamoxifen in stage II breast cancer. *Proceedings of the American Society of Clinical Oncology, 21*, Abstract 182.

Solimando, D.A., Jr. (Ed.). (2007). *Drug information handbook for oncology* (6th ed.). Hudson, OH: Lexi-Comp.

Stanford, B.L., Zondor, S.D., & Jumper, C.A. (2005). Chemotherapy administration sequences—Review of the literature and administration recommendations. *Journal of Clinical Oncology, 2005 ASCO Annual Meeting Proceedings, 23*(16S), 6121.

Trigg, M.E. (2004). Hematopoietic stem cells. *Pediatrics, 113*(4), 1051–1057.

Womer, R.B., Tracy, E., Soo-Hoo, W., Bickert, B., DiTaranto, S., & Barnsteiner, J.H. (2002). Multidisciplinary systems approach to chemotherapy safety: Rebuilding processes and holding the gains. *Journal of Clinical Oncology, 20*(24), 4705–4712.

Zitella, L.J., Friese, C.R., Hauser, J.H., Gobel, B.H., Woolery, M., O'Leary, C., et al. (2006). Putting Evidence Into Practice: Preventing infection. *Clinical Journal of Oncology Nursing, 10*(6), 739–750.

C. Pretreatment: Follow institutional guidelines regarding documentation of assessment and provision of care. Appendices 1 and 2 provide sample flow sheets.
  1. Nursing assessment and case review
    a) Patient history
      (1) Review recent treatment(s), including surgery, radiation therapy, prior cytotoxic therapy, hormonal therapy, and complementary therapies (e.g., acupuncture, chiropractic, nutritional).
      (2) Review and document medical, psychiatric, and surgical history.
      (3) Document drug, food, latex, and environmental allergies.
      (4) Document pregnancy and reproductive status, including date of last menstrual period when applicable.
      (5) Obtain an accurate list of all medications and supplements that the patient uses, including prescription, over-the-counter (OTC), herbs, and vitamins. According to the National Center for Complementary and Alternative Medicine (2007), 37% of adults in the United States use complementary and alternative medicine. Patients may only disclose use of these products when directly questioned in a nonjudgmental fashion.
      (6) *Age-specific concerns:* Older adults often have multiple comorbidities for

which they take multiple medications. Be aware of the potential for drug interactions with chemotherapy agents (Hood, 2003).
      b) Signs and symptoms of underlying disease process and any previous treatments
        (1) Symptom screening during the pretreatment phase is crucial to successful symptom management.
        (2) Poorly controlled symptoms affect patients' QOL and can interfere with delivery of chemotherapy and other treatment modalities (Dodd, Miaskowski, & Paul, 2001; Houldin, 2000), as well as adherence to the treatment regimen.
  2. Screening tools
    a) Assess performance status by using scales such as the Karnofsky, Zubrod, or ECOG scales (see Table 4).
    b) Assess pain using an age-appropriate scale (e.g., 0–10 scale, facial expressions, visual analog).
    c) Assess for fatigue using an appropriate scale, such as the Brief Fatigue Inventory (Mendoza et al., 1999), the Piper Fatigue Scale (Piper et al., 1998), or the Schwartz Cancer Fatigue Scale (Schwartz, 1998).
    d) *Age-specific concerns:* The number of instruments or scales available to measure physical symptoms in children with cancer is limited. Direct observation measures are used in assessment of young children; children as young as age seven can report symptoms accurately (Linder, 2005).
  3. Patient data
    a) Obtain and document the patient's **actual** height and weight; compare with previous visits as well as the patient's precancer weight.
    b) Compare current and previous lab values. *Age-specific concerns:* Assess for age-related changes in pulmonary, renal, and cardiac function in older adults.
    c) Review diagnosis, tumor type, grade, and staging of current malignancy and any previous cancers.
    d) Obtain treatment records from past encounters to determine symptom management strategies that were employed.
    e) Assess cultural and spiritual issues that may affect the treatment plan.
    f) Assess psychosocial problems such as transportation.
    g) Determine the need for referral to a social worker, spiritual care provider, dietitian, physical therapist, and other member of

the multidisciplinary team as needed. *Age-specific concerns:* When caring for pediatric patients, consult play therapists and child-life specialists. If a school-age youth is going to be out of school for a prolonged time, explore options for continued study available through the appropriate school district (e.g., home study, online programs).

h) If the patient is pregnant, anticipate collaboration with the maternal fetal medicine team before chemotherapy is started.

(1) Establish accurate gestational age because chemotherapy is contraindicated during the first trimester (Rimes, Gano, Hahn, Ramirez, & Milbourne, 2006).

(2) The key goals of multidisciplinary care for the pregnant patient with cancer include keeping the patient as comfortable as possible and not harming the fetus.

(3) Allow at least three weeks between the last dose of chemotherapy and delivery to allow blood counts to recover.

(4) Chemotherapy is not recommended after 35 weeks to avoid delivery during a period of bone marrow suppression and the lack of drug excretion from immature fetal organs.

(5) Breastfeeding is contraindicated during chemotherapy treatment.

4. Patient education: Oncology nurses are responsible for educating new patients. Learning about cancer and the treatment plan can help patients to regain some control and mitigate the fear of the unknown (Mueller & Glennon, 2006). Identify information and learning needs of patients and families (Houldin, 2000).

a) Determine the preferred language for verbal and written instruction.

b) Assess speaking fluency and reading literacy.

c) Review patients' goals for education; some may want information given to their significant others rather than themselves, whereas others will want very detailed information.

d) Assess level of understanding of the disease and treatment.

e) Identify the preferred learning style.

f) Provide information regarding the following.

(1) Drugs, side effects, and symptom management

(2) When and how to call the nurse and/or doctor

(3) Body fluid precautions for 48 hours after chemotherapy

(4) Sexual relations and contraception

(5) Follow-up care and labs

(6) How to access support services

5. Treatment plan (Santell, Protzel, & Cousins, 2004)

a) Read the written orders in their entirety, and then scrutinize each line for the following.

(1) Name of drug ordered

(2) Drug dose

(3) Method of determining dose (e.g., treatment protocol, clinical trial)

(4) Route of administration

(5) Rate of administration

(6) Frequency and/or date(s) of administration

(7) Premedications for hypersensitivity and/or nausea

(8) Hydration, if applicable

(9) Protocol or reference

(10) Documentation of IC to receive chemotherapy

b) Assess orders for completeness (e.g., hydration, premedications).

c) Review the patient's actual height and weight; double-check the patient's BSA.

d) Have two individuals independently recalculate the drug dose and compare to the ordered dose (ASHP, 2002). Follow institutional policy for who can double-check doses (e.g., two RNs, RN and pharmacist).

e) Verify that the dose is appropriate for the patient, diagnosis, and treatment plan. If in doubt, clarify. Consult a pharmacist and/or physician.

f) Determine the vesicant and irritant potential of the drug(s).

g) Follow institutional policy regarding having patients sign an IC document for treatment document prior to starting the chemotherapy.

h) Assess the patient's prior experience with cytotoxic therapy (e.g., adequacy of symptom management, delayed side effects, willingness to proceed).

i) Immediately before administration, verify the order, the drug names, calculations, expiration dates and times, appearance of the drugs, and accuracy of two different patient identifiers.

(1) Informed patients and their family members are a vital component of patient safety programs, as they can review the agents with the nurse before administration as well as express concerns about chemotherapy administration safety (Sheridan-Leos, 2007).

(2) Error prevention in chemotherapy administration is an ongoing quality improvement process that requires continuous evaluation and review of systems involved in the chemotherapy process (Sheridan-Leos, 2007).

D. Treatment

1. Patient preparation

a) Provide explanation to the patient and family/caregivers regarding who will administer the chemotherapy, the route, and the planned sequence of events.

b) Involve the patient and family in safety practices by teaching them about indicators used to verify patient identity and medications. Encourage them to ask questions.

c) Describe the plan for symptom management. Provide information regarding the following (Polovich & Gullatte, 2007; Vandergrift, 2001).

(1) Premedications

(2) Hydration

(3) Intake and output assessment

(4) Laboratory monitoring

(5) Diet during chemotherapy

(6) Potential side effects of chemotherapeutic and adjunct medications and the importance of reporting the experience of side effects

(7) Baseline vital signs as indicated

2. Staff preparation

a) Review all physician orders.

b) Have a spill kit, extravasation equipment, and emergency drugs/equipment available as needed (Otto, 2004; Polovich & Gullatte, 2007).

c) *Age-specific concerns:* If administering chemotherapy to a child, patient-specific dosing information and emergency equipment must be available. Calculate emergency drug doses before they are needed.

d) Obtain monitoring equipment as indicated.

e) Obtain infusion pumps and other devices as needed. *Age-specific concerns:* Use a volumetric pump to administer chemotherapy to pediatric patients (Frey, 2001; Infusion Nurses Society [INS], 2006).

3. Routes of administration

a) Oral: The role of oral chemotherapy agents is expanding, with many new drugs in development, reflecting a new paradigm in which cancer is treated as a chronic disease with long-term management (Bedell, 2003). Few studies have looked at adherence with oral chemotherapy regimens (Winkeljohn, 2007).

(1) Advantages

(a) Convenience and sense of control for patients

(b) Ease and portability of administration

(c) Increased sense of patient independence

(2) Disadvantages

(a) Difficulties with adherence, safety, patient teaching, and access to oral chemotherapy agents can hinder treatment (Winkeljohn, 2007) as well as a patient's inability to swallow tablets or capsules.

(b) The error rate for oral chemotherapy at home has been documented at approximately 10%, including errors of dosing or failure to take the medication.

(c) Inconsistency of absorption

(d) Potential loss of drug in the event of emesis

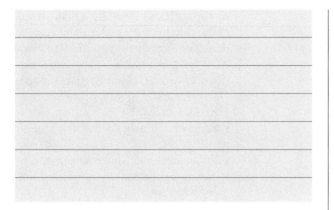

(e) Potential for drug–herb–diet interactions (e.g., grapefruit juice interacts with CYP enzymes in the liver) (Winkeljohn, 2007)

(f) Issue of medication adherence: Taking too much or too little

(g) Cost/reimbursement concerns (Birner, 2003): Newer drugs are very expensive, possibly resulting in large out-of-pocket expenses for patients.

(3) Potential complications

(a) Drug-specific

(b) Related to drug–drug interactions

(c) Related to swallowing difficulties; do not crush oral agents because of exposure potential.

(4) Nursing implications

(a) Age-specific concerns: Young children may require liquid preparations. For older adult patients, evaluate ability to swallow pills intact plus ability to self-manage a medication regimen (Hartigan, 2000).

(b) Patient education is key to promoting medication regimen adherence. Provide verbal and written instructions, including name of the medication, dose and schedule, a calendar to show on which days the medication is taken and when there are breaks, how the drug is taken, and safety (storage and handling).

(c) Teach patients to bring the pill bottle to office or clinic visits for pill counts to monitor adherence to the medication plan.

(d) Teach patients and family to use disposable gloves to handle the oral chemotherapy pills and how to dispose of them properly.

(e) Teach patients and family about pharmaceutical patient assistance programs to help with medication costs.

(f) Ideally, oral chemotherapy orders should be preprinted rather than handwritten and should incorporate a process for double-checking order accuracy.

b) Subcutaneous (SC) or intramuscular (IM) injection (Camp-Sorrell, 2004; Hayden & Goodman, 2005)

(1) Advantages

(a) Ease of administration

(b) Decreased side effects

(2) Disadvantages

(a) Inconsistency of absorption

(b) Requires adequate muscle mass and tissue for absorption

(3) Potential complications

(a) Pain/discomfort

(b) Infection

(c) Bleeding

(4) Nursing implications

(a) Wear appropriate PPE (Polovich & Gullatte, 2007).

(b) Monitor platelet count and absolute neutrophil count (ANC).

(c) Use smallest needle possible; some solutions may come with pre-prepared syringes (follow manufacturer's instructions).

(d) Follow institutional policy for site antisepsis and documentation.

(e) Assess previous injection sites for signs and symptoms of infection or bleeding.

c) Intra-arterial: Delivers medication directly into an organ (e.g., brain, liver, head and neck, pelvis) or tumor by means of three types of access devices. Refer to the Oncology Nursing Society's *Access Device Guidelines: Recommendations for Nursing Practice and Education* (Camp-Sorrell, 2004) for more detailed information.

(1) Types of devices

(a) Short-term percutaneous catheters inserted via femoral or brachial artery (frequently placed by interventional radiologists)

(b) Long-term catheters placed during surgery and used as an external catheter or attached to an implanted pump

(c) Implanted ports for long-term therapy

(2) Advantages

(a) Increased exposure of tumor to drug resulting in greater tumor response with decreased systemic side effects

(b) Considered a local treatment, as the drug's first major site of action is the target lesion, thereby avoiding the first pass effect (i.e., concentration of drug is greatly reduced before reaching the systemic circulation).

(c) Decreased surgical complications resulting from decreased tumor bulk if therapy is planned as neo-adjuvant

(3) Disadvantages

(a) Increased risk for distant metastases because of less systemic circulation of the chemotherapy

(b) Requires surgical procedure or special radiography equipment for catheter or port placement

(c) Requires specialized nursing education for arterial pumps

(d) May sharply limit patient's mobility for three to seven days if treatment is given by percutaneous catheter

(4) Potential complications

(a) Bleeding

(b) Embolism

(c) Pain

(d) Pump occlusion or malfunction

(e) Hepatic artery injury

(f) Arterial catheter leak or break

(g) Skin reaction to tape or dressing

(h) Catheter migration/dislodgment

(5) Nursing implications

(a) Wear appropriate PPE (Polovich & Gullate, 2007).

(b) Monitor for signs/symptoms of bleeding, including monitoring prothrombin time (PT)/partial thromboplastin time (PTT).

(c) Monitor catheter site for infection, bleeding, and signs of catheter migration/dislodgment, including epigastric pain, nausea, vomiting, diarrhea, edema, diminished peripheral pulse, and inability to infuse.

(d) Monitor for signs of occlusion, including inability to flush or withdraw fluid, abdominal pain, or change in color/pulse/temperature of involved extremity. If patient is going home with infusion, provide patient education regarding pump and catheter care. Follow pump manufacturer's recommendations for implanted pumps (Barber & Fabugais-Nazario, 2003; Hagle, 2003).

d) IT/intraventricular (Camp-Sorrell, 2004; Polovich & Gullatte, 2007). **Note: Vinca alkaloids such as vincristine are never given intrathecally because of potentially lethal neurotoxicity.**

(1) Advantages

(a) Affords more consistent drug levels in cerebrospinal fluid

(b) Bypasses the blood-brain barrier

(c) Can be used to sample cerebrospinal fluid and to administer opiates and antibiotics

(2) Disadvantages

(a) Requires lumbar puncture or surgical placement of implanted intraventricular device (e.g., Ommaya reservoir)

(b) Generally requires a physician or specially trained RN to access and administer chemotherapy via this route

(3) Potential complications: Increased intracranial pressure, headaches, confusion, lethargy, nausea and vomiting, seizures, and infection

(4) Nursing implications

(a) Wear appropriate PPE (Polovich & Gullatte, 2007).

(b) Observe site for signs of infection.

(c) Assess patient for headache or other signs of increased intracranial pressure (Kosier & Minkler, 1999).

(d) Accessing the Ommaya reservoir is a sterile procedure. Medication

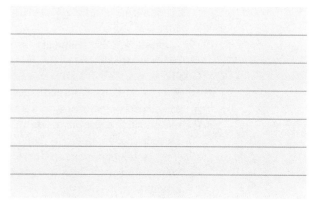

to be instilled must be preservative free.
- (e) Do not use a Vacutainer® to withdraw cerebrospinal fluid: Rapid withdrawal of fluid could damage the choroid plexus of the ventricle. Avoid air embolism.
- e) Intraperitoneal (IP) (Camp-Sorrell, 2004; Hayden & Goodman, 2005): According to NCI (2008), IP plus IV chemotherapy postoperatively is an option for treating advanced ovarian cancer. Other conditions with potential applications of IP chemotherapy include malignant peritoneal mesothelioma, appendiceal malignancy, peritoneal dissemination from primary pancreatic cancer, and peritoneal carcinomatosis (Marin, Oleszewski, & Muehlbauer, 2007).
  - (1) Advantages
    - (a) Provides direct exposure of intra-abdominal metastases to the drug(s), resulting in higher drug concentrations at the disease site(s)
    - (b) Bypasses the cellular enclosure of the peritoneal cavity, which may prevent systemic chemotherapy from reaching the structures within the cavity
    - (c) Allows instillation of radioactive or colloid materials intraperitoneally
    - (d) Allows for cyclic treatments over a long period of time
  - (2) Disadvantages
    - (a) Requires placement of a peritoneal catheter or intraperitoneal port during initial or subsequent surgical procedure
    - (b) Requires small enough tumor volume to permit adequate drug penetration
  - (3) Potential complications
    - (a) Abdominal pain and cramping
    - (b) Distention due to the requisite fluid volume > 1,500 ml
    - (c) Severe nausea and vomiting
    - (d) Bleeding
    - (e) Ileus
    - (f) Intestinal perforation
    - (g) Infection
    - (h) Anaphylaxis
    - (i) Dyspnea secondary to abdominal distention
  - (4) Nursing implications
    - (a) Wear appropriate PPE (Polovich & Gullatte, 2007).
    - (b) Peritoneal port is accessed with a 19–20-gauge, 1–2", 90° noncoring Huber needle, using sterile technique.
    - (c) Warm chemotherapy to body temperature (Otto, 2004) using in-line fluid warmer or water bath. *Never* microwave.
    - (d) Check patency of catheter or port according to institutional policy. Once accessed, it should flush without difficulty. The placement of the port is in the peritoneal cavity, not in a vessel. Therefore, no blood can be withdrawn; do not attempt to aspirate to verify placement.
    - (e) Premedicate for nausea; IV lorazepam and opioids may be ordered to relieve cramping.
    - (f) Instill solution according to protocol: Infuse drug, and reposition patient for maximum surface exposure to drug, usually every 15 minutes for two hours after the fluid is infused.
- f) Intrapleural: Instills sclerosing agents such as mechlorethamine, bleomycin, or 5-FU, or sterile talc into the pleural space (Hayden & Goodman, 2005); also may instill radioactive colloidal materials.
  - (1) Advantage: Scleroses the pleural lining to prevent recurrence of effusions
  - (2) Disadvantages
    - (a) Requires insertion of a thoracotomy tube
    - (b) Must be administered by a physician
  - (3) Potential complications
    - (a) Pain
    - (b) Infection
  - (4) Nursing implications

(a) Wear appropriate PPE (Polovich & Gullate, 2007).

(b) The effusion must be completely drained from the pleural cavity before instillation of the drug (thoracentesis).

(c) Following instillation, clamp the tubing and reposition the patient every 10–15 minutes for two hours, or as ordered (Otto, 2004).

(d) Assess for and treat pain and anxiety.

g) Intravesicular (Hayden & Goodman, 2005; Washburn, 2007): Incidence of urinary bladder cancer is increasing and is expected to continue to do so as the population ages, thereby increasing use of intravesicular chemotherapy, including instillation immediately following transurethral resection of bladder tumors.

(1) Advantage: Provides direct exposure of nonmuscle-invasive tumors of the bladder to drugs, such as thiotepa, mitomycin, epirubicin, doxorubicin, and mitoxantrone

(2) Disadvantages: Requires placement of a Foley catheter

(3) Potential complications

(a) Urinary tract infection

(b) Cystitis

(c) Bladder contracture

(d) Urinary urgency

(e) Flu-like symptoms following instillation of bacillus Calmette-Guérin (BCG)

(f) Potential extravasation of vesicant agents; can result in peritoneal necrosis, fistula formation, and chronic pain

(4) Nursing implications

(a) Maintain sterile technique during Foley insertion.

(b) Follow physician orders or protocol for schedule of repositioning the patient and clamping and unclamping the catheter after instilling the chemotherapy.

(c) Wear appropriate PPE, including a mask, when administering BCG (Polovich & Gullate, 2007). Healthcare workers with weakened immune systems should avoid working with or near BCG.

(d) If pain is not relieved by pain medication following vesicant agent administration, suspect extravasation. Release the agent and urine and notify the physician immediately.

h) IV (Camp-Sorrell, 2004; Hayden & Goodman, 2005)

(1) Advantages

(a) Consistent absorption

(b) Required for vesicant and many other agents

(2) Disadvantages

(a) Requires considerable nursing and patient time in a healthcare facility

(b) Interferes with patient's activities; causes sclerosing of veins over time

(c) May require surgical procedure for central line placement

(3) Potential complications

(a) Infection

(b) Phlebitis

(c) Infiltration

(d) Extravasation (INS, 2006)

(e) Local discomfort

(f) Drug-specific concerns

(4) Nursing implications will be discussed in the following section.

4. IV cytotoxic administration: Most cytotoxic agents are given intravenously. Refer to *Access Device Guidelines: Recommendations for Nursing Practice and Education* (Camp-Sorrell, 2004) for a complete discussion of IV access.

a) Peripheral IV access

(1) Existing IV site

(a) Avoid using a site that is more than 24 hours old.

(b) Assess the insertion site for signs of inflammation and infiltration, and consider the patient's statements about comfort. Use another access site if there is any doubt about the integrity of the IV site.

(c) Assess blood return and patency.

(2) New IV site: Avoid use of steel needles for vesicant administration (Centers for Disease Control and Prevention, 2002). Select the smallest gauge and shortest length catheter to accommodate the prescribed therapy (INS, 2006). Consider use of dermal anesthesia to minimize pain during IV insertion.

(a) In adults (Camp-Sorrell, 2004; Hayden & Goodman, 2005)

   i) Identify an appropriate IV site by assessing the patient's arms carefully. Veins of choice are smooth and pliable; the large veins of the forearm are preferred.

   ii) Avoid establishing an IV site in the following.
- Injured or sclerosed veins
- Areas of flexion
- Small, fragile, tortuous veins
- An extremity with altered venous return or lymphedema
- An extremity with decreased sensation or paresthesia
- The lower extremities

   iii) Perform venipuncture per institutional policy and procedure.

   iv) Establish blood return and patency.

   v) Secure the IV device appropriately, in a manner that allows a clear view of the site.

   vi) If venipuncture is unsuccessful, use the opposite arm for the next attempt. If it is not possible to use the opposite arm, select a site proximal to the first venipuncture.

(b) *Age-specific concerns:* In children, select an appropriate site, following institutional policies and the guidelines that follow (Sievers & Andam, 2004).

   i) If possible, do not use the feet or dominant hand of an infant or toddler as an IV site.

   ii) The veins of the scalp of a child younger than 12 months old can be used as an IV site; however, do not use a scalp vein to administer a vesicant.

   iii) Stabilize the extremity, if necessary, while inserting and securing the IV.

b) Central venous catheters (CVCs): CVCs include percutaneous subclavian catheters, tunneled subclavian catheters, and peripherally inserted central catheters (PICCs). (A midline catheter is considered a peripheral line because it ends in the middle of the upper arm.) An implanted port, although technically a CVC, is unique and will be addressed later. Most CVCs require the use of syringes larger than 10 cc to minimize pressure (pounds per square inch [psi]) on delicate catheter walls (Camp-Sorrell, 2004). Follow manufacturers' and institutional guidelines carefully to avoid catheter rupture. After CVC insertion and before administering the agent, perform the following.

(1) Verify that the catheter's placement is correct prior to initial use per institutional guidelines.

(2) Inspect exit site for evidence of erythema, swelling, drainage, and leakage.

(3) Inspect ipsilateral chest for signs of venous thrombosis (INS, 2006).

(4) Aspirate the line to verify blood return. If blood return is not evident,

(a) Flush the catheter with saline, gently using the push-pull method as described in *Access Device Guidelines: Recommendations for Nursing Practice and Education* (Camp-Sorrell, 2004).

(b) Reposition the patient as appropriate.

(c) Ask the patient to cough.

(d) Explain to the patient why delaying therapy is necessary. Although patients may report that lack of blood return from their catheter is common, DO NOT administer cytotoxic therapy.

    (e) Obtain a physician's order for a declotting procedure; follow institutional protocol.

    (f) Use x-rays or dye studies to confirm proper CVC placement per institutional policy and rule out catheter malfunction or migration in the absence of a blood return.

c) Implanted ports: Implanted ports are available that allow venous, peritoneal, arterial, and epidural access. Ascertain which type is being used. Some patients have more than one type.

  (1) Assess initial line placement by using the results of x-ray or fluoroscopic dye studies.

  (2) Choose a noncoring needle (Hayden & Goodman, 2005) with a length that is appropriate to the depth of the port and size of the patient (i.e., the amount of SC tissue or fat located above the port).

  (3) Prepare the patient's skin according to institutional policy.

  (4) Access the port, ensuring proper placement of the needle in the reservoir.

  (5) Establish blood return and patency. If blood return is not evident, repeat steps listed for CVCs. (Blood return is not expected with epidural or peritoneal access devices.)

  (6) Inspect the needle insertion site for needle dislodgment, leakage of IV fluid, drainage, or edema.

  (7) Examine the ipsilateral chest for signs and symptoms of venous thrombosis.

  (8) Apply an occlusive dressing to stabilize the needle. The dressing should be transparent to allow a clear view of the insertion site. Experts disagree about other dressing characteristics that are desirable (Camp-Sorrell, 2004). Padding the undersides of the butterfly wings of the access needle may be necessary if the needle does not lie securely on the skin.

  (9) Extravasation can occur with CVC devices and is less obvious. Common symptoms include pain in the neck or shoulder, chest pain, chest palpitations, ipsilateral fluid wave in chest or neck, and cough depending on the position

of the catheter and the location of the extravasated fluid.

d) Piggy-back or short-term infusion

  (1) Verify blood return and IV patency prior to hanging the infusion. Do not pinch the IV catheter to determine blood return because the resulting dramatic change in pressure within the vein may cause a rupture. Preferred methods of verifying patency are the following.

    (a) Use a syringe inserted at the injection port closest to the patient to gently aspirate the line, while pinching off fluid from the bag.

    (b) Use a gravity check by removing the bag from the pump, lowering it below the patient's IV site, and watch for blood return.

  (2) Attach the secondary tubing to the appropriate injection port, using a needleless, Luer lock connector (INS, 2006).

  (3) Initiate flow rate according to the physician's orders and observe the patient closely for any reactions.

  (4) When administering a vesicant drug by short infusion using a peripheral vein,

    (a) Avoid using an IV pump in order to decrease pressure on the veins.

    (b) Remain with the patient during the infusion. Visually monitor the site for signs of extravasation while verifying blood return every 5–10 minutes.

    (c) Avoid infusing vesicant agents peripherally for more than 30–60 minutes.

    (d) Note: Confirming extravasation of vesicants during chemotherapy administration can be difficult because manifestations can vary

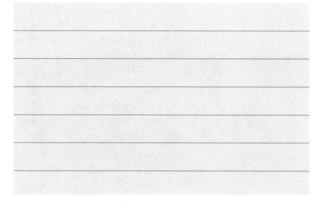

from no immediate signs to pain, swelling, and loss of blood return, as well as differentiating extravasation from flare and recall reactions.

(5) Once the short infusion is complete, check vein patency and flush the line with a compatible IV solution.

e) Continuous infusion

(1) Follow guidelines for checking blood return and IV patency.

(2) The cytotoxic agent may be connected directly to the IV catheter or into a compatible line of maintenance solution, according to institutional policy.

(3) Secure all connections with Luer locking devices.

(4) Monitor the IV site throughout the infusion according to institutional policy and procedure. Monitor the patient closely for any reactions, such as signs or symptoms of hypersensitivity (Otto, 2004).

(5) When administering a vesicant (Chu & DeVita, 2005; Vandergrift, 2001)

(a) DO NOT use a peripheral IV site for continuous vesicant administration.

(b) Use a central venous access catheter or implanted access device to administer any vesicant infusing for longer than 30–60 minutes.

(c) Check for blood return and patency periodically, according to institutional policy.

(6) Once the infusion is complete, check vein patency and flush the line with a compatible IV solution (Otto, 2004).

f) IV push: Refer to physician orders and/or pharmacy guidelines for suggested IV push rates, diluents, and other drug-specific details (Hayden & Goodman, 2005; INS, 2006; Vandergrift, 2001).

(1) Free-flow method (side-arm technique)

(a) Attach the syringe with the drug at the injection port closest to the patient.

(b) Aspirate the line to verify IV patency.

(c) Allow IV solution to flow freely.

(d) Slowly administer the chemotherapy agent as an IV push, allowing the flush solution to dilute the drug. Unless otherwise indicated, administer the agent at a rate of 1–2 ml/min.

(e) When administering a vesicant, verify blood return every 2–5 ml.

(f) Once the IV push is completed, check vein patency and flush the line with a compatible IV solution.

(2) Direct push method: Some institutions may require that certain cytotoxic agents be administered as an IV push directly into the IV device (Hayden & Goodman, 2005; Temple & Poniatowski, 2005; Vandergrift, 2001).

(a) Select an appropriate vein, and prepare the skin according to policy.

(b) Establish a patent IV, flushing the new line with sterile IV solution (typically normal saline [NS] or 5% dextrose in water [D5W]).

(c) Verify blood return by aspirating the line gently.

(d) Detach the flush syringe, and attach the syringe containing the cytotoxic agent. Maintain sterile technique and minimize blood loss.

(e) Slowly administer the agent, aspirating for blood return every 2–5 ml.

(f) Upon completion of the IV push, disconnect the cytotoxic syringe. Avoid blood loss; the blood will contain the cytotoxic agent.

(g) Connect a syringe containing sterile flush solution; gently flush the catheter.

(h) Cap or discontinue the IV access device, as indicated.

References

American Society of Health-System Pharmacists. (2002). ASHP guidelines on preventing medication errors with antineoplastic agents. *American Journal of Health-System Pharmacy, 59*(17), 1648–1668.

Barber, F.D., & Fabugais-Nazario, L.E. (2003). What's old is new again: Patients receiving hepatic arterial infusion chemotherapy. *Clinical Journal of Oncology Nursing, 7*(6), 647–652.

Bedell, C.H. (2003). A changing paradigm for cancer treatment: The advent of new oral chemotherapy agents. *Clinical Journal of Oncology Nursing, 7*(Suppl. 6), 5–9.

Birner, A. (2003). Safe administration of oral chemotherapy. *Clinical Journal of Oncology Nursing, 7*(2), 158–162.

Camp-Sorrell, D. (Ed.). (2004). *Access device guidelines: Recommendations for nursing practice and education* (2nd ed.). Pittsburgh, PA: Oncology Nursing Society.

Centers for Disease Control and Prevention. (2002). Guidelines for prevention of intravascular catheter-related infections. *Morbidity and Mortality Weekly Report, 51*(32), 1–29.

Chu, E., & DeVita, V.T., Jr. (2005). *Physicians' cancer chemotherapy drug manual.* Sudbury, MA: Jones and Bartlett.

Dodd, M.J., Miaskowski, C., & Paul, S.M. (2001). Symptom clusters and their effect on the functional status of patients with cancer. *Oncology Nursing Forum, 28*(3), 465–470.

Frey, A.M. (2001). Intravenous therapy in children. In J. Hankins, R.A.W. Lonsway, C. Hedrick, & M. Perdue (Eds.), *Infusion therapy in clinical practice* (2nd ed., pp. 561–591). St. Louis, MO: Saunders.

Hagle, M.E. (2003). Arterial access devices. *Clinical Journal of Oncology Nursing, 7*(6), 669–674.

Hartigan, K. (2000). Patient education: The cornerstone of successful oral chemotherapy treatment. *Clinical Journal of Oncology Nursing, 7*(Suppl. 6), 21–24.

Hayden, B.K., & Goodman, M. (2005). Chemotherapy: Principles of administration. In C.H. Yarbro, M.H. Frogge, & M. Goodman (Eds.), *Cancer nursing: Principles and practice* (6th ed., pp. 351–411). Sudbury, MA: Jones and Bartlett.

Hood, L.E. (2003). Chemotherapy in the elderly: Supportive measures for chemotherapy-induced myelotoxicity. *Clinical Journal of Oncology Nursing, 7*(2), 185–190.

Houldin, A.D. (2000). *Patients with cancer: Understanding the psychological pain.* Philadelphia: Lippincott Williams & Wilkins.

Infusion Nurses Society. (2006). Infusion nursing standards of practice. *Journal of Infusion Nursing, 23*(Suppl. 6), S1–S88.

Kosier, M.B., & Minkler, P. (1999). Nursing management of patients with an implanted Ommaya reservoir. *Clinical Journal of Oncology Nursing, 3*(2), 63–67.

Linder, L.A. (2005). Measuring physical symptoms in children and adolescents with cancer. *Cancer Nursing, 28*(1), 16–26.

Marin, K., Oleszewski, K., & Muehlbauer, P. (2007). Intraperitoneal chemotherapy: Implications beyond ovarian cancer. *Clinical Journal of Oncology Nursing, 11*(6), 881–890.

Mendoza, T.R., Wang, X.S., Cleeland, C.S., Morrissey, M., Johnson, B.A., Wendt, J.K., et al. (1999). The rapid assessment of fatigue severity in cancer patients: Use of the Brief Fatigue Inventory. *Cancer, 85*(5), 1186–1196.

Mueller, P.S., & Glennon, C.A. (2006). A self-developed prechemotherapy education checklist. *Clinical Journal of Oncology Nursing, 11*(5), 715–719.

National Cancer Institute. (2008). *Ovarian epithelial cancer treatment (PDQ®).* Retrieved June 28, 2008, from http://www.cancer.gov/cancertopics/pdq/treatment/ovarianepithelial/healthprofessional

National Center for Complementary and Alternative Medicine. (2007). *The use of complementary and alternative medicine in the United States.* Retrieved November 11, 2008, from http://nccam.nih.gov/news/camsurvey_fs1.htm#use

Otto, S. (2004). *Oncology nursing clinical reference.* St. Louis, MO: Mosby.

Piper, B.F., Dibble, S.L., Dodd, M.J., Weiss, M.C., Slaughter, R.E., & Paul, S.M. (1998). The revised Piper Fatigue Scale: Psychometric evaluation in women with breast cancer. *Oncology Nursing Forum, 25*(4), 677–684.

Polovich, M., & Gullatte, M.M. (2007). Principles and standards of chemotherapy administration. In M.M. Gullatte (Ed.), *Clinical guide to antineoplastic therapy: A chemotherapy handbook* (2nd ed., pp. 39–56). Pittsburgh, PA: Oncology Nursing Society.

Rimes, S., Gano, J., Hahn, C., Ramirez, M., & Milbourne, A. (2006). Caring for pregnant patients with breast cancer. *Oncology Nursing Forum, 33*(6), 1065–1069.

Santell, J.P., Protzel, M.M., & Cousins, D. (2004). Medication errors in oncology practice. *U.S. Pharmacist, 29*(4). Retrieved July 4, 2008, from http://www.uspharmacist.com/index.asp?show=article&page=8_1259.htm

Schwartz, A.L. (1998). The Schwartz Cancer Fatigue Scale: Testing reliability and validity. *Oncology Nursing Forum, 25*(4), 711–717.

Sheridan-Leos, N. (2007). A model of chemotherapy education for novice oncology nurses that supports a culture of safety. *Clinical Journal of Oncology Nursing, 11*(4), 545–552.

Sievers, T.D., & Andam, R. (2004). Chemotherapy administration and immediate postadministration issues. In N.E. Kline (Ed.), *The pediatric chemotherapy and biotherapy curriculum* (pp. 75–97). Glenview, IL: Association of Pediatric Oncology Nurses.

Temple, S.V., & Poniatowski, B.D. (2005). Nursing implications of antineoplastic therapy. In J.K. Itano & K.N. Taoka (Eds.), *Core curriculum for oncology nursing* (4th ed., pp. 785–802). St. Louis, MO: Elsevier Saunders.

Vandergrift, K.V. (2001). Oncologic therapy. In J. Hankins, R.A.W. Lonsway, C. Hedrick, & M.B. Perdue (Eds.), *Infusion therapy in clinical practice* (2nd ed., pp. 248–275). St. Louis, MO: Saunders.

Washburn, D.J. (2007). Intravesical antineoplastic therapy following transurethral resection of bladder tumors: Nursing implications from the operating room to discharge. *Clinical Journal of Oncology Nursing, 11*(4), 553–560.

Winkeljohn, D.L. (2007). Oral chemotherapy medications: The need for a nurse's touch. *Clinical Journal of Oncology Nursing, 11*(6), 793–797.

V. Immediate Complications of Cytotoxic Therapy

The oncology nurse must be alert for immediate complications of cytotoxic therapy. The information in this section covers complications that may be experienced by patients during chemotherapy administration or shortly thereafter. Terms used in this section include

- *Extravasation:* "A passage or escape into the tissues" (*Mosby's Dictionary of Medicine, Nursing and Health Professions,* 2006, p. 697).
- *Vesicants (also referred to as "blistering agents"):* "Chemicals that cause blistering of the skin or mucous membranes" (*Mosby's,* 2006, p. 228).
- *Irritant:* "An agent that produces inflammation or irritation" (*Mosby's,* 2006, p. 1019).
- *Flare reaction:* "A red blush on the skin at the periphery of an urticarial lesion seen in immediate hypersensitivity reactions" (*Mosby's,* 2006, p. 743).
- *Hypersensitivity reaction:* "An inappropriate and excessive response of the immune system to a sensitizing antigen, called an allergen" (*Mosby's,* 2006, p. 923).
- *Anaphylaxis:* "An exaggerated, life-threatening hypersensitivity reaction to a previously encountered antigen. The reaction may consist of a localized wheal and flare of generalized itching, hyperemia, angioedema, and in severe cases vascular collapse, bronchospasm, and shock" (*Mosby's,* 2006, p. 93).

A. Extravasation
   1. Pathophysiology: Tissue damage secondary to vesicant extravasation occurs as a result of one of two major mechanisms.
      a) The vesicant binds to nucleic acids in the DNA of healthy cells in the tissue, causing cell death. Complexes are released from the dead cells and taken up by adjacent healthy cells. This process of cellular uptake of extracellular substances sets up a continuing cycle of tissue damage as the DNA-binding vesicant is retained and recirculated in the tissue for a long period of time (Luedke, Kennedy, & Rietschel, 1979). Examples of DNA-binding vesicants include the anthracyclines (daunorubicin, doxorubicin, epirubicin, idarubicin), dactinomycin, mechlorethamine (nitrogen mustard), and mitomycin.
      b) The vesicant does not bind to cellular DNA. The vesicant has an indirect rather than direct effect on the cells in healthy tissue. It is eventually metabolized in the tissue and is more easily neutralized than DNA-binding vesicants (Ener, Meglathery, & Styler, 2004). Examples of non-DNA-binding vesicants include paclitaxel and the plant alkaloids (vinblastine, vincristine, vindesine, vinorelbine).
   2. Extent of tissue damage: Factors that affect the degree of tissue damage include
      a) The type of vesicant that extravasates (DNA-binding or nonbinding)
      b) The concentration and amount of the vesicant in the tissue
      c) The location of the extravasation
      d) Patient factors, such as older age, comorbidity (e.g., diabetes), and impaired immunocompetence influence the extent of tissue damage and patients' responses to vesicant extravasation treatment (Ener et al., 2004; Schulmeister, 2007a).
   3. Risk factors for peripheral extravasation (Goolsby & Lombardo, 2006; Sauerland, Engelking, Wickham, & Corbi, 2006)
      a) Small, fragile veins
      b) Previous multiple venipunctures
      c) Prior treatment with irritating or sclerosing drugs, such as chemotherapy
      d) Sensory deficits
      e) Limited vein selection because of lymph node dissection, lymphedema, or limb removal
      f) Somnolence, impaired cognition, altered mental status
      g) Probing during IV catheter insertion
      h) Inadequately secured IV catheter
      i) Administration site in areas with minimal overlying tissue (e.g., dorsum of the hand, wrist, or antecubital area)
      j) Use of rigid IV devices (e.g., steel-winged "butterfly" needles)
   4. Possible etiologies of peripheral extravasations (Sauerland et al., 2006)
      a) Vein wall puncture, piercing, or trauma
      b) Dislodgment of the catheter from the vein
      c) Administration of a vesicant in a vein below a recent venipuncture site (< 24 hours)
      d) Administration of a vesicant in a vein below a recent or nonhealed vesicant extravasation site

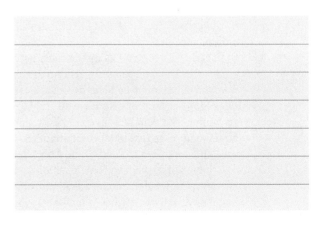

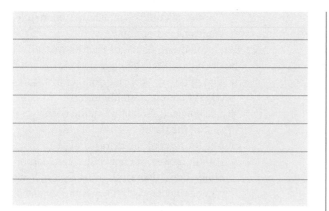

e) Inadvertent IM or SC vesicant administration

5. Risk factors for extravasation from central venous access devices (Sauerland et al., 2006)

   a) Difficulty encountered during device insertion (e.g., probing during venipuncture, inability to advance guide wire and/or catheter)

   b) Inadvertent slicing, piercing, or nicking of catheter prior to or during insertion

   c) Device misplacement with catheter tip outside of the venous system

   d) Inadequately secured noncoring needles (implanted ports)

   e) Deeply implanted ports

   f) Presence of a fibrin sheath or thrombus at the catheter tip

   g) Catheter migration

   h) Long device dwell time (increases risk of catheter fracture secondary to compression or "pinch-off" between the clavicle and first rib)

6. Possible etiologies of extravasations from central venous access devices (Sauerland et al., 2006)

   a) Vein perforation

   b) Catheter leakage, rupture, or fracture

   c) Separation of the catheter from a portal body (implanted ports)

   d) Incomplete insertion of a noncoring needle into an implanted port

   e) Noncoring needle dislodgment from an implanted port

   f) Backflow of vesicant along the catheter to the venotomy site secondary to fibrin sheath or thrombus at the catheter tip

7. Signs and symptoms of vesicant extravasation: Irritation of the vein and flare reactions may mimic some of the signs and symptoms of vesicant extravasation (see Table 10 and Appendix 4). Irritation of the vein and flare reactions are unique to peripheral chemotherapy administration; they do not occur when chemotherapy is

administered via central venous access devices because the chemotherapy is rapidly diluted in large veins (Wickham, Engelking, Sauerland, & Corbi, 2006). Signs and symptoms of vesicant extravasation include the following (Ener et al., 2004).

   a) Swelling (common)

   b) Redness

   c) Stinging, burning, or pain at the vesicant administration site (not always present)

   d) Loss of a blood return from the IV device

   e) IV flow rate that slows or stops

   f) Leaking around the IV catheter or implanted port needle

8. Possible consequences of vesicant extravasation (Ener et al., 2004; Goolsby & Lombardo, 2006)

   a) Blistering (typically occurs one to two weeks post-extravasation)

   b) Peeling and sloughing of skin (usually begins within two weeks post-extravasation)

   c) Tissue necrosis (usually evident two to three weeks post-extravasation)

      (1) DNA-binding vesicants remain in the tissue for long periods of time. The area of tissue necrosis becomes progressively larger in size and deeper in depth over time.

      (2) Non-DNA-binding vesicants are more easily metabolized in the tissue. Tissue necrosis is generally localized and improves over time.

   d) Damage to tendons, nerves, and joints

   e) Functional and sensory impairment of the affected area

   f) Disfigurement

   g) Loss of limb

9. Vesicant extravasation management: A suspected vesicant extravasation is best assessed and managed using a systematic and collaborative approach that involves the patient, the nurse administering the vesicant, and the oncologist treating the patient.

   a) Initial management of extravasation: When a vesicant extravasation occurs or is suspected (Goolsby & Lombardo, 2006; Schulmeister, 2007a),

      (1) Immediately STOP administering the vesicant and IV fluids.

      (2) Disconnect the IV tubing from the IV device. Do not remove the IV device or noncoring port needle.

      (3) Attempt to aspirate residual vesicant from the IV device or port needle using a small (1–3 cc) syringe.

      (4) Remove the peripheral IV device or port needle.

Table 10. Signs and Symptoms Associated With Vesicant Extravasation, Venous Irritation, and Flare Reaction

Signs and Symptoms	Vesicant Extravasation		Irritation of the Vein	Flare Reaction
	Immediate Manifestations	**Delayed Manifestations**		
Pain	Pain typically occurs and is described as burning, stinging, or a sensation of coolness at and around the vesicant administration site. However, some patients do not experience pain when a vesicant extravasates.	Pain usually increases in intensity over time.	Aching and tightness along a peripheral vein, above the administration site, occurs as the drug infuses.	No pain; the skin overlying the vein may itch.
Redness	Redness in the area of the vesicant administration site commonly occurs but is not always present or may be difficult to detect if the extravasation is occurring deeper in the tissue (e.g., as a result of needle dislodgment from implanted port).	Redness generally intensifies over time.	The vein may appear reddened or darkened.	Immediate blotches or streaks develop along the vein, which usually subside within a few minutes. Wheals may appear along the vein.
Swelling	Swelling commonly is observed and is easier to detect when extravasation is superficial (e.g., from a peripheral vein) rather than deep in the tissue (e.g., implanted ports).	Swelling typically increases over time.	Swelling does not occur.	Swelling does not occur.
Blood return	Loss of blood return from IV device occurs.	–	Blood return should be present. If loss of blood return occurs, suspect infiltration of irritant.	Blood return is present.
Ulceration	Skin integrity is intact.	If vesicant extravasation is not treated, blistering and sloughing begins within 1–2 weeks, followed by tissue necrosis that may require surgical debridement and skin grafting or flap placement.	Ulceration does not occur.	Ulceration does not occur.

Note. Based on information from Goolsby & Lombardo, 2006; Sauerland et al., 2006; Schulmeister, 2007a.

(5) Assess the site of the suspected extravasation.
(6) Assess symptoms experienced by the patient (e.g., pain, impairment of range of motion of extremity).
(7) Notify the physician or advanced practice nurse.
(8) Initiate appropriate management measures in accordance with Table 11 and institutional policies.

b) Vesicant extravasation antidotes and treatments
   (1) Efficacy: The efficacy of extravasation antidotes and treatments is unknown, with the exception of dexrazoxane for injection (Totect®), which has a 98.2% overall efficacy. In two European studies, 53 of 54 patients with biopsy-confirmed anthracycline extravasations did not require surgical intervention. The median baseline extravasation area was 25 cm² (range 1–253 cm²), and 11 patients had extravasation areas exceeding 75 cm². Thirteen patients had late sequelae at the event site such as site pain, fibrosis, atrophy, and local sensory disturbance; all were judged as mild (Mouridsen et al., 2006; Schulmeister, 2007b).

   (2) Anecdotal reports: No clinical (human) studies have been conducted on the efficacy of dimethyl sulfoxide, growth factors, early surgical intervention, saline washout, or hyperbaric oxygen in treating biopsy-confirmed vesicant extravasations. Information about these

Table 11. Vesicant Extravasation Management Guidelines

Drug Classification and Medication Name	Immediate Topical Therapy	Antidote or Treatment	Antidote or Treatment Administration, Patient Monitoring, and Follow-Up
Alkylating agents • Mechlorethamine hydrochloride (nitrogen mustard, Mustargen®)	Apply ice for 6–12 hours following sodium thiosulfate antidote injection (Merck and Co., Inc., 2005).	<u>Antidote:</u> Sodium thiosulfate <u>Mechanism of action:</u> Neutralizes mechlorethamine to form nontoxic thioesters that are excreted in the urine <u>Preparation:</u> Prepare 1/6 molar solution. • If 10% sodium thiosulfate solution: Mix 4 ml with 6 ml sterile water for injection. • If 25% sodium thiosulfate solution: Mix 1.6 ml with 8.4 ml sterile water. <u>Storage:</u> Store at room temperature between 15°–30°C (59°–86°F).	Inject 2 ml of the sodium thiosulfate solution for each milligram of mechlorethamine suspected to have extravasated. Inject the solution subcutaneously into the extravasation site using a 25-gauge or smaller needle (change needle with each injection). Assess the extravasation area for pain, blister formation, and skin sloughing periodically as needed or in accordance with institutional policy. Instruct the patient to monitor the extravasation site and report fever, chills, blistering, skin sloughing, and worsening pain. Instruct patients with peripheral extravasations to report arm or hand swelling and stiffness.
Anthracyclines • Daunorubicin (Cerubidine®) • Doxorubicin (Adriamycin®) • Epirubicin (Ellence®) • Idarubicin (Idamycin®)	Apply ice pack (but remove at least 15 minutes prior to Totect® treatment).	<u>Treatment:</u> Totect Note: Totect is a patent-protected, U.S. Food and Drug Administration (FDA)-approved treatment for anthracycline extravasation (TopoTarget USA, 2007). Zinecard® and generic dexrazoxane are neither indicated nor FDA-approved for anthracycline extravasation treatment. There are no therapeutic equivalents to Totect (FDA, 2007). <u>Mechanism of action:</u> Unknown <u>Dose:</u> The recommended dose of Totect is based on the patient's body surface area: • Day one: 1,000 mg/m² • Day two: 1,000 mg/m² • Day three: 500 mg/m² The maximum recommended dose is 2,000 mg on days one and two and 1,000 mg on day three. The dose should be reduced 50% in patients with creatinine clearance values < 40 ml/minute. <u>Preparation:</u> Each vial of Totect 500 mg must be mixed with 50 ml diluent. The patient's dose of Totect is then added to a 1,000 ml normal saline infusion bag for administration. <u>Storage:</u> The Totect emergency treatment kit contains 10 vials of Totect 500 mg and 10 vials of 50 ml diluent and is stored at 25°C (77°F).	The first Totect infusion should be initiated as soon as possible and within 6 hours of the anthracycline extravasation. Totect should be infused over 1–2 hours in a large vein in an area other than the extravasation area (e.g., opposite arm). The same arm should be used only when the patient's clinical status (e.g., lymphedema, loss of limb) precludes use of the unaffected arm, and a large vein distal to the extravasation site should be used for Totect administration. Dimethyl sulfoxide should not be applied to the extravasation area. Assess the extravasation area for pain, blister formation, and skin sloughing periodically as needed or in accordance with institutional policy. Instruct the patient to monitor the extravasation site and report fever, chills, blistering, skin sloughing, and worsening pain. Instruct patients with peripheral extravasations to report arm or hand swelling and stiffness. Instruct the patient about Totect treatment side effects (e.g., nausea/vomiting, diarrhea, stomatitis, bone marrow suppression, elevated liver enzyme levels, infusion site burning). Monitor the patient's complete blood count and liver enzyme levels.

(Continued on next page)

Table 11. Vesicant Extravasation Management Guidelines *(Continued)*

Drug Classification and Medication Name	Immediate Topical Therapy	Antidote or Treatment	Antidote or Treatment Administration, Patient Monitoring, and Follow-Up
Antitumor antibiotics • Mitomycin (Mutamycin®) • Dactinomycin (actinomycin D, Cosmegen®)	Apply ice pack for 15–20 minutes at least four times a day for the first 24 hours.	No known antidotes or treatments	Assess the extravasation area for pain, blister formation, and skin sloughing periodically as needed or in accordance with institutional policy. In collaboration with the physician or advanced practice nurse, refer the patient for specialized care when indicated or needed (e.g., plastic or hand surgery consult, physical therapy, pain management, rehabilitation services).
Plant alkaloid or microtubular inhibiting agents • Vinblastine (Velban®) • Vincristine (Oncovin®) • Vindesine • Vinorelbine (Navelbine®)	Apply warm pack for 15–20 minutes at least four times per day for the first 24–48 hours. Elevate extremity (peripheral extravasations).	Antidote: Hyaluronidase Mechanism of action: Degrades hyaluronic acid and promotes drug diffusion Preparation: Available hyaluronidase preparations are • Amphadase™ [bovine] (hyaluronidase injection (Amphastar Pharmaceuticals, 2005). – Vial contains 150 units per 1 ml. Do not dilute. Use solution as provided. – Store in refrigerator at 2°–8°C (36°–46°F). • Hydase™ (hyaluronidase injection) – Vial contains 150 units per 1 ml. Do not dilute. Use solution as provided. Store in refrigerator at 2°–8°C (36°–46°F). • Hylenex® [recombinant] (hyaluronidase human injection (Baxter Healthcare Corporation, 2006) – Vial contains 150 units per 1 ml. Do not dilute. Use solution as provided. Store in refrigerator at 2°–8°C (36°–46°F). • Vitrase® [ovine] (hyaluronidase injection (ISTA Pharmaceuticals, 2007) – Vial contains 200 units in 2 ml vial. Dilute 0.75 ml of solution with 0.25 ml of 0.9% sodium chloride (final concentration is 150 units per 1 ml). Store in refrigerator at 2°–8°C (36°–46°F).	Administer 1 ml of the hyaluronidase solution as five separate injections, each containing 0.2 ml of hyaluronidase, subcutaneously into the extravasation site using a 25-gauge or smaller needle (change needle with each injection). Assess the extravasation area for pain, blister formation, and skin sloughing periodically as needed or in accordance with institutional policy. Instruct the patient to monitor the extravasation site and report fever, chills, blistering, skin sloughing, and worsening pain. Instruct patients with peripheral extravasations to report arm or hand swelling and stiffness.
Taxanes • Docetaxel (Taxotere®) • Paclitaxel (Taxol®)	Apply ice pack for 15–20 minutes at least four times a day for the first 24 hours.	No known antidote or treatment. Docetaxel extravasation may cause hyperpigmentation, redness, and tenderness (Sanofi-Aventis, 2007). Paclitaxel is a mild vesicant; extravasation may cause induration, blistering, and rarely tissue necrosis (Bristol-Myers Squibb, 2003; Stanford & Hardwicke, 2003).	Assess the extravasation area for pain, blister formation, and skin sloughing periodically as needed or in accordance with institutional policy. Instruct the patient to monitor the extravasation site and report fever, chills, blistering, skin sloughing, and worsening pain. Instruct patients with peripheral extravasations to report arm or hand swelling and stiffness.

antidotes and treatments is anecdotal and based on case reports (Goolsby & Lombardo, 2006; Schrijvers, 2003; Wickham et al., 2006).

10. Documentation of vesicant extravasation and treatment: Key elements that may be included in vesicant extravasation documentation are listed in Figure 17.
    a) Assessment of findings
    b) Concentration and amount of vesicant suspected to have extravasated
    c) Nursing interventions (e.g., topical cooling or heating, notification of physician or advanced practice nurse)
    d) Extravasation treatments/antidotes utilized
    e) Follow-up recommendations
    f) Patient teaching in accordance with institutional guidelines
    g) Measurements and photographs of the extravasation site per institutional policy

11. Patient follow-up: Dependent upon individual patient needs and institutional policies
    a) Periodically assess the patient's response to extravasation treatment.
    b) Assessment may include inspection and measurement of the extravasation area, skin integrity, presence of pain or other

symptoms, arm/hand mobility (for peripheral extravasations), and sensation.
    c) Obtain follow-up photographs that include the date and time in the photograph per institutional policy.
    d) In collaboration with the physician or advanced practice nurse, refer the patient for specialized care when indicated (e.g., plastic or hand surgery consult, physical therapy, pain management, rehabilitation services).
    e) Instruct the patient to protect the extravasation area from sunlight, monitor the site, and report fever, chills, blistering, skin sloughing, and worsening pain.

B. Irritation
1. Irritants: Chemotherapy agents that may inflame and irritate the peripheral veins include bleomycin, carboplatin, carmustine, dacarbazine, etoposide, gemcitabine, ifosfamide, irinotecan, liposomal daunorubicin, liposomal doxorubicin, and melphalan (Ener et al., 2004).
2. Irritants with vesicant properties
    a) Oxaliplatin (Eloxatin®)
       (1) Classified as a nonvesicant; however, case reports of local pain, inflammation, and tissue necrosis suggest that it is at least an irritant (de Lemos & Walisser, 2005; Kennedy, Donahue, Hoang, & Boland, 2003) and may be a vesicant (Baur, Kienzer, Rath, & Dittrich, 2000).
       (2) Because cold packs cause local vasoconstriction, they may precipitate or worsen the cold neuropathy associated with oxaliplatin.
       (3) A warm compress applied to an oxaliplatin extravasation site is preferable and may reduce local pain and inflammation (Foo, Michael, Toner, & Zalcberg, 2003).
       (4) High-dose dexamethasone (8 mg twice daily for up to 14 days) also has been reported to reduce oxaliplatin extravasation-related inflammation (Kretzschmar et al., 2003).
    b) Vinorelbine (Navelbine®)
       (1) This drug is classified as both a vesicant (Ener et al., 2004; Goolsby & Lombardo, 2006; Hadaway, 2007; Sauerland et al., 2006) and an irritant (de Lemos, 2005; Rittenberg, Gralla, & Rehmeyer, 1995)
       (2) The manufacturer of vinorelbine states that it is an irritant, and extravasation

---

Figure 17. Key Elements of Vesicant Extravasation Documentation

- Date and time that extravasation occurred or was suspected
- Type and size of peripheral venous access device or type of central venous access device and gauge/length of noncoring needle (implanted ports)
- Location and patency of peripheral or central venous access device
- Number and location(s) of venipuncture attempts (for peripheral vesicant administration)
- Description and quality of a blood return before and during vesicant administration
- Vesicant administration technique (e.g., bolus, infusion)
- Concentration and estimated amount of extravasated vesicant
- Symptoms reported by patient (e.g., burning, pain)
- Description of administration site appearance including measurement of edema and/or redness if present
- Photographs of administration site that include date and time in the photograph field
- Assessment of extremity (if applicable) for range of motion and discomfort with movement
- Immediate nursing interventions (e.g., topical cooling or heating, physician notification)
- Follow-up recommendations (e.g., referral to plastic surgery, return appointments)
- Patient teaching (e.g., skin assessment, temperature monitoring, reporting pain)

Note. From "Extravasation Management," by L. Schulmeister, 2007, *Seminars in Oncology Nursing, 23*(3), p. 185. Copyright 2007 by Elsevier Inc. Reprinted with permission.

may cause local tissue necrosis and/or thrombophlebitis (Bedford Labs, 2005).

(3) Data suggest that rapid IV infusion over 6–10 minutes followed by a flush of > 75–124 ml of IV fluid may reduce vinorelbine-induced irritation (de Lemos, 2005).

c) Melphalan (Alkeran®)

(1) Conflicting information exists in the literature about the risk of extravasation associated with melphalan. The drug is listed as neither an irritant nor a vesicant by Dorr (1986) and Camp, Gilmore, Gullatte, and Hutcherson (2007), as an irritant by Ener et al. (2004) and Goolsby and Lombardo (2006), and as a vesicant by Sauerland et al. (2006).

(2) Prescribing information from the package insert states that IV melphalan "may cause local tissue damage should extravasation occur" (GlaxoSmithKline, 2008). It is recommended that the drug is not administered by direct injection into a peripheral vein but rather by injecting it slowly into a fast-running IV infusion via an injection port. In cases of poor peripheral access, melphalan should be administered by central venous line (GlaxoSmithKline).

3. Risk factors for irritation
   a) Small veins
   b) Prior treatment with irritating or sclerosing drugs, such as chemotherapy

4. Possible etiologies of venous irritation
   a) Low pH of infused drug
   b) Concentrated drugs or infusion solutions

5. Signs and symptoms of venous irritation (see Table 10)

6. Management of venous irritation
   a) Application of heat (warm pack) may reduce local discomfort.
   b) Restarting the peripheral IV in a larger vein in another location may be indicated.
   c) Consult with pharmacist to explore diluting irritating medications.
   d) Instruct patients to report the development of a hard cord along the vein, pain, and temperature elevation.

C. Flare reaction: Flare reaction is distinguishable from extravasation by the lack of pain or swelling and the presence of a good blood return (Hayden & Goodman, 2005). In the event of a flare reaction,

1. Verify presence of blood return.
2. Flush the vein slowly with saline and watch for resolution of flare.
3. If resolution does not occur, get a physician's order to administer hydrocortisone. For adults, the dose is 25–50 mg IV followed by a saline flush.
4. Once the flare reaction has resolved if blood return continues to be present, slowly resume infusion of the drug (Hayden & Goodman, 2005).
5. If the drug is to be administered again at a later date, consider premedication with antihistamines and/or corticosteroids. Slowing infusion rates may be helpful (Hayden & Goodman, 2005).
6. Document the episode, including all treatment and the patient's responses, according to institutional policy.

D. Acute infusion reactions: Hypersensitivity, anaphylaxis, and cytokine-release syndrome
   1. Pathophysiology
      a) Hypersensitivity and anaphylaxis related to chemotherapy agents are allergic reactions mediated by the immune system—usually by immunoglobulin E. These reactions may be triggered by the therapeutic agent, the diluent, or the delivery vehicle (solution). Symptoms may range from itching at the injection site to systemic shock. The response usually occurs within 5–30 minutes of the initiation of chemotherapy (Gobel, 2005).
      b) Cytokine-release syndrome, which is commonly referred to as infusion reaction, is a symptom complex that occurs most frequently when MoAbs are administered. This reaction is related to the release of cytokines such as IL-2, IFN, and TNF from the targeted cells and other recruited immune cells, such as lymphocytes (Breslin, 2007).
   2. Risk factors for hypersensitivity and anaphylaxis (Gobel, 2005)

       a) A chemotherapy agent known to cause hypersensitivity reactions (see Figure 18)
       b) Preexisting allergies, such as to foods, drugs, bee stings (Grosen, Siitari, Larrison, Giggelaar, & Roecker, 2000), blood products, and radiographic contrast media
       c) Previous exposure to the agent
       d) Failure to administer known effective prophylactic premedications
  3. Risk factors for cytokine-release syndrome: See Figure 19 (Breslin, 2007; Gobel, 2007; Lenz, 2007).
       a) First infusion of MoAbs
       b) Chemotherapy-naïve patients receiving MoAbs
       c) Patients with leukemia or lymphoma, especially those having high circulating lymphocyte counts (> 25,000/mm³)

Figure 18. Immediate Hypersensitivity Reactions: Predicted Risk of Chemotherapy

High Potential
- L-asparaginase
- Taxanes
  - Paclitaxel
  - Docetaxel
- Platinum compounds
  - Cisplatin
  - Carboplatin
  - Oxaliplatin
- Epipodophyllotoxins
  - Etoposide
  - Teniposide

Occasional Potential
- Anthracyclines
  - Doxorubicin
  - Daunorubicin
  - Idarubicin
  - Epirubicin
- Mercaptopurine
- Azathioprine

Rare Potential
- Bleomycin
- Chlorambucil and melphalan
- Cyclophosphamide and ifosfamide
- Cytarabine and fludarabine
- Dacarbazine
- Dactinomycin
- 5-fluorouracil
- Hydroxyurea
- Methotrexate
- Polyethylene glycol-modified *E. coli asparaginase*
- Vincristine and vinblastine

Note. From "Chemotherapy-Induced Hypersensitivity Reactions," by B.H. Gobel, 2005, *Oncology Nursing Forum, 32*(5), p. 1028. Copyright 2005 by Oncology Nursing Society. Reprinted with permission.

Figure 19. Biotherapy Drugs Associated With Hypersensitivity Reactions and Cytokine-Release Syndromes

Interferon
- Interferon alfa
- Interferon beta (1A and 1B)
- Interferon gamma

Interleukin
- Aldesleukin
- Denileukin diftitox

Monoclonal antibodies (murine)
- Ibritumomab tiuxetan
- Tositumomab

Monoclonal antibodies (chimeric)
- Cetuximab
- Rituximab

Monoclonal antibodies (humanized)
- Alemtuzumab
- Bevacizumab
- Gemtuzumab ozogamicin
- Trastuzumab

Monoclonal antibodies (fully human)
- Panitumumab

Note. Based on information from Gobel, 2007; Lenz, 2007.

  4. Preadministration guidelines: Implement the following steps to prevent and manage hypersensitivity reactions, anaphylaxis, and infusion reactions.
       a) Obtain and record baseline vital signs.
       b) Review the patient's allergy history (e.g., food, medication, environment).
       c) Administer premedications as ordered. Common premedications include an H₁ blocker (diphenhydramine), H₂ blocker (such as cimetidine), acetaminophen (for MoAbs), and dexamethasone.
       d) Ensure that emergency equipment and medications are readily available.
       e) Obtain physician's orders for emergency treatment before drug administration. Written standing orders for management of hypersensitivity and infusion reactions are recommended (Gobel, 2005, 2007; Lenz, 2007; Timoney, Eagan, & Sklarin, 2003).
       f) Instruct the patient to report symptoms of hypersensitivity and infusion reaction.
       g) Monitor for reactions with each treatment; hypersensitivity reactions can occur with a patient's repeated exposure to a drug and at any time during the infusion or the treatment cycle. For example, the incidence of carboplatin hypersensitivity may increase with multiple doses and can occur after the

drug has infused (Gobel, 2005; Winkeljohn & Polovich, 2006).

h) Perform a scratch test or intradermal skin test, or administer a test dose before the initial dose of the drug to a patient who has a high likelihood of a hypersensitivity reaction. For a patient receiving repeated doses of carboplatin, a skin test is suggested after the seventh dose (Markman et al., 2003; Winkeljohn & Polovich, 2006).

  (1) Observe the patient for any local or systemic reaction for a minimum of 30 minutes. If no sign of hypersensitivity is evident, proceed with the initial dosing.

  (2) When administering an IV bolus drug that is associated with hypersensitivity, infuse the drug slowly and continue to observe the patient for signs and symptoms of hypersensitivity.

    (a) Any patient who has had a severe anaphylactic reaction accompanied by hypotension should not be treated again with that agent unless special circumstances exist (Weiss, 2001).

    (b) Avoid administering subsequent doses if a patient is considered sensitized to the drug. If the drug is considered critical to the treatment plan, premedication with antihistamines and/or corticosteroids may prevent a recurrent hypersensitivity reaction (Gobel, 2005; Lenz, 2007; Timoney et al., 2003; Weiss, 2001).

5. Clinical manifestations of hypersensitivity and anaphylaxis (Gobel, 2005)

a) Uneasiness or agitation

b) Tightness in the chest

c) Shortness of breath, with or without wheezing

d) Hypotension

e) Urticaria (hives) or rash

f) Localized or generalized itching

g) Periorbital or facial edema

h) Lightheadedness or dizziness

i) Abdominal cramping, diarrhea, nausea, vomiting (less common)

6. Clinical manifestations of cytokine-release syndrome (severe reactions are characterized by rapid onset and more severe symptoms) (Breslin, 2007)

a) Fever or chills

b) Nausea

c) Hypotension

d) Tachycardia

e) Asthenia

f) Headache

g) Rash

h) Tongue and throat swelling

i) Dyspnea

7. Emergency management of anaphylaxis: The need for emergency management usually arises within 30 minutes of initial administration or an increase in the infusion rate (Gobel, 2005; Timoney et al., 2003). Immediate action is imperative.

a) STOP drug infusion immediately.

b) Maintain an IV line with NS or another appropriate solution.

c) Stay with the patient. Have another staff member notify the physician and emergency team or, if outside the hospital setting, call the local emergency medical service.

d) Place the patient in a supine position if not short of breath or vomiting. Elevate legs for shock (systolic blood pressure < 60 mm/Hg).

e) Monitor vital signs (pulse, respirations, blood pressure, oxygen saturation) every 2 minutes until the patient is stable, then every 5 minutes for 30 minutes, then every 15 minutes.

f) Maintain airway, assessing the patient for increasing edema of the respiratory tract. Administer oxygen if needed. Anticipate the need for cardiopulmonary resuscitation.

g) Administer emergency medications based on symptoms (see Table 12).

h) Provide emotional support to the patient and family.

i) Document all treatments and the patient's response in the medical record.

j) Symptoms of anaphylaxis may recur hours after initial intervention; therefore, patients who have experienced a severe reaction should be hospitalized and monitored closely for 24 hours (Sampson et al., 2006).

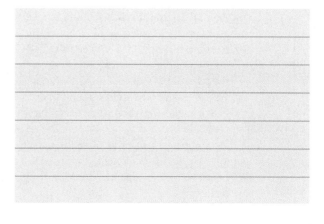

Table 12. Emergency Drugs for Use in Case of Hypersensitivity or Anaphylactic Reaction[a]

Indication	Drug	Dose	Comments
Bronchial constriction (dyspnea, wheezing, stridor)	Epinephrine	0.1–0.5 mg IM into thigh (0.1–0.5 ml of 1:1000 solution or EpiPen® 0.3 mg automatic device)	IM administration is preferred over IV to minimize adverse cardiac effects. Anterior-lateral thigh is preferable to deltoid (may also be administered by inhalation or subcutaneously). May repeat every 5–10 minutes if needed.
Shortness of breath, tachypnea (rate > 20) or decreased oxygen saturation	Oxygen	6–10 L/min by face mask	Patients who are hemodynamically unstable may also benefit from oxygen.
	Albuterol	2.5 mg by inhalation (3 ml of 0.083% inhalation solution) by nebulizer	Hold if heart rate is > 110.
Hypotension (> 30% decrease in systolic blood pressure from baseline)	Epinephrine	0.1–0.5 mg IM into thigh (0.1–0.5 ml of 1:1,000 solution or EpiPen® 0.3 mg automatic device or 5–10 mcg IV bolus (0.2 mcg/Kg) for hypotension (0.5–1.0 ml of 1:10,000 solution)	IM administration is preferred over IV to minimize adverse cardiac effects, except in the presence of cardiovascular collapse. Cardiac monitoring is recommended.
	Normal saline IV	500 ml fluid bolus	Over 10 minutes x 1, then as ordered. Multiple fluid boluses may be required if patient remains hypotensive despite epinephrine.
Hives, itching, flushing, swollen lips or tongue	Diphenhydramine	25–50 mg IVP	To counteract the multiple effects of histamine release, both H_1 and H_2 blockers should be administered.
	Famotidine -OR-	20 mg IV	
	Ranitidine	50 mg IV	
To prevent delayed reaction	Methylprednisolone Hydrocortisone injection Dexamethasone	30–50 mg IV 100–500 mg IV 10–20 mg IV	Limited evidence is available to support this recommendation, although steroids have been used frequently.

[a] Additional emergency medications (e.g., sodium bicarbonate, furosemide, lidocaine, naloxone hydrochloride, sublingual nitroglycerine) and emergency supplies (e.g., oxygen, suction machine with catheters, Ambu® bag) should be available in case of medical emergency. IM—intramuscular; IV—intravenous; IVP—intravenous push

Note. Based on information from Sampson et al., 2006.

8. Clinical management of cytokine-release syndrome (Gobel, 2007; Lenz, 2007)
   a) Stop infusion and observe patient until symptoms resolve, usually within 30 minutes.
   b) Administer additional histamine blockers as ordered.
   c) Resume infusion at a slower rate (50%) after resolution of symptoms, and titrate the rate slowly.
   d) If severe symptoms occur, administer emergency medications according to symptoms (see Table 12).
9. Clinical management of localized hypersensitivity (Hayden & Goodman, 2005)
   a) Observe and evaluate symptoms (e.g., urticaria).

   b) Administer diphenhydramine, cimetidine, and/or corticosteroids per physician's order or according to protocol.
   c) Monitor vital signs at least every 15 minutes for 1 hour or as the patient's condition requires.
   d) Document the episode, including all treatments and the patient's response, according to institutional policies.

E. Patient and family education
   1. Before cytotoxic therapy, inform the patient and family that chemotherapy and biotherapy agents have the potential for immediate complications and instruct them

to immediately report signs and symptoms of extravasation, flare, hypersensitivity, or infusion reactions.

2. Document all patient teaching. Schulmeister and Camp-Sorrell (2000) stated that "plaintiffs in extravasation lawsuits typically deny being informed of the risk of extravasation or state that they were led to believe that the risk was minuscule" (p. 532).

3. After therapy, instruct the patient and family about the importance of immediately reporting symptoms of any delayed reaction.

References

Amphastar Pharmaceuticals. (2005). Amphadase (hyaluronidase injection) [Package insert]. Rancho Cucamonga, CA: Author.

Baur, M., Kienzer, H.R., Rath, T., & Dittrich, C. (2000). Extravasation of oxaliplatin (Eloxatin®)—Clinical course. *Onkologie, 23*(5), 468–471.

Baxter Healthcare Corporation. (2006). Hylenex recombinant (hyaluronidase human injection) [Package insert]. Deerfield, IL: Author.

Bedford Labs. (2005). Vinorelbine [Package insert]. Bedford, OH: Author.

Breslin, S. (2007). Cytokine-release syndrome: Overview and nursing implications. *Clinical Journal of Oncology Nursing, 11*(Suppl. 1), 37–42.

Bristol-Myers Squibb. (2003). Taxol [Package insert]. Princeton, NJ: Author.

Camp, M.J., Gilmore, J.W., Gullatte, M.M., & Hutcherson, D.A. (2007). Antineoplastic agents. In M.M. Gullatte (Ed.), *Clinical guide to antineoplastic therapy: A chemotherapy handbook* (2nd ed., pp. 77–362). Pittsburgh, PA: Oncology Nursing Society.

de Lemos, M.L. (2005). Vinorelbine and venous irritation: Optimal parenteral administration. *Journal of Oncology Pharmacy Practice, 11*(2), 79–81.

de Lemos, M.L., & Walisser, S. (2005). Management of extravasation of oxaliplatin. *Journal of Oncology Pharmacy Practice, 11*(4), 159–162.

Dorr, R.T., Alberts, D.S., & Soble, M. (1986). Lack of experimental vesicant activity for the anticancer agents cisplatin, melphalan, and mitoxantrone. *Cancer Chemotherapy and Pharmacology, 16*(2), 91–94.

Ener, R.A., Meglathery, S.B., & Styler, M. (2004). Extravasation of systemic hemato-oncological therapies. *Annals of Oncology, 15*(6), 858–862.

Foo, K.F., Michael, M., Toner, G., & Zalcberg, J. (2003). A case report of oxaliplatin extravasation. *Annals of Oncology, 14*(6), 961–962.

Gobel, B.H. (2005). Chemotherapy-induced hypersensitivity reactions. *Oncology Nursing Forum, 32*(5), 1027–1035.

Gobel, B.H. (2007). Hypersensitivity reactions to biological drugs. *Seminars in Oncology Nursing, 23*(3), 191–200.

Goolsby, T.V., & Lombardo, F.A. (2006). Extravasation of chemotherapeutic agents: Prevention and treatment. *Seminars in Oncology, 33*(1), 139–143.

Grosen, E., Siitari, E., Larrison, E., Giggelaar, C., & Roecker, E. (2000). Paclitaxel hypersensitivity reactions related to bee-sting allergy. *Lancet, 355*(9200), 288–289.

Hadaway, L. (2007). Infiltration and extravasation. Preventing a complication of IV catheterization. *American Journal of Nursing, 107*(8), 64–72.

Hayden, B.K., & Goodman, M. (2005). Chemotherapy: Principles of administration. In C.H. Yarbro, M.H. Frogge, & M. Goodman (Eds.), *Cancer nursing: Principles and practice* (6th ed., pp. 351–411). Sudbury, MA: Jones and Bartlett.

ISTA Pharmaceuticals. (2007). Vitrase [Package insert]. Irvine, CA: Author.

Kennedy, J.G., Donahue, J.P., Hoang, B., & Boland, P.J. (2003). Vesicant characteristics of oxaliplatin following antecubital extravasation. *Clinical Oncology, 15*(5), 237–239.

Kretzschmar, A., Pink, D., Thuss-Patience, P., Dörken, B., Reichart, P., & Eckert, R. (2003). Extravasation of oxaliplatin. *Journal of Clinical Oncology, 21*(21), 4068–4069.

Lenz, H. (2007). Management and preparedness for infusion and hypersensitivity reactions. *Oncologist, 12*(5) 601–609.

Luedke, D.W., Kennedy, P.S., & Rietschel, R.L. (1979). Histopathogenesis of skin and subcutaneous injury induced by Adriamycin. *Plastic and Reconstructive Surgery, 63*(4), 463–465.

Markman, M., Zanotti, L., Peterson, G., Kulp, B., Webster, K., & Belinson, J. (2003). Expanded experience with an intradermal skin test to predict for the presence or absence of carboplatin hypersensitivity. *Journal of Clinical Oncology, 21*(24), 4611–4614.

Merck and Co., Inc. (2005). Mustargen [Package insert]. Whitehouse Station, NJ: Author.

Mosby's dictionary of medicine, nursing and health professions (7th ed.). (2006). St. Louis, MO: Elsevier Mosby.

Mouridsen, H.T., Langer, S.W., Buter, J., Eidtmann, H., Rosti, G., de Wit, M., et al. (2006). Treatment of anthracycline extravasation with Savene (dexrazoxane). Results from two prospective clinical multicentre studies. *Annals of Oncology, 18*(3), 546–550.

Rittenberg, C.N., Gralla, R.J., & Rehmeyer, T.A. (1995). Assessing and managing venous irritation associated with vinorelbine tartrate (Navelbine). *Oncology Nursing Forum, 22*(4), 707–710.

Sampson, H.A., Munoz-Furlong, A., Campbell, R.L., Adkinson, N.F., Bock, S.A., Branum, A., et al. (2006). Second symposium on the definition and management of anaphylaxis: Summary report—Second National Institute of Allergy and Infectious Disease/Food Allergy and Anaphylaxis Network symposium. *Journal of Allergy and Clinical Immunology, 117*(2), 391–397.

Sanofi-Aventis. (2007). Taxotere [Package insert]. Bridgewater, NJ: Author.

Sauerland, C., Engelking, C., Wickham, R., & Corbi, D. (2006). Vesicant extravasation part I: Mechanisms, pathogenesis, and nursing care to reduce risk. *Oncology Nursing Forum, 33*(6), 1134–1141.

Schrijvers, D.L. (2003). Extravasation: A dreaded complication of chemotherapy. *Annals of Oncology, 14*(Suppl. 3), 26–30.

Schulmeister, L. (2007a). Extravasation management. *Seminars in Oncology Nursing, 23*(3), 184–190.

Schulmeister, L. (2007b). Totect™: A new agent for treating anthracycline extravasation. *Clinical Journal of Oncology Nursing, 11*(3), 387–395.

Schulmeister, L., & Camp-Sorrell, D. (2000). Chemotherapy extravasation from implanted ports. *Oncology Nursing Forum, 27*(3), 531–538.

Stanford, B.L., & Hardwicke, F. (2003). A review of clinical experience with paclitaxel extravasations. *Supportive Care in Cancer, 11*(5), 270–277.

Timoney, J.P., Eagan, M.M., & Sklarin, N.T. (2003). Establishing clinical guidelines for the management of acute hypersensitivity reactions secondary to the administration of chemotherapy/biologic therapy. *Journal of Nursing Care Quality, 18*(1), 80–86.

TopoTarget USA. (2007). Totect [Package insert]. Rockaway, NJ: Author.

U.S. Food and Drug Administration. (2007). *Drugs@FDA drug details: Totect.* Retrieved October 16, 2007, from http://www.accessdata.fda.gov/scripts/cder/drugsatfda/index.cfm?fuseaction=Search.DrugDetails

Weiss, R.B. (2001). Hypersensitivity reactions. In M.C. Perry (Ed.), *The chemotherapy source book* (3rd ed., pp. 436–452). Philadelphia: Lippincott Williams & Wilkins.

Wickham, R., Engelking, C., Sauerland, C., & Corbi, D. (2006). Vesicant extravasation part II: Evidence-based management and continuing controversies. *Oncology Nursing Forum, 33*(6), 1143–1150.

Winkeljohn, D., & Polovich, M. (2006). Carboplatin hypersensitivity reactions. *Clinical Journal of Oncology Nursing, 10*(5), 595–598.

VI. Care of the Patient Receiving Cancer Therapy

A. Patient education
  1. Definitions
     a) Rankin and Stallings (2001) identified patient education as "the most effective means of returning control to the patient by reducing feelings of helplessness and enhancing the ability to be the chief decision-maker in the management of one's health and illness problems" (p. 4).
     b) Patient education, as defined by Bartlett (1985), is "a planned learning experience using a combination of methods such as teaching, counseling, and behavioral modification techniques, which influence patients' knowledge and health behavior" (pp. 323–324).
     c) Aujoulat, d'Hoore, and Deccache (2006) acknowledged that patient education should be directed at empowering the patient and, by definition, must be patient-centered. The process of patient education includes a continuous relationship between the provider and the patient.
  2. Patient teaching is dependent on the following (Blecher, 2004).
     a) Expertise in terms of the information to be given
     b) An understanding of the different ways in which individuals learn
     c) The variety of strategies available for patient education
     d) Matching appropriate strategies to specific content and specific learners
  3. Outcomes of patient education include the following (Blecher, 2004).
     a) Empowering active participation in health care
     b) Explanation of diagnosis and treatment options
     c) Identifying signs and symptoms that need to be reported
     d) Demonstration of the ability to perform self-care and/or adapt to potential limitations
     e) Promoting coping with a life-threatening condition
     f) Enabling autonomous decision making regarding treatment or no treatment
     g) Identification and use of community resources
  4. Methods of patient teaching should be selected based on patients' preferences and abilities (e.g., auditory, visual, by demonstration).

  5. Barriers to patient education
     a) Barriers to learning should be assessed on an individual basis. The following are some common barriers to comprehension (JCAHO, 2004).
        (1) Lack of knowledge of diagnosis and treatment plan
        (2) Expectations regarding treatment, patient/significant other, and healthcare team
        (3) Concerns/misconceptions about therapy because of prior experience or the experience of a friend or relative, which may prevent the patient from undergoing treatment
        (4) Language barriers
        (5) Educational barriers
        (6) Physical barriers: Visual, hearing, and cognitive impairments, as well as the inability to speak, can interfere with patients' comprehension of teaching. Patients may have multiple barriers to comprehension.
     b) Methods of overcoming barriers
        (1) Allow patients to express concerns.
        (2) Correct any misconceptions concerning treatment and follow-up care.
        (3) Provide access to translators, in person or through telecommunications. Note: Significant others are not recommended as translators because of role conflicts or inability to communicate complex medical terminology (Lipson, 1996).
        (4) Cancer-related Spanish-language educational literature is available through NCI at www.cancer.gov.
        (5) Teaching should be tailored to the patient's level of understanding.
        (6) Patients should be assessed individually and information taught at the appropriate level.

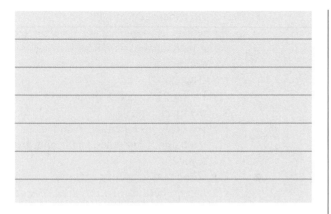

(7) Cancer-related literature for patients with low literacy is available through NCI at www.cancer.gov.

6. Documentation: Nurses need to assess and document patients' understanding of content after instruction takes place to meet regulatory (JCAHO) standards, manage risk, and enhance staff communication (Janousek, Heermann, & Eilers, 2005; JCAHO, 2004; Stolfi, Dudley, Moore, & Johnson, 2007).

B. Adherence to therapy
1. With the increasing numbers of oral therapies available, adherence to the prescribed medication regimen is becoming a concern.
   a) Oral therapies provide greater patient flexibility and are more convenient for patients.
   b) Studies of adherence have identified adherence to oral chemotherapy as a problem (Bendell, 2003; Partridge, Avorn, Wang, & Winer, 2002; Weingart et al., 2007).
2. Additional barriers to adherence
   a) Cost
   b) Complexity of regimen
   c) Side effects
   d) Poor understanding of the importance of adherence
   e) Lack of acceptance of illness because of current state of feeling well (asymptomatic)
3. Optimizing adherence (Partridge et al., 2002; Saca-Hazboun, 2007; Viele, 2007)
   a) Provide patient education.
      (1) Assess readiness to learn.
      (2) Identify necessary information.
      (3) Provide multiple resources, including verbal education, Internet material, and printed materials.
   b) Employ behavior modification.
   c) Use reminder systems.

(1) Pill boxes
(2) Calendars
(3) Diaries
(4) Follow-up telephone calls
   d) Discuss medications at each intervention.
   e) Count pills.
   f) Include caregivers in all discussions.

C. Toxicity management
1. General principles of toxicity management
   a) Cancer therapies can cause side effects.
   b) Combined modality therapy has potential for more side effects than single modality treatment.
   c) Side effects may be exacerbated if the patient
      (1) Has impaired renal or hepatic function
      (2) Has comorbid conditions
      (3) Has protein-calorie malnutrition
      (4) Is younger than one year old or is elderly
      (5) Has a tumor with high growth fractions, which are most affected by cytotoxic therapy, including
         (a) Bone marrow
         (b) Mucosal cells of the gastrointestinal (GI) tract
         (c) Hair follicles and skin
         (d) Organs of the reproductive system.
2. Grading toxicities
   a) Grading toxicities provides an objective assessment.
   b) Accurate grading permits evaluation of interventions implemented to treat toxicities.
   c) Grade of toxicity is the rationale for dosage adjustments or delays.
   d) Most toxicity scales range from 0 to 5; 0 equals no toxicity and 5 indicates severe or life-threatening toxicity.
   e) See Figure 20 for an example of the NCI CTEP CTCAE grading scale for GI symptoms. This scale and others can be accessed via the Internet.
      (1) NCI CTCAE: http://ctep.cancer.gov/forms/CTCAEv3.pdf
      (2) WHO Grading of Acute and Subacute Toxicities: http://whqlibdoc.who.int/offset/WHO_OFFSET_48.pdf
      (3) ECOG Common Toxicity Criteria: www.ecog.org/general/common_tox.html

Figure 20. National Cancer Institute Common Terminology Criteria for Adverse Events: Selected Gastrointestinal Symptoms

Adverse Event	Short Name	Grade				
		1	2	3	4	5
Diarrhea	Diarrhea	Increase of < 4 stools per day over baseline; mild increase in ostomy output compared to baseline	Increase of 4–6 stools per day over baseline; IV fluids indicated < 24 hrs; moderate increase in ostomy output compared to baseline; not interfering with ADL	Increase of ≥ 7 stools per day over baseline; incontinence; IV fluids ≥ 24 hrs; hospitalization; severe increase in ostomy output compared to baseline; interfering with ADL	Life-threatening consequences (e.g., hemodynamic collapse)	Death

Remark: Diarrhea includes diarrhea of small bowel or colonic origin and/or ostomy diarrhea.
Also consider: Dehydration; Hypertension.

Adverse Event	Short Name	Grade				
		1	2	3	4	5
Mucositis/ stomatitis (clinical exam) • Select: – Anus – Esophagus – Large bowel – Larynx – Oral cavity – Pharynx – Rectum – Small bowel – Stomach – Trachea	Mucositis (clinical exam) • Select	Erythema of the mucosa	Patchy ulcerations or pseudomembranes	Confluent ulcerations or pseudomembranes; bleeding with minor trauma	Tissue necrosis; significant spontaneous bleeding; life-threatening consequences	Death

Remark: Mucositis/stomatitis (functional/symptomatic) may be used for mucositis of the upper aerodigestive tract caused by radiation, agents, or GVHD.

Adverse Event	Short Name	Grade				
		1	2	3	4	5
Mucositis/stomatitis (functional/ symptomatic) • Select: – Anus – Esophagus – Large bowel – Larynx – Oral cavity – Pharynx – Rectum – Small bowel – Stomach – Trachea	Mucositis (functional/ symptomatic) • Select	Upper aerodigestive tract sites: Minimal symptoms, normal diet; minimal respiratory symptoms but not interfering with function Lower GI sites: Minimal discomfort, intervention not indicated	Upper aerodigestive tract sites: Symptomatic but can eat and swallow modified diet; respiratory symptoms interfering with function but not interfering with ADL Lower GI sites: Symptomatic, medical intervention indicated but not interfering with ADL	Upper aerodigestive tract sites: Symptomatic and unable to adequately aliment or hydrate orally; respiratory symptoms interfering with ADL Lower GI sites: Stool incontinence or other symptoms interfering with ADL	Symptoms associated with life-threatening consequences	Death

(Continued on next page)

Figure 20. National Cancer Institute Common Terminology Criteria for Adverse Events: Selected Gastrointestinal Symptoms (Continued)

| Adverse Event | Short Name | Grade | | | | |
		1	2	3	4	5
Nausea	Nausea	Loss of appetite without alteration in eating habits	Oral intake decreased without significant weight loss, dehydration or malnutrition; IV fluids indicated < 24 hrs	Inadequate oral caloric or fluid intake; IV fluids, tube feedings, or TPN indicated ≥ 24 hrs	Life-threatening consequences	Death

Also consider: Anorexia; Vomiting.

| Adverse Event | Short Name | Grade | | | | |
		1	2	3	4	5
Vomiting	Vomiting	1 episode in 24 hrs	2–5 episodes in 24 hrs; IV fluids indicated < 24 hrs	≥ 6 episodes in 24 hrs; IV fluids, or TPN indicated ≥ 24 hrs	Life-threatening consequences	Death

Also consider: Dehydration.

Note. From *Common Terminology Criteria for Adverse Events* (Version 3.0), by the National Cancer Institute Cancer Therapy Evaluation Program, 2006. Retrieved October 3, 2008, from http://ctep.cancer.gov/forms/CTCAEv3.pdf

References

Aujoulat, I., d'Hoore, W., & Deccache, A. (2006). Patient empowerment in theory and practice: Polysemy or cacophony? *Patient Education and Counseling, 66*(1), 13–20.

Bartlett, E.E. (1985). At last, a definition [Editoral]. *Patient Education and Counseling, 7*(4), 323–324.

Bendell, C.H. (2003). A changing paradigm for cancer treatment: The advent of new oral chemotherapy agents. *Clinical Journal of Oncology Nursing, 7*(Suppl. 6), 5–24.

Blecher, C.S. (Ed.). (2004). *Standards of oncology education: Patient/significant other and public* (3rd ed.). Pittsburgh, PA: Oncology Nursing Society.

Janousek, L., Heermann, J., & Eilers, J. (2005). Tracking patient education documentation across time and care settings. *American Medical Informatics Association Annual Symposium Proceedings, 2005,* 993.

Joint Commission on Accreditation of Healthcare Organizations. (2004). *Comprehensive accreditation manual for hospitals: The official handbook.* Oakbrook Terrace, IL: Author.

Lipson, J.G. (1996). Culturally competent nursing care. In J.G. Lipson, S. Dibble, & P.A. Minarik (Eds.), *Culture and nursing care: A pocket guide* (pp. 1–6). San Francisco: University of California San Francisco Nursing Press.

Partridge, A.H., Avorn, J., Wang, P., & Winer, E.P. (2002). Adherence to therapy with oral antineoplastic agents. *Journal of the National Cancer Institute, 94*(9), 652–661.

Rankin, S.H., & Stallings, K.D. (2001). *Patient education: Principles and practice* (4th ed.). Philadelphia: Lippincott Williams & Wilkins.

Saca-Hazboun, H. (2007). Empowering patients with knowledge. An update on trends in patient education. *ONS Connect, 22*(5), 8–12.

Stolfi, A., Dudley, G., Moore, K., & Johnson, G. (2007, April). *Enhancing patient assessment, care, and documentation through technology.* Poster presented at the 32nd Annual Oncology Nursing Society Congress, Las Vegas, NV.

Viele, C.S. (2007). Managing oral chemotherapy: The healthcare practitioner's role. *American Journal of Health-System Pharmacy, 64*(9, Suppl. 5), S25–S32.

Weingart, S.N., Flug, J., Brouillard, D., Morway, L., Partridge, A., Bartel, S., et al. (2007). Oral chemotherapy safe practices at US cancer centres: Questionnaire survey. *BMJ, 334*(7590), 407.

VII. Side Effects of Cancer Therapy

A. Myelosuppression: A condition where there is a significant decrease in the neutrophils, megakaryocytes, and erythrocytes within the bone marrow (Gobel & O'Leary, 2007). Terms used in this discussion include the following.
- *Neutropenia:* The condition where there is a marked decrease in circulating neutrophils. Generally defined as an ANC of < 1,500 cells/mm^3 and profound neutropenia (grade 4) as an ANC < 500 cells/mm^3 (Camp-Sorrell, 2005). Neutropenia is further defined by the Infectious Diseases Society of America as an ANC of < 500/mm^3 or an ANC of 500–1,000/mm^3 for patients expected to have further decline (Gobel & O'Leary, 2007; Hughes et al., 2002).
- *Anemia:* A reduction (< 12 g/dl) in normal concentration of hemoglobin (Hgb) or red blood cells (RBCs) in the blood. A decrease in the hematocrit (Hct) or number of RBCs can also be used to define anemia, but Hgb is the value used most often because it reflects the physiologic consequences of anemia (Gobel & O'Leary, 2007).
- *Thrombocytopenia:* The decrease in circulating platelet count below 100,000/mm^3 (Gobel & O'Leary, 2007)
- *Cytopenia:* The lack of cellular elements in circulating blood
- *Nadir:* Following cytotoxic therapy, the time or level at which the lowest blood cell count is reached. The nadir varies with individual agents but usually occurs 7–10 days after treatment (Otto, 2007). Nurses need to be cognizant of cytotoxic therapies with a prolonged nadir, such as the nitrosoureas. Platelet and white blood cell (WBC) counts usually are the first to drop (Gobel & O'Leary, 2007).
- *Hematopoiesis:* The formation and development of blood cells, a process that involves proliferation, differentiation, and maturation (see Figure 21). In adults, most hematopoiesis occurs in the bone marrow, in myeloid tissue.
  - The process begins with hematopoietic stem cells (HSCs), also called pluripotent stem cells (Ososki & O'Riley, 2007). These are the most primitive type of blood cell and the source of all hematopoietic cells. Pluripotent stem cells are able to self-renew and maintain their numbers because they have the capacity to proliferate, differentiate, and mature into all cell lines. With each stem cell division, one daughter cell stays in the stem cell pool while the other daughter cell leaves the stem cell pool and becomes committed to a distinct cell line. These committed progenitor cells differentiate and mature in the bone marrow. Whether the HSCs proliferate or differentiate is determined by the body's needs in response to exogenous (e.g., high altitude) or endogenous (e.g., stress, infection, hemorrhage, drug therapy) influences.
  - Most chemotherapy agents cause some degree of myelosuppression. The degree and duration of chemotherapy-related myelosuppression is related to the agent's mechanism of action (e.g., cell-cycle–specific drugs are associated with rapid cytopenias) (Gobel & O'Leary, 2007). Myelosuppression is known to be more severe in patients whose disease originates in the bone marrow because tumor cells in the marrow physically crowd out progenitor blood cells. Life spans of blood cells vary greatly (see Table 13). Maturation time will vary depending on the cell line.
1. Neutropenia: Chemotherapy-induced neutropenia (CIN) is the primary dose-limiting toxicity associated with systemic chemotherapy (Lyman, 2005). It has significant negative clinical consequences for patients with cancer, including life-threatening infections, prolonged hospital stays, dose reductions, and dose delays.
   a) Normal physiology of neutrophils (see Figure 21)
      (1) Neutrophils and monocytes stem from the colony-forming unit–granulocyte macrophage progenitor cell. The earliest identifiable cell of the neutrophil lineage is the myeloblast. Differentiation from myeloblast to segmented neutrophil takes 7–14 days. Normal bone marrow can produce 60–400 × 10^7 neutrophils each day (Smith, 2006).
      (2) Locations of neutrophils (Gobel & O'Leary, 2007)
         (a) The bone marrow of a healthy adult contains a large number of both

Table 13. Life Spans of Blood Components

Blood Component	Typical Life Span
Red blood cell	90–120 days
Platelet	7–8 days
Neutrophil	7–12 hours
Monocyte	3 days
Macrophage	3 days
Eosinophil	3–8 hours
Basophil	7–12 hours
Tissue mast cell	7–12 hours
B lymphocyte	Depends on type and subtype
T lymphocyte	Depends on type and subtype
Natural killer cell	Unknown

mature and immature neutrophils. It takes 7–14 days for neutrophils to mature in the bone marrow.

(b) Mature and immature neutrophils also exist in the bloodstream. These cells are the body's first line of defense against invading bacteria. Circulating neutrophils have a half-life of six to nine hours.

(c) Marginated neutrophils function as reserve cells by adhering to blood vessel walls and migrating into tissue. Neutrophils stored in extravascular tissue can survive for up to two days (Smith, 2006).

(3) Pathophysiology (Camp-Sorrell, 2005)

(a) The bone marrow must constantly produce neutrophils because the life span of a neutrophil is estimated at only six to eight hours. Chemotherapeutic agents suppress bone marrow activity and damage stem cells; therefore, chemotherapy decreases the neutrophil count as mature neutrophils die and are not replaced.

(b) The WBC nadir depends on the specific drugs and dosages used. A prolonged nadir may occur if the stem cell population fails to repopulate quickly following high-dose chemotherapy (Camp-Sorrell, 2005).

i) Cell-cycle–specific agents (e.g., antimetabolites) produce rapid nadirs in 7–14 days, with neutrophil recovery within 7–21 days (Barton-Burke, Wilkes, & Ingwersen, 2001; Scott, 2004).

ii) Cell-cycle–nonspecific agents (e.g., antitumor antibiotics) cause neutropenia in 10–14 days, with recovery at 21–24 days (Barton-Burke et al., 2001).

iii) Some cell-cycle–nonspecific agents (e.g., nitrosoureas) produce a delayed and prolonged neutropenia.

   • For adults, nadir occurs at 26–63 days, with recovery at 35–89 days (Barton-Burke et al., 2001).

   • For children, nadir occurs at 21–35 days, with recovery at 42–50 days (Scott, 2004).

iv) Agents such as docetaxel can result in an early, short-lasting type of neutropenia at a dose of > 100 mg/m² when infused over one hour every three weeks (Camp-Sorrell, 2005).

(4) Incidence: The incidence of neutropenia varies according to agents, doses, and administration schedule as well as patient factors (e.g., previous treatment, bone marrow involvement) (Camp-Sorrell, 2005).

(5) Risk factors for neutropenia (NCCN, 2008a)

(a) Preexisting neutropenia resulting from disease (Ozer et al., 2000) such as myelodysplastic syndrome (MDS)

(b) Treatment with a highly myelosuppressive chemotherapy regimen

(c) Tumor involvement in the bone marrow

(d) Degeneration of the immune system, which can occur in physiologically elderly patients

(e) Low neutrophil count at the beginning of a chemotherapy cycle

(f) History of febrile neutropenia

(g) Hepatic or renal dysfunction, which may lead to decreased metabolism and excretion of chemotherapeutic agent

Figure 21. Schema of Hematopoiesis

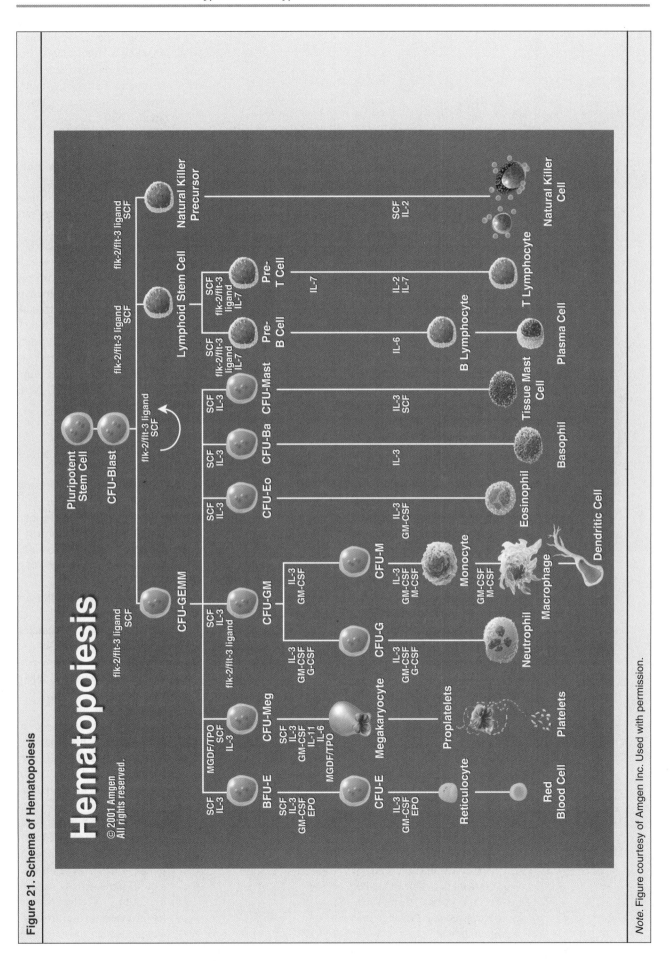

Note. Figure courtesy of Amgen Inc. Used with permission.

        (h) Protein-calorie malnutrition, which decreases the body's ability to manufacture and repair the normal cells destroyed by chemotherapy

        (i) Concurrent use of the following drugs or types of drugs: phenothiazides, diuretics, immunosuppressive agents

        (j) History of radiation therapy

(6) Clinical manifestations of infection in patients with neutropenia (Wujcik, 2004)

    (a) A fever of > 38°C (100.4°F) is the most reliable, and often the only, sign of infection in patients with neutropenia. Normally, WBCs cause the classic signs of infection (e.g., redness, edema, pus). Extremely neutropenic patients, however, may not be able to manifest the usual signs—not even a fever.

    (b) Common sites of infection and corresponding signs and symptoms of infection in neutropenic patients are the following (NCCN, 2008a; Wujcik, 2004).

      i) GI tract: Abdominal pain, alimentary mucositis (mucositis at any level of the digestive tract), or diarrhea

      ii) Respiratory tract: Fever, cough, dyspnea on exertion, and adventitious breath sounds

      iii) Urinary tract: Fever, dysuria, frequency, hematuria, and cloudy urine

      iv) Indwelling devices (e.g., vascular access devices [VADs], ventricular peritoneal shunts): Fever, erythema, pain or tenderness, edema, drainage, and induration at site

      v) Skin and mucous membranes: Erythema, tenderness, hot skin, and edema (especially in axilla, buttocks, mouth, sinuses, or perineal or rectal area)

      vi) Central nervous system (CNS) symptoms: Mental status changes, headache, or seizures (NCCN, 2008b)

    (c) Septic shock associated with neutropenia has a high mortality rate (Lichtman, 2006).

(7) Assessment: Use laboratory data to assess the presence of neutropenia by calculating ANC. Note that neutropenia can occur when the total WBC count is within a normal range (4,000–10,000/mm^3) (Gobel & O'Leary, 2007). Consequently, calculating the ANC is essential to achieving a correct assessment of neutrophil status (Camp-Sorrell, 2005). To calculate ANC, ANC = % (polys + bands) × WBC.

    (a) Obtain complete WBC count, including differential.

    (b) Add neutrophils (polys [segs] and bands).

    (c) Convert sum from (2) to percentage.

    (d) Multiply total WBC count by total neutrophil percentage (polys + bands). ANC calculation example: WBC count = 1,600, polys = 48, bands = 5.

      i) Add polys and bands: 48 + 5 = 53.

      ii) Convert sum to percentage: 53 ÷ 100 = 0.53 = 53%.

      iii) Multiply WBC count by percentage to find ANC: 1,600 × 0.53 = 848.

(8) Collaborative management

    (a) Nurses play an important role in preventing infection in patients with cancer through evidence-based nursing practice, research, and patient education (Zitella et al., 2006).

      i) Proper hand hygiene reduces the risk of healthcare-associated infections by decreasing person-to-person transmission of pathogens (Zitella et al., 2006). Protective isolation has no effect on the host's endogenous flora and no impact on organisms transmitted by water or food.

ii) Diet: There have been no recent studies linking neutropenic diets (restricting fresh fruits and vegetables) with lower risk of infection for neutropenic patients with cancer. Dietary precautions regarding the omission of fresh fruits and vegetables remain unsupported (Gardner, 2007; Wilson, 2002; Zitella et al., 2006). Basic safe food handling practices—such as avoiding uncooked meats, seafood, eggs, and unwashed fruits and vegetables—should be employed (Wilson).

iii) Environment (Zitella et al., 2006)
- Patients with airborne respiratory viruses including varicella and tuberculosis (TB) should be in rooms with an anteroom to maintain proper air balance. HEPA filters are to be used for air recirculation. Use portable HEPA filters if anteroom not available.
- Protective or strict isolation studies reveal no significant differences in documented infections, febrile episodes, or antibiotic use for patients with CIN.

iv) Plants (Zitella et al., 2006)
- Because fresh or dried flowers could expose patients with cancer to *Aspergillus*, they should be kept out of patient rooms.
- If plants must be present, plant care should be done by staff not directly caring for patients.
- If patient care staff are unable to avoid plant care, they should wear gloves and perform hand hygiene after removing gloves.
- Water in vases should be changed every two days, emptying water outside the patient's room.
- Vases should be disinfected after use.

v) Treatment with colony-stimulating factors (CSFs) (see Table 14): The development of CSFs has had an enormous impact on reducing the incidence of infection related to chemotherapy.
- Filgrastim and pegfilgrastim are approved by the FDA for the prevention of CIN. These drugs are recommended when the risk of febrile neutropenia is > 20% (Amgen Inc., 2007b; NCCN, 2008b).
- Sargramostim (granulocyte macrophage–CSF [GM-CSF]) is FDA approved only for acceleration of bone marrow recovery (recovery of myeloid cells) after autologous or allogeneic BMT (Bayer HealthCare, 2008).
- Both G-CSF and GM-CSF are indicated for use following induction chemotherapy in acute myeloid leukemia (AML), for mobilization of peripheral blood progenitor cells (PBPCs), following transplantation of autologous PBPCs, and in BMT failure or engraftment delay (Wilkes & Barton-Burke, 2006).
- The manufacturer recommends initiation of G-CSF no earlier than 24 hours following chemotherapy and continuing daily up to

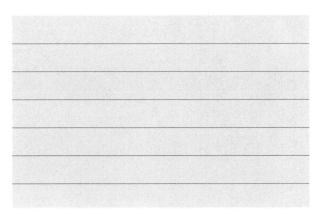

Table 14. Growth Factors

Classification	Mechanism of Action	Medication Name(s)	Route of Administration	Indications	Side Effects	Nursing Considerations
Colony-stimulating factor	Stimulates erythropoiesis via the same mechanism as endogenous erythropoietin	Darbepoetin (Aranesp®)	SC	Treatment of anemia associated with chronic renal failure whether or not the patient is receiving dialysis Treatment of anemia in patients with nonmyeloid malignancies where anemia is caused by concomitantly administered chemotherapy	Hypertension, skin rash, urticaria, pure red cell aplasia, myalgia, infection, fatigue edema, diarrhea, thrombotic events	Increased risk of death and serious cardiovascular events exists when administered if hemoglobin is greater than 12 g/dl. Ensure adequate iron stores in patients prior to and during use. Agent may be administered every 1, 2, or 3 weeks but should maintain consistent dosing schedule. Use lowest effective dose. Do not shake vials or syringes containing drug. Store in refrigerator. Do not freeze.
	Stimulates erythropoiesis via the same mechanism as endogenous erythropoietin	Epoetin alfa (Procrit®)	SC	Treatment of anemia associated with chronic renal failure whether or not the patient is receiving dialysis Treatment of anemia associated with treatment using zidovudine in HIV-infected patients Treatment of anemia in patients with nonmyeloid malignancies where anemia is caused by concomitant use of chemotherapy Treatment of anemia in patients scheduled to undergo elective noncardiac, nonvascular surgery to reduce the need for allogeneic red blood cell transfusions	Hypertension, skin rash, urticaria, pure red cell aplasia, myalgia, infection, fatigue edema, diarrhea, thrombotic events	Increased risk of death and serious cardiovascular events exists when administered if hemoglobin is greater than 12 g/dl. Ensure adequate iron stores in patients prior to and during use. Agent may be given three times weekly or once weekly. Use lowest effective dose. Do not shake vials or syringes containing drug. Store in refrigerator. Do not freeze.

(Continued on next page)

Table 14. Growth Factors (Continued)

Classification	Mechanism of Action	Medication Name(s)	Route of Administration	Indications	Side Effects	Nursing Considerations
Colony-stimulating factor (cont.)	Regulates the production of neutrophils within the bone marrow	Filgrastim (G-CSF, Neupogen®)	SC, IV	Used to decrease the incidence of infection in patients with neutropenic fever associated with myelosuppressive anticancer treatments for nonmyeloid malignancies Used to reduce the time to neutrophil recovery and duration of fever following induction or consolidation chemotherapy in patients with AML Used to reduce the duration of neutropenia and associated sequelae in patients receiving myeloablative chemotherapy prior to marrow transplant Used to mobilize hematopoietic progenitor cells into peripheral blood for collection via leukapheresis Used for chronic administration to reduce the incidence and duration of sequelae of neutropenia in patients with congenital neutropenia, cyclic neutropenia, or idiopathic neutropenia	Allergic reactions including urticaria, rash, and facial edema; risk of rare splenic rupture; adult respiratory distress syndrome, nausea, vomiting, bone pain secondary to rapid growth of myeloid cells in the bone marrow, fever	Store in refrigerator. Do not freeze. Agent may be diluted with 5% dextrose in water. Do not dilute with saline solutions. Do not shake.
	Stimulates keratinocyte growth factor receptor resulting in proliferation, differentiation, and migration of epithelial cells	Palifermin (rHuKGF, Kepivance®)	IV	Used to decrease the incidence and duration of severe oral mucositis in patients with hematologic malignancies receiving myelosuppressive chemotherapy prior to hematopoietic stem cell transplant	Skin rash, skin erythema, pruritus, fever, dysesthesia, tongue discoloration, tongue thickening, alteration of taste, pain arthralgias, elevated serum amylase, elevated serum lipase	Do not use within 24 hours before, during, or after administration of myelosuppressive chemotherapy. Administer for 3 days before and then 3 days after myelosuppressive chemotherapy. Do not shake reconstituted solution. Reconstituted product should not be used if stored at room temperature for more than 1 hour. Do not filter reconstituted solution.

(Continued on next page)

Table 14. Growth Factors (Continued)

Classification	Mechanism of Action	Medication Name(s)	Route of Administration	Indications	Side Effects	Nursing Considerations
Colony-stimulating factor (cont.)	Regulates the production of neutrophils within the bone marrow	Pegfilgrastim (Neulasta®)	SC	Decreases the incidence of infection related to neutropenia in patients with nonmyeloid malignancies receiving myelosuppressive chemotherapy	Allergic reactions including urticaria, rash, facial edema; risk of rare splenic rupture; adult respiratory distress syndrome, nausea, vomiting, bone pain secondary to rapid growth of myeloid cells in the bone marrow, fever	Pegfilgrastim has reduced renal clearance and prolonged persistence compared to filgrastim. Do not administer in the period beginning 14 days before until 24 hours after administration of myelosuppressive chemotherapy. Administer as a single 6 mg injection once per chemotherapy cycle. The 6 mg fixed dose should not be administered to children or adolescents weighing less than 45 kg. Store in refrigerator. Do not freeze. Do not shake.
	Induces committed progenitor cells to divide and differentiate in the granulocyte-macrophage pathways including neutrophils, monocytes/macrophages, and myeloid-derived dendritic cells	Sargramostim (GM-CSF, Leukine®)	SC, IV	Used following induction chemotherapy in patients with AML to shorten neutrophil recovery and reduce incidence of infection. Used in patients for the mobilization of hematopoietic progenitor cells for collection via leukapheresis and to speed engraftment following autologous transplantation of progenitor cells. Used to accelerate myeloid recovery following allogeneic BMT. Used in patients with failure of engraftment following BMT	Edema, capillary leak syndrome, pleural or pericardial effusions, dyspnea, fever, abdominal pain, headache, chills, diarrhea, bone pain secondary to rapid growth of myeloid cells in the bone marrow	Dilution for IV use should be in NS solution. Store in refrigerator. Do not freeze. Do not shake. Do not administer through in-line filter.

(Continued on next page)

Table 14. Growth Factors (Continued)

Classification	Mechanism of Action	Medication Name(s)	Route of Administration	Indications	Side Effects	Nursing Considerations
Thrombopoietic growth factor	Stimulation of megakaryocytopoiesis and thrombopoiesis	Oprelvekin (IL-11, Neumega®)	SC	Prevents severe thrombocytopenia and reduces the need for platelet transfusions in patients receiving chemotherapy	Anaphylaxis, dilutional anemia, diarrhea, dizziness, fever, fluid retention resulting in peripheral edema, pulmonary edema, dyspnea, capillary leak syndrome, atrial arrhythmias, and exacerbation of preexisting pulmonary effusions, headache, nausea, vomiting, insomnia, rhinitis	Store in refrigerator but do not freeze. Reconstitute with sterile water. Should be used within 3 hours of reconstitution. Do not shake or freeze following reconstitution. Protect from light.

AML—acute myeloid leukemia; BMT—bone marrow transplant; G-CSF—colony-stimulating factor; GM-CSF—granulocyte macrophage–colony-stimulating factor; IV—intravenous; NS—normal saline; SC—subcutaneous

Note. Based on information from manufacturers' prescribing information.

14 days, until post-nadir ANC > 10,000/mm^3 is achieved (Amgen Inc., 2007a, 2007b).

- Pegfilgrastim is administered as a single 6 mg injection once per chemotherapy cycle and should not be administered in the period between 14 days before and 24 hours after chemotherapy (Amgen Inc., 2007a).

vi) Prevent trauma to the patient's skin and mucous membranes (Gobel & O'Leary, 2007).

- Provide meticulous care to all indwelling devices.
- Prevent pressure sores and constipation.
- Cleanse and protect wounds as directed.
- Change water in pitchers, denture cups, and nebulizers at least daily.
- Consider risk-benefit ratio for invasive procedures (e.g., thoracentesis, paracentesis, percutaneous endoscopic gastrostomy tube placement, VAD placement).

vii) Teach neutropenic patients protective measures that they can employ (Camp-Sorrell, 2005; Gobel & O'Leary, 2007; Zitella et al., 2006).

- Personal hygiene
  - Wash hands frequently with soap and water or an antiseptic hand rub. Hands may remain colonized with microorganisms if they are not dried properly after hand washing.
  - Bathe daily.
  - Protect skin from cuts and burns. Immediately cleanse and treat any wound that breaks the skin.
  - Wear gloves when working in the garden.
  - Perform frequent oral care (at least three to four times per day).

- Cleanse the perineal area after voiding and bowel movements.
- Use only an electric razor to shave unwanted body hair.
- Avoid/manage exposure to pathogens (e.g., wear a surgical face mask).
- Avoid people with colds or contagious illnesses (e.g., chicken pox, herpes zoster, influenza).
- Consider obtaining influenza and pneumonia vaccines.
- Avoid contact with people who have been vaccinated with a live vaccine within the past 30 days (Centers for Disease Control and Prevention, 1993).
- Do not share food utensils.
- Do not provide direct care for pets or farm animals; avoid contact with animal feces, saliva, urine, litter box contents, and barns.
- Refrain from direct or indirect contact with reptiles, fish, and birds.
- Do not receive live vaccinations (e.g., oral vaccination for polio, varicella, smallpox; nasal flu vaccine).
- Avoid exposure to fresh or dried plants and flowers because of risk of *Aspergillus* infection.

Plant care may be done by staff not directly providing care to patient.
- Do not enter, travel through, or stay in areas of construction/renovation or where construction material/debris have been placed or where fields have recently been plowed.
- Do not eat meat or any food that has not been either cooked or washed. Adhere to safe food handling practices, and avoid consuming food when safety of preparation, storage, or serving is not guaranteed.

(b) Management of neutropenic fever: Data regarding the efficacy of CSFs after a patient is diagnosed with febrile neutropenia are inconclusive (Camp-Sorrell, 2005). To manage neutropenic fever, the clinician should
  i) Culture the following (NCCN, 2008b).
    • Urine: If symptomatic, with catheter, or if urinalysis abnormal
    • Blood: Two sets (one set includes two bottles). If patient has a central VAD (CVAD), options include
      - One peripheral and one CVAD
      - Both peripheral or both CVAD
      - Other suspected sources of infection.
    • Stool: For diarrhea, obtain *Clostridium difficile* assay and enteric pathogen screen.
    • Skin: Aspirate/biopsy skin lesions.
    • VAD cutaneous site: Consider routine fungal/*Mycobacterium* culture if inflammation is present.
    • Vesicular/ulcerated lesions for viral cultures
    • Throat/nasopharynx when respiratory viral symptoms

are present, especially during seasonal outbreaks

ii) Conduct site-specific history and physical in an attempt to identify the source of infection (NCCN, 2008b).

- Assess VADs, skin, lungs, sinus, mouth, pharynx, esophagus, bowel, rectum, and perivaginal and perirectal areas for signs and symptoms of infection.
- Obtain historical data including comorbidities, date and regimen of last chemotherapy, previous infections, recent antibiotic therapy/prophylaxis, medications, and HIV status. Explore exposure risks including anyone at home with similar symptoms, pets, travel, recent blood product administration, or TB exposure.

iii) For all adults, obtain a chest x-ray (CXR) when respiratory symptoms present. For children, obtain a CXR only if the patient's condition warrants.

iv) Administer empiric antibiotics, which should include coverage for gram-positive and gram-negative organisms as ordered until organism source is identified.

v) Monitor blood culture reports daily.

(c) Patient and family education

i) Teach patients and significant others to report the following.

- Temperature elevation > 38°C (100.4°F)
- Shaking chills (rigors)
- Dysuria
- Dyspnea
- Respiratory congestion or sputum production
- Pain

ii) Reinforce the need for meticulous hygiene.

iii) Teach patients and significant others SC injection technique for G-CSF or GM-CSF administration if applicable.

References

Amgen Inc. (2007a). Neulasta [Package insert]. Thousand Oaks, CA: Author.

Amgen Inc. (2007b). Neupogen [Package insert]. Thousand Oaks, CA: Author.

Barton-Burke, M., Wilkes, G.M., & Ingwersen, K.C. (2001). *Cancer chemotherapy: A nursing process approach* (3rd ed.). Sudbury, MA: Jones and Bartlett.

Bayer HealthCare. (2008). Leukine [Package insert]. Seattle, WA: Author.

Camp-Sorrell, D. (2005). Chemotherapy toxicities and management. In C.H. Yarbro, M.H. Frogge, & M. Goodman (Eds.), *Cancer nursing: Principles and practice* (6th ed., pp. 412–457). Sudbury, MA: Jones and Bartlett.

Centers for Disease Control and Prevention. (1993). Recommendations of the Advisory Committee on Immunization Practices (ACIP): Use of vaccines and immune globulins in persons with altered immunocompetence. *Morbidity and Mortality Weekly Report, 42*(No. RR-4). Retrieved October 1, 2008, from http://www.cdc.gov/mmwr/preview/mmwrhtml/00023141.htm

Gardner, A. (2007, April). *Neutropenic diet with leukemia patients.* Paper presented at the 32nd Annual Congress of the Oncology Nursing Society, Las Vegas, NV.

Gobel, B.H., & O'Leary, C. (2007). Bone marrow suppression. In M.E. Langhorne, J.S. Fulton, & S.E. Otto (Eds.), *Oncology nursing* (5th ed., pp. 488–504). St. Louis, MO: Elsevier Mosby.

Hughes, W.T., Armstrong, D., Bodey, G.P., Bow, E.J., Brown, A.E., Calandra, T., et al. (2002). 2002 guidelines for the use of antimicrobial agents in neutropenic patients with cancer [Electronic version]. *Clinical Infectious Diseases, 34*(6), 730–751.

Lichtman, M.A. (2006). Classification and clinical manifestations of neutrophil disorders. In M.A. Lichtman, E. Beutler, J.K. Thomas, U. Seligsohn, K. Kawshansky, & J.T. Prchal (Eds.), *Williams hematology* (7th ed., pp. 899–905). Columbus, OH: McGraw-Hill.

Lyman, G.H. (2005). Guidelines of the National Comprehensive Cancer Network on the use of myeloid growth factors with cancer chemotherapy: A review of the evidence. *Journal of the National Comprehensive Cancer Network, 3*(4), 557–571.

National Comprehensive Cancer Network. (2008a). *NCCN Clinical Practice Guidelines in Oncology™: Myeloid growth factors* [v.1.2008]. Retrieved October 24, 2008, from http://www.nccn.org/professionals/physician_gls/PDF/myeloid_growth.pdf

National Comprehensive Cancer Network. (2008b). *NCCN Clinical Practice Guidelines in Oncology™: Prevention and treatment of cancer-related infections* [v.1.2008]. Retrieved October 24, 2008, from http://www.nccn.org/professionals/physician_gls/PDF/infections.pdf

Ososki, R.E., & O'Riley, K. (2007). Leukemia. In M.E. Langhorne, J.S. Fulton, & S.E. Otto (Eds.), *Oncology nursing* (5th ed., pp. 232–257). St. Louis, MO: Elsevier Mosby.

Otto, S. (2007). Chemotherapy. In M.E. Langhorne, J.S. Fulton, & S.E. Otto (Eds.), *Oncology nursing* (5th ed., pp. 362–376). St. Louis, MO: Elsevier Mosby.

Ozer, H., Armitage, J.O., Bennett, C.L., Crawford, J., Demetri, G.D., & Pizzo, P.A. (2000). 2000 update of recommendations for the use of hematopoietic colony-stimulating factors: Evidence-based, clinical practice guidelines. American Society of Clinical Oncology Growth Factors Expert Panel. *Journal of Clinical Oncology, 18*(20), 3558–3585.

Scott, T.E. (2004). Neutropenia. In N.E. Kline (Ed.), *Essentials of pediatric oncology nursing: A core curriculum* (2nd ed., pp. 67–69). Glenview, IL: Association of Pediatric Oncology Nurses.

Smith, C.W. (2006). Production, distribution, and fate of neutrophils. In M.A. Lichtman, E. Beutler, J.K. Thomas, U. Seligsohn, K. Kawshansky, & J.T. Prchal (Eds.), *Williams hematology* (7th ed., pp. 855–861). Columbus, OH: McGraw-Hill.

Wilkes, G.M., & Barton-Burke, M. (2006). *2006 oncology nursing drug handbook.* Sudbury, MA: Jones and Bartlett.

Wilson, B.J. (2002). Dietary recommendations for neutropenic patients. *Seminars in Oncology Nursing, 18*(2), 44–49.

Wujcik, D. (2004). Infection. In C.H. Yarbro, M.H. Frogge, & M. Goodman (Eds.), *Cancer symptom management* (3rd ed., pp. 252–267). Sudbury, MA: Jones and Bartlett.

Zitella, L., Friese, C., Gobel, B.H., Woolery-Antill, M., O'Leary, C., Hauser, J., et al. (2006). Putting Evidence Into Practice: Prevention of infection. *Clinical Journal of Oncology Nursing, 10*(6), 739–750.

2. Anemia
   a) Erythropoiesis: Normal production and role of RBCs
      (1) Erythropoietin (EPO), produced mostly in the kidneys, is the primary growth factor for the production of RBCs. RBCs are produced in the bone marrow and then reside in the sternum, ribs, vertebrae, pelvis, and proximal end of the femur and humerus. The Hgb molecule transports oxygen from the lungs to body tissue(s). Carbon dioxide is then returned from the tissues to the lungs (Gillespie & Berger, 2004; Spivak, 2002).
      (2) In response to hypoxia, EPO interacts with the progenitor stem cells to increase RBC production (Amgen Inc., 2008a).
   b) Iron is necessary for the normal production of RBCs. It is carried to the precursor cells by transferrin, where it is then incorporated into a heme molecule and stored as ferritin in various tissues. Daily dietary sources of iron are needed to maintain iron stores (Kogut & Luthringer, 2005; Loney & Chernecky, 2000). The major steps of erythropoiesis follow (see Figure 21).
      (1) A pluripotent stem cell develops into a progenitor cell committed to the development of RBCs.
      (2) The stem cell divides and matures to form a reticulocyte.
      (3) Hgb synthesis begins at the erythroblast stage. RBCs develop increased amounts of Hgb as they mature in the bone marrow. Approximately 25% of Hgb is synthesized after reticulocytes leave the marrow (Bron, Meuleman, & Mascaux, 2001; Dessypris, 1999; Spivak, 2002).

   c) The role of EPO in erythropoiesis: EPO is a glycoprotein cytokine produced chiefly by the interstitial cells of the kidney in response to hypoxia (Gillespie & Berger, 2004). More than 90% of EPO is produced in the kidneys, with a very small amount produced in the liver. When EPO is secreted into the plasma, erythrocyte precursor cells in the bone marrow are stimulated and RBC production and maturation are accelerated (Loney & Chernecky, 2000). Because EPO is essential for erythropoiesis, even a slight underproduction of this glycoprotein can result in anemia (Gillespie & Berger). Although erythropoiesis was originally thought to be the sole physiologic function of EPO, it is now known that EPO receptors in tissue are not limited to hematopoietic cells. Active EPO receptors also have been identified on endothelial, renal, neuronal, and cardiac cells in vitro (Smith, 2004). This fact helps to explain many of the neuropathic toxicities experienced by patients with anemia. EPO stimulates increased production of RBCs by
      (1) Increasing the number of stem cells committed to the red cell line
      (2) Shortening the time a stem cell takes to become a mature RBC (Erickson, 1996).
   d) RBC mass and volume: EPO production and erythropoiesis usually are orderly and continuous processes that result in a constant circulating RBC mass for each individual, but this volume may vary by more than 10% in people of the same age and gender (Loney & Chernecky, 2000).
   e) RBC life span: A typical RBC can survive 90–120 days. This span, longer than that of a neutrophil or platelet, is the primary reason anemia occurs later after chemotherapy than do neutropenia and thrombocytopenia.
   f) Pathophysiology
      (1) Isolating the cause of anemia to a single factor in patients with cancer often is difficult. Various mechanisms that interfere with bone marrow functioning, erythropoiesis, RBC destruction, and maintenance of a stable blood volume often are involved (Loney & Chernecky, 2000).
      (2) Classifications of anemia (Gillespie & Berger, 2004; Hurter & Bush, 2007)
         (a) Normocytic: Normal-sized red blood cells (mean corpuscular

volume [MCV] 80–100 femtoliters [fL]); caused by nutritional deficiency, hemolytic anemia, aplastic anemia, and chronic disease. Chemotherapy or radiation therapy may directly decrease RBC production. These treatments induce bone marrow suppression, which, in turn, causes depletion in the pluripotent stem cells. Severe catabolism associated with cancer also may impair protein production, causing the bone marrow to produce inadequate numbers of RBCs. Although the numbers are low, the size of the cells remains normal.

(b) Microcytic: Small RBCs (MCV < 80–100 fL); caused by iron deficiency, thalassemia (a genetic underproduction of Hgb), sideroblastic anemia, and anemia of chronic disease states. In patients with cancer, the most frequent causes of iron deficiency are inadequate absorption, excessive loss of iron due to blood loss, or other cancer-related effects, such as poor dietary intake of iron. As described by Hurter and Bush (2007), "malignancies and other conditions such as chronic infections, inflammatory conditions, and congestive heart failure contribute to a common state of factors resulting in anemia and are referred to as anemia of chronic disease" (p. 350).

(c) Macrocytic: Large RBCs (MCV > 100 fL); alcohol and drug exposure, liver disease, anorexia, malabsorption syndromes, vitamin B_{12} deficiency, folate deficiency; vitamin B_{12} and folic acid deficiencies interfere with DNA synthesis necessary for RBC precursor production. In patients with cancer, certain medications may lead to folic acid deficiencies, such as anticonvulsants and folic acid antagonists (methotrexate, hydroxyurea, and pemetrexed).

(3) Chemotherapy not only suppresses bone marrow functioning and erythropoiesis, but it also may cause poor dietary intake of iron, RBC lysis, and microangiopathic bleeding (Kogut &

Luthringer, 2005; Loney & Chernecky, 2000).

(4) Chemotherapy-induced anemia is associated with bone marrow suppression resulting in decreased numbers of RBCs. Cytotoxic chemotherapeutic agents prohibit stem cells from developing into erythrocytes. RBCs have a longer life than WBCs or platelets. As a result, the RBC depression may not be evident for up to six weeks following the treatment (Loney & Chernecky, 2000).

g) Alteration in erythroblast development: DNA cell-cycle–specific agents inhibit the overall production of DNA, resulting in the alteration of erythrocyte development.

h) Peripheral macrocytosis: An increase in the size of erythrocytes. Vitamin B_{12} and folate deficiencies are common causes of megaloblastic macrocytic anemia. These deficiencies interfere with DNA synthesis of erythrocyte precursor cells and disrupt the normal maturation of RBCs in the marrow (Gillespie & Berger, 2004). Methotrexate can cause folic acid depletion potentially leading to anemia.

i) Because the kidneys produce more than 90% of EPO, any nephrotoxic agents (e.g., cisplatin, carboplatin) have the potential to deplete EPO levels. The usual constant level of EPO in circulation is lost, and a greater degree of hypoxia is needed to stimulate the EPO response (Loney & Chernecky, 2000).

j) Increased RBC destruction can occur as a result of the following mechanisms.

(1) Antimetabolites triggering mechanical RBC lysis (e.g., 5-FU, hydroxyurea, methotrexate, gemcitabine, capecitabine)

(2) Enzyme deficiency: People with a hereditary glucose-6-phosphate-dehy-

drogenase deficiency lack an enzyme needed for antioxidant protection of RBCs. Without the enzyme, exposure to oxidizing agents (e.g., chemotherapy and viral or bacterial infections) can damage RBC, Hgb, and cell membranes (Loney & Chernecky, 2000). This is one type of hemolytic anemia. Sickle cell disease is another type of hemolytic anemia (Gillespie & Berger, 2004; Hurter & Bush, 2007).

(3) In anemia of cancer, as with anemia of chronic disease, the problem lies with inflammatory cytokines. TNF-alpha, IL-1, IL-6, and IFN-gamma irregularities are the most likely causative factors. These cytokines interfere with erythrocyte production and cause blunted iron metabolism. Patients have a "functional iron deficiency." In this form of anemia, erythrocyte survival is shortened as well (Gillespie & Berger, 2004).

k) Incidence
  (1) The degree of chemotherapy-induced anemia is related to drug, dose, and frequency of treatment regimens as well as the extent of the disease. Patients treated with cytotoxic therapy for lymphomas, lung tumors, and gynecologic or genitourinary tumors experience a high rate of anemia (Rogers, 2008).
  (2) Up to 60% of patients with solid tumors and lymphoma may experience anemia, and those receiving myelosuppressive chemotherapy and/or radiation therapy have an even higher incidence (70%–90%) (Rogers, 2008).

l) Risk factors
  (1) Drugs that cause hypoproliferation (i.e., decreased RBC production related to either bone marrow suppression or

impaired EPO response) (Loney & Chernecky, 2000)
  (a) Known nephrotoxic agents: Platinum drugs or platinum-based regimens
  (b) Combination therapy with cyclophosphamide, methotrexate, and 5-FU (a combination known to result in anemia as long as five years after initial treatment) (Rogers, 2008)
  (c) Antimicrotubular agents (e.g., taxanes, vinorelbine)
  (d) Camptothecins (e.g., irinotecan, topotecan)
  (e) Biotherapies (e.g., IL, IFN, imatinib, sunitinib) (Rogers, 2008)
  (f) Patients who have undergone high-dose chemotherapy with stem cell transplant or radiation therapy to areas of prolific bone marrow (e.g., pelvis, sternum) (Rogers, 2008)
  (g) Patients treated with repeated cycles of myelosuppressive chemotherapy (Rogers, 2008)
(2) Tumor infiltration of bone marrow, resulting in decreased RBC precursors
(3) Previous chemotherapy/biotherapy with or without concomitant radiation exposure to bone marrow and associated fibrosis. In adults, fibrosis in the sternum, long bones, or sacrum is a risk factor for anemia. In children, fibrosis in the spine or pelvis is a risk factor.
(4) Acute bleeding or hemorrhaging, which may cause a rapid drop in Hgb and progressive hypoxia; the hematologic effects of acute blood loss are most profound in older adults (Penninx, Cohen, & Woodman, 2007).
(5) Age
  (a) Patients younger than age five are more tolerant of chemotherapy because their marrow contains more hematopoietic cells and a lower percentage of fat than does the marrow of older patients (Hoagland, 1992; Penninx et al., 2007).
  (b) Although data on anemia in the older adult population are limited, anemia occurs more often in older individuals, and the prevalence increases with age. Anemia is likely to be a comorbid condition prior to the initiation of any therapy in an older adult patient. Age-related

reductions in hematopoietic stem cell reserves and proliferative capacity also contribute to the potential for increased anemia in the older adult population (Penninx et al., 2007).

(6) Poor nutrition: Poor dietary intake related to the toxicities associated with chemotherapy can greatly alter the reabsorption of iron and diminish available iron stores. Patients with a negative nitrogen balance and associated weight loss are unable to repair cells damaged by chemotherapy (Loney & Chernecky, 2000). Vitamin B_{12} and folate deficiencies will interfere with the production of RBCs by interfering with the synthesis of DNA and disrupting the formation of new cells (Cope & Reb, 2006; Gillespie & Berger, 2004; Kogut & Luthringer, 2005; Van Cleave, 2006).

(7) Comorbidities (NCCN, 2008)
   (a) Cardiac history/decompensation
   (b) Chronic pulmonary disease
   (c) Cerebral vascular disease

(8) Use of certain drugs (Shelton, 2006; Worrall, Tompkins, & Rust, 1999)
   (a) Alcohol
   (b) Aspirin and nonsteroidal anti-inflammatory drugs (NSAIDs)
   (c) Anticonvulsants (e.g., phenytoin sodium, primidone, carbamazepine)
   (d) Antidysrhythmics
   (e) Antiretroviral agents
   (f) Oral contraceptives
   (g) Oral hypoglycemics
   (h) Antibiotics
   (i) Tranquilizers
   (j) Antimicrobials

m) Clinical manifestations: See Table 15.
n) Collaborative management
   (1) Patients with cancer have rated fatigue as the leading complaint, superseding nausea and vomiting, as having the greatest impact on their energy and activity levels. Fatigue may be the first indication of anemia. QOL issues become paramount for patients. However, until recently, the symptom of fatigue has been inadequately assessed (Cella, 2006; Gillespie, 2003; Tchekmedyian, 2002). A research tool called the Functional Assessment of Cancer Therapy—Anemia (FACT-An) consists of the FACT-G (General) instrument

in addition to 13 fatigue-related questions and 7 nonfatigue anemia-related questions. It provides information to researchers to help to determine specific issues related to patients and their QOL while anemic. It classifies patients based on Hgb and fatigue levels (Cella).

(2) Identify the underlying cause of the anemia.

(3) Implement iron supplementation only for patients with anemia related to iron deficiency. In general, serum ferritin levels less than 100 mcg/L or transferrin saturation levels less than 20% are taken as evidence of functional iron deficiency, and oral supplementation may be warranted (NCCN, 2008).

(4) Address symptoms related to hypoxia. Improving Hgb and, thus, oxygen levels

Table 15. Symptoms of Anemia		
Hgb Levels	**Classification**	**Common Clinical Findings**
10–11 mg/dl	Mild anemia	• Activity intolerance • Constipation, slowed peristalsis • Difficulty concentrating or reasoning • Fatigue • Headache
8–10 mg/dl	Moderate anemia	• Asthenia, profound fatigue, weariness, altering activities of daily living or health maintenance • Somnolence • Tachycardia, irritable beats (e.g., premature ventricular beats)
< 8 mg/dl	Severe anemia	• Altered level of consciousness (e.g., somnolence or coma) • Cyanosis • Decreased urine output • Dyspnea • Dysrhythmias, life-threatening (e.g., ventricular tachycardia, ventricular fibrillation, heart block) • Hypothermia • Hypoxia • Inability to provide self-care

Hgb—hemoglobin

Note. From "Therapeutic Options for Patients With Cancer- and Treatment-Related Anemia," by B.K. Shelton, 2006, *Johns Hopkins Advanced Studies in Nursing, 4*(5), p. 111. Copyright 2006 by Galen Publishing. Reprinted with permission.

has a positive impact on treatment—both chemotherapy and radiation. Anoxic tumor cells are two to three times more resistant to radiation therapy than are normally oxygenated cells (Weiss, 2003).

  (a) Encourage patients to rest to conserve energy. This recommendation only is made if the patient is hypoxic and benefits from the use of oxygen. The new paradigm regarding exercise for patients receiving treatment and at all levels of health and illness is based on the positive influence of exercise on QOL (Mock, 2003).

  (b) Encourage the use of or administer oxygen if oxygen saturation is less than 90%.

(5) Compare laboratory results with important indices. Table 16 presents results that are considered in the normal range for healthy men and women. If a patient's results are abnormal, take appropriate action.

(6) Administer erythropoiesis-stimulating agents (ESAs) for chemotherapy-induced anemia. ESAs are indicated for the treatment of anemia associated with concomitant administration of chemotherapy based on studies that have shown a reduction in the need for RBC transfusions in patients with nonmyeloid malignancies (Amgen Inc., 2008a).

  (a) Two types of ESAs are indicated for use with patients with nonmyeloid malignancies experiencing chemotherapy-induced anemia. Erythropoietin alfa (Procrit®) and darbepoetin alfa (Aranesp®). (Note: A third ESA, epoetin beta, is available in Europe but not commercially available in the United States.) The American Society of Clinical Oncology (ASCO) and the American Society of Hematology recently collaborated on a committee to determine the appropriate use of ESAs in the clinical setting. The results of their efforts are substantial, including the following information.

    i) "The use of ESA therapy is recommended as a treatment option for patients with chemotherapy-induced

anemia and a Hgb that is approaching, or has fallen below, 10 g/dl, to increase Hgb and decrease transfusions. RBC transfusion is an option depending on the severity of the anemia or the clinical circumstances" (Rizzo et al., 2008, p. 134).

    ii) For patients with less severe anemia, Hgb levels > 10 but < 12 g/dl, the decision of when to start an ESA should be determined by clinical circumstances; in particular, older adult patients with "limited cardiopulmonary reserve, coronary artery dis-

Table 16. Laboratory Assessment of Anemia: Normal Values (Adults)

Laboratory Test	Normal Value
Red blood cell count	Male: 4.7–6 m/µl; female: 4.2–5.4 m/µl
Hemoglobin	Male: 13.5–18 g/dl; female: 12–16 g/dl
Hematocrit	Male: 42%–52%; female: 37%–47%
Mean corpuscular volume	78–100 fL
Mean corpuscular hemoglobin	27–31 pg/cell
Red cell distribution width	11.5%–14%
Reticulocyte count	0.5%–1.85% of erythrocytes
Ferritin	Male: 20–300 ng/ml; female: 15–120 ng/ml
Serum iron	Male: 75–175 µg/dl; female: 65–165 µg/dl
Total iron binding capacity	250–450 µg/dl
Serum erythropoietin level	Male: 17.2 mIU/ml; female: 18.8 mIU/ml
Coomb's test (direct and indirect)	Negative
Serum B$_{12}$	190–900 mg/ml
Serum folate	> 3.5 µg/l

Note. From "Overview of Anemia" (p. 791), by M.P. Lynch in D. Camp-Sorrell and R.A. Hawkins (Eds.), *Clinical Manual for the Oncology Advanced Practice Nurse* (2nd ed.), 2006, Pittsburgh, PA: Oncology Nursing Society. Copyright 2006 by the Oncology Nursing Society. Reprinted with permission.

ease, symptomatic angina, or substantially reduced exercise capacity, energy, or ability to carry out activities of daily living (ADLs)" (Rizzo et al., 2008, p. 134). RBC transfusion remains an option as well.

iii) Risks associated with ESA use include increased mortality, serious cardiovascular and thromboembolic events, and increased risk of tumor progression or recurrence. These warnings are contained in a "black box" seen at the top of the package insert for the products. Care should be taken to monitor patients for any untoward events related to these products. ESAs are not indicated in any patient with uncontrolled hypertension nor for patients receiving potentially curative therapy. Transfusion is an option to correct anemia (NCCN, 2008). Physicians are expected to discuss both the risks and the benefits of the proposed treatment to alleviate anemia.

iv) The FDA-approved starting dose of epoetin alfa is 150 U/ kg or 40,000 U weekly administered SC. Darbepoetin alfa's starting dose is 2.25 mcg/kg weekly or 500 mcg every three weeks subcutaneously. Treatment should continue toward a target Hgb of 10 g/dl but should not exceed 10 g/dl. Dose reductions are indicated if the Hgb rises > 1 g/dl in any two-week period (Rizzo et al., 2008). Acceptable alternative dosing includes a darbepoetin alfa 100 mcg fixed dose administered SC weekly, a 200 mcg fixed dose SC every two weeks, or 300 mcg SC every three weeks (NCCN, 2008). Alternative regimens for epoetin alfa are 80,000 units SC every two weeks or 120,000 units SC every three weeks (NCCN).

v) "Baseline and periodic monitoring of iron, total iron binding capacity, transferrin saturation, and ferritin, and use of iron repletion, when indicated, may be valuable in limiting the need for epoetin, maximizing symptomatic improvement, and determining the reason for failure to respond adequately to epoetin therapy" (Rizzo et al., 2008, p. 135).

vi) Strong evidence exists against the use of ESAs in patients with anemia associated with malignancy alone (not treatment) or the anemia of cancer among patients with solid or nonmyeloid malignancies who are not receiving chemotherapy. This is consistent with the black box warning that was added to the prescribing information of the ESAs in March 2007 (Rizzo et al., 2008). The FDA required a labeling change, including the black box warning in 2008 following the completion of the review of information in 2007 from eight separate studies that showed an unfavorable risk-benefit profile for the products. Physicians are expected to discuss the goals of therapy and the risks and benefits of ESA use (NCCN, 2008). To summarize,

- ESAs are not indicated for use in patients receiving hormonal agents, therapeutic biologic products, or radiotherapy unless they

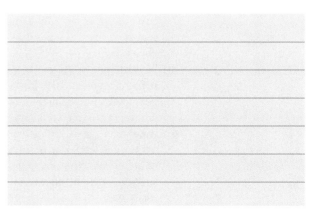

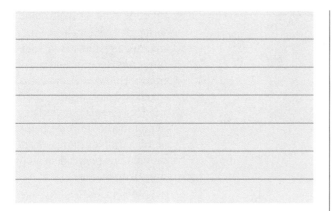

are receiving concomitantly myelosuppressive chemotherapy treatment.

- ESAs are not indicated for patients receiving myelosuppressive chemotherapy when the anticipated outcome is cure.
- ESAs are not indicated to improve symptoms of anemia, QOL, fatigue, or patient well-being.

(b) Although darbepoetin alfa is closely related to epoetin alfa, it has five N-linked carbohydrate chains, which give it a much heavier molecular weight and confer a longer half-life than epoetin alfa. It may, thus, be administered less frequently (Amgen Inc., 2008a). In 2006, Amgen received FDA approval for every-three-week administration of darbepoetin alfa. The results of a clinical trial showed that every-three-week administration of darbepoetin alfa was as effective as weekly dosing (Canon et al., 2006).

   i) The authors found that every-three-week dosing was effective in treating both mild and moderate anemia caused by chemotherapy.
   ii) This simplifies the management of anemia, in that many chemotherapy regimens are administered on an every-three-week basis, so darbepoetin alfa could, therefore, be administered at the same time the patient comes for treatment.

iii) Monitoring
- After initiation of ESA therapy, monitor Hgb at least weekly. The dose should be adjusted to maintain the lowest Hgb level sufficient to avoid an RBC transfusion (NCCN, 2008). If the Hgb level rises more than 1 g/dl in a two-week period or the Hgb reaches a level needed to avoid a transfusion, the dose should be reduced by 40% of the previous dose. If the Hgb exceeds a level needed to avoid a transfusion, the ESA should be temporarily held until the Hgb falls to a level where transfusion may be required. At this point, the dose should be reinstated at a dose 40% below the previous dose (Amgen Inc., 2008a; Ortho Biotech, 2007).
- Once the target Hgb has been achieved, monitor Hgb weekly until stabilized and then at regular intervals (Amgen Inc., 2008a). At no time should the Hgb target exceed 10 g/dl (Lyman & Glaspy, 2006).
- ESAs require at least two weeks of treatment before an increase in the number of RBCs is seen. If there is no response after four weeks of epoetin alfa or six weeks of darbepoetin alfa, the dose should be titrated upward (NCCN, 2008).
- In the absence of an Hgb response, even after dose escalation, discontinue therapy after six to eight weeks (Lyman & Glaspy, 2006).
- Instruct patients to call the physician if they experience pain or swelling in the legs, new or worsening shortness of breath, increase in blood pressure, dizziness or loss of consciousness, or extreme fatigue (NCCN, 2008).

- If Hct falls below 25%, Hgb drops below 8 g/dl, or cardiopulmonary symptoms develop, administer 1–2 units packed RBCs over 2–3 hours as ordered by the physician.
- When determining whether a patient is a candidate for ESAs, the clinician must carefully consider the risk-benefit ratio. As studies are ongoing, the use of ESAs must only be initiated by a clinician with current knowledge of the indications, black box warnings, and toxicity profile (NCCN, 2008).
- Monitor patients for "functional" iron deficiency, which can follow ESA therapy. Supplemental iron will be required eventually for most patients to maintain optimal erythropoiesis. Rapid ESA stimulation of RBC production pulls from the usable iron stores. In addition, inflammatory cytokines in the tumor setting can delay iron release. Together, these situations slow the adequate EPO response to anemia (NCCN, 2008). Baseline iron studies should be performed prior to initiating ESA therapy: serum iron, total iron binding capacity, and serum ferritin. These studies should be repeated periodically during the course of treatment (NCCN). Iron can be administered in the oral formulation or parenteral form. Current studies have shown superiority of IV over oral dosing (NCCN).

o) Patient and family education
   (1) Encourage patients to set short-term goals for ADLs to conserve energy (Loney & Chernecky, 2000).
   (2) Encourage patients to change positions slowly to prevent dizziness secondary to postural hypotension.

   (3) Acknowledge patients' reports of symptoms such as fatigue as real, even if stated in vague terminology (Loney & Chernecky, 2000).
   (4) Discuss the potential for anemia and the signs and symptoms of anemia when teaching patients about the side effects of chemotherapy and/or radiation.
   (5) Help patients and caregivers to develop mechanisms for managing persistent symptoms of anemia (e.g., fatigue, shortness of breath, decreased stamina).
   (6) Provide instruction regarding the self-administration of EPO, including written materials.
   (7) When applicable, encourage patients to maintain an optimal level of physical activity, allowing for rest periods as needed (Shelton, 2006).
   (8) Remind patients to maintain a well-balanced diet, adding iron-rich foods to improve the quality of the diet.
   (9) Teach patients and caregivers about the hazards, risks, and benefits of blood transfusions.

3. Thrombocytopenia (Camp-Sorrell, 2005; Shuey, 1996)
   a) Normal physiology of platelets: See Figure 21 (Psaila & Bussel, 2007)
      (1) Platelets, or thrombocytes, are small anucleate cell particles that are released into the bloodstream by megakaryocytes.
      (2) Megakaryocyte development occurs by an intricate cascade of events organized by cytokines and growth factors.
      (3) Thrombopoietin is the primary regulator of thrombopoiesis, promoting megakaryocyte differentiation from HSCs.
      (4) A normal platelet count is 150,000–400,000 cells/mm^3. The average life

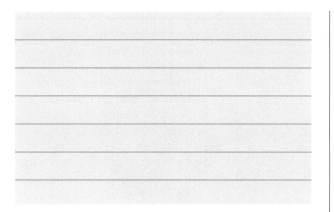

span of a platelet is 7–10 days. Platelets are not stored in bone marrow but may sequester in the spleen.

(5) Following an initial insult to a blood vessel, platelets adhere to collagen along the subendothelial surface and release several compounds, including serotonin and adenosine diphosphate. These compounds cause the recruitment of more platelets, which adhere to collagen and stick together. This leads to the formation of a clot, a large platelet aggregate, or a hemostatic plug. The entire process normally occurs within three to five minutes.

(6) Secondary hemostasis occurs when factors VII and XII are activated as a result of proteins on the platelet surface coming into contact with the damaged endothelial cells.

(7) When the extrinsic and intrinsic pathways are activated, they converge at the common pathway, producing activated factor that converts prothrombin to thrombin. Thrombin converts fibrinogen to fibrin, leading to a stable clot.

(8) Fibrinolysis is the mechanism by which clots are broken down. The factors responsible for fibrinolysis (plasminogen activators) are present in most body fluids and normal and neoplastic tissue (Gobel, 2005).

b) Pathophysiology (Camp-Sorrell, 2005)
(1) Bone marrow suppression caused by acute or delayed effects of chemotherapy decreases platelet production.
(2) Thrombocytopenia usually occurs with neutropenia.
(3) Indices vary by institution and protocol, but a general rule of thumb for solid tumors is to hold chemotherapy if the platelet count is < 100,000/mm^3

(Camp-Sorrell, 2005). Check with the patient's physician before holding chemotherapy. Treatment may be administered with lower counts. The physician then may decide to support the patient with platelet transfusions or growth factors if it becomes necessary. Thrombocytopenia in a child receiving chemotherapy may necessitate dosing changes and a delay in treatment (Felgenhauer et al., 2000).

(4) The following drugs are known to cause thrombocytopenia as a dose-limiting toxicity (Wilkes, Ingwersen, & Barton-Burke, 2008).
  (a) Platinums (carboplatin and cisplatin)
  (b) Dacarbazine
  (c) Daunorubicin
  (d) Doxorubicin
  (e) Bortezomib
  (f) Gemcitabine
  (g) Lomustine
  (h) Mitomycin
  (i) Thiotepa
  (j) Trimetrexate
  (k) Taxanes

(5) A cumulative and delayed onset of thrombocytopenia has been observed with the following (Roesser, 2007; Wilkes et al., 2008).
  (a) Carmustine
  (b) Dactinomycin
  (c) Fludarabine
  (d) Lomustine
  (e) Mitomycin
  (f) Paclitaxel
  (g) Docetaxel
  (h) Streptozocin
  (i) Thiotepa
  (j) 6-thioguanine

c) Incidence
(1) Chemotherapy commonly causes thrombocytopenia. The use of growth factors (e.g., G-CSF) allows for the administration of higher doses of chemotherapeutic drugs. In turn, this causes the incidence of dose-limiting thrombocytopenia to increase (Kurzrock, 2000).
(2) Incidence varies depending on the agent used.

d) Risk factors (Gobel, 2005; Lynch, 2006)
(1) Myelosuppressive chemotherapy, concurrent chemotherapy and radiation, or radiation therapy alone
(2) Disease infiltration of bone marrow

(3) Disseminated intravascular coagulation (DIC)

(4) Elevated temperature leading to destruction of platelets (Fuller, 1990)

(5) Concomitant diseases (Gobel, 2005; Lynch, 2006)
 (a) Cirrhosis or metastasis to the liver
 (b) Diabetes mellitus
 (c) Infection, sepsis, HIV
 (d) Scleroderma, systemic lupus erythematosus, sarcoidosis
 (e) Aplastic anemia

(6) Nutritional deficiencies (vitamin B_{12}, folate) (Kogut & Luthringer, 2005)

(7) Drug therapy known to affect platelet production or function (Wilkes et al., 2008)
 (a) Antibiotics
 (b) Anticoagulants
 (c) Antidepressants
 (d) Aspirin
 (e) Codeine
 (f) Ethanol
 (g) Indomethacin
 (h) NSAIDs
 (i) Sulfa drugs
 (j) Amphotericin B in children

e) Clinical manifestations (Camp-Sorrell, 2005; Gobel, 2005; Roesser, 2007)

(1) Petechiae (tiny purplish-red dots) and ecchymoses (purplish bruises) indicate capillary microvascular bleeding in the soft tissue such as waist, soft palate, and skin beneath eyebrows.

(2) Overt bleeding (e.g., nosebleeds, bleeding from gums, wounds, body orifices, or around existing tubes). Mucous membranes (i.e., nasopharynx, oral mucosa, GI and urinary tracts, upper airways) have capillaries close to the surface, so they bleed easily.

(3) Enlarged and tender liver or spleen indicates that the organ may be capturing enlarged or fragmented cells (e.g., sequestering platelets).

(4) Occult or overt blood in stool or urine

(5) Headaches (may indicate intracranial bleeding)

(6) Hypotension or tachycardia in adults; hypotension and tachycardia do not occur in cases of thrombocytopenia in children.

(7) Prolonged menstruation and an increased number of pads saturated during menses

f) Laboratory indicators

(1) Platelet count and risk of bleeding (Kasper et al., 2005)
 (a) ≤ 100,000/mm³: Injury or surgery may provoke excess bleeding.
 (b) ≤20,000/mm³: Spontaneous bleeding may occur.
 (c) ≤10,000/mm³: Often is associated with serious hemorrhage.

(2) Hgb and Hct: Monitor for signs of blood loss in thrombocytopenic patients, such as signs or symptoms of anemia.

(3) Assessment of coagulation tests (e.g., PT, activated PTT, thrombin time, platelet aggregation) to determine if patient has disseminated intravascular coagulation.

(4) Monitor for occult blood in the urine, stool, or emesis. The stool of patients taking iron supplements may falsely test guaiac-positive.

g) Collaborative management (Roesser, 2007)

(1) Maintain and reinforce bleeding precautions when the platelet count is < 50,000/mm³.

(2) Decrease patient's activity to prevent injury (e.g., falls, bumping into objects). Discourage activities that pose a high risk of injury (e.g., bicycle riding, contact sports).

(3) Maintain a safe environment; use nonskid rugs, and a night light to help prevent falls.

(4) Maintain the integrity of skin (Roesser, 2007).
 (a) Use electric versus straight-edged razors.
 (b) Use an emery board versus metal file for nail care, or use metal nail clippers.
 (c) Ensure that the patient knows to avoid wearing restrictive clothing

(especially restrictive undergarments).

(d) Do not use tourniquets.

(e) Minimize invasive procedures such as needlesticks and injections (especially IM injections).

(5) Maintain integrity of mucous membranes (Gobel, 2005; Roesser, 2007).

(a) Encourage patients to

i) Blow their nose gently (e.g., with their mouth open to prevent increased intracranial pressure).

ii) Use a water-based lubricant before sexual intercourse.

iii) Use only a soft toothbrush or sponge-tipped applicator, and rinse the mouth with a mild saltwater solution rather than a commercial mouthwash.

(b) Discourage patients from

i) Having dental care until platelets normalize

ii) Using oral irrigation tools

iii) Using dental floss if gum bleeding occurs

iv) Using tampons

v) Having anal intercourse

vi) Having sexual intercourse if the platelet count is < 50,000/mm^3.

(6) Maintain the integrity of the genitourinary tract (Gobel, 2005; Petursson, 1998; Roesser, 2007; Shelton, 1998).

(a) Increase patients' hydration, and avoid the use of indwelling catheters whenever possible. If catheterization becomes necessary, use only a small-lumen catheter and ample lubrication.

(b) Encourage patients to increase fluid intake to two to three liters per day.

(7) Maintain the integrity of the GI tract (Gobel, 2005; Petursson, 1998; Roesser, 2007; Shelton, 1998).

(a) Remind patients to take steroids with food.

(b) Use prophylactic stool softeners and stimulants to avoid constipation; avoid using enemas, suppositories, harsh laxatives, or rectal thermometers.

(c) Avoid spicy, hot, and acidic foods. Allow food to cool before attempting to eat.

(8) Maintain optimal nutritional status (Gobel, 2005; Kogut & Luthringer, 2005; Petursson, 1998; Shelton, 1998).

(a) Encourage consumption of protein-containing foods; protein is needed for megakaryocyte production.

(b) Encourage patients to consume a soft diet and avoid foods that are irritating (e.g., hot foods, acidic foods, spicy foods).

(c) Discourage alcohol use.

(9) Avoid all medications that have the potential to induce bleeding (e.g., aspirin, NSAIDs). The anti-inflammatory drug choline magnesium trisalicylate is platelet-sparing. It is indicated for osteoarthritis, analgesia, and antipyresis.

(10) Administer appropriate medications and treatments.

(a) Administer platelet transfusions prophylactically to adults when the platelet count is 10,000–20,000/mm^3 or when the patient is symptomatic (bleeding), based on institutional guidelines or protocol. Platelet levels need to be kept higher (e.g., 50,000/mm^3) when patients are having an invasive procedure or at 20,000/mm^3 for minor procedures (Brant et al., 2006). Patients with brain tumors usually receive platelet transfusions if the count drops below 50,000/mm^3. Platelet administration for counts < 10,000/mm^3 is a nursing priority (Roesser, 2007).

(b) Administer stool softeners or laxatives to avoid constipation.

(c) Consider administering IL-11, also known as oprelvekin,

to minimize chemotherapy-induced thrombocytopenia (Wyeth Pharmaceuticals Inc., 2006). The FDA approved IL-11 as a growth factor for megakaryocytes in nonmyeloid malignancies and nonmyeloblative chemotherapy regimens (Camp-Sorrell, 2005). IL-11 stimulates the proliferation of HSCs and megakaryocyte progenitor cells, thereby inducing the maturation of megakaryocytes and increased platelet production. Presently, a safe and effective dose has not been established in children. IL-11 may reduce platelet transfusion requirements; however, the role of this growth factor in prevention of bleeding has not been established (Brant et al., 2006).

i) The potential exists for hypersensitivity and anaphylaxis from oprelvekin. This information is contained in a black box warning at the beginning of the package insert. Other side effects of IL-11 are related to a shift in plasma volume and may include weight gain, atrial arrhythmias, and transient anemia. Some patients experience visual disturbances. Be cautious when administering IL-11 to patients with a history of fluid retention, congestive heart failure (CHF), atrial arrhythmias, or coronary artery disease. Patients who are at risk for developing any of the preceding symptoms, such as older adults, or patients who are heavily pretreated with anthracyclines should be monitored carefully (Camp-Sorrell, 2005; Wyeth Pharmaceuticals Inc., 2006).

ii) The recommended dose of IL-11 is 50 mcg/kg SC once daily beginning 6–24 hours after completion of chemotherapy. The drug is to be continued until the post-nadir platelet count is ≥ 50,000/mm^3. Dosing beyond 21 days per treatment cycle is not recommended (Barbour & Crawford, 2007).

iii) Monitor patients daily for fluid status changes, especially dyspnea, pleural effusion, weight gain, and edema, and for eye irritation or discomfort. These side effects are thought to result from an increase in renal sodium retention and plasma volume expansion, which cause an increase in intravascular fluid (Roesser, 2007).

(d) Next generation thrombopoietic agents (Psaila & Bussel, 2007)

i) Romiplostim (Nplate™) was approved by the FDA in 2008. It is an Fc-peptide fusion protein, called a *peptibody*. The peptide sequence binds and activates the thrombopoietin receptor, causing megakaryocyte differentiation, proliferation, and platelet production. Romiplostim is indicated for the treatment of thrombocytopenia in patients with chronic immune thrombocytopenic purpura (ITP) who have had an insufficient response to corticosteroids, immunoglobulins, or splenectomy. Romiplostim is given as a weekly SC injection. The starting dose is 1 mcg/kg and should only be used for patients with ITP

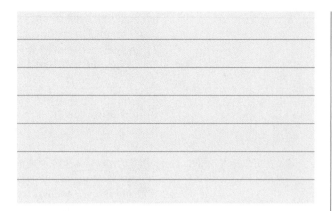

whose thrombocytopenia puts them at risk for bleeding. The weekly dose is adjusted to achieve and maintain a platelet count of ≥ 50,000. Romiplostim is not intended to normalize platelet counts. The most common side effects are headache, arthralgias, and dizziness. The package insert contains a warning that romiplostim increases the risk for bone marrow reticulin deposition. Clinical trials have not ruled out the possibility that reticulin and other fiber deposition may result in bone marrow fibrosis and cytopenias. When romiplostim is discontinued, worsening of the thrombocytopenia may occur (Amgen Inc., 2008b).

ii) Eltrombopag is an oral nonpeptide platelet growth factor. It interacts with the transmembrane domain of the thrombopoietin receptor, inducing phosphorylation of the signaling pathways to promote megakaryocyte differentiation, proliferation, and platelet production (Akhtari, 2007). Eltrombopag is being tested in hepatitis C–associated thrombocytopenias, relapsed refractory ITP, as well as other trials in sarcoma and metastatic disease, renal impairment, and hepatic impairment (Psaila & Bussel, 2007).

iii) Other thrombopoietic agents are in development. Studies are ongoing to establish efficacy in ITP, chemotherapy-induced thrombocytopenia, and other indications (Psaila & Bussel, 2007).

h) Patient and family education (Camp-Sorrell, 2005; Shelton, 1998)

(1) Instruct patients and significant others regarding signs and symptoms of thrombocytopenia.

(2) Tell patients and significant others to immediately notify the nurse or physician of signs and symptoms of bleeding.

(3) Instruct patients about the signs and symptoms of transfusion reaction.

(4) Reinforce the need to avoid injuries; list the activities that patients should avoid to prevent injury.

(5) Provide instruction on interventions to manage bleeding (e.g., the use of ice packs and application of pressure, institution of a bowel program including stool softeners and laxatives to avoid constipation) (Roesser, 2007).

(6) Provide healthcare providers' names and telephone numbers, and instruct patients to call if any of the following occur.

(a) Bleeding from any body orifice

(b) New petechiae or bruising

(c) Headache

(d) Change in level of consciousness

(7) Provide an inclusive list of medications that may interfere with megakaryocyte production.

References

Akhtari, M. (2007). Updates on thrombocytopenia, mobilizing hematopoietic stem cells, erythropoiesis-stimulating agents, neutropenia, and oral mucositis. *Meniscus Special Report: Supportive Care Issues in Cancer,* Issue 2, pp. 5–17.

Amgen Inc. (2008a). Aranesp [Package insert]. Thousand Oaks, CA: Author.

Amgen Inc. (2008b). Nplate [Package insert]. Thousand Oaks, CA: Author.

Barbour, S., & Crawford, J. (2007). Hematopoietic growth factors. In R. Padjur, L. Coia, W. Hoskins, & L. Wagman (Eds.), *Cancer management: A multidisciplinary approach. Medical, surgical and radiation oncology* (10th ed.). Melville, NY: PRR, Inc. Retrieved November 2, 2008, from http://www.cancernetwork.com/cancer-management/chapter40,article,10165/1172173?pageNumber+4

Brant, J., Damron, B., Friend, P., Lacher, M., Schaal, A., & Samsonow, S. (2006). *Putting Evidence Into Practice: Prevention of bleeding*. Pittsburgh, PA: Oncology Nursing Society.

Bron, D., Meuleman, N., & Mascaux, C. (2001). Biological basis of anemia. *Seminars in Oncology, 28*(2, Suppl. 8), 1–6.

Camp-Sorrell, D. (2005). Chemotherapy toxicities and management. In C.H. Yarbro, M.H. Frogge, & M. Goodman (Eds.), *Cancer nursing: Principles and practice* (6th ed., pp. 412–457). Sudbury, MA: Jones and Bartlett.

Canon, J., Vansteenkiste, J., Gyorgy, B., Mateos, M., Bastit, L., Ferreira, I., et al. (2006). Randomized double-blind, active-controlled trial of every-3-week darbepoietin alfa for the treatment of chemotherapy-induced anemia. *Journal of the National Cancer Institute, 98*(4), 273–284.

Cella, D. (2006). Quality of life and clinical decisions in chemotherapy-induced anemia. *Oncology, 20*(8). Retrieved January 9, 2008, from http://www.cancernetwork.com/article/showArticle.jhtml?articleId=191801189

Cope, D.G., & Reb, A.M. (Eds.). (2006). *An evidence-based approach to the treatment and care of the older adult with cancer*. Pittsburgh, PA: Oncology Nursing Society.

Dessypris, E.N. (1999). Erythropoiesis. In G.R.M. Lee, J. Foester, J. Lukens, F. Paraskevas, J.P. Greer, & G.M. Rodgers (Eds.), *Wintrobe's clinical hematology* (10th ed., pp. 169–192). Baltimore: Williams & Wilkins.

Erickson, J.M. (1996). Anemia. *Seminars in Oncology Nursing, 12*(1), 2–14.

Felgenhauer, J., Hawkins, D., Pendergrass, T., Lindsley, K., Conrad, E.U., III, & Miser, J.S. (2000). Very intensive, short-term chemotherapy for children and adolescents with metastatic sarcomas. *Medical and Pediatric Oncology, 34*(1), 29–38.

Fuller, A.K. (1990). Platelet transfusion therapy for thrombocytopenia. *Seminars in Oncology Nursing, 6*(2), 123–128.

Gillespie, T.W. (2003). Anemia in cancer: Therapeutic implications and interventions. *Cancer Nursing, 26*(2), 119–128.

Gillespie, T.W., & Berger, A.M. (2004). The mechanics of cancer-related anemia. *Anemia Management Institute, 1*, 1–16.

Gobel, B.H. (2005). Bleeding. In C.H. Yarbro, M.H. Frogge, & M. Goodman (Eds.), *Cancer nursing: Principles and practice* (6th ed., pp. 723–740). Sudbury, MA: Jones and Bartlett.

Hoagland, H.C. (1992). Hematologic complications of cancer chemotherapy. In M.C. Perry (Ed.), *The chemotherapy source book* (2nd ed., pp. 498–507). Baltimore: Williams & Wilkins.

Hurter, B., & Bush, N. (2007). Cancer-related anemia: Clinical review and management update. *Clinical Journal of Oncology Nursing, 11*(3), 349–358.

Kasper, D., Braunwald, E., Fauci, A., Houser, S., Longo, D., & Jameson, J. (2005). *Harrison's manual of medicine* (16th ed., pp. 275–280). New York: McGraw-Hill.

Kogut, V., & Luthringer, S. (Eds.). (2005). *Nutritional issues in cancer care*. Pittsburgh, PA: Oncology Nursing Society.

Kurzrock, R. (2000). RhIL-11 for the prevention of dose-limiting chemotherapy-induced thrombocytopenia. *Oncology (Williston Park), 14*(9, Suppl. 8), 9–11.

Loney, J., & Chernecky, C. (2000). Anemia. *Oncology Nursing Forum, 27*(6), 951–964.

Lyman, G., & Glaspy, J. (2006). Advances in the clinical management of chemotherapy-induced anemia and its treatment. *American Journal of Oncology Review, 5*(4), 236–241.

Lynch, M.P. (2006). Overview of anemia. In D. Camp-Sorrell & R.A. Hawkins (Eds.), *Clinical manual for the oncology advanced practice nurse* (2nd ed., pp. 787–788). Pittsburgh, PA: Oncology Nursing Society.

Mock, V. (2003). Clinical excellence through evidence-based practice: Fatigue management as a model. *Oncology Nursing Forum, 30*(5), 787–796.

National Comprehensive Cancer Network. (2008). *NCCN Clinical Practice Guidelines in Oncology™: Cancer and treatment-related anemia* [v.2.2009]. Jenkintown, PA: Author.

Ortho Biotech. (2007). Procrit [Package insert]. Raritan, NJ: Author.

Penninx, B., Cohen, H., & Woodman, R. (2007). Anemia and cancer in older persons. *Journal of Supportive Oncology, 5*(3), 107–113.

Petursson, C.T. (1998). Bleeding due to thrombocytopenia. In J.M. Yasko (Ed.), *Nursing management of symptoms associated with chemotherapy* (4th ed., pp. 127–134). Bala Cynwyd, PA: Meniscus Health Care Communications.

Psaila, B., & Bussel, J. (2007). *Recent insights into chemotherapy-induced thrombocytopenia*. Retrieved January 20, 2008, from http://www.medscape.com/viewprogram/6989_pnt

Rizzo, J., Somerfield, M., Hagerty, K., Seidenfeld, J., Bohlius, J., Bennett, C., et al. (2008). The use of epoetin and darbepoetin in patients with cancer: 2007 American Society of Clinical Oncology/American Society of Hematology clinical practice guideline update. *Journal of Clinical Oncology, 26*(1), 132–149.

Roesser, K. (2007). Symptom management. In M. Gullatte (Ed.), *Clinical guide to antineoplastic therapy: A chemotherapy handbook* (2nd ed., pp. 597–599). Pittsburgh, PA: Oncology Nursing Society.

Rogers, G. (2008). Managing patients with chemotherapy-induced anemia. *Johns Hopkins Advanced Studies in Medicine, 8*(10), 346–351.

Shelton, B.K. (1998). Bleeding disorders. In C.R. Ziegfeld, B.G. Lubejko, & B.K. Shelton (Eds.), *Oncology fact finder* (pp. 244–261). Philadelphia: Lippincott.

Shelton, B.K. (2006). Therapeutic options for patients with cancer- and treatment-related anemia. *Johns Hopkins Advanced Studies in Nursing, 4*(5), 109–114.

Shuey, K.M. (1996). Platelet-associated bleeding disorders. *Seminars in Oncology Nursing, 12*(1), 15–27.

Smith, R.E., Jr. (2004). Erythropoietic agents in the management of cancer patients. Part 2: Studies on their role in neuroprotection. *Journal of Supportive Oncology, 2*(1), 39–49.

Spivak, J. (2002). Iron and anemia of chronic disease. *Oncology, 16*(9, Suppl. 10), 25–33. Retrieved November 7, 2008, from http:/www.cancernetwork.com/display.article/10165/80513?Number=1

Tchekmedyian, M.S. (2002). Anemia in cancer patients: Significance, epidemiology, and current therapy. *Oncology, 16*(9, Suppl. 10), 17–24.

Van Cleave, J.H. (2006). The older adult with myelosuppression and anemia. In D.G. Cope & A.M. Reb (Eds.), *An evidence-based approach to the treatment and care of the older adult with cancer* (pp. 325–347). Pittsburgh, PA: Oncology Nursing Society.

Weiss, M.J. (2003). New insights into erythropoietin and epoetin alfa: Mechanisms of action, target tissues, and clinical applications. *Oncologist, 8*(Suppl. 3), 18–29.

Wilkes, G.M., Ingwersen, K., & Barton-Burke, M. (2008). *2008 oncology nursing drug handbook*. Sudbury, MA: Jones and Bartlett.

Worrall, L.M., Tompkins, C.A., & Rust, D.M. (1999). Recognizing and managing anemia. *Clinical Journal of Oncology Nursing, 3*(4), 153–160.

Wyeth Pharmaceuticals Inc. (2006). Neumega [Package insert]. Philadelphia: Author.

B. GI and mucosal side effects
   1. Nausea and vomiting: Studies suggest that healthcare providers perceive that patients have less acute and delayed CINV than they actually do and that patients do not receive adequate preventive antiemetics (Fabi et al., 2003; Grunberg, Hansen, Deuson, & Mavros, 2002; Grunberg et al., 2004; Liau et al., 2005; Valle et al., 2006). Oncology nurses must be knowledgeable and proactive when treating CINV. Terms used in this discussion include the following.
      • *Nausea:* Nausea is an unpleasant subjective experience that is described as a "wavelike" feeling occurring in the stomach and/or the back of the throat that may be accompanied by vomiting (NCI, 2008b). The autonomic nervous system is involved in the development of nausea and vomiting. Physical manifestations include tachycardia, diaphoresis, lightheadedness, dizziness, pallor, excess salivation, and weakness (Camp-Sorrell, 2005).
      • *Retching:* A rhythmic contraction involving the esophagus, diaphragm, and abdominal muscles in an attempt to eject stomach contents. Retching in the absence of vomiting is known as dry heaves (Camp-Sorrell, 2005).
      • *Vomiting:* The forceful expulsion of gastric, duodenum, or jejunum contents through the mouth (NCI, 2008b).
      a) Pathophysiology
         (1) Mechanisms of emesis (see Figure 22): Nausea, retching, and vomiting are independent phenomena that can occur sequentially or as separate entities. The subjective nature of nausea prevents a clear understanding of it; however, mechanisms of vomiting related to chemotherapy administration are becoming better understood.
            (a) Vomiting results from the stimulation of a complex process that involves the activation of various pathways and neurotransmitter receptors (see Figures 22 and 23).
            (b) Vomiting occurs when certain neural structures in the brain stem,

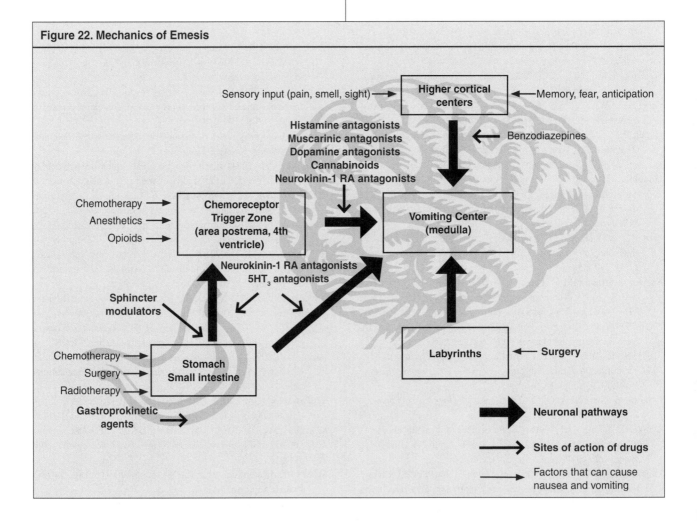

Figure 22. Mechanics of Emesis

Figure 23. Neurotransmitter Receptors

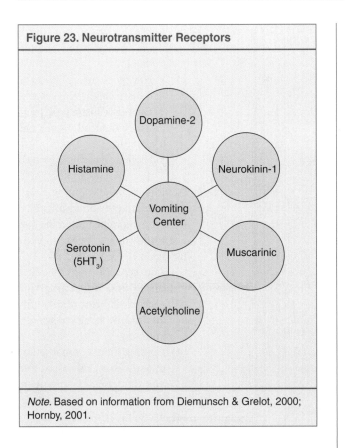

Note. Based on information from Diemunsch & Grelot, 2000; Hornby, 2001.

collectively called the vomiting center (VC), are stimulated. The VC is activated by the visceral and vagal afferent pathways from the GI tract, the chemoreceptor trigger zone (CTZ), the vestibular apparatus (VA), and the cerebral cortex. Decreased motility and reverse motility occur when the VC is stimulated (Camp-Sorrell, 2005).

(c) Chemotherapy and radiation to the gut stimulate enterochromaffin cells, causing them to release serotonin (5-hydroxytryptamine-3 [5HT$_3$]). The vagus nerve plays a key role in emesis caused by chemotherapy, radiation therapy to the epigastrium, and abdominal distention or obstruction. Serotonin release causes the activation of the vagus nerve, which stimulates vomiting through either the CTZ or the VC (O'Bryant, Gonzales, & Bestul, 2004). Serotonin is primarily involved in acute nausea and vomiting.

(d) The CTZ, a highly vascular area, lies at the surface of the fourth ventricle, close to the VC. The

CTZ is not confined within the blood-brain barrier. Therefore, it can detect chemical stimuli in the cerebrospinal fluid and the blood. The CTZ plays a role in nausea and vomiting associated with chemotherapy as well as in emesis associated with other causes such as anesthetics and opioids.

(e) Substance P is found in vagal afferent neurons and binds to neurokinin-1 receptors, causing vomiting. The study of this specific mechanism of vomiting has led to the development of a new class of antiemetics, neurokinin-1 receptor antagonists (Campos et al., 2001; Hesketh, 2001).

(f) Motion sickness and labyrinthitis are the most common stimuli to the VA of the inner ear that induce nausea and vomiting. The VA may play a minor role in CINV. Surgery can also induce vomiting through stimulation of the vestibular system.

(g) Memory, fear, anticipation, pain, and a distasteful smell can trigger nausea and vomiting at the cerebral cortex.

(h) Factors that can cause nausea and vomiting include chemotherapy, biotherapy, targeted therapy, radiation therapy, surgery, opioids, and other medications.

(2) Patterns of therapy-related emesis (NCCN, 2008b)

(a) Anticipatory nausea and vomiting: A conditioned response that occurs most commonly before treatment and can be triggered by a particular smell, taste, or sight

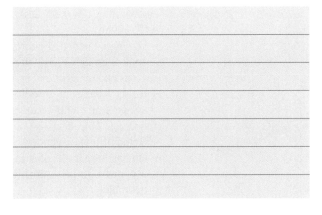

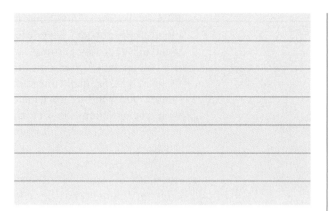

i) Anticipatory nausea and vomiting can occur during treatment and may last one to two days after therapy. This usually is a result of a previous unpleasant experience(s) with uncontrolled nausea and vomiting, and it may be worse in patients with high levels of anxiety. Anticipatory nausea usually occurs after two or three cycles of chemotherapy. To minimize the risk of this side effect, adequate antiemetic control with initial treatments is essential. Infants and young children usually do not experience anticipatory nausea and vomiting.

ii) Incidence: Anticipatory nausea and vomiting occurs in 18%–54% of patients as a result of classical conditioning from stimuli associated with chemotherapy (e.g., odors, tastes of drugs, visual cues) (NCCN, 2008b).

iii) Risk factors: The factors that follow may increase susceptibility to anticipatory nausea and vomiting (Hesketh, 2005; NCI, 2008b).
  • Having a history of poorly controlled CINV with previous encounters
  • Being young or middle-aged (i.e., patients younger than age 50)
  • Being of female gender
  • Having high levels of anxiety prior to and during treatment

• Feeling warm, hot, dizzy, or sweaty after chemotherapy
• Having a susceptibility to motion sickness
• Having a history of pregnancy-induced nausea and vomiting
• Feeling generalized weakness after chemotherapy

(b) Acute nausea and vomiting: Starts within minutes to hours after chemotherapy administration and may last up to 24 hours, depending upon the agent (NCCN, 2008b)

i) The type of chemotherapy, dose, and administration schedule influence the severity and risk of acute nausea and vomiting.

ii) Combination chemotherapy causes more nausea and vomiting than single-agent therapy.

iii) The duration of chemotherapy administration affects nausea and vomiting, with shorter infusions being associated with more nausea and vomiting than continuous infusions.

iv) Incidence is determined by the emetogenicity of the chemotherapy agents (see Table 17) and whether pretreatment with an antiemetic agent occurred (Camp-Sorrell, 2005).

v) Risk factors: The following factors increase susceptibility to acute nausea and vomiting (Hesketh, 2005; NCI, 2008b).
  • Type and dose of antitumor treatment used (see Table 17)
  • Gender: Women experience more acute nausea and vomiting than do men.
  • Age: Patients older than age 50 experience less nausea and vomiting than patients younger than 50.
  • Alcohol use: Patients with a history of chronic or high alcohol intake generally have less severe nausea than do those without such a history.

- Advanced-stage disease
- Fatigue
- Pain
- Tumor burden
- Concomitant medical conditions (e.g., obstruction, pancreatitis, hepatic metastases)
- Presence of strong taste disturbances during chemotherapy
- A high level of pretreatment anxiety
- Susceptibility to GI distress
- Poor performance status

- A history of hyperemesis during pregnancy or morning sickness throughout pregnancy

(c) Delayed nausea and vomiting: Occurs at least 24 hours after chemotherapy administration and may last up to six days (O'Bryant et al., 2004)

  i) The peak of delayed nausea is approximately 48–72 hours after chemotherapy is started (Tipton et al., 2005).

  ii) Chemotherapy metabolites may cause increased delayed nausea and vomiting because

Table 17. Emetogenic Potential of Various Chemotherapeutic Drugs

Incidence	Level	Agent	Onset (hours)	Duration (hours)
Very high (> 90%)	5	Cisplatin (> 50 mg/m^2)	1–6	24–48+
		Dacarbazine	1–3	1–12
		Mechlorethamine	0.5–2	8–24
		Melphalan: high-dose	0.3–6	6–12
		Streptozocin	1–6	12–24
		Cytarabine: high-dose (> 1 g/m^2)	1–4	12–48
High (60%–90%)	4	Carmustine (> 100 mg/m^2)	2–4	4–24
		Cyclophosphamide (600 mg/m^2)	4–12	12–24
		Procarbazine	24–27	variable
		Etoposide: high-dose	4–6	24+
		Semustine	1–5	12–24
		Lomustine	4–6	12–24
		Dactinomycin	2–5	24
		Plicamycin	1–6	12–24
		Methotrexate: high-dose	1–12	24–72
		Actinomycin D	1–12	24–48
		Cytarabine (500 mg/m^2)	1–12	24–48
		Epirubicin	6–12	24+
		Idarubicin	6–12	24+
		Oxaliplatin	1–6	24
Moderate (30%–60%)	3	Doxorubicin (> 50–75 mg/m^2)	4–6	6+
		Mitoxantrone	4–6	6+
		5-fluorouracil	3–6	24+
		Mitomycin-C	1–4	48–72
		Carboplatin	4–6	12–24
		Daunorubicin (< 50 mg/m^2)	2–6	24
		L-asparaginase	1–4	2–12
		Topotecan	6–12	24–72
		Ifosfamide (< 1.5 g/m^2)	3–6	24–72
		Irinotecan	6–12	24+
		Epirubicin	–	–
		Idarubicin	–	–

(Continued on next page)

Table 17. Emetogenic Potential of Various Chemotherapeutic Drugs *(Continued)*

Incidence	Level	Agent	Onset (hours)	Duration (hours)
Low (10%–30%)	2	Bleomycin	3–6	–
		Cytarabine (20 mg/m²)	6–12	3–12
		Etoposide	3–8	–
		Melphalan	6–12	–
		6-mercaptopurine	4–8	–
		Methotrexate (< 100 mg/m²)	4–12	3–12
		Vinblastine	4–8	–
		Hydroxyurea	–	–
		Teniposide	–	–
		Gemcitabine	–	–
		Vinorelbine	–	–
		Fludarabine	–	–
		Topotecan	–	–
		Capecitabine	–	–
		Trimetrexate	–	–
		Imatinib mesylate	–	–
Very low (< 10%)	1	Vincristine	4–8	–
		Chlorambucil	48–72	–
		Busulfan	–	–
		Thioguanine	–	–
		Hormones	–	–
		Paclitaxel	4–8	–
		Docetaxel	–	–
		Thiotepa	–	–
		Bortezomib	–	–
		Temozolomide	–	–
		Valrubicin	–	–
		Tretinoin	–	–
		Gefitinib	–	–

Note. From "Chemotherapy: Toxicity Management" (p. 428), by D. Camp-Sorrell in C.H. Yarbro, M.H. Frogge, and M. Goodman (Eds.), *Cancer Nursing: Principles and Practice* (6th ed.), 2005, Sudbury, MA: Jones and Bartlett. Copyright 2005 by Jones and Bartlett. Reprinted with permission.

of an ongoing effect on the CNS and/or GI tract (Camp-Sorrell, 2005).

iii) Cisplatin is associated with the highest incidence of delayed nausea and vomiting.

iv) In a multisite, longitudinal, descriptive study of patients with breast cancer by Dibble, Israel, Nussey, Casey, and Luce (2003), younger, heavier women experienced delayed nausea more frequently than other women. In addition, this study found that women who had a history of experiencing nausea with stressful situations were more likely to have delayed nausea after receiving cyclophosphamide.

b) Risk factors
(1) Cisplatin-containing regimens (60%–90% of patients) (Jordan, Sipple, & Schmoll, 2007)
(2) High-dose chemotherapy
(3) Cyclophosphamide, ifosfamide, doxorubicin
(4) Poor control of acute nausea and vomiting

c) Assessment: Determine the potential causes of nausea and vomiting, the specific type(s), and the level of emetogenicity.

(1) Chemotherapy: Utilizing the emetogenic levels as described by Hesketh (2005), the emetogenic potential of a particular regimen can be estimated.
  (a) Begin with the most highly emetogenic agent in the regimen and then add levels based on the other agents in the regimen.
  (b) In general, level 1 agents do not add to the emetogenicity of a regimen.
  (c) As one or more level 2 chemotherapy agents are added to a regimen, the emetogenicity of the regimen should be increased by one level.
  (d) Each level 3 or 4 agent added to the regimen increases the emetogenicity of the regimen by one level.
(2) Biotherapy (IFN or IL-2)
  (a) Patients receiving biologic agents may experience nausea and/or vomiting as part of a flu-like syndrome.
  (b) Biotherapy involving the infusion of MoAbs may be associated with nausea and/or vomiting during the infusion; the cause seems related to the infusion process, not the antibodies.
  (c) When nausea or vomiting occurs, it usually does so during the first infusion (e.g., an infusion with rituximab) (Kosits & Callaghan, 2000).
(3) Targeted therapies: Many targeted drugs, which are primarily in pill form, have emerged in the last decade. Each one is unique in terms of mechanism of action and side effects. The majority of currently FDA-approved targeted drugs are associated with mild nausea and vomiting (Hesketh, 2005).
(4) Physical causes: Tumor obstruction, constipation, increased intracranial pressure, brain metastasis, vestibular dysfunction, uncontrolled pain
(5) Metabolic causes: Hypercalcemia, hyponatremia, hyperglycemia, uremia, increased creatinine
(6) Other medications (e.g., opioids, antibiotics)
(7) Psychological causes: Anxiety, fear, emotional distress

d) Potential complications of nausea and vomiting
  (1) Discomfort
  (2) Delay of treatment
  (3) Interference with QOL (e.g., impaired mobility, fatigue)
  (4) Dehydration
  (5) Metabolic disturbances
  (6) Anorexia and weight loss
  (7) Physical debilitation from malnutrition
  (8) Straining of abdominal muscles
  (9) Increased intracranial pressure
  (10) Danger of aspiration
e) Collaborative management—Pharmacologic actions: See Table 18.
  (1) Prevention of nausea and vomiting is the primary goal.
    (a) Choose antiemetics appropriate to the chemotherapeutic regimen.
    (b) Consider level of emetogenicity based on route of administration and dose administered.
    (c) Consider cumulative chemotherapy emetogenicity.
    (d) Administer antiemetics to cover the expected emetogenic period of the chemotherapy agent, considering duration and pattern of emesis.
    (e) Note: Steroids may be contraindicated for patients receiving biotherapy agents because of their immunosuppressive effects. This is agent-specific and should be a consideration prior to use. The benefit of steroids for minimizing hypersensitivity reactions or treating nausea and vomiting may outweigh the risks related to immunosuppression (Genentech, 2007; Kang & Saif, 2007).

Table 18. Select Pharmacologic Agents for the Prevention and Treatment of Chemotherapy-Induced Nausea and Vomiting

Class	Mechanism of Action	Medication Name	Route, Dose, and Schedule	Indications	Side Effects	Nursing Considerations
Antipsychotic	Action in multiple CINV receptor sites	Olanzapine	2.5–5 mg PO BID	Breakthrough nausea/vomiting	Dry mouth, weight gain, dizziness, sedation	Drug is contraindicated in older adult patients with dementia.
Anxiolytic	CNS depressant, interferes with afferent nerves from cerebral cortex causing sedation	Alprazolam	0.5–2 mg PO TID, for anticipatory nausea/vomiting 0.5–2 mg PO TID, beginning the night before treatment	Prevention of anticipatory nausea/vomiting	Sedation, confusion, hyperactivity, agitation, dizziness, lightheadedness, hallucinations	Decrease starting dose to 0.25 mg PO BID or TID in older adult patients, patients with advanced liver disease, or patients with other comorbidities that are pertinent.
	CNS depressant, interferes with afferent nerves from cerebral cortex causing sedation	Lorazepam	0.5–2 mg PO or sublingual; 0.5–2 mg IV every 4–6 hr, for anticipatory nausea/vomiting 0.5–2 mg PO beginning the night prior to treatment and the morning of treatment	Prevention of anticipatory nausea/vomiting In combination with other antiemetics as needed for acute or delayed nausea/vomiting	Sedation, confusion, hyperactivity, agitation, dizziness, lightheadedness, hallucinations	Use with caution in older adult patients or those with hepatic or renal dysfunction. Give first dose the night before treatment and the morning of chemotherapy for anticipatory nausea/vomiting.
Cannabinoid	Interacts with cannabinoid receptors	Dronabinol	5–10 mg PO TID or QID	Treatment of CINV after standard antiemetics have failed	Sedation, vertigo, euphoria, dysphoria, dry mouth, tachycardia, orthostasis	Incidence of paranoid reactions or abnormal thinking increases with maximum doses. Use with caution in patients with history of psychiatric illness.
		Nabilone	1–2 mg PO BID Maximum recommended dose is 6 mg given in divided doses TID.	Treatment of CINV after standard antiemetics have failed	Sedation, vertigo, euphoria, dysphoria, dry mouth, tachycardia, orthostasis	Incidence of paranoid reactions or abnormal thinking increases with maximum doses. Use with caution in patients with history of psychiatric illness.
Corticosteroid	Anti-prostaglandin synthesis activity	Dexamethasone	12 mg IV or PO day 1 of chemotherapy; 8 mg PO or IV days 2–4 of chemotherapy	Prevention of nausea and vomiting caused by high and moderately emetogenic chemotherapy Prevention of delayed nausea or vomiting	Administer slowly over at least 10 min to prevent perianal or vaginal burning or itching. Insomnia, anxiety, acne	Adding a corticosteroid increases the efficacy of antiemetic regimens by 15%–25%. Add dexamethasone to 5HT$_3$ regimens.
Dopamine antagonist	Blocks dopamine receptors	Haloperidol	1–2 mg PO every 4–6 hr or 1–3 mg IV every 4–6 hr	Prevention of delayed nausea/vomiting or treatment of breakthrough nausea/vomiting	Sedation, extrapyramidal symptoms, dystonia, dizziness, orthostasis	Administering haloperidol with diphenhydramine 25–50 mg PO or IV prevents extrapyramidal symptoms; occurs more commonly in younger patients. Drug is highly sedating.

(Continued on next page)

Table 18. Select Pharmacologic Agents for the Prevention and Treatment of Chemotherapy-Induced Nausea and Vomiting (Continued)

Class	Mechanism of Action	Medication Name	Route, Dose, and Schedule	Indications	Side Effects	Nursing Considerations
		Metoclopramide	20–40 mg PO every 4–6 hr; 1–2 mg/kg IV every 3–4 hr	Prevention of nausea/vomiting caused by moderately emetogenic chemotherapy; Prevention of delayed nausea/vomiting or treatment of breakthrough nausea/vomiting	Sedation, extrapyramidal symptoms, dystonia, dizziness, orthostasis	Incidence of drowsiness is greater with high doses. Drug may cause diarrhea.
		Prochlorperazine	Doses vary: 10 mg PO or IV every 4–6 hr; Also available: 25 mg suppositories every 12 hr	Prevention of delayed nausea/vomiting or treatment of breakthrough nausea/vomiting	Sedation, extrapyramidal symptoms, dystonia, dizziness, orthostasis	Drug is not used for pediatric patients. Drug is highly sedating.
Neurokinin-1 antagonist	Neurokinin-1 receptor antagonist	Aprepitant	Capsules: 125 mg PO day 1 of chemotherapy, then 80 mg PO days 2 and 3	Prevention of acute and delayed CINV in combination with other antiemetics; Approved for initial and repeated courses of highly emetogenic chemotherapy	Constipation, hiccups, loss of appetite, diarrhea, fatigue	Drug is given in combination with corticosteroid and $5HT_3$ antagonists on day 1 and a corticosteroid on days 2 and 3. Consider a 50% dose reduction of oral methylprednisolone and dexamethasone and a 25% dose reduction of IV methylprednisolone. (Aprepitant increases the AUC of steroids 1–3-fold.) Use with caution in patients receiving chemotherapy that is primarily metabolized through CYP3A4. The efficacy of oral contraceptives during administration of aprepitant may be compromised. Coadministration of aprepitant and warfarin may decrease INR; monitor closely.
Serotonin antagonist	Serotonin receptor antagonist	Dolasetron	100 mg PO, or 100 mg IV, 30 min before chemotherapy	Prevention of CINV	Headache, diarrhea, dizziness, fatigue, abnormal LFTs	Dolasetron precipitates with dexamethasone in D5W. Dolasetron can be administered as a rapid IV bolus.
		Granisetron	2 mg PO up to 1 hr before chemotherapy; 1 mg PO or 10 mcg/kg IV 30 min before chemotherapy	Prevention of nausea and vomiting during chemotherapy at initial and repeated cycles; Approved for use with high-dose cisplatin	Headache, asthenia, diarrhea, constipation, fever, somnolence	Granisetron can be administered by rapid bolus. Instruct patients to take oral formulation with milk or food.

(Continued on next page)

Table 18. Select Pharmacologic Agents for the Prevention and Treatment of Chemotherapy-Induced Nausea and Vomiting (Continued)

Class	Mechanism of Action	Medication Name	Route, Dose, and Schedule	Indications	Side Effects	Nursing Considerations
		Granisetron transdermal (Sancuso®)	Transdermal patch containing 34.3 mg of granisetron; one patch delivers 3.1 mg per 24 hr. Apply a single patch to the upper outer arm a minimum of 24 hr before chemotherapy. Patch can be worn for up to 7 days (depending upon the duration of the regimen). Remove patch a minimum of 24 hr after completion of chemotherapy.	Prevention of nausea and vomiting in patients receiving moderately and/or highly emetogenic chemotherapy for up to 5 consecutive days	Constipation; may mask a progressive ileus and/or gastric distention caused by the underlying condition Headache, skin rash, QTc prolongation	Drug is contraindicated in patients with known hypersensitivity to granisetron or any of the components of the patch. Remove patch if severe skin reactions occur (allergic rash, or erythematous, macular, papular rash or pruritus). Avoid direct exposure of patch to natural or artificial light while wearing the patch and for 10 days after removing it.
		Ondansetron	8–32 mg IV once; infuse over 15 min; give 30 min before chemotherapy. Oral doses vary, ranging from 8–24 mg/day. With moderately emetogenic therapy, administer 8 mg BID 30 min before chemotherapy and continuing for 1–2 days after chemotherapy. With highly emetogenic chemotherapy, administer 24 mg PO 30 min before chemotherapy. Orally disintegrating tablet formulation: 8 mg	Prevention of nausea/vomiting associated with single-day highly and moderately emetogenic chemotherapy in adults	Headache, diarrhea, fever, constipation, transient increase in serum SGOT, SGPT, hypotension	Ondansetron and dexamethasone are compatible.
		Palonosetron	0.25 mg fixed IV dose; infuse over 30 sec. Give 30 min prior to chemotherapy.	Prevention of acute nausea and vomiting associated with initial and repeated courses of moderately and highly emetogenic chemotherapy and the prevention of delayed nausea and vomiting associated with initial and repeat courses of moderately emetogenic chemotherapy	Headache, constipation	Mean terminal elimination half-life is approximately 40 hr. Palonosetron is the first $5HT_3$ approved for delayed nausea/vomiting. Repeat dosing within a 7-day interval is not recommended until further evaluated. Drug is not currently used for pediatric patients.

AUC—area under the plasma concentration versus time curve; BID—two times daily; CINV—chemotherapy-induced nausea and vomiting; CNS—central nervous system; D5W—5% dextrose in water; $5HT_3$—hydroxytryptamine-3; hr—hour; INR—international normalized ratio; IV—intravenous; LFT—liver function test; mcg—microgram; mg—milligram; min—minute; PO—oral; QID—four times daily; QTc—QT interval corrected; sec—second; SGOT—serum glutamic-oxaloacetic transaminase; SGPT—serum glutamic-pyruvic transaminase; TID—three times daily

Note. Based on information from Camp-Sorrell, 2005; Massaro & Lenz, 2005; Merck & Co., Inc., 2008; National Comprehensive Cancer Network, 2008b; Tipton et al., 2005.

(2) To manage acute nausea and vomiting (NCCN, 2008b) (Tipton et al., 2005)

(a) For patients at high risk (level 5): Use a combination of a $5HT_3$ antagonist, a neurokinin-1 (NK-1) antagonist, plus a corticosteroid before chemotherapy. Lorazepam also may be used in combination with the aforementioned antiemetics to improve control in high-risk regimens.

   i) Administration of a corticosteroid with a $5HT_3$ antagonist has been found to improve the control of nausea and vomiting when compared to a $5HT_3$ antagonist alone and is recommended for acute nausea in highly emetogenic regimens by NCCN, ASCO, and the Multinational Association of Supportive Care in Cancer (MASCC) (Jordan, Sippel, et al., 2007).

   ii) If the antitumor regimen contains steroids as part of the treatment regimen (e.g., CHOP), additional steroids may not be needed (NCCN, 2008b).

   iii) A recent meta-analysis demonstrated no difference in efficacy between IV and PO $5HT_3$ antagonists (Jordan, Grothey, et al., 2007).

(b) For patients at moderate risk (levels 3–4): Use a combination of a corticosteroid and a $5HT_3$ antagonist. Consider adding an NK-1 antagonist for patients at high risk (e.g., patients receiving anthracycline and cyclophosphamide regimens). The addition of lorazepam may be considered in select patients.

(c) For patients at low risk (level 2): Use a daily single agent such as a corticosteroid, prochlorperazine, metoclopramide, or $5HT_3$ antagonist. Lorazepam also may be added.

(d) For patients at minimal risk (level 1): No routine prophylaxis. Ongoing assessment for the occurrence of nausea and/or vomiting should be performed. If nausea and vomiting occurs, treat per low-risk guidelines.

(e) For patients undergoing multiple consecutive days of chemotherapy: Each day, use antiemetics appropriate to the risk category of the chemotherapy to be administered that day.

(3) To manage delayed nausea and vomiting (NCCN, 2008b)

(a) Delayed nausea and vomiting is a significant problem for patients with cancer who are receiving chemotherapy, and prevention is the primary goal. New approaches such as NK-1 antagonists and longer-acting $5HT_3$ antagonists continue to be investigated in an attempt to improve management of nausea and vomiting in this setting (Massaro & Lenz, 2005).

(b) For patients at risk for delayed nausea and vomiting (e.g., patients receiving cisplatin)

   i) Utilize an NK-1 antagonist on days 1–3 for delayed nausea and vomiting in combination with a corticosteroid.

   ii) Utilize a single agent such as a corticosteroid, a $5HT_3$ antagonist, or a dopamine antagonist.

   iii) Utilize a combination of the previously listed antiemetics based on patient-specific needs (see Table 18).

   iv) Note: Metoclopramide rarely is used for pediatric patients.

(4) To manage anticipatory nausea and vomiting: Use the most active antiemetic regimens appropriate to the chemotherapy being given. Such regimens must be used with the initial chemotherapy rather than after assess-

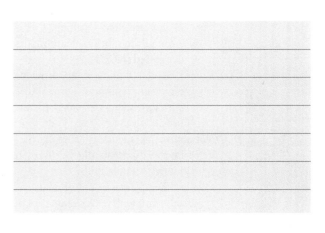

ment of the patient's emetic response to less-effective treatment.

   (a) Benzodiazepines (lorazepam or alprazolam) are the primary drugs used for the treatment of anticipatory nausea and vomiting (Aapro, Molassiotis, & Olver, 2004).

   (b) Consider the addition of nonpharmacologic interventions, which can be helpful in this type of nausea (see section *f*) (Tipton et al., 2005).

(5) For patients experiencing breakthrough nausea and vomiting despite optimal prophylaxis in current or prior cycles, ascertain that the best regimen is being given based on the emetogenic potential of the regimen (NCCN, 2008b).

   (a) Conduct a careful evaluation of risk, antiemetic agents, disease, concurrent conditions, and medication factors.

   (b) Consider adding an antianxiety agent to the regimen.

   (c) Consider adding other antiemetic agents from different drug classifications, using caution to avoid overlapping side effects (see Table 18).

   (d) Multiple agents used in combination may be required to gain control over nausea and vomiting.

   (e) Around-the-clock scheduling is suggested (NCCN, 2008b).

   (f) Consider adding nonpharmacologic interventions in conjunction with antiemetics per patient preference.

f) Collaborative management—Nonpharmacologic interventions should be used in conjunction with antiemetics.

(1) Music therapy is the controlled use of music to influence physiologic, psy-chological, and emotional responses. Music therapy often is used in conjunction with other techniques.

   (a) In a randomized study of 33 BMT recipients receiving high-dose chemotherapy, music therapy was found to significantly reduce the incidence of nausea and vomiting.

   (b) It has been suggested that music therapy may decrease the patient's perception of the degree of vomiting (Ezzone, Baker, & Terrepka, 1998). However, this has not been firmly established and requires further study.

(2) Moderate aerobic exercise may be beneficial in improving the relief of nausea (Tipton et al., 2005). Additional research is needed in this area.

(3) Acupressure wristbands have been used with some success. Acupressure is a form of massage using pressure to localized areas to reduce symptoms such as nausea and vomiting (NCI, 2008b).

   (a) In a recent Cochrane Database systematic review (Ezzo, Streitberger, & Schneider, 2006), acupressure was found to have no significant benefit for delayed nausea and vomiting. This review found acupressure to have some benefit in acute nausea but not vomiting.

   (b) Dibble et al. (2007) studied acupressure in patients with breast cancer undergoing chemotherapy and found a benefit when utilizing acupressure at the p6 point (medial aspect of the forearm) for delayed CINV. Additional studies are warranted.

(4) Acupuncture and electroacupuncture currently are being studied for the treatment of CINV.

   (a) Acupuncture is the insertion of fine-gauge needles at specific points.

   (b) Electroacupuncture is the use of electric pulses with acupuncture needles to increase stimulation.

   (c) Research is needed to determine which of these treatments may be more beneficial, as well as the efficacy when combined with current pharmacologic interventions (Ezzo et al., 2006).

(5) Behavioral interventions such as self-hypnosis, progressive muscle relaxation, biofeedback, guided imagery, cognitive distraction, and systematic desensitization have been used either alone or in combination with pharmacologic agents to prevent or control CINV. These behavioral methods have been used with success and may be used as adjunct therapies with pharmacologic interventions.

(6) Dietary interventions (Tipton et al., 2005; Wickham, 2008)

  (a) Encourage patients to eat small, frequent meals.

  (b) Medicate patients prior to meals so that the antiemetic effect is active during, and immediately after, eating.

  (c) Encourage patients to avoid fatty, spicy, and highly salted foods, and foods with strong odors.

  (d) Determine and repeat past measures that have been effective in controlling nausea and vomiting.

  (e) Encourage patients to eat cold or room-temperature foods because these emit fewer odors than do hot foods.

  (f) Suggest that patients cook meals between chemotherapy regimens, when they are not nauseated, and freeze the meals for later use, or suggest that another family member cook meals.

  (g) Encourage patients to eat favorite foods when not experiencing nausea and vomiting to prevent permanent dislike of these foods (NCI, 2008b).

  (h) Utilize ginger for CINV only per patient preference.

    i) In a systematic review of six randomized, controlled clinical trials (RCCTs) performed to assess the efficacy of ginger for nausea and vomiting, there was insufficient evidence to show benefit (Ernst & Pittler, 2000).

    ii) In another randomized study of gynecologic patients receiving cisplatin, ginger did not prove beneficial (Manu-sirivithaya et al., 2004).

    iii) Additional RCCTs with patients receiving chemotherapy are needed to prove safety and benefit.

  g) Patient and family education

    (1) Instruct adult patients to notify the staff if nausea and vomiting persist for more than 24 hours or if they are unable to maintain fluid intake. Ensure that parents of pediatric patients know to notify staff if vomiting persists for more than two hours. In children, just a few hours of vomiting can cause dehydration.

    (2) Remind patients as necessary to take antiemetics before arriving for treatment. Ensure that antiemetics have been taken prior to administration of chemotherapy.

    (3) Follow up 24–48 hours after outpatient treatment to ensure adherence to or effectiveness of the antiemetic regimen (Camp-Sorrell, 2005).

2. Diarrhea

  a) Pathophysiology

    (1) Diarrhea is defined as loose or watery stools. Diarrhea resulting from administration of chemotherapy or specific biotherapy agents is a frequent problem. Left untreated or inadequately treated, diarrhea can lead to severe dehydration, hospitalizations, chemotherapy delays, dose reductions, and even death (Dranitsaris, Maroun, & Shah, 2005).

    (2) The pathophysiology and etiology of diarrhea in patients with cancer can be multifaceted. All possible causes of diarrhea need to be considered to treat the patient appropriately. The most common mechanisms of chemotherapy-induced diarrhea are osmotic, secretory, and exudative (NCI, 2008a).

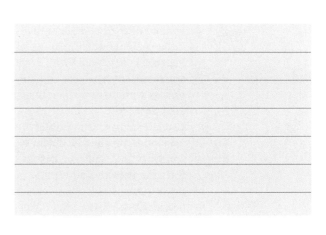

(a) Osmotic diarrhea: Osmotic diarrhea usually is related to injury to the gut, dietary factors, or problems with digestion. Unabsorbable substances draw water into the intestinal lumen by osmosis, resulting in increased stool volume and weight (Field, 2003). Lactose intolerance is an example of this type of diarrhea, which can occur in patients undergoing cancer treatment (Roy, 2006). Osmotic diarrhea is associated with large stool volumes and sometimes is improved with fasting or elimination of the causative factor (e.g., lactose, glucose) (Vogel, Viele, & Stern, 2004).

(b) Secretory diarrhea: The small and large intestines secrete more fluids and electrolytes than can be absorbed. Infection and inflammation of the gut; damage to the gut caused by chemotherapy, radiation, or graft-versus-host disease (GVHD); and certain endocrine tumors can cause secretory diarrhea. The imbalance between absorption and secretion leads to the production of a large volume of fluid and electrolytes in the small bowel. This type of diarrhea is associated with large volumes and usually is not improved with fasting (Engelking, 2004).

(c) Exudative diarrhea: Caused by alterations in mucosal integrity, epithelial loss, enzyme destruction, and defective absorption of the colon. Mucosal inflammation and ulceration caused by inflammatory diseases, cancers, and cancer treatment may result in the outpouring of plasma, proteins, mucus, and blood into the stool, all of which can result in exudative diarrhea. This type of diarrhea is characterized by > six stools per day (Field, 2003).

b) Chemotherapy agents presenting the highest risk of diarrhea (Weaver & Buckner, 2007)
   (1) Irinotecan
   (2) 5-FU
   (3) Paclitaxel
   (4) Dactinomycin
   (5) Dacarbazine
   (6) Capecitabine

c) Examples of chemotherapy agents that may cause diarrhea
   (1) Fludarabine
   (2) Cytarabine
   (3) Idarubicin
   (4) Mitoxantrone
   (5) Pentostatin
   (6) Floxuridine
   (7) Topotecan
   (8) Cisplatin
   (9) Oxaliplatin
   (10) Docetaxel
   (11) Pemetrexed
   (12) Hydroxyurea

d) Biotherapy agents that may cause diarrhea
   (1) IL-2
   (2) IFNs

e) Targeted agents that may cause diarrhea
   (1) MoAbs
   (2) Imatinib mesylate
   (3) Dasatinib
   (4) Erlotinib
   (5) Bortezomib
   (6) Lapatinib
   (7) Gefitinib
   (8) Sunitinib malate
   (9) Temsirolimus
   (10) Revlimid and thalidomide
   (11) Vorinostat

f) Incidence of diarrhea following cytotoxic therapy
   (1) The incidence of diarrhea varies greatly depending upon the agent(s) used. The incidence of chemotherapy-induced diarrhea is < 80% with specific agents or combinations of agents (Arnold et al., 2005).
   (2) The specific agent, dose, schedule, and combination with other anticancer

therapies all influence the severity of chemotherapy-induced diarrhea.

g) Clinical manifestations and consequences: If manifestations are severe, the course of action may be to modify or hold the chemotherapeutic agent, which could compromise the benefit of the regimen. The clinical manifestations of diarrhea include the following (Arnold et al., 2005; Benson et al., 2004; Vogel et al., 2004).

(1) Dehydration: Diarrhea dehydrates pediatric patients very quickly.
(2) Orthostasis
(3) Life-threatening hypokalemia, metabolic acidosis, hypercalcemia, malnutrition
(4) Cardiovascular or renal compromise
(5) Impaired immune function following frequent episodes of chemotherapy-induced diarrhea
(6) Perianal skin breakdown and/or infection
(7) Reduced absorption of oral medications
(8) Pain (abdominal cramping)
(9) Anxiety
(10) Exhaustion
(11) Decreased QOL

h) Risk factors

(1) Radiation therapy to the pelvis, abdomen, or lower thoracic and lumbar spine. This can lead to destruction of the cells of the lumen of the bowel and can be an acute or chronic toxicity.
(2) 5-FU in combination with high-dose leucovorin (500 mg/m²) or 5-FU administered as a weekly bolus (versus continuous infusion) (Goldberg, Sargent, et al., 2004). Irinotecan is associated with both acute and delayed diarrhea. Irinotecan combined with bolus 5-FU and leucovorin is associated with increased morbidity and mortality related to diarrhea (Benson et al., 2004).
(3) Immunosuppression
(4) Intestinal resection or gastrectomy
(5) Manipulation of bowel during surgery, which may cause diarrhea or ileus
(6) Intestinal infection secondary to mucositis and neutropenia (e.g., infection with Rotavirus, *Escherichia coli, Shigella, Salmonella, Giardia,* or *Clostridium difficile*)

(7) GVHD
(8) Dietary causes (e.g., lactose intolerance; ingestion of caffeine, alcohol, or spicy or fatty foods; use of hyperosmotic dietary supplements)
(9) Inflammatory conditions, such as diverticulitis, irritable bowel syndrome, or ulcerative colitis
(10) Malabsorption, partial bowel obstruction, bowel edema, motility disruption
(11) Anxiety and stress

i) Assessment: Accurate assessment is vital in determining the cause and type of diarrhea; knowing the cause and type can be crucial to proper treatment.

(1) Mistakenly using an antidiarrheal to treat diarrhea caused by infection can intensify diarrhea severity and infectious complications (Curry, Hospenthal, & Lee, 2007).
(2) Irinotecan causes two distinct forms of diarrhea (early onset and late onset), and each requires a different management strategy (Pfizer Oncology, 2007).
(3) Assess stools.
   (a) Assess the pattern of elimination and stool character in relation to treatments (e.g., onset, duration, frequency, consistency, amount, odor, color). Chemotherapy-induced diarrhea usually consists of frequent, watery to semisolid stools with an onset of 24–96 hours after chemotherapy administration (Engelking, 2004).
   (b) Assess for presence of nocturnal diarrhea, which can be associated with diabetic autonomic neuropathy or infections. Loss of sleep or interrupted sleep during the night also may increase fatigue.

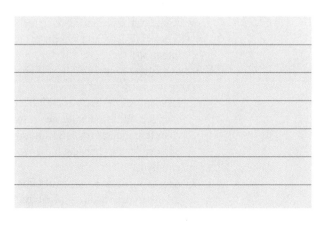

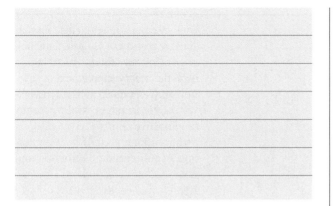

(c) Grade the diarrhea according to NCI CTCAE criteria (NCI CTEP, 2006).

(d) Watch for the presence of blood or mucus in the stools.

(e) Monitor the patient for incontinence.

(4) Conduct a physical examination: The presence of fever, blood in the stool, abdominal pain, weakness, or dizziness warrants medical attention to rule out infection, bowel obstruction, or dehydration (Benson et al., 2004). The steps of a physical examination follow.

(a) Auscultate for bowel sounds.

(b) Palpate and assess the abdomen.

(c) Assess for fecal impaction. Use caution with thrombocytopenic and neutropenic patients.

(d) Look for signs of malnutrition, dehydration, electrolyte imbalance, and infectious process.

(e) Ask about pain experienced during or after defecation.

(f) Assess for fever, weakness, and dizziness.

(g) Determine if blood has been present in the stool (occult or gross).

(h) Assess perianal area for skin breakdown and signs and symptoms of infection.

(5) Take a diet history (Engelking, 2008).

(a) Determine if dietary habits have changed. Be especially aware of clues that indicate that the amount of fiber in the diet has increased rapidly.

(b) Assess for intake that could contribute to diarrhea (e.g., irritating foods, alcohol, coffee, fiber, fruit, lactose-containing foods/fluids, sorbitol-based gum, candy, or other foods).

(c) Assess for food or lactose intolerance or allergies.

(6) Take a medication history: Assess for use of the following (Engelking, 2008).

(a) Antacids (especially those containing magnesium)

(b) Antibiotics

(c) Antihypertensives

(d) Potassium or calcium supplements

(e) Diuretics

(f) Caffeine

(g) Theophylline

(h) NSAIDs

(i) Antiarrhythmic drugs

(j) Laxatives or stool softeners

(k) Promotility agents (metoclopramide)

(l) Magnesium oxide

(m) Opioids (withdrawal)

(7) Assess for other possible contributing factors.

(a) Travel history (outside the United States)

(b) Use of alternative therapies (e.g., dietary supplements, herbal remedies)

(8) Take objective measurements (Engelking, 2008).

(a) Monitor intake and output.

(b) Monitor weight.

(c) Monitor laboratory data.

i) Check stool culture results to determine the presence of infection.

ii) Check serum chemistries to determine if electrolyte imbalance, specifically potassium, exists. Albumin also may be decreased with diarrhea.

iii) Assess complete blood count (CBC) to determine if neutropenia and/or infection are present.

(d) Check skin turgor.

(e) Check vital signs.

j) Collaborative management

(1) Monitor number, amount, and consistency of bowel movements. For patients with colostomies, an increase in the number of loose

stools daily should be monitored to assess for chemotherapy-induced diarrhea.

(2) Replace fluid and electrolytes, including potassium. Electrolytes and fluids are absorbed in the small intestine. When diarrhea occurs, these substances quickly pass through the small intestine without absorbing. This can cause severe fluid and electrolyte disturbances.

(3) Administer antidiarrheal medication as appropriate once an infection has been ruled out. This will reduce stool frequency, volume, and peristalsis. Reassess the severity of chemotherapy-induced diarrhea at the appropriate interval after antidiarrheal medication. Table 19 lists antidiarrheal medications.

(4) Consider the use of antibiotics for patients with persistent diarrhea and signs of infection (Benson et al., 2004).

(5) See Figure 24 for an example of chemotherapy-induced diarrhea treatment guidelines.

k) Patient and family education (Engelking, 2008; NCI, 2008a): Instruct patients to

(1) Know when to start antidiarrheal medications (e.g., with certain chemotherapeutic agents, antidiarrheal medication should be provided so that patients can self-administer at the onset).

(2) Add to diet foods containing pectin, such as bananas, avocados, or beets; unspiced applesauce; and peeled apples. Pectin is a natural fiber that can reduce diarrhea.

(3) Eliminate from the diet foods that are stimulating or irritating to the GI tract (e.g., whole-grain products, nuts, seeds, popcorn, pickles, relishes, rich pastries, raw vegetables).

(4) Eat a low-residue, low-roughage, low-fat diet that includes potassium-rich foods, such as the BRAT diet (bananas, rice, applesauce or apples [peeled], and toast [dry]).

(5) Avoid alcohol, caffeine-containing products, and tobacco.

(6) Avoid greasy foods, spicy foods (e.g., curry, chili powder, garlic), and fried foods.

(7) Maintain fluid intake by drinking 8–10 large glasses each day of clear fluids (e.g., bouillon; weak, tepid tea; gelatin; sports drinks). Water alone lacks the needed electrolytes and vitamins. Carbonated and caffeinated drinks contain relatively few electrolyes and may worsen diarrhea. Fluids with glucose are useful because glucose absorption drives sodium and water back into the body.

(8) Avoid prune juice and orange juice.

(9) Eat food at room temperature. Hot and cold foods may aggravate diarrhea.

(10) Avoid milk and dairy products.

(11) Avoid hyperosmotic supplements (e.g., Ensure®), which can contribute to the production of loose, high-volume stools (Wadler, 2004).

(12) Clean the rectal area with mild soap and water after each bowel movement, rinse well, and pat dry with a soft towel. Cleaning decreases the risk of infection and skin irritation.

(13) Apply moisture-barrier ointment to protect perianal skin.

(14) Take warm sitz baths to relieve pain related to perianal inflammation. Anesthetic creams or sprays also may help to relieve pain related to inflammation.

(15) Know when diarrhea can be self-managed and when to seek help.

(16) Report excessive thirst, fever, dizziness or lightheadedness, palpitations, rectal spasms, excessive cramping, watery or bloody stools, and continued diarrhea in spite of antidiarrheal treatment. These symptoms can be life-threatening.

Table 19. Common Antidiarrheal Medications

Class	Mechanism of Action	Medication Name	Route, Dose, and Schedule*	Side Effects*	Nursing Considerations*
Absorbent agent	Bulk-forming laxative	Calcium polycarbophil (FiberCon®, Equalactin®)	Adults: 1 g 1–4 times daily or as needed; do not exceed 6 g in 24 hr	Abdominal distention, flatulence	Contraindicated in patients with blood or mucus in the stool and for patients with fecal impaction or intestinal obstruction May interfere with absorption of some medications Adequate water intake must be ensured (at least 8 ounces with each dose).
Antimotility agent	Slows GI transit time and promotes reabsorption of water from bowel; antiperistaltic	Diphenoxylate HCl with atropine sulfate (Lomotil®)	Adults: Individualize dosage. Initial dose is 10 mg followed by 5 mg PO QID; maximum dose is 20 mg/day.	Dry mouth, urinary retention, confusion, sedation, restlessness	Invasive bacterial diarrhea, pseudomembranous colitis In patients with advanced liver disease, drug may precipitate hepatic coma. Do not use in children younger than age two.
		Loperamide (Imodium® A-D)	Adults: 4 mg PO initially, followed by 2 mg PO after each unformed stool; do not exceed 16 mg/day. Exception: Doses are higher for late-onset irinotecan-induced diarrhea (2 mg every 2 hr).	Constipation, fatigue, urinary retention, drowsiness, dizziness	Invasive bacterial diarrhea Should not be used in children younger than age two
Antisecretory agent	Binds bacterial toxins, stimulates absorption of fluid and electrolytes	Bismuth subsalicylate (Pepto-Bismol®)	Adults: 2 tablets or 30 ml every 30 minutes for 1 hr, as needed, up to 8 doses in 24 hr	Many formulations exist; check packaging for appropriate dosing guidelines.	Drug interacts with warfarin and tetracycline. Use caution with concomitant aspirin/salicylates. Each tablespoon of regular-strength Pepto-Bismol contains 120 mg of salicylate and should be avoided in patients with thrombocytopenia. Drug can darken stool and tongue.
Somatostatin analog	Inhibits growth hormone, glucagon, and insulin; prolongs intestinal transit time; increases sodium and water absorption	Octreotide (Sandostatin®)	Adults: IV/IM and SC doses for chemotherapy-induced diarrhea vary.	Abdominal discomfort, flatulence, constipation, diarrhea, nausea, dizziness, headache, cardiac dysrhythmias, bradycardia	Drug may interact with insulin, oral hypoglycemic medications, beta-blockers, or calcium channel blockers. Insulin requirements may be decreased. Observe for hyperglycemia/hypoglycemia. Drug may decrease levels of cyclosporine when given concurrently. Drug may increase risk of developing gallstones.

(Continued on next page)

Table 19. Common Antidiarrheal Medications (Continued)

Class	Mechanism of Action	Medication Name	Route, Dose, and Schedule*	Side Effects*	Nursing Considerations*
Anticholinergic	Antagonist of acetylcholine	Atropine	Adults: Used for early-onset cholinergic diarrhea (e.g., irinotecan induced) 0.25–1 mg PO or SC	Dry mouth, blurred vision, photophobia, constipation, xerostomia, tachyarrhythmia	Antacids interfere with absorption of atropine. Drug is contraindicated in patients with closed-angle glaucoma.
	Antagonist of acetylcholine	Belladonna	Consult product information for dosing.	Dry mouth, blurred vision, photophobia	Many formulations exist. Belladonna causes many drug interactions.
	Tropane alkaloid drug with muscarinic antagonistic effects	Scopolamine (transdermal scopolamine patch)	1.5 mg patch lasts 72 hr. Used for nausea/vomiting associated with motion sickness	Dry mouth, blurred vision, photophobia, restlessness	Apply to the postauricular area. Do not apply to irritated skin. Wash hands after applying and removing patch. Apply at least 4 hr before desired effect. Drug is contraindicated in children and lactating women.

*Consult product information for complete list of contraindications, drug interactions, and dosage ranges.

GI—gastrointestinal; hr—hour; IM—intramuscular; IV—intravenous; PO—oral; QID—four times daily; SC—subcutaneous

Note. Based on information from Benson et al., 2004; Engelking, 2008; Micromedex, 2007; Rosenoff, 2004; Spratto & Woods, 2007; Wadler, 2004; and manufacturers' prescribing information.

3. Mucositis: Mucositis is a common complication of both systemic cytotoxic therapy and radiation therapy. It can be a dose-limiting toxicity of hyperfractionated radiotherapy and concurrent chemotherapy and radiation (NCI, 2008c; Sonis, 2007). Severe mucositis is associated with decreased QOL, increased risk of infections, hospitalizations, opioid use, parenteral nutrition, and dose reductions and delays (Murphy, 2007; Rosenthal, 2007). Terms used in this discussion include the following.

  • *Mucositis:* A general term referring to inflammation of any mucosal membranes, including the oral cavity

  • *Stomatitis or oral mucositis:* Any inflammatory condition of oral tissue including mucosa, dentition, periapices, and periodontium (Eilers & Million, 2007). Stomatitis includes oral infections.

  a) Pathophysiology: Oral mucositis traditionally has been attributed to the direct effects of cytotoxic drugs or radiation on epithelial stem cells. More recently, evidence has suggested that microvascular injury and connective tissue damage in the submucosa precede epithelial damage. Oral mucositis is now described as having five phases (Sonis, 2007).

   (1) Initiation: Stomatotoxic drugs or radiation therapy generate reactive oxygen species that damage DNA, resulting in cell, tissue, and blood vessel damage in the mucosa.

   (2) Upregulation and generation of messenger signals: Nuclear factor-κB (NF-κB) is activated by chemotherapy or radiation therapy. This results in the upregulation of a large number of genes and the release of proinflammatory cytokines, such as TNF-alpha (TNF-α), IL-1 beta (IL-1β), and IL-6. These and other cytokines are responsible for tissue injury and apoptosis.

   (3) Signaling and amplification: In addition to direct tissue damage caused by the proinflammatory cytokines, they activate the production of tissue-damaging TNF-α, IL-1β, and IL-6, and other cytokines that alter the tissues in the mucosa.

   (4) Ulceration: Tissue injury in the oral mucosa appears as ulcers that penetrate through the epithelium to the submucosa. Bacteria penetrate the submucosa and stimulate macrophage activity, which increases the release of pro-

Figure 24. Proposed Algorithm for the Assessment and Management of Treatment-Induced Diarrhea

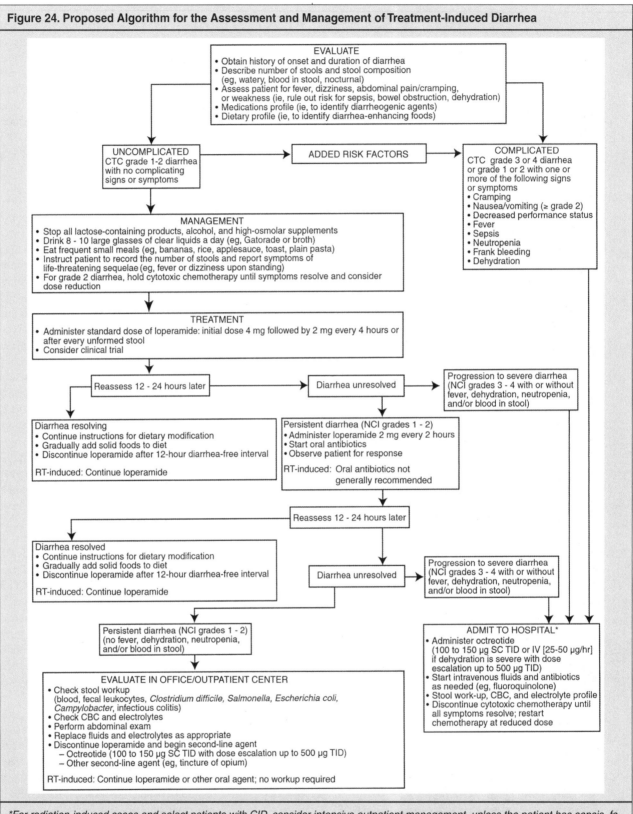

For radiation-induced cases and select patients with CID, consider intensive outpatient management, unless the patient has sepsis, fever, or neutropenia. CTC, Common Toxicity Criteria; NCI, National Cancer Institute; RT, radiotherapy; SC, subcutaneous; tid, three times per day; IV, intravenous; CBC, complete blood count; CID, chemotherapy-induced diarrhea.

Note. Based on information from Benson et al., 2004.
From "Management of Cancer Treatment–Related Diarrhea Issues and Therapeutic Strategies," by S.M. Kornblau, A.B. Benson, III, R. Catalano, R.E. Champlin, C. Engelking, M. Field, et al., 2000, *Journal of Pain and Symptom Management, 19*(2), p. 125. Copyright 2000 by Elsevier. Adapted with permission.

inflammatory cytokines. Angiogenesis also is stimulated.

(5) Healing: Signals from the extracellular tissues stimulate epithelial proliferation until the mucosa returns to its normal thickness. Tissues do not return completely to normal, however, placing them at increased risk for future injury.

b) Incidence: Oral mucositis occurs in

(1) 30%–40% of patients receiving standard-dose chemotherapy (Goldberg, Chiang, Selina, & Hamarman, 2004; NCI, 2008c; Rubenstein et al., 2004)

(2) 80% of stem cell transplant recipients (NCI, 2008c)

(3) Up to 100% of patients undergoing head and neck radiation therapy (NCI, 2008c).

c) Risk factors

(1) Chemotherapeutic agents that affect DNA synthesis are the most stomatotoxic (Dodd, 2004), but the drug class alone does not predict mucositis risk (NCI, 2008c). The following classes of chemotherapy agents have been associated with mucositis.

   (a) Antimetabolites

   (b) Antitumor antibiotics

   (c) Alkylating agents

   (d) Plant alkaloids

(2) Biologic agents, particularly IL-2 and IFN

(3) Neutropenia

(4) Drugs or therapies that alter mucous membranes (Beck, 2004)

   (a) Oxygen therapy: Dries out the mucosal lining

   (b) Anticholinergics: Decrease salivary flow

   (c) Phenytoin: Causes gingival hyperplasia

   (d) Steroids: Can result in fungal overgrowth

(5) Total body irradiation (TBI) or radiation therapy to the head or neck

(6) Dental disease and poor oral hygiene (Beck, 2004)

(7) Ill-fitting dentures: Ill-fitting dentures irritate the mucosa and break integrity (Beck, 2004).

(8) Advanced age and youth

   (a) Further study is needed to determine if age is a conclusive risk factor in the development of oral mucositis (NCCN, 2008a).

   (b) Older adult patients may be at risk because of degenerative

changes, decreased salivary flow, diminished keratinization of mucosa, and increased prevalence of gingivitis. Younger patients are more prone to develop oral mucositis more frequently than older patients because of their increased rate of basal cell turnover (Woo & Treister, 2006).

(9) History of alcohol and/or tobacco use: Alcohol and tobacco irritate the mucosa (Beck, 2004).

(10) Poor nutrition

   (a) Reduced nutritional intake delays healing.

   (b) A diet high in refined sugars promotes dental decay (Beck, 2004).

(11) Consumption of irritating foods: Acidic or spicy foods inflame and traumatize mucosa (Beck, 2004).

(12) Dehydration: Dehydration alters mucosal integrity.

(13) Head and neck cancer: Patients with head and neck cancer are at especially high risk if they have surgery followed by radiation therapy.

(14) Leukemia, lymphoma, stem cell transplant: These conditions put patients at risk because their treatment involves drugs with a great potential to produce oral mucositis and cause prolonged neutropenia.

(15) Methotrexate for prophylaxis of GVHD and the presence of GVHD following stem cell transplant (Brennan, Bultizingslower, Schubert, & Keefe, 2006; Cutler et al., 2005)

(16) Hepatic or renal impairment: Inadequate metabolism or excretion of certain mucosatoxic cytotoxic agents

(17) Multimodal therapies that traumatize the mucosa (Beck, 2004)

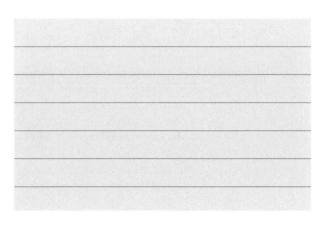

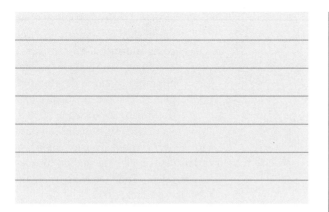

d) Clinical manifestations
  (1) The pattern of mucositis varies both by drug regimen and by individual. Intensity and duration vary by type of drug, and by dose and frequency of administration (Keefe et al., 2007).
    (a) Visible signs of oral mucositis are evident four to five days following standard-dose chemotherapy.
    (b) Stem cell transplant recipients experience mucositis three to five days following the conditioning regimen.
    (c) In patients receiving head and neck radiation therapy, mucositis is clinically evident during week two of therapy.
  (2) Intensity increases with higher doses of cytotoxic drugs. Drugs that are not usually stomatotoxic at standard doses (e.g., cyclophosphamide) can cause cellular damage to the mucosa at high doses (Keefe et al., 2007).
  (3) The duration of mucositis may be prolonged with frequent drug administration because there is no time for cellular recovery and healing (Beck, 2004).
  (4) Signs and symptoms include
    (a) Changes in taste and ability to swallow
    (b) Hoarseness or decreased voice strength
    (c) Pain when swallowing or talking
    (d) Changes in the color of the oral mucosa (e.g., pallor, erythema of varying degrees, white patches, discolored lesions or ulcers) (Beck, 2004)
    (e) Changes in oral moisture (e.g., amount of saliva, quality of secretions)
    (f) Edema of oral mucosa and tongue
    (g) Mucosal ulcerations.
  e) Assessment
    (1) Use a standardized assessment tool or scale when performing a physical examination. Scales designed for clinical use take into account symptoms, signs, and functional disturbances associated with oral mucositis and assign an overall score. Three common tools are
      (a) Oral Assessment Guide: This tool contains eight categories that reflect oral health and function (see Table 20).
      (b) Oral Cavity Assessment: This tool uses a numeric rating, 1–4, in each of five categories (lips, gingival/oral mucosa, tongue, teeth, and saliva). The total score represents the level of dysfunction: mild (6–10), moderate (11–15), or severe (16–20) (Beck, 2004).
      (c) NCI CTCAE: The NCI CTEP tool consists of a 0–4 grading index that is associated with descriptions of mucosal changes. This scale includes a clinical examination and a functional/symptomatic grading tool (NCI CTEP, 2006).
    (2) Examine the lips, tongue, and oral mucosa after removing dental appliances for color, moisture, integrity, and cleanliness (Beck, 2004).
    (3) Assess the patient for changes in taste, voice, ability to swallow, and comfort during swallowing (Beck, 2004).
    (4) Examine the saliva for amount and quality (Beck, 2004).
  f) Collaborative management: Currently no standard of care exists for the prevention and treatment of oral mucositis. MASCC, in collaboration with the International Society for Oral Oncology, issued clinical practice guidelines in 2004 with suggestions and recommendations based on literature published between 1966 and 2001. The guidelines were revised in 2005 and again in 2007 and include the following.
    (1) Oral care protocols, including patient education, should be instituted in an attempt to reduce the severity of oral mucositis from chemotherapy and radiation therapy (Rubenstein et al., 2004). Patient education may improve compliance with oral care,

Table 20. Oral Assessment Guide

Category	Tools for Assessment	Methods of Measurement	Numeric and Descriptive Ratings		
			1	2	3
Voice	Auditory	Converse with patient.	Normal	Deeper or raspy	Difficulty talking or painful
Swallow	Observation	Ask patient to swallow. To test gag reflex, gently place blade on back of tongue and depress. Observe result.	Normal swallow	Some pain on swallow	Unable to swallow
Lips	Visual/palpatory	Observe and feel tissue.	Smooth and pink and moist	Dry or cracked	Ulcerated or bleeding
Tongue	Visual and/or palpation	Feel and observe appearance of tissue.	Pink and moist and papillae present	Coated or loss of papillae with a shiny appearance with or without redness	Blistered or cracked
Saliva	Tongue blade	Insert blade into mouth, touching the center of the tongue and the floor of the mouth.	Watery	Thick or ropy	Absent
Mucous membranes	Visual	Observe appearance of tissue.	Pink and moist	Reddened or coated (increased whiteness) without ulcerations	Ulcerations with or without bleeding
Gingiva	Tongue blade and visual	Gently press tissue with tip of blade.	Pink and stippled and firm	Edematous with or without redness	Spontaneous bleeding or bleeding with pressure
Teeth or dentures (or denture-bearing area)	Visual	Observe appearance of teeth or denture-bearing area.	Clean and no debris	Plaque or debris in localized areas (between teeth if present)	Plaque or debris generalized along gum line or denture-bearing area

Note. Table courtesy of June Eilers, PhD, APRN-CNS, BC, The Nebraska Medical Center. Used with permission.

frequency, and ability to cope with mucositis.

(a) Provide patient education, which is essential in promoting good oral hygiene (Dodd, 2004).

(b) Conduct a pretreatment dental evaluation with attention to potentially irritating teeth surfaces, underlying gingivitis, periodontal infection, and ill-fitting dentures (Dodd, 2004). Crucial dental work should be done before chemotherapy begins. Once therapy begins, neutropenia and thrombocytopenia contraindicate corrective dental work (Beck, 2004). Removing braces may be necessary in adult and pediatric patients if they are to undergo transplantation or if prolonged periods of neutropenia are anticipated.

(c) Emphasize intake of high-protein foods and plenty of fluids (> 1,500 ml/day) to encourage oral mucous membrane regeneration (Vannice, 2008).

(2) Prevention of oral mucositis (MASCC, 2005; Rubenstein et al., 2004)

(a) Oral cryotherapy (ice chewing) is recommended for patients receiving bolus 5-FU for GI malignancies and for patients receiving high-dose melphalan.

(b) Chlorhexidine and acyclovir should not be used to prevent oral mucositis resulting from head and neck radiation or chemotherapy or to treat established mucositis.

(c) Consider use of a keratinocyte growth factor for patients with hematologic malignancies undergoing high-dose chemotherapy and TBI.

(d) GM-CSF mouthwashes should not be used in the prevention of oral mucositis in patients receiving hematopoietic stem cell transplant (HSCT).

(3) Prevention of GI mucositis (MASCC, 2005; Rubenstein et al., 2004)

(a) Either ranitidine or omeprazole is recommended for the prevention of epigastric pain after treatment with cyclophosphamide, methotrexate and 5-FU, or 5-FU with or without folinic acid.

(b) Amifostine has been suggested for reducing the severity of esophagitis caused by the combination of chemotherapy and radiation therapy for NSCLC (MASCC, 2005). However, ASCO does not recommend the routine use of amifostine for the prevention of esophagitis in patients receiving concurrent chemotherapy because of insufficient evidence (Hensley et al., 2009).

(c) Glutamine is not recommended for the prevention of GI mucositis.

(4) Treatment: Currently, there are no evidence-based recommendations for the treatment of established oral mucositis. Interventions are aimed at symptom relief and preventing further tissue damage. These interventions may include the following (MASCC, 2005).

(a) Encourage the use of oral agents to promote cleansing, moisture, and comfort (see Table 21).

(b) Encourage the patient to brush, floss, and rinse to maintain mucosal health.

(c) Administer systemic pain medications for mucositis pain. The MASCC guidelines recommend the use of patient-controlled analgesia in stem cell transplant recipients experiencing oral mucositis pain (Rubenstein et al., 2004).

(d) Culture mucosal lesions so that appropriate antimicrobial agents can be prescribed. Candidal lesions look like whitish or cream-colored plaques on the mucosa and often are treated while cultures are pending.

g) Patient and family education: Stress the goals of keeping the oral cavity clean, moist, and intact to prevent further damage to the mucosa during mucosatoxic therapy (Harris, Eilers, Cashavelly, Maxwell, & Harriman, 2007). To do this, patients should

(1) Perform a daily oral self-examination and report signs and symptoms of mucositis.

(2) Comply with an oral hygiene program: Oral hygiene should be performed after every meal and at bedtime. If mild to moderate dysfunction is present, the frequency of oral hygiene should be increased to every two to four hours. If the condition progresses to a more severe dysfunction, hourly care may be indicated. The program should include the following.

(a) Flossing the teeth with dental tape at least once daily or as advised by clinician (Harris et al., 2007); patients who do not regularly floss should not do so while immunosuppressed.

(b) Brushing the teeth with a soft toothbrush for at least 90 seconds at least twice daily (Harris et al., 2007); sponge swabs are not as effective as toothbrushes and should be avoided except in patients who cannot tolerate a toothbrush because of severe pain with mucositis.

(c) Cleansing the oral cavity after meals, at bedtime, and at other times by vigorously swishing the mouth with an appropriate cleans-

Table 21. Oral Mucositis Management: Available Agents

Agent	Efficacy	Comments
Bland rinses		
0.9% saline solution	Formal evaluation is lacking.	Relatively innocuous and economical rinsing solution
Sodium bicarbonate	Formal evaluation is lacking.	Creates an alkaline environment that promotes bacterial microflora Unpleasant taste may affect adherence. Recommended by NCI
0.9% saline/sodium bicarbonate	Formal evaluation is lacking. ½ teaspoon salt mixed with 2 tablespoons sodium bicarbonate with 32 ounces of water	Inexpensive rinsing solution Unpleasant taste may affect adherence. Recommended by NCI
Rinse, multiagent	Data demonstrating efficacy are lacking for prevention/treatment of mucositis.	Various agents exist that include antihistamines, lidocaine, and Mylanta®. May be useful for pain or discomfort only Patients may experience numbness, which can cause potential injury. Alcohol-based elixirs should be avoided.
Other		
Cryotherapy (ice chips)	Demonstrates consistent reduction in incidence and severity of oral mucositis among patients receiving bolus 5-FU Also recommended for bolus edatrexate chemotherapy infusion	Not recommended in patients with head and neck cancers Also recommended by MASCC (2005) for high-dose melphalan Apply ice chips to mouth 5 minutes before bolus 5-FU therapy and continue for 30 minutes after. Not recommended in patients receiving capecitabine or oxaliplatin because of potential discomfort with exposure to coldness (Harris et al., 2007)
L-glutamine	Essential amino acid, poorly absorbed Not recommended systemically for the prevention of GI mucositis	Has not been shown to prevent mucositis
Coating agents, mucosal protectants		
Sucralfate suspension	Most data demonstrate no statistically significant difference in oral mucositis severity, pain intensity scores, and other subjective symptoms (e.g., taste alteration, dry mouth).	Mucosal coating agent Has not demonstrated benefit Poor tolerability and potential for GI side effects (Harris et al., 2007)
Gelclair®	Bioadherant oral gel forms coating to make a barrier. Provides moisture and is flavorful Not recommended for the prevention or treatment of oral mucositis	May be helpful for improvement of swallowing and pain scores
Tissue protectants		
Amifostine	Recommended for reduction of esophagitis induced by simultaneous chemotherapy and radiation therapy in patients with non–small cell lung cancer (MASCC, 2005). However, ASCO does not recommend the routine use of amifostine for the prevention of esophagitis in patients receiving concurrent chemotherapy because of insufficient evidence (Hensley et al., 2009).	Tissue protector Studies needed to determine role in prevention of oral mucositis

(Continued on next page)

Table 21. Oral Mucositis Management: Available Agents *(Continued)*

Agent	Efficacy	Comments
Antiseptic agents		
Chlorhexidine	Overall, data demonstrate no significant change in oral mucositis severity or suppression of any type of oral microflora.	Contains alcohol Reports of rinse-induced discomfort, taste alteration Not recommended for oral mucositis (MASCC, 2005) Can turn teeth brown
Hydrogen peroxide	Mixed results: Linked to exacerbation or dryness, stinging, pain, and nausea; some reports of intensification of symptoms as a result of glossodynia	Repeated use as a rinse is not recommended; long-term use is discouraged. At full potency, it may break down new granulation tissue and disrupt normal oral flora due to potential for damage of fibroblasts and keratinocytes.
Povidone-iodine	Possesses antiviral, antibacterial, and antifungal efficacy; less tolerable than normal saline	Potency limits use in patients with new granulation tissue. Swallowing is contraindicated. Further study is needed.
Antimicrobial agents		
Acyclovir (and its analogs)	Antiviral Not recommended for prevention of oral mucositis	—
Antimicrobial lozenges	Not recommended for prevention of radiation-induced oral mucositis	More research is needed.
Anti-inflammatory agents		
Kamillosan liquidum rinse	Unfavorable results in clinical trials	Most patients appear to develop mucositis despite treatment.
Chamomile	Lacks data demonstrating its efficacy	Anti-inflammatory, antipeptic properties reported Inexpensive, readily available, and innocuous
Oral corticosteroids	No significant difference in degree of mucositis compared to placebo	Data are limited; definitive conclusions cannot be drawn.
Benzydamine	Nonsteroidal anti-inflammatory analgesic Anti–tumor necrosis factor activity	Only recommended for the prevention of oral mucositis in patients with solid tumors of the head and neck receiving radiotherapy
Analgesics		
Topical lidocaine	Limited data; may provide significant relief of limited duration	Requires frequent application; may lead to decreased sensitivity and additional trauma, and may impair taste perception Prophylaxis is not recommended.
Topical capsaicin	Pilot data demonstrated marked reduction in oral pain.	Clinical potential possibility linked to re-epithelization and elevation of pain threshold Further study is warranted.
Morphine	Topical morphine has limited utility. Patient-controlled analgesia utilizing morphine recommended for patients undergoing hematopoietic stem cell transplant	Oral alcohol-based formulations may cause burning. Comprehensive pain assessments should be performed to adequately treat pain associated with mucositis.

(Continued on next page)

Table 21. Oral Mucositis Management: Available Agents *(Continued)*

Agent	Efficacy	Comments
Antiproliferative, mucosal protectant, cytokine-like agents and growth factors		
GM-CSF	Some data indicate reduction in oral mucositis severity and pain; others do not. No evidence of benefit with duration or severity of oral mucositis	Oral mouthwashes are not recommended use; high rate of drug discontinuation because of intolerable side effects, including local skin reaction, fever, bone pain, and nausea when administered subcutaneously
G-CSF	Limited data; some indication of significant reductions of oral mucositis severity in BMT recipients and oral mucositis occurrence in patients undergoing radiation therapy when used prophylactically	Further study is needed to draw any conclusion.
Keratinocyte growth factor-1: Palifermin	Approved for the prevention of oral mucositis in autologous stem cell transplant recipients receiving high-dose chemotherapy or total body irradiation	60 mcg/kg/day IV for 3 days prior to the preparatory regimen and 3 days post-transplant Further study is needed in other patient populations.

ASCO—American Society of Clinical Oncology; BMT—bone marrow transplant; 5-FU—5-fluorouracil; G-CSF—granulocyte-colony-stimulating factor; GI—gastrointestinal; GM-CSF—granulocyte macrophage-colony-stimulating factor; IV—intravenous; MASCC—Multinational Association of Supportive Care in Cancer; NCI—National Cancer Institute

Note. Based on information from Bensinger et al., 2008; Harris et al., 2007; MASCC, 2005; NCI, 2007.

From "Nursing Interventions and Supportive Care for the Prevention and Treatment of Oral Mucositis Associated With Cancer Treatment," by J. Eilers, 2004, *Oncology Nursing Forum, 31*(Suppl. 4.), pp. 19–20. Copyright 2004 by Oncology Nursing Society. Adapted with permission.

---

ing agent (see Table 21); oral rinsing should be done to remove excess debris. Patients should use one tablespoon of rinse to swish in the oral cavity for 30 seconds and then expectorate (Harris et al., 2007).

(d) Avoiding use of oral irrigators, which may force microorganisms into ulcerated and compromised gingival tissue, leading to bacteremia (Madeya, 1996)

(e) Avoiding irritating agents, including commercial mouthwashes containing phenol, astringents, or alcohol; highly abrasive toothpastes; acidic, hot, or spicy foods and beverages; rough foods; alcohol; tobacco; poorly fitting dentures; braces; and lemon-glycerin swabs and solutions

4. Anorexia
   a) Pathophysiology
      (1) Definitions
         (a) Anorexia is an abnormal loss of appetite for food (NCI, n.d.).
         (b) Cachexia is a wasting syndrome characterized by the substantial loss of adipose and muscle tissue (Illman et al., 2005).
      (2) The two entities are interrelated. Lack of food intake is one factor that contributes to weight loss, muscle wasting, and malnutrition.
      (3) Anorexia/cachexia results from a complicated process involving numerous physiologic and psychological factors.
         (a) Tumor effect (Inui, 2002)
            i) Obstruction of the GI tract can lead to nutrient malabsorption, nausea, vomiting, and pain.
            ii) Proinflammatory cytokines such as IL-6, IL-1, TNF-α and IFN-alfa may be released by the tumor and cause satiety and metabolic abnormalities. These agents also may serve as tumor promoters and thus contribute to a negative prognosis (MacDonald, 2007).
            iii) Metabolic abnormalities may lead to elevated blood glucose, amino acid, and free fatty acid levels, resulting

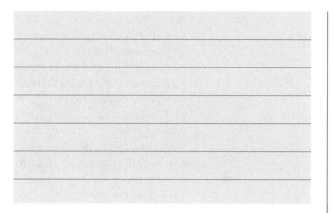

in early satiety and appetite suppression.

    iv) Neurohormonal abnormalities may directly affect the hypothalamic appetite center.

    v) Hypercalcemia secondary to bony involvement may lead to nausea, vomiting, and anorexia.

(b) Treatment effects (Mattox, 2005)

    i) Surgery may result in malabsorption, obstruction, and fluid and electrolyte abnormalities.

    ii) Chemotherapy and radiation therapy side effects include nausea, vomiting, mucositis, taste changes, constipation, and diarrhea.

    iii) Combination therapy results in greater number of adverse effects.

(c) Psychosocial effects

    i) Cancer-related depression often coincides with uncontrolled appetite loss and eventually cachexia, especially with patients who are at a late stage or have multiple symptoms (Illman et al., 2005).

    ii) The prevalence of depression among patients with cancer is estimated to be 10%–30%, compared to 5%–10% in the general medical population (Illman et al., 2005).

    iii) Anxiety, fear, grief, fatigue, pain, and the patient's reaction to change in body image may also contribute to anorexia.

(4) Cachexia results in decreased survival and adherence to chemotherapy and an increase in treatment toxicity (Del Fabbro, Dalal, Delgado, Freer, & Bruera, 2007).

b) Incidence: Overall incidence of anorexia/cachexia in patients with cancer is about 50%, increasing to 80% before death (Inui, 2002).

c) Risk factors (Del Fabbro, Dalal, & Bruera, 2006)

    (1) Advanced cancer

    (2) Solid tumor: Most common types are GI and lung.

    (3) Chronic illness such as pulmonary disease and CHF

    (4) Increased prevalence in the very young and older adults

    (5) Multimodal therapies

d) Clinical manifestations (Strasser & Breuera, 2002)

    (1) Involuntary weight loss of more than 5% of usual weight

    (2) Lack of appetite

    (3) Loss of muscle mass

    (4) Loss of adipose tissue

    (5) Fatigue and weakness

e) Assessment

    (1) Monitor weight: Compare with pretreatment weight.

    (2) Obtain a diet history or have patient complete a food diary for several days.

    (3) Measure body composition.

        (a) Triceps skin fold thickness estimates body fat.

        (b) Mid-arm muscle circumference estimates muscle mass.

    (4) Evaluate laboratory results (Bender et al., 2002).

        (a) Serum albumin measures visceral protein stores. Less than 3.5 g/dl indicates recent protein depletion.

        (b) Serum prealbumin less than 15 mg/dl indicates protein depletion.

        (c) Serum transferrin less than 200 mg/dl reflects a decrease in the body's ability to make serum proteins.

    (5) Assess functional status (Chang, Xia, & Kasimis, 2005; Ottery, 1994).

        (a) The Patient-Generated Subjective Global Assessment and the Functional Assessment of Anorexia/Cachexia Therapy are easy-to-use tools that patients complete in the clinical setting.

(b) Functional status tools include symptom distress and QOL questions.

f) Collaborative management: The extent of nutrition intervention depends on the cause of weight loss and overall goals of the patient, family, and the healthcare team.

(1) Treatment of the cancer is the primary objective.

(2) Symptom management: Management of the symptoms such as nausea and vomiting, mucositis, diarrhea, taste changes, fatigue, and dysphagia may improve anorexia. (See the discussion of management in the specific sections of this publication.)

(3) Pharmacologic intervention: Progestins and corticosteroids are the only two classes of drugs to have limited effectiveness as appetite stimulants (Jatoi, 2006).

(a) Progestins (Berenstein & Ortiz, 2008)

i) Megestrol acetate is most commonly used.

ii) Mechanism of action is not known.

iii) Optimal dose is not defined but ranges from 100–1,600 mg/day.

iv) Side effects include deep vein thrombosis, edema, impotence in men, and GI disturbances.

(b) Corticosteroids (Mattox, 2005)

i) Mechanism of action is unknown but may be related to euphoric and anti-inflammatory effects.

ii) Effects are short-lived.

iii) Many side effects, both short- and long-term, can occur, including immunosuppression, hyperglycemia, and muscle wasting.

(c) Cannabinoids (Mattox, 2005)

i) Indicated for AIDS-related anorexia and CINV.

ii) Synthetic form of tetrahydrocannabinol is administered orally.

iii) Side effects include increased heart rate, conjunctival reddening, drowsiness, anxiety, delusions, and hallucinations at higher doses.

(4) Nonpharmacologic interventions (Brown, 2002; Del Fabbro et al., 2006)

(a) Interventions may not increase weight or length of survival but may improve QOL.

(b) Refer to a dietitian for nutritional counseling. This has been shown to improve dietary intake.

(c) Provide high-calorie/high-protein oral supplements as needed and tolerated.

(d) Enteral feedings (Strasser & Bruera, 2002)

i) Routine use is not indicated; generally used as a preoperative intervention.

ii) Patients must have a functioning bowel.

iii) Complications include aspiration pneumonia, electrolyte abnormalities, diarrhea, and infection.

(e) Parenteral feedings (Nelson, 2000)

i) Use is limited to preoperative treatment in patients who are surgical candidates for cure or have an obstruction.

ii) Complications include high infection rate.

g) Patient education (Kellner, 2004; McClement, 2005)

(1) Provide written handouts, stressing high-calorie/high-protein foods (see Figure 25).

(2) Monitor and record weight weekly, using the same scale at the same time of the day.

(3) Encourage small, frequent meals.

(4) Provide an attractive setting for meals.

(5) Encourage physical activity.

(6) Use measures to control nausea and vomiting, mucositis, dry mouth, taste changes, and other side effects of treatment.

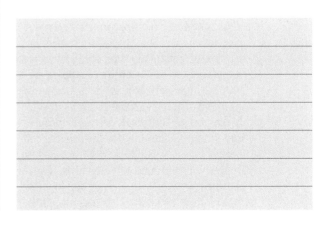

Figure 25. High-Calorie/High-Protein Diet Patient Handout

High-Calorie and High-Protein Diet

The following foods are high in calories and/or protein.

Main Dishes	Fruits	Dairy	Nondairy	Snacks	Miscellaneous
Eggs, meat, poultry, fish, beans, peanut butter, hot cereal with milk, pizza, fast foods, stews, casseroles, cream-based soups, chunky soups	Juice, nectar, dried fruit, fruit in heavy syrup, frozen fruit	Whole milk, high-protein milk (see recipe below), cream, ice cream, custard, cheese, cottage cheese, milkshakes or shakes, instant breakfast powder, pudding	Soy milk, rice milk, almond milk	Potato chips, corn chips, nachos with cheese, popcorn with butter or parmesan cheese, crackers with peanut butter, fruit or vegetables with dip (such as cream cheese, black bean, hummus), pastries, candy, cookies, cake, roasted nuts, seeds	Margarine, butter, gravy, mayonnaise, sour cream, cream cheese

High-Protein Milk

By the quart:
1 quart whole milk
1 cup instant nonfat dry milk powder

By the cup:
1 cup whole milk
¼ cup instant nonfat dry milk powder

Mix well and chill. For extra flavor, add fruit syrup, vanilla or coffee extract, chocolate, strawberry, or maple syrup. Use in cream soups, desserts, hot cereal, and cocoa.

You may use a multi-vitamin supplement that provides no more than 100% of the U.S. RDA. More than 100% could interfere with your treatment.

If you would like more information, or if you are on a special diet (low salt, diabetic, or low fiber) or are unable to follow these suggestions, please contact the Oncology Nutrition Service.

Note. Copyright 2006 by Sidney Kimmel Comprehensive Cancer Center at Johns Hopkins. Used with permission.

(7) Include patients in family activities to avoid isolation, even if patients have no appetite. Do not force patients to eat.
(8) Remind families that patients' lack of appetite is caused by the effects of the disease. It is not their fault.
(9) Refer to community resources as needed, such as home care and Meals on Wheels.
5. Constipation: Constipation is defined as excessively hard and dry bowel movements that are infrequent and a result of a decrease in rectal emptying or filling (Camp-Sorrell, 2005). Constipation may be a presenting symptom of the cancer diagnosis, a side effect of therapy, or the result of tumor progression. It may be unrelated to the cancer or the therapy (Massey, Haylock, & Curtiss, 2004). Depression and anxiety caused by cancer treatment or pain can lead to constipation, either alone or with other functional and

physiologic disorders. The most common causes are inadequate fluid intake and pain medications (NCI, 2008a).
a) Pathophysiology: Decreased motility of the large intestine is the primary cause of constipation. Mechanisms of constipation include altered strength of contractions within the intestines, poor muscle tone within the colon, and sensory changes relating to the rectum and anus (Pace, 1999).
(1) Agents that decrease motility
(a) Vinca alkaloids: Autonomic nervous system dysfunction can result in upper colon impaction, colicky abdominal pain, and paralytic ileus. Rectal emptying is decreased when nonfunctional afferent and efferent pathways from the sacral cord are interrupted (Camp-Sorrell, 2005).
i) Vincristine, vinorelbine, and vinblastine can cause neuro-

toxicity that affects the smooth muscles of the GI tract, leading to decreased peristalsis or paralytic ileus.

    ii) Vincristine may damage the myenteric plexus of the colon.

(2) Certain chemotherapy agents that cause nausea and vomiting may contribute to constipation in that they cause the patient to decrease oral intake, slowing peristaltic push-down in the GI tract. In the absence of food intake, fewer stool are produced, transit time increases, and the stool becomes hard and difficult to eliminate.

(3) Opioids profoundly impact the bowel's ability to maintain appropriate motility. They are the primary cause of medication-induced constipation (Robinson et al., 2000).

b) Incidence

(1) Clinically, constipation is a common problem for patients with cancer. Constipation occurs in approximately 50% of patients with cancer and can increase to 75% and 90% for patients who are terminally ill or receiving opioids, respectively (Engelking, 2008). It is more common in older adult patients than in others and may lead to bowel obstruction (Engelking).

(2) Constipation has been reported in 20%–35% of patients receiving vinblastine, especially in high doses or after prolonged treatment (Engelking, 2008)

(3) Constipation, abdominal pain, and paralytic ileus are common side effects of vincristine (Chu & DeVita, 2004).

(4) Vinorelbine may cause severe (grades 3 and 4) constipation, with an overall incidence of all grades of 35% (Glaxo-SmithKline, 2007).

(5) Constipation occurs in up to 55% of patients receiving thalidomide (Celgene, 2007b) and approximately 35% of patients receiving lenalidomide (Celgene, 2007a).

(6) Bortezomib causes constipation in 41% of patients (Millennium, 2007).

c) Clinical consequences

(1) Abdominal or rectal discomfort or pain

(2) Nausea and/or vomiting

(3) Anorexia

(4) Impaction

(5) Ileus

(6) Anal fissures

(7) Hemorrhoids

(8) Ruptured bowel and life-threatening sepsis

d) Risk factors (Massey et al., 2004)

(1) Mechanical pressure on the bowel (e.g., bowel obstruction secondary to tumor in the GI tract, pressure from ascites)

(2) Damage to the spinal cord from T8 to L3, which causes compression of nerves that innervate the bowel

(3) Decreased mobility

(4) Dehydration

(5) Low dietary fiber intake

(6) Metabolic and endocrine disorders (NCI, 2008a)

    (a) Hypercalcemia

    (b) Addison disease

    (c) Hypothyroidism and hyperthyroidism

    (d) Cushing syndrome

    (e) Hypokalemia

    (f) Diabetes mellitus

(7) Use of certain medications (Massey et al., 2004)

    (a) Neurotoxic chemotherapy drugs

    (b) Anticholinergic medications

    (c) Diuretics

    (d) Opioids

    (e) Aluminum- and calcium-based antacids

    (f) Calcium and iron supplements

    (g) Tricyclic antidepressants

    (h) Antihypertensives

    (i) Anxiolytics

    (j) $5HT_3$ antagonists

    (k) NSAIDs

(8) Overuse of laxatives

e) Assessment

(1) Assess patterns of elimination, including the amount and frequency of elimination and the urge to defecate, character of the stool, volume of stool, chronic use of laxatives or stool softeners, other measures to enhance bowel function (Pace, 1999).
(2) Assess patients' usual dietary patterns, focusing on fluid and fiber intake.
(3) Assess mobility, activity level, and functional status.
(4) Assess abdominal pain or cramping.
(5) Determine facts about the patient's last bowel movement (e.g., when, amount, consistency, color, presence of blood).
(6) Determine current medication usage.
(7) Use laboratory results to assist in metabolic evaluation.
(8) Perform abdominal palpation and rectal examination if appropriate. A rectal examination is not routinely performed in pediatric patients. Rectal or stoma manipulation, for examinations, enemas, or suppositories, should be avoided in myelosuppressed patients (Bisanz et al., 2008).
(9) Use radiographs to differentiate between mechanical obstruction and decreased motility from an ileus (Massey et al., 2004).
f) Collaborative management
(1) Pharmacologic interventions
(a) Bulk-forming laxatives (e.g., methylcellulose, psyllium): Cause water to be retained in the stool; of limited use for patients who cannot tolerate fluids; must be taken with at least 200–300 ml of water (Bisanz et al., 2008)
(b) Lubricants and emollients (e.g., mineral oil, glycerin supposito-

ries): Coat and soften the stool; excessive doses can lead to rectal seepage and perianal irritation.
(c) Saline laxatives (magnesium salts, sodium phosphate): Contain magnesium or sulfate ions; act by drawing water into the gut; of little use in a daily prevention program; used most often for acute evacuation of the bowel
(d) Osmotic laxatives (e.g., lactulose, sorbitol): Attract and retain water in the bowel, resulting in softer stool; effective onset usually is within 24–72 hours after the drug has reached the colon; adverse reactions include abdominal pain, gas, and abdominal distention (Avila, 2004).
(e) Polyethylene glycol with or without electrolytes has been found to be effective in the non-oncology population. NCCN (2008) recommends this as an alternative for patients with cancer who have persistent constipation.
(f) Detergent laxatives (e.g., docusate sodium): Have a direct action on the intestines by allowing water and fats to penetrate into dry stool; decrease electrolyte and water absorption from the colon; appropriate for short-term use when straining is to be avoided
(g) Stimulant laxatives: (e.g., bisacodyl, senna): Act directly on the colon to stimulate motility and are activated by bacterial degradation in the intestine; the most commonly used in a prophylactic plan
(h) Suppositories: Stimulate the intestinal nerve plexus and cause rectal emptying; not indicated for long-term bowel management
(i) Prokinetic agents (e.g., metoclopramide): May be used for delayed gastric emptying; the appropriate dose is taken prior to meals and at bedtime; the onset of action is within 60 minutes of the oral dose (Avila, 2004). Avoid prokinetic agents in patients with large abdominal tumors or bowel obstruction (Bisanz et al., 2008).
(j) Methylnaltrexone is a novel drug recently approved for opioid-in-

duced constipation in patients with advanced illness who are receiving palliative care. Methylnaltrexone is a peripherally acting opioid receptor antagonist. This drug has shown efficacy in preventing opioid-induced constipation without diminishing pain palliation or precipitating opioid withdrawal (Yuan, 2004). The most common adverse effects reported were flatulence, abdominal pain, and nausea. This drug is contraindicated if there is known or suspected mechanical GI obstruction (Wyeth, 2008).

(k) Use a combination laxative-stool softener prophylactically for patients receiving vinca alkaloids (Engelking, 2008).

(2) Other

(a) Include an increase in physical activity or passive exercise as appropriate in a bowel-retraining regimen. These promote the urge to defecate by helping to move feces into the rectum.

(b) Help patients to maintain usual bowel habits during hospitalization. Provide privacy and comfort.

(c) Increase fluid and fiber intake, and begin management with oral medications to help constipated patients with neutropenia or thrombocytopenia.

(d) Do not perform rectal examinations or use suppositories or enemas in patients who are myelosuppressed; doing so may increase the risk of infection and bleeding. This could introduce bacteria into the rectum or lead to anal tears, fissures, or abscesses (Engelking, 2008).

(e) Rotating opioids may decrease constipation (e.g., switching from a long-acting oral morphine to a transdermal fentanyl patch) (Bisanz et al., 2008).

g) Patient and family education

(1) Increase fluid intake: Encourage patients to drink at least eight eight-ounce glasses of fluid daily unless medically contraindicated. Drinking warm liquids before a defecation attempt may be helpful to stimulate

bowel movement. Consumption of coffee, tea, and grapefruit juice usually is discouraged because these beverages act as diuretics (Engelking, 2008).

(2) Increase fiber in diet: Fiber causes feces to pass through intestines more rapidly and decreases the occurrence of fecal impaction.

(a) High-fiber foods include bran, popcorn, corn, raisins, dates, vegetables, fruits, and whole grains.

(b) Advise patients that they may experience abdominal discomfort, flatulence, or a change in bowel habits in the first few weeks after increasing fiber intake. Fiber tolerance will develop, and such effects can be minimized by slowly titrating fiber consumption, start by adding 3–4 g/day and increasing to 6–10 g/day. This approach is contraindicated in cases of structural bowel blockage because increasing bulky intraluminal contents may increase the obstruction (Engelking, 2008).

(c) Fiber should not be recommended in patients with cancer who have inadequate fluid intake (Bisanz et al., 2007).

(3) Encourage patients to exercise regularly. Regular exercise stimulates GI motility.

(4) Teach diaphragmatic breathing and abdominal muscle exercises; these help to increase muscle tone, which assists with defecation (Engelking, 2008).

(5) Help patients to develop a regular bowel program.

(6) Instruct patients to report constipation and to be aware of the complications

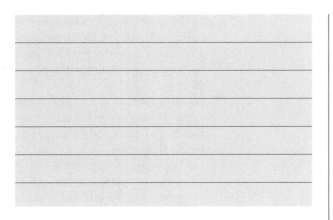

associated with constipation, such as fecal impaction.

(7) Stress that patients should call a physician if three days pass without a bowel movement to initiate a bowel program.

6. Perirectal cellulitis: Inflammation and edema of the perineal and rectal area

  a) Pathophysiology

    (1) Minimal tears of the anorectal mucosa allow infection. The most common infective organisms include gram-negative aerobic bacilli, enterococci, and bowel anaerobes (Alexander, Walsh, Freifeld, & Pizzo, 2002).

    (2) Infection starting as a local abscess can lead to systemic sepsis.

  b) Incidence: Overall incidence has decreased in the past decade, presumably because of the early use of empiric antibiotics in febrile neutropenic patients. Perirectal infection has been reported in 5% of patients with hematologic malignancies (Bodey, 2000).

  c) Risk factors

    (1) Neutropenia or thrombocytopenia that is chronic (the condition lasts for more than seven days) or profound (ANC < 100/mm³) places patients at high risk for developing infection (Alexander et al., 2002; Wujcik, 2004).

    (2) Constipation: The passage of hard stool causes trauma to the rectal mucosa.

    (3) Diarrhea: Caustic fluid irritates and breaks down perirectal tissue.

    (4) Perirectal mucositis caused by chemotherapy and/or radiation therapy

    (5) Any rectal trauma, such as rectal stimulation or the use of rectal thermometers or suppositories

    (6) Hemorrhoids or anal fissures/abscesses

  d) Assessment

    (1) Ask patients if they are experiencing perineal and/or rectal discomfort. Fear of defecation may not be reported and may increase risk of constipation and pain. A large majority of patients with rectal abscess will complain of dull, aching or throbbing pain, which may worsen when sitting or before defecation (Fenton, 2008).

    (2) Monitor for the presence of fever.

    (3) Perform a physical examination of the perineal area.

      (a) The entrance site for the infective agent may be a small tear that shows minimal irritation. Conversely, gross swelling and inflammation of the perirectal area may be observed. Obtain a culture for identification of infectious organism(s).

      (b) Look for and document tissue sloughing and necrosis.

  e) Collaborative management (Alexander et al., 2002; Kline, 2002; NCCN, 2008a)

    (1) Ensure that antibiotic coverage includes a specific antianaerobic agent, such as clindamycin or metronidazole, in addition to broad-spectrum aerobic coverage. Consider *Enterococcus* or *Candida* coverage if appropriate (NCCN, 2008a).

    (2) Administer antipyretic medications to relieve fever.

    (3) Teach and encourage patients to take sitz baths or use perineal irrigation.

    (4) Administer stool softeners and encourage patients to eat a low-bulk diet. Consult a dietitian as needed.

    (5) Inspect the perirectal mucosa frequently for any signs of irritation or skin breakdown.

  f) Patient and family education

    (1) Teach patients and significant others to

      (a) Maintain meticulous perineal hygiene, especially in the presence of neutropenia.

      (b) Apply appropriate barrier creams and medicated creams.

      (c) Monitor carefully for any signs of infection or worsening of tissue integrity.

    (2) Ensure that patients and significant others are able to

(a) Identify the risk factors for perirectal cellulitis.

(b) Implement measures that minimize the risk of developing perirectal cellulitis.

(c) Identify situations that require prompt professional intervention (Wujcik, 2004).

    i) Pain, redness, or swelling in the affected area

    ii) Body temperature > 38.0°C (100.4°F)

References

Aapro, M.S., Molassiotis, A., & Olver, I. (2004). Anticipatory nausea and vomiting. *Supportive Care in Cancer, 13*(2), 117–121.

Alexander, S.W., Walsh, T.J., Freifeld, A.G., & Pizzo, P.A. (2002). Infectious complications in pediatric cancer patients. In P.A. Pizzo & D.G. Poplack (Eds.), *Principles and practice of pediatric oncology* (4th ed., pp. 1239–1283). Philadelphia: Lippincott Williams & Wilkins.

Arnold, R.J., Gabrail, N., Raut, M., Kim, R., Sung, J., & Zhou, Y. (2005). Clinical implications of chemotherapy-induced diarrhea in patients with cancer. *Journal of Supportive Oncology, 3*(3), 227–232.

Avila, J. (2004). Pharmacologic treatment of constipation in cancer patients. *Cancer Control, 11*(3), 10–18.

Beck, S. (2004). Mucositis. In C.H. Yarbro, M.H. Frogge, & M. Goodman (Eds.), *Cancer symptom management* (3rd ed., pp. 276–287). Sudbury, MA: Jones and Bartlett.

Bender, C.M., McDaniel, R.W., Murphy-Ende, K., Pickett, M., Rittenberg, C.N., Rogers, M.P., et al. (2002). Chemotherapy-induced nausea and vomiting. *Clinical Journal of Oncology Nursing, 6*(2), 94–102.

Bensinger, W., Schubert, M., Ang, K., Brizel, D., Brown, E., Eilers, J., et al. (2008). NCCN Task Force report: Prevention and management of mucositis in cancer care. *Journal of the National Comprehensive Cancer Network, 6*(Suppl. 1), S-1–S-19.

Benson, A.B., Ajani, J.A., Catalano, R.B., Engelking, C., Kornblau, S., Martensen, J., et al. (2004). Recommended guidelines for the treatment of cancer treatment–induced diarrhea. *Journal of Clinical Oncology, 22*(14), 2918–2926.

Berenstein, E.G., & Ortiz, Z. (2008). Megestrol acetate for the treatment of anorexia-cachexia syndrome. *Cochrane Database of Systematic Reviews* 2008, Issue 3. Art. No.: CD004310. DOI: 10.1002/14651858.CD004310.pub2.

Bisanz, A., Palmer, J.L., Reddy, S., Cloutier, L., Dixon, T., Cohen, M.Z., & Bruera, E. (2008). Characterizing postoperative paralytic ileus as evidence for future research and clinical practice. *Gastroenterology Nursing, 31*(5), 336–344.

Bodey, G. (2000). Unusual presentation of infection in neutropenic patients. *International Journal of Antimicrobial Agents, 16*(2), 93–95.

Brennan, M., Bultizingslower, I., Schubert, M., & Keefe, D. (2006). Alimentary mucositis: Putting the guidelines into practice. *Supportive Care in Cancer, 14*(6), 573–579.

Brown, J.K. (2002). A systematic review of the evidence on symptom management of cancer-related anorexia and cachexia. *Oncology Nursing Forum, 29*(3), 517–532.

Campos, D., Pereira, J.R., Reinhardt, R.R., Carracedo, C., Poli, S., Vogel, C., et al. (2001). Prevention of cisplatin-induced emesis by the oral neurokinin-1 antagonist, MK-869, in combination with granisetron and dexamethasone or with dexamethasone alone. *Journal of Clinical Oncology, 19*(6), 1759–1767.

Camp-Sorrell, D. (2005). Chemotherapy: Toxicity management. In C.H. Yarbro, M.H. Frogge, & M. Goodman (Eds.), *Cancer nursing: Principles and practice* (6th ed., pp. 425–427). Sudbury, MA: Jones and Bartlett.

Celgene Corporation. (2007a). Revlimid [Package insert]. Summit, NJ: Author.

Celgene Corporation. (2007b). Thalidomid [Package insert]. Summit, NJ: Author.

Chang, V.T., Xia, Q., & Kasimis, B. (2005). The Functional Assessment of Anorexia/Cachexia Therapy (FAACT) appetite scale in veteran cancer patients. *Journal of Supportive Oncology, 3*(5), 377–382.

Chu, E., & DeVita, V.T. (2007). *Physician's cancer chemotherapy drug manual 2007.* Sudbury, MA: Jones and Bartlett.

Curry, J., Hospenthal, D.R., & Lee, J. (2007). *Pseudomembranous colitis.* Retrieved October 29, 2008, from http://www.emedicine.com/med/TOPIC1942.HTM

Cutler, C., Li, S., Kim, H.T., Laglenne, P., Szeto, K.C., Hoffmeister, L., et al. (2005). Mucositis after allogeneic hematopoietic stem cell transplantation: A cohort study of methotrexate and nonmethotrexate containing graft-versus-host disease prophylaxis regimens. *Biology of Blood and Marrow Transplantation, 11*(5), 383–388.

Del Fabbro, E., Dalal, S., & Bruera, E. (2006). Symptom control in palliative care—Part II: Cachexia/anorexia and fatigue. *Journal of Palliative Medicine, 9*(2), 409–421.

Del Fabbro, E., Dalal, S., Delgado, M., Freer, G., & Bruera, E. (2007). Secondary vs. primary cachexia in patients with advanced cancer. *Journal of Clinical Oncology, 25*(Suppl. 18), 9128.

Dibble, S.L., Israel, J., Nussey, B., Casey, K., & Luce, J. (2003). Delayed chemotherapy-induced nausea in women treated for breast cancer [Online exclusive]. *Oncology Nursing Forum, 30*(2), E40–E47.

Dibble, S.L., Luce, J., Cooper, B.A., Israel, J., Cohen, M., Nussey, B., et al. (2007). Acupressure for chemotherapy-induced nausea and vomiting: A randomized clinical trial. *Oncology Nursing Forum, 34*(4), 813–820.

Diemunsch, P., & Grelot, L. (2000). Potential of substance P antagonists as antiemetics. *Drugs, 60*(3), 533–546.

Dodd, M.J. (2004). The pathogenesis and characterization of oral mucositis associated with cancer therapy. *Oncology Nursing Forum, 31*(Suppl. 4), 5–23.

Dranitsaris, G., Maroun, J., & Shah, A. (2005). Severe chemotherapy-induced diarrhea in patients with colorectal cancer: A cost of illness analysis. *Supportive Care in Cancer, 13*(5), 318–324.

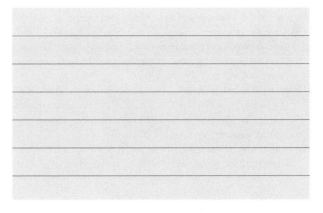

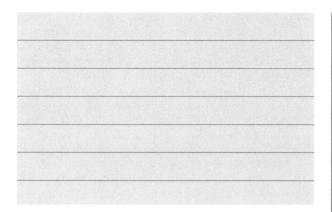

Eilers, J., & Million, R. (2007). Prevention and management of oral mucositis in patients with cancer. *Seminars in Oncology Nursing, 23*(3), 201–212.

Engelking, C. (2004). Diarrhea. In C.H. Yarbro, M.H. Frogge, & M. Goodman (Eds.), *Cancer symptom management* (3rd ed., pp. 528–555). Sudbury, MA: Jones and Bartlett.

Engelking, C. (2008). Diarrhea and constipation. In R.A. Gates & R.M. Fink (Eds.), *Oncology nursing secrets* (3rd ed., pp. 372–397). St. Louis, MO: Elsevier Mosby.

Ernst, E., & Pittler, M.H. (2000). Efficacy of ginger for nausea and vomiting: A systematic review of randomized clinical trials. *British Journal of Anaesthesia, 84*(3), 367–371.

Ezzo, J., Streitberger, K., & Schneider, A. (2006). Cochrane systematic reviews examine P6 acupuncture-point stimulation for nausea and vomiting. *Journal of Alternative and Complementary Medicine, 12*(5), 489–495.

Ezzone, S., Baker, R., & Terrepka, E. (1998). Music as an adjunct to antiemetic therapy. *Oncology Nursing Forum, 25*(9), 1551–1556.

Fabi, A., Barduagni, M., Lauro, S., Portalone, L., Mauri, M., Marinis, F., et al. (2003). Is delayed chemotherapy-induced emesis well managed in oncological clinical practice? An observational study. *Supportive Care in Cancer, 11*(3), 156–161.

Fenton, D. (2008). *Perirectal abscess.* Retrieved October 20, 2008, from http://www.emedicine.com/emerg/topic494.htm

Field, M. (2003). Intestinal ion transport and the pathophysiology of diarrhea. *Journal of Clinical Investigation, 111*(7), 931–943.

Genentech. (2007). Rituximab [Package insert]. South San Francisco, CA: Author.

GlaxoSmithKline. (2007). Navelbine [Package insert]. Research Triangle Park, NC: Author.

Goldberg, R.M., Sargent, D.J., Morton, R.F., Fuchs, C.S., Ramanathan, R.K., Williamson, S.K., et al. (2004). A randomized controlled trial of fluorouracil plus leucovorin, irinotecan, and oxaliplatin combinations in patients with previously untreated and metastatic colorectal cancer. *Journal of Clinical Oncology, 22*(1), 23–30.

Goldberg, S.L., Chiang, L., Selina, N., & Hamarman, S. (2004). Patient perceptions about chemotherapy-induced oral mucositis: Implications for primary/secondary prophylaxis strategies. *Supportive Care in Cancer, 12*(7), 526–530.

Grunberg, S.M., Deuson, R.R., Mavros, P., Geling, O., Hansen, M., Gruciani, G., et al. (2004). Incidence of chemotherapy-induced nausea and emesis after modern antiemetics: Perception versus reality. *Cancer, 100*(10), 2261–2268.

Grunberg, S.M., Hansen, M., Deuson, R., & Mavros, P. (2002). Incidence and impact of nausea/vomiting with modern antiemetics: Perception vs. reality [Abstract 996]. *Proceedings of the American Society of Clinical Oncology, 21,* 250a.

Harris, D.J., Eilers, J.G., Cashavelly, B.J., Maxwell, C.L., & Harriman, A. (2007). *Putting evidence into practice: Mucositis.* Pittsburgh, PA: Oncology Nursing Society.

Hensley, M.L., Hagerty, K.L., Kewalramani, T., Green, D.M., Meropol, N.J., Wasserman, T.H., et al. (2009). American Society of Clinical Oncology 2008 clinical practice guideline update: Use of chemotherapy and radiation therapy protectants. *Journal of Clinical Oncology, 27*(1), 127–145.

Hesketh, P.J. (2001). Potential role of NK1 receptor antagonists in chemotherapy-induced nausea and vomiting. *Supportive Care in Cancer, 9*(5), 350–354.

Hesketh, P.J. (2005). *Management of nausea and vomiting in cancer and cancer treatment.* Sudbury, MA: Jones and Bartlett.

Hornby, P.J. (2001). Receptors and transmission in the brain-gut axis: II. Excitatory amino acid receptors in the brain-gut axis. *American Journal of Physiology—Gastrointestinal and Liver Physiology, 280*(6), 1055–1060.

Illman, J., Corringham, R., Robinson, D., Davis, H., Rossi, J., Cella, D., et al. (2005). Are inflammatory cytokines the common link between cancer-associated cachexia and depression? *Journal of Supportive Oncology, 3*(1), 37–50.

Inui, A. (2002). Cancer anorexia-cachexia syndrome: Current issues in research and management. *CA: A Cancer Journal for Clinicians, 52*(2), 72–91.

Jatoi, A. (2006). Pharmacologic therapy for the cancer anorexia/weight loss syndrome: A data-driven, practical approach. *Journal of Supportive Oncology, 4*(10), 499–502.

Jordan, K., Hinke, A., Grothey, A., Voigt, W., Arnold, D., Wolf, H.H., et al. (2007). A meta-analysis comparing the efficacy of five 5-HT3-receptor antagonists for acute chemotherapy-induced emesis. *Supportive Care in Cancer, 15*(9), 1023–1033.

Jordan, K., Sipple, C., & Schmoll, H. (2007). Guidelines for antiemetic therapy for chemotherapy-induced nausea and vomiting. *Oncologist, 12*(9), 1143–1150.

Kang, S.P., & Saif, M.W. (2007). Infusion-related and hypersensitivity reactions of monoclonal antibodies used to treat colorectal cancer—Identification, prevention, management. *Journal of Supportive Oncology, 5*(9), 451–457.

Keefe, D.M., Schubert, M.M., Elting, L.S., Sonis, S.T., Epstein, J.B., Raber-Durlacher, J.E., et al. (2007). Updated clinical practice guidelines for the prevention and treatment of mucositis. *Cancer, 109*(5), 820–831.

Kellner, T. (2004). Nutritional problems. In B.K. Shelton, C.R. Ziegfeld, & M.M. Olsen (Eds.), *Manual of cancer nursing* (pp. 407–427). Philadelphia: Lippincott Williams & Wilkins.

Kline, N.E. (2002). Prevention and treatment of infections. In C.R. Baggott, K.P. Kelly, D. Fochtman, & G.V. Foley (Eds.), *Nursing care of children and adolescents with cancer* (3rd ed., pp. 266–278). Philadelphia: Saunders.

Kosits, C., & Callaghan, M. (2000). Rituximab: A new monoclonal antibody therapy for non-Hodgkin lymphoma. *Oncology Nursing Forum, 27*(1), 51–59.

Liau, C., Chu, N., Liu, H., Deuson, R., Lien, J., & Chen, J. (2005). Incidence of chemotherapy-induced nausea and vomiting in Taiwan: Physicians' and nurses' estimation vs. patients' reported outcomes. *Supportive Care in Cancer, 13*(5), 277–286.

MacDonald, N. (2007). Cancer cachexia and targeting chronic inflammation: A unified approach to cancer treatment and palliative/supportive care. *Journal of Supportive Oncology, 5*(4), 157–162.

Madeya, M. (1996). Oral complications from cancer therapy: Part 2—Nursing implications for assessment and treatment. *Oncology Nursing Forum, 23*(5), 808–819.

Manusirivithaya, S., Sripramote, M., Tangjitgamol, S., Sheanakul, C., Leelahakorn, S., Thavaramara, T., et al. (2004). Antiemetic effect of ginger in gynecologic oncology patients receiving cisplatin. *International Journal of Gynecological Cancer, 14*(6), 1063–1069.

Massaro, A.M., & Lenz, K.L. (2005). Aprepitant: A novel antiemetic for chemotherapy-induced nausea and vomiting. *Annals of Pharmacotherapy, 39*(1), 77–85.

Massey, R.L., Haylock, P.J., & Curtiss, C. (2004). Constipation. In C.H. Yarbro, M.H. Frogge, & M. Goodman (Eds.), *Cancer symptom management* (3rd ed., pp. 512–527). Sudbury, MA: Jones and Bartlett.

Mattox, T.W. (2005). Treatment of unintentional weight loss in patients with cancer. *Nutrition in Clinical Practice, 20*(4), 400–410.

McClement, S. (2005). Cancer anorexia-cachexia syndrome: Psychological effect on the patient and family. *Journal of Wound, Ostomy, and Continence Nursing, 32*(4), 264–268.

Merck & Co., Inc. (2008). Emend [Package insert]. Whitehouse Station, NJ: Author.

Micromedex. (2007). *Micromedex® healthcare series 2007* (version 5.1) [Intranet]. Greenwood Village, CO: Thomas Healthcare.

Millennium Pharmaceuticals. (2007). Velcade [Package insert]. Cambridge, MA: Author.

Multinational Association of Supportive Care in Cancer. (2005). *Summary of evidence-based clinical practice guidelines for care of patients with oral and gastrointestinal mucositis.* Retrieved November 14, 2007, from http://www.mascc.org/content/338 .html

Murphy, B. (2007). Clinical and economic consequences of mucositis induced by chemotherapy and/or radiation therapy. *Journal of Supportive Oncology, 5*(9, Suppl. 4), 13–21.

National Cancer Institute. (2008a). *Gastrointestinal complications (PDQ®).* Retrieved July 17, 2008, from http://www.cancer.gov/ cancertopics/pdq/supportivecare/gastrointestinalcomplications/ HealthProfessional/page2

National Cancer Institute. (2008b). *Nausea and vomiting (PDQ®).* Retrieved July 16, 2008, from http://www.cancer.gov/cancertopics/ pdq/supportivecare/nausea/HealthProfessional/page3

National Cancer Institute. (2008c). *Oral complications of chemotherapy and head and neck radiation (PDQ®).* Retrieved July 17, 2008, from http://www.cancer.gov/cancertopics/pdq/ supportivecare/oralcomplications/healthprofessional

National Cancer Institute. (n.d.). *National Cancer Institute dictionary of cancer terms.* Retrieved July 14, 2008, from http://www .cancer.gov/dictionary

National Cancer Institute Cancer Therapy Evaluation Program. (2006). *Common terminology criteria for adverse events* (version 3.0). Bethesda, MD: National Cancer Institute. Retrieved October 4, 2008, from http://ctep.cancer.gov/reporting/ctc_v30 .html

National Comprehensive Cancer Network. (2008a). *NCCN Clinical Practice Guidelines in Oncology™: Prevention and treatment of cancer-related infections* [v.1.2008]. Jenkintown, PA: Author.

National Comprehensive Cancer Network. (2008b). *NCCN Clinical Practice Guidelines in Oncology™: Prevention and treatment of cancer-related infections: Antiemesis* [v.3.2008]. Jenkintown, PA: Author.

Nelson, K.A. (2000). The cancer anorexia-cachexia syndrome. *Seminars in Oncology, 27*(1), 64–68.

O'Bryant, C.L., Gonzales, J.A., & Bestul, D. (2004). Guide to the prevention and management of nausea and vomiting in the oncology setting. *Oncology Special Edition, 7,* 67–74.

Ottery, F.D. (1994). Rethinking nutritional support of the cancer patient: The new field of nutritional oncology. *Seminars in Oncology, 21*(6), 770–778.

Pace, J. (1999). Symptom management. In C. Miaskowski & P.C. Buchsel (Eds.), *Oncology nursing: Assessment and clinical care* (pp. 275–304). St. Louis, MO: Mosby.

Pfizer Oncology. (2007). Camptosar [Packet insert]. Retrieved November 10, 2007, from http://www.pfizer.com/files/products/ uspi_camptosar.pdf

Robinson, C., Fritch, M., Hullett, L., Petersen, M., Sikkema, S., Theuninck, L., et al. (2000). Development of a protocol to prevent opioid-induced constipation in patients with cancer: A research utilization project. *Clinical Journal of Oncology Nursing, 4*(2), 79–84.

Rosenoff, S.H. (2004). Octreotide LAR resolves severe chemotherapy-induced diarrhea (CID) and allows continuation of full-dose therapy. *European Journal of Cancer Care, 13*(4), 380–383.

Rosenthal, D. (2007). Consequences of mucositis-induced treatment breaks and dose reductions on head and neck cancer treatment outcomes. *Journal of Supportive Oncology, 5*(9, Suppl. 4), 23–31.

Roy, P. (2006). *Lactose intolerance.* Retrieved November 1, 2007, from http://www.emedicine.com

Rubenstein, E.B., Peterson, D.E., Schubert, M., Keefe, D., McGuire, D., Epstein, J., et al. (2004). Clinical practice guidelines for the prevention and treatment of cancer therapy-induced oral and gastrointestinal mucositis. *Cancer, 100*(Suppl. 9), 2026–2046.

Sonis, S.T. (2007). Pathobiology of oral mucositis: Novel insights and opportunities. *Journal of Supportive Oncology, 5*(9, Suppl. 4), 3–11.

Spratto, G.R., & Woods, A.L. (2007). *2008 PDR nurse's drug handbook.* Montvale, NJ: Thomson Healthcare.

Strasser, F., & Bruera, E.D. (2002). Update on anorexia and cachexia. *Hematology/Oncology Clinics of North America, 16*(3), 1–23.

Tipton, J., McDaniel, R., Barbour, L., Johnston, M., LeRoy, P., Kayne, M., et al. (2005). *Putting evidence into practice: Chemotherapy-induced nausea and vomiting.* Pittsburgh, PA: Oncology Nursing Society.

Valle, E.A., Wisniewski, T., Vadillo, F., Burke, T.A., & Corona, M. (2006). Incidence of chemotherapy-induced nausea and vomiting in Mexico: Healthcare provider predictions versus observed. *Current Medical Research and Opinion, 22*(12), 2403–2410.

Vannice, S. (2008). Mucositis. In R.A. Gates & R.M. Fink (Eds.), *Oncology nursing secrets* (3rd ed., pp. 372–397). St. Louis, MO: Elsevier Mosby.

Vogel, W., Viele, C., & Stern, J. (2004, April). *Cancer treatment–induced diarrhea: Interventions to minimize the roller coaster ride* [Continuing education program]. Ancillary event presented at the 29th Annual Congress of the Oncology Nursing Society, Anaheim, CA.

Wadler, S. (2004). Treatment guidelines for chemotherapy-induced diarrhea. *Oncology Special Edition, 7,* 83–87.

Weaver, C., & Buckner, C.D. (2007). *Managing side effects: Chemotherapy-induced diarrhea.* Retrieved November 1,

2007, from http://patient.cancerconsultants.com/SideEffects
.aspx?TierId=1090&LinkId=54146&DocumentId=1002
#a6

Wickham, R. (2008). Nausea and vomiting. In R.A. Gates & R.M.
Fink (Eds.), *Oncology nursing secrets* (3rd ed., pp. 372–397).
St. Louis, MO: Elsevier Mosby.

Woo, S., & Treister, N.S. (2006). *Chemotherapy-induced oral mucositis.* Retrieved October 20, 2008, from http://www.emedicine
.com/derm/topic682.htm

Wujcik, D. (2004). Infection. In C.H. Yarbro, M.H. Frogge, & M.
Goodman (Eds.), *Cancer symptom management* (3rd ed., pp.
252–272). Sudbury, MA: Jones and Bartlett.

Wyeth. (2008). Relistor [Package insert]. Madison, NJ: Author.

Yuan, C. (2004). Clinical status of methylnaltrexone, a new agent
to prevent and manage opioid-induced side effects. *Journal of
Supportive Oncology, 2*(2), 111–117.

C. Cutaneous toxicity: Patients receiving chemo-
therapy/biotherapy may experience a variety
of cutaneous complications (Goodman, 2004).
Recently, the use of targeted therapies such as
EGFR inhibitors (EGFRIs) has come to the
forefront in the treatment of specific types of
cancer (e.g., colorectal, lung, head and neck).
Although most targeted therapies are devoid of
hematopoietic and nonspecific (e.g., GI) toxicities
common with conventional chemotherapy, they
are characterized by the development of dermatologic reactions, which occur in the majority
of patients (Lacouture, Basti, Patel, & Benson,
2006).
1. Rash terminology
   a) Described in phenotypic (observable traits)
      terms related to its appearance and location
      (Perez-Soler et al., 2005)
   b) Recommended terms are *pustular/papular
      rash, pustular eruption, or follicular,* and
      intrafollicular pustular eruption.
   c) Accurate rash description is essential for
      proper treatment. See Figure 26.
2. Pathophysiology
   a) The exact role of human epidermal recep-
      tor/EGFR (HER1/EGFR) in skin is not
      fully understood although it is involved
      in many normal epidermal processes,
      and abnormal expression is implicated
      in epithelial tumor formation and epider-
      mal hyperproliferation disorders such as
      psoriasis.
   b) HER1/EGFR is expressed in epidermal
      and follicular keratinocytes, sebaceous
      epithelium, eccrine epithelium, dendritic
      antigen-presenting cells, and various
      connective tissues (Perez-Soler et al.,
      2005).
   c) The histologic findings show that, in
      agreement with clinical observation, the

rash has a strong inflammatory element.
However, the sebaceous glands are not
affected.
d) More studies are required to define the
   exact histology of the rash, key structures
   involved, primary cellular mediators, and
   extent/incidence of secondary infection
   (Perez-Soler et al., 2005).
e) The pathology and etiology of the rash
   associated with HER1/EGFR-targeted
   agents are unclear yet are distinct from
   acne vulgaris.
f) The rash associated with HER1/EGFR-
   targeted agents is dominated by pustules that
   develop an impetiginous, honey-combed
   crust in serious cases.
g) Noninflammatory comedones (black-
   heads and whiteheads) have not been
   described.
h) In rash associated with HER1/EGFR-
   targeted agents, microcomedones (the
   smallest form of acne lesion, it is the very
   beginning of pore blockage) and comedones
   are not seen.
i) Pustules show an intrafollicular collection of neutrophils—the hallmark of an
   infectious folliculitis (Perez-Soler et al.,
   2005).
j) Avoid using terms such as *acne, acne-like,*
   or *acneform* when communicating with
   patients.
k) Differentiation of rash etiology and characteristics
   (1) Do not confuse the rash associated
       with HER1/EGFR-targeted agents
       with acne vulgaris, steroid-induced
       rash, or cellulitis; the rashes are
       separate entities and vary in their
       characteristics.
   (2) Acne vulgaris has a unique pathology.
       Acne is characterized clinically by both
       noninflammatory lesions known as
       comedones, as well as inflammatory
       papules, pustules, and nodules (Perez-
       Soler et al., 2005).
   (3) Patients taking steroids for their
       cancer may develop steroid-induced
       acne. Steroid-induced acne is a mono-
       morphous eruption with widespread,
       2–3 mm firm, erythematous papules
       primarily on the trunk. Any attempt to
       open and culture will not reveal any
       purulent material (Perez-Soler et al.,
       2005).
   (4) Do not mistake EGFR rash for cel-
       lulitis. Cellulitis typically presents
       with a localized area of warmth,

Figure 26. Acneform Eruption

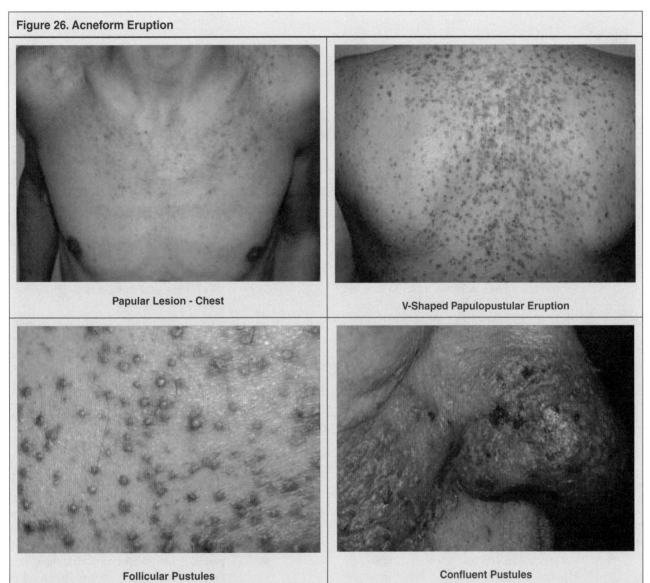

Papular Lesion - Chest

V-Shaped Papulopustular Eruption

Follicular Pustules

Confluent Pustules

Note. From "Clinical Signs, Pathophysiology and Management of Skin Toxicity During Therapy With Epidermal Growth Factor Inhibitors," by S. Segaert and E. Van Cutsem, 2005, *Annals of Oncology, 16*(9), p. 1427. Copyright 2005 by Oxford University Press. Reprinted with permission.

erythema, and tenderness and can be associated with fever (Perez-Soler et al., 2005).

3. Incidence
   a) Patients treated with agents that inhibit HER1/EGFR exhibit a high incidence of rash (Luu, Lai, Patel, Guitart, & Lacouture, 2007). Rash commonly occurs within the first two weeks of treatment. Time to first rash appearance may be related to the agent and dose (Perez-Soler et al., 2005).
      (1) Papulopustular rash (45%–100%)
      (2) Xerosis (7%–35%)
      (3) Periungual inflammation (12%–16%)
      (4) Alopecia (12%–14%)
      (5) Ocular reactions (4%–12%) are characteristic of EGFR inhibitors resulting in significant ocular discomfort and potential visual blur (Lacouture, 2007).
         (a) Trichomegaly
         (b) Conjunctivitis
         (c) Keratoconjunctivitis sicca
         (d) Lacrimation

4. Grading rash severity: The grading system should be used as a guide only, with emphasis on early intervention as the key to controlling the overall outcome (Rhee, Oishi, Garey, & Kim, 2005). The standard grading of dermatologic toxicity employs the NCI CTCAE (NCI CTEP,

2006) or the ECOG grading systems (see Table 22).

a) **Grade 1** reactions consist of an asymptomatic, nonconfluent, maculopapular rash in an acneform distribution (head, chest, and upper back area) (Rhee et al., 2005).

b) **Grade 2** reactions are similar to those of grade 1, except for associated symptoms of pruritus, dryness, or edema, and have the beginnings of confluence or pustules (i.e., worse-appearing rash than grade 1) (Rhee et al., 2005).

c) **Grade 3** lesions are confluent and symptomatic, with possible associated pain and ulceration (Rhee et al., 2005).

d) **Grade 4** lesions consist of exfoliative or ulcerating dermatitis. Although grades 3 and 4 rashes prompt a discontinuation of therapy with the EGFR agent, they are uncommon (Perez-Soler et al., 2005).

5. Cutaneous reactions may lead to dose reduction, dose interruption, or treatment cessation when considered intolerable by the patient or oncologist (Perez-Soler et al., 2005). However, there are anecdotal reports of rash improving or resolving spontaneously in spite of continued treatment (Perez-Soler et al.).

6. Nursing interventions: Treatment of rash is largely dependent on the patient's symptoms. Many patients are asymptomatic, and current treatments are not consistently effective in eliminating or improving dermatologic toxicities (Rhee et al., 2005). See Table 23.

a) Suggest covering rash with makeup. A dermatologist-approved cover-up (e.g., Dermablend®) can be used, although any type of foundation may be useful.

b) Instruct patient to remove makeup with a hypoallergenic liquid cleanser (e.g., Neutrogena®, Cetaphil®, Dove®, Ivory Skin Cleansing Liquid Gel®) (Perez-Soler et al., 2005).

c) Instruct patient *not* to use OTC medications that are used to treat acne vulgaris, such as benzoyl peroxide and topical retinoids. These will cause excessive dryness and may aggravate the rash (Meniscus Ltd., 2006).

d) Recommend emollients free of perfume, alcohol, and petroleum jelly (e.g., Neutrogena Norwegian Formula® hand cream or Vaseline Intensive Care® Advanced Healing Lotion) to prevent skin dryness (Meniscus Ltd., 2006).

e) Instruct patient to avoid sun exposure and use sunscreens containing zinc oxide with a sun protection factor of at least 15 (Lynch et al., 2007) (e.g., Anthelios®). Wear hats and sunglasses, and cover exposed skin.

f) Suggest use of an antihistamine such as diphenhydramine or hydroxyzine hydrochloride, which may be helpful for pruritus (Perez-Soler et al., 2005).

g) Infected skin rash should be treated with a short course of oral antibiotics such as tetracyclines because of their effectiveness against *Staphylococcus* (Meniscus Ltd., 2006).

h) Consider prescribing standard analgesia if the rash is painful, before reducing the dose of the HER1/EGFR-targeted agent. If the pain is localized or becomes more severe, then cellulitis should be considered (Perez-Soler et al., 2005). The benefit of topical corticosteroids is unclear; however, they may have some efficacy when used to treat mild rashes.

7. Management of skin rash

a) The optimal management of rash in patients receiving anti-EGFR therapy remains somewhat anecdotal; this is a result of imprecise classification of rash as well as the lack of prospective clinical trials to determine the most appropriate treatment algorithm for these patients (Perez-Soler et al., 2005).

b) Perez-Soler et al. (2005) formulated an algorithm through the HER1/EGFR Inhibitor Rash Management Forum. The algorithm was developed based on available information, knowledge of the rash's inflammatory nature, and the unpublished experience of the oncologists and dermatologists present at the forum to develop broad suggestions to assist when patients present with HER1/EGFR-associated rash. See Figure 27.

Table 22. National Cancer Institute Common Terminology Criteria for Adverse Events (Version 3.0ᵃ) Categories Relevant to Epidermal Growth Factor Receptor Inhibitor–Associated Dermatologic Toxicity

Adverse Event	Grade 1	Grade 2	Grade 3	Grade 4	Grade 5
Dry skin	Asymptomatic	Symptomatic, not interfering with ADLs	Interfering with ADLs	–	–
Nail changes	Discoloration, ridging, pitting	Partial or complete loss of nails, pain in nailbed(s)	Interfering with ADLs	–	–
Pruritus/itching	Mild or localized	Intense or widespread	Intense or widespread and interfering with ADLs	–	–
Rash/desquamation	Macular or papular eruption or erythema without associated symptoms	Macular or papular eruption or erythema with pruritus or other associated symptoms, localized desquamation or other lesions covering < 50% BSA	Severe, generalized erythroderma or macular, papular, or vesicular eruption; desquamation covering > 50% BSA	Generalized exfoliative, ulcerative, or bullous dermatitis	Death
Rash; acne/acneiform	Intervention not indicated	Intervention indicated	Associated with pain, disfigurement, ulceration, or desquamation	–	Death
Dermatology/skin—other	Mild	Moderate	Severe	Life-threatening, disabling	Death

ᵃ Version 2.0 of the National Cancer Institute Common Toxicity Criteria was used in trials prior to 2006.

ADLs—activities of daily living; BSA—body surface area

Note. From *Common Terminology Criteria for Adverse Events* (Version 3.0), by National Cancer Institute Cancer Therapy Evaluation Program, 2006. Retrieved December 11, 2007, from http://ctep.cancer.gov/reporting/ctc_v30.html

c) Patients should be referred to a dermatologist if lesions have an uncharacteristic appearance or distribution, or if there is necrosis, blistering, or petechial purpuric lesions (Segaert & Van Cutsem, 2005).

8. Secondary infection: Signs of secondary infection can be subtle, especially in patients who are neutropenic or taking systemic steroids (Perez-Soler et al., 2005).

a) The pustules associated with HER1/EGFR inhibitors are notably sterile with negative cultures or staining for bacteria, fungi, and yeast (Segaert & Van Cutsem, 2005).

b) Inflammatory-based pustules should be sterile, but experience shows that secondary infections are common.

(1) The most common presentation of a secondary infection is recognized only by an increase in pustules.

(2) Significant oozing of fluid from lesions or an abrupt change in their appearance may be present.

(3) Some organisms (e.g., *Staphylococcus [S.] aureus*) produce a classic impetigo appearance, indicated by a yellowish/brown crust overlying inflammatory lesions.

(4) Inspect rash regularly, culturing pustules in early-onset rash to find if *S. aureus* is present.

(5) Frequent culturing enables assessment of the extent of secondary infection, the type of colonizing bacteria, and treatments.

(6) If antibiotic resistance is suspected, culture the pustules to determine bacterial strain before treating.

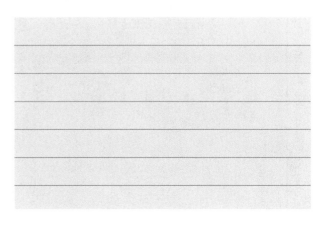

Table 23. Cutaneous Reactions to Chemotherapy and Biotherapy

Cutaneous Reaction	General Comments	Chemotherapy	Biotherapy
Hair changes	A number of chemotherapy drugs can cause hair changes and hair loss. Dose, route of administration, combination of drugs, and other individual characteristics all will have an impact on whether hair loss occurs, as well as the degree of hair loss experienced. Hair changes may occur 2–3 months after initiation of EGFR therapy, with hair thinning and developing a dry, brittle, or curly texture (Segaert & Van Cutsem, 2005).	Doxorubicin, carboplatin, cisplatin, cyclophosphamide, dactinomycin, etoposide, hexamethamelamine, ifosfamide, paclitaxel, vincristine, and bexarotene (Targretin®) (Ligand Pharmaceuticals, 1999)—alopecia: 3%–6% Other chemotherapy agents associated with lesser degree of hair loss include bleomycin, 5-FU, and methotrexate (OncoLink, 2001).	Cetuximab (Erbitux®) (ImClone Systems and Bristol-Myers Squibb, 2006)—alopecia: 4% grades 1–4, 0% grades 2–4 Sunitinib (Sutent®) (Pfizer Labs, 2007)—hair color changes: 16% all grades, 0% grades 3 and 4
Trichomegaly (see Figure 28)	Increased hair growth of the eyelashes and eyebrows can occur, although rare (Segaert & Van Cutsem, 2005). Excessive length can cause conjunctival irritation. Although many researchers (Braiteh et al., 2008; Eaby et al., 2008; Esper et al., 2007; Segaert & Van Cutsem, 2007) agree that patients experiencing trichomegaly should see an ophthalmologist if eye irritations occur and that eyelashes may be carefully and safely trimmed, only Basti (2007) advises patients to not cut their lashes or have them cut. Waxing or electrolysis may be recommended (Braiteh et al., 2008; Segaert & Van Cutsem, 2005).	Gemcitabine, IFN alfa-2b, cyclosporine, gefitinib (Bouche et al., 2005)	Panitumumab (Vectibix®) (Amgen Inc., 2006)—growth of eyelashes: 6% all grades Cetuximab (Erbitux®) (ImClone Systems & Bristol-Myers Squibb, 2006)—6% all grades
Paronychia (see Figure 29)	Painful inflammation of tissue around fingernails and toenails; more commonly seen in the great toe and thumbs Often delayed, developing after 4–8 weeks of treatment (Segaert & Van Cutsem, 2005) May be prevented by wearing shoes that are not tight-fitting; avoid friction. Hot soaks and cushioning provide comfort; Epsom salt soaks promote drainage of the affected area. Use of topical antiseptic or antibiotic ointments may help (Segaert & Van Cutsem, 2005).	Bleomycin, cyclophosphamide, doxorubicin, and hydroxyurea; docetaxel and methotrexate	Cetuximab (Erbitux®) (ImClone Systems & Bristol-Myers Squibb, 2006)—nail disorders including paronychia: 16% grades 1–4, < 1% grades 3 and 4 Panitumumab (Vectibix®) (Amgen Inc., 2006)—paronychia: 25% all grades, 2% grades 3 and 4
Nail shedding	Involuntary release of the nail from the nail bed	Bleomycin, cisplatin, docetaxel, doxorubicin, melphalan, and vincristine	—
Dystrophy	Transverse midline linear groove in the nail plate	Bleomycin and hydroxyurea	—
Beau's lines	Transverse groove in the nail plate	Bleomycin, cisplatin, docetaxel, doxorubicin, melphalan, vincristine	—

(Continued on next page)

Table 23. Cutaneous Reactions to Chemotherapy and Biotherapy (Continued)

Cutaneous Reaction	General Comments	Chemotherapy	Biotherapy
Hyperpigmentation (see Figure 30)	Sun exposure should be avoided or effective sun barrier preparations should be used to minimize the risk of hyperpigmentation. Sun exposure aggravates hyperpigmentation. Bleaching creams are not helpful; the hyperpigmentation will fade spontaneously with time (months) (Segaert & Van Cutsem, 2005). Occurs most commonly in people of Mediterranean descent The drugs are thought to stimulate the melanocytes to produce more melanin. Darkening may occur within 2–3 weeks of chemotherapy/biotherapy and persist for months following the completion of therapy. Hyperpigmentation may involve the nail beds, oral mucosa, tongue, and palms and soles, may appear along veins, and may be generalized to involve the surface of the skin (Goodman, 2004). Post-inflammatory hyperpigmentation is seen following acneform eruption or other causes of skin inflammation such as eczema or an inflamed sebaceous cyst (Segaert & Van Cutsem, 2005).	Bleomycin, busulfan, cyclophosphamide, dacarbazine, daunorubicin, docetaxel, doxorubicin, etoposide, 5-FU, hydroxyurea, melphalan, methotrexate, nitrogen mustard, nitrosourea, and paclitaxel (Vassallo et al., 2001) Flagellate streaks caused by nail scratching the skin have been reported with parenteral and intrapleural administration of bleomycin (Goodman, 2004). Temsirolimus (Torisel®) (Wyeth Pharmaceuticals, 2007)—nail disorders: 14% all grades, 0% grades 3 and 4	—
Rash	—	Docetaxel and paclitaxel (Hetherington et al., 2007)	Panitumumab (Vectibix®) (Amgen Inc., 2006)—skin rash: 22% all grades; 1% grades 3 and 4 Lapatinib (Tykerb®) (GlaxoSmithKline, 2007)—rash: 28% all grades, 2% grade 3, 0% grade 4 when given in combination with capecitabine (Xeloda®) (Roche Pharmaceuticals, 2008); dry skin: 10% all grades, 0% grades 3 and 4 when given in combination with capecitabine
Blistering of the skin	—	Vinblastine, 5-FU, and IL-2 (White & Cox, 2006)	—
Xerosis	Abnormal dryness of the skin, mucous membranes, or conjunctiva (Segaert & Van Cutsem, 2005) Hydration of the skin with the use of bath oil or shower oil may help to alleviate symptoms. Alcohol-containing gels, lotions, and soaps should be avoided, as they may exacerbate dryness. Dryness can be alleviated by using emollient (oil in water) creams (Segaert & Van Cutsem, 2005).	Temsirolimus (Torisel®) (Wyeth Pharmaceuticals, 2007)—dry skin: 11% all grades, 1% grades 3 and 4; rash: 47% all grades, 10% grades 3 and 4 Bexarotene (Targretin®) (Ligand Pharmaceuticals, 1999)—dry skin: 9.4%–10.7%; rash: 12%–14%; exfoliative dermatitis: 8%–18%	Erlotinib (Tarceva®) (Genentech, Inc., 2007)—rash: 75% any grade, 8% grade 3, <1% grade 4; dry skin: 12% any grade, 0% grades 3 and 4 Gefitinib (Iressa®) (AstraZeneca, 2004)—dry skin: 13% all grades, 12% grade 1, 1% grade 2, 0% grades 3 and 4 Sunitinib (Sutent®) (Pfizer Labs, 2007)—dry skin: 18% all grades, <1% grades 3 and 4; skin discoloration/yellow skin: 19% all grades, 0% grades 3 and 4; rash: 27% all grades, 1% grades 3 and 4

(Continued on next page)

Table 23. Cutaneous Reactions to Chemotherapy and Biotherapy *(Continued)*

Cutaneous Reaction	General Comments	Chemotherapy	Biotherapy
Painful fissures	May develop on the fingers and toes, in nail folds, and over the interphalangeal joints (Segaert & Van Cutsem, 2005) Fissures can be treated with propylene glycol 50% solution under plastic occlusion, salicylic acid 10% ointment, a hydrocolloid dressing, flurandrenolone tape, or liquid cyanoacrylate glue. Liquid bandage formulations may be helpful in protecting the fissures (Segaert & Van Cutsem, 2005).	—	Panitumumab (Vectibix®) (Amgen Inc., 2006)—20% all grades, 1% grades 3 and 4
Telangiectasia	Veins appear as eruptions under the skin (Goodman, 2004). Chronic dilation of groups of capillaries leads to elevated dark red blotches on the skin. May be seen in early-onset of rash, with symptoms appearing on the face, nose, chest, back, and limbs around a follicular pustule (Segaert & Van Cutsem, 2005) Telangiectasia caused by treatment with EGFRIs, unlike spontaneous telangiectasia, will gradually disappear over months. In selected cases, electrocoagulation or pulsed dye laser therapy can be applied to accelerate disappearance (Segaert & Van Cutsem, 2005). Radiation may cause telangiectasis, which is thought to be related to the destruction of the capillary bed (Goodman, 2004).	Telangiectasias associated with chemotherapy are not harmful but can be disturbing for the patient depending on where they are located. They generally are considered a permanent change in the vessel but can fade over time (Goodman, 2004). Topical carmustine and mechlorethamine cause vessel fragility and destruction (Goodman, 2004).	Scattered telangiectasia can be seen with the development of any acneform eruption caused by EGFRIs.
Ocular changes	Adverse effects vary, from seemingly mild changes such as dry eyes and blurred vision, to more severe and sometimes permanent changes, such as retinal damage, glaucoma, and cataracts (Meniscus Ltd., 2006). Ocular irritation manifests as dry eyes, progressing to erythematous lids and crusting in the eyelash follicules with the use of EGFRIs (looks like blepharitis or conjunctivitis). Ocular irritation is rare, but if it occurs, it is usually within the first 4 weeks of EGFRI therapy (Segaert & Van Cutsem, 2005). Treatment may consist of ophthalmic ointment, warm soaks, and natural tears. Lid hygiene is very important. Treatment should be done under the care of an eye doctor (Segaert & Van Cutsem, 2005).	Changes in visual fields and acuity have been attributed to chemotherapy agents such as the antimetabolites, alkylating agents, taxanes, and platinum agents. 5-FU may cause dry eyes and/or excessive tearing (Meniscus Ltd., 2006). With systemic 5-FU, the prevalence of blepharitis was 3.8%; eyelid dermatitis: 5.8%; tearing: 26.9%; punctalcanalicular stenosis: 5.8%; conjunctivitis: 5.8%; keratitis: 3.8%; blurred vision: 11.5%. Excessive tearing resolves on cessation of treatment with 5-FU (Omoti & Omoti, 2006). Corneal opacities have been reported with the use of tamoxifen. Posterior subcapsular cataract can occur with busulfan, methotrexate, and tamoxifen. Combination chemotherapy of cyclophosphamide, methotrexate, and 5-FU can cause pruritus and/or burning sensation.	Panitumumab (Vectibix®) (Amgen Inc. 2006)—conjunctivitis: 4%; ocular hyperemia: 3%; increased lacrimation: 2%; eye/eyelid irritation: 1% Cetuximab (Erbitux®) (ImClone Systems & Bristol-Myers Squibb, 2006)—conjunctivitis: 7% grades 1–4, < 1% grades 3 and 4 Erlotinib (Tarceva®) (Genentech, Inc., 2007)—conjunctivitis: 12% any grade, < 1% grade 3, 0% grade 4; keratoconjunctivitis sicca: 12% any grade, 0% grades 3 and 4

(Continued on next page)

Table 23. Cutaneous Reactions to Chemotherapy and Biotherapy (Continued)

Cutaneous Reaction	General Comments	Chemotherapy	Biotherapy
Ocular changes (cont.)		Combination chemotherapy for acute lymphocytic leukemia with standard dose of vincristine, cyclophosphamide or teniposide, cytarabine, and asparaginase has been associated with corneal toxicity. Tamoxifen and IFN can cause marked irreversible visual loss even at therapeutic doses (Omoti & Omoti, 2006).	—
Acral erythema (see Figures 31 and 32)	Generally presents as dysesthesia (altered sensation of the skin) with tingling in the hands and feet progressing to pain. After 4 or 5 days of intense edematous erythema and even fissures of the palms, soles, and digital joints, progression to desquamation and re-epithelialization occurs. Resolves 5–7 days after therapy is discontinued. The etiology is not clear but may be related to concentration of the drug in the eccrine glands of the palms and soles. Applying cold compresses and elevating the hands and feet during drug administration may minimize incidence and degree of toxicity. Skin care and comfort measures are instituted as soon as symptoms are evident. Supportive care may include wound dressings, analgesia (pain relief), and cold compresses. Acral erythema may be the presenting symptom of GVHD (Goodman, 2004).	Acral erythema may be worsened by cyclosporine or trimethoprim-sulfamethoxazole (Goodman, 2004). High-dose cytarabine, cyclophosphamide, docetaxel, doxorubicin, hydroxyurea, methotrexate, mercaptopurine, mitoxantrone, paclitaxel, vinorelbine, 5-FU, capecitabine, daunorubicin, vincristine, vinblastine, and etoposide (Goodman, 2004)	
Palmar-plantar erythrodysesthesia (see Figure 33)	First appears as mild redness on the palms and soles with tingling sensations in the hands, usually at the fingertips; symptoms progress to a more intense burning pain and tenderness. Palms and soles appear edematous, and patients may have difficulty walking or grasping objects. Ulceration may occur if therapy is not stopped. Incidence and severity of symptoms are related to protracted exposure of cells to the drug. Early recognition and cessation of drug administration are critical to symptom management (Goodman, 2004). Symptoms also may include flaking, swelling, small blisters, or small sores. Prevention and treatment include reducing exposure of hands and feet to friction and heat by having patients avoid • Hot water (washing dishes, long showers, hot baths) • Impact on their feet (jogging, aerobics, walking, jumping) • Using tools that require them to squeeze their hand on a hard surface (garden tools, household tools, kitchen knives) • Rubbing (applying lotion, massaging).	Infusional therapy of 5-FU, doxorubicin, capecitabine, liposomal encapsulated doxorubicin, cytarabine, floxuridine, idarubicin (Goodman, 2004)	Lapatinib (Tykerb®) (GlaxoSmithKline, 2007)—palmar-plantar erythrodysesthesia when given with capecitabine: 53% all grades, 12% grade 3, 0% grade 4

(Continued on next page)

Table 23. Cutaneous Reactions to Chemotherapy and Biotherapy *(Continued)*

Cutaneous Reaction	General Comments	Chemotherapy	Biotherapy
Photosensitivity	Sunburn occurring after minimal sun exposure. Appears as an erythematous response to ultraviolet radiation; skin appears red with erythema, edema, and possibly vesicles. Patients are instructed to wear a wide-brim hat, cover their extremities while in the sun, and avoid direct sunlight when possible. They should wear a sunscreen with an SPF of at least 15 (Goodman, 2004).	High-dose methotrexate, 5-FU, dactinomycin, doxorubicin, bleomycin, dacarbazine, hydroxyurea, and vinblastine (Goodman, 2004)	Cetuximab (Erbitux®) (ImClone Systems & Bristol-Myers Squibb, 2006) Panitumumab (Vectibix®) (Amgen Inc., 2006)
Transient erythema or urticaria	Urticaria is characterized as multiple swollen, raised areas on the skin that are intensely itchy. They appear primarily on the chest, back, extremities, face, or scalp. It usually occurs within hours of chemotherapy and disappears within a few hours. It may be generalized or local at the site of chemotherapy or along the vein.	Doxorubicin can cause an erythematous flare with pruritus at the IV site and along the vein. Mechlorethamine can cause erythema and urticaria (Goodman, 2004). Cytarabine can cause transient erythema. Bleomycin causes erythema over pressure points and hyperpigmentation (Goodman, 2004). Cyclophosphamide causes generalized urticaria (Goodman, 2004). Chlorambucil, methotrexate, melphalan, and thiotepa can cause urticaria and angioedema. Asparaginase can cause urticaria, fever, chills, and hypotension (skin testing is advised). Aldesleukin can cause a diffuse erythematous reaction that may progress into a pruritic papular rash (Goodman, 2004). IFN alfa-2a and IFN alfa-2b can cause a dry, scaling skin or pruritic maculopapular reaction (Goodman, 2004). Filgrastim can cause transient erythematous eruptions and pruritus (Goodman, 2004).	Panitumumab (Vectibix®) (Amgen Inc., 2006)—erythema: 65% all grades, 5% grades 3 and 4 When combining chemotherapy and biologic response modifiers, it is important to note the occurrence of cutaneous reactions with each new agent to determine the offending agent. The drug may need to be discontinued if the reaction is severe or associated with systemic reactions such as a generalized rash (Goodman, 2004).
Erythema multiforme	Condition generally presents as a macular-papular erythematous lesion that may progress to vesicles; can progress to Stevens-Johnson syndrome and toxic epidermal necrolysis Record description, presentation, and severity (use a grading scale). Consult with physician regarding possible etiology. Consider discontinuing offending agent. Examine areas of tissue breakdown, and attend to comfort measures with skin care and pain management strategies (Goodman, 2004).	Occurs with high-dose therapy of hydroxyurea, mechlorethamine, busulfan, etoposide, chlorambucil, procarbazine, bleomycin, methotrexate, cytarabine, and 5-FU (Goodman, 2004) Can occur with phenytoin sodium, carbamazepine, allopurinol, and various antibiotics (Goodman, 2004)	–

(Continued on next page)

Table 23. Cutaneous Reactions to Chemotherapy and Biotherapy (Continued)

Cutaneous Reaction	General Comments	Chemotherapy	Biotherapy
Acneiform eruptions	Generally presents as a diffuse erythema over the face and body, progressing to follicular papules and pustules resembling acne. Causative (chemotherapy) agent should be discontinued. Causative EGFRIs may not need to be discontinued. Area should be kept clean with a gentle soap to avoid infection. Eruptions usually heal within five days. Macular hyperpigmentation may be present (Goodman, 2004).	Dactinomycin, high-dose methotrexate, and cyclosporine are generally the causative agents. Long-term steroids can also cause papules and pustules over shoulders, chest, back, and upper arms (Goodman, 2004). Temsirolimus (Torisel®) (Wyeth Pharmaceuticals, 2007)—acne: 10% all grades, 0% grades 3 and 4	Cetuximab (Erbitux®) (ImClone Systems & Bristol-Myers Squibb, 2006)—acneform rash: 90% grades 1–4, 8% grades 3 and 4 Panitumumab (Vectibix®) (Amgen Inc., 2006)—acne dermatitis: 57% all grades, 7% grades 3 and 4; acne: 13% all grades, 1% grades 3 and 4 Lapatinib (Tykerb®) (GlaxoSmithKline, 2007)—dermatitis acneform: < 1% grade 3 Gefitinib (Iressa®) (AstraZeneca, 2004)—acne: 25% all grades, 19% grade 1, 6% grade 2, 0% grades 3 and 4 Trastuzumab (Herceptin®) (Genentech, Inc., 2000)—rash: 18%; herpes simplex: 2%; acne: 2%
Pruritus or itching	May be localized or generalized; symptoms may be worsened with dehydration. Patients should be encouraged to drink 8–10 glasses of fluid per day and minimize salt and alcohol intake. Recommended skin care includes the use of mild cleansers such as Aveeno® oatmeal bath and Neutrogena®, Ivory®, and Basis® soaps. Apply moisturizing lotions such as Aquaphor®, Lubriderm®, Alpha-Keri®, Cetaphil®, or Nivea® following the bath (Goodman, 2004). Wearing of loose-fitting clothing and clothing made of cotton or other soft fabrics can alleviate pruritus. Use antibiotics if pruritus is secondary to infection. Use oral antihistamines, with increased doses at bedtime. Use of distraction, relaxation, positive imagery, or cutaneous stimulation is encouraged (National Cancer Institute, 2008).	Alkylating agents, antimetabolites, antibiotics, plant alkaloids, and nitrosoureas The agents most associated with hypersensitivities include doxorubicin, daunorubicin, cytarabine, L-asparaginase, paclitaxel, and cisplatin (National Cancer Institute, 2008). Asparaginase, cisplatin, carboplatin, cytarabine, etoposide, teniposide, IFN alfa-2a and IFN alfa-2b, doxorubicin, melphalan, and daunorubicin can all cause a rash. Gemcitabine has been associated with a perianal pruritus (Goodman, 2004). Temsirolimus (Torisel®, Wyeth Pharmaceuticals, 2007)—pruritus: 19% all grades, 1% grades 3 and 4	Cetuximab (Erbitux®) (ImClone Systems & Bristol-Myers Squibb, 2006)—pruritus: 11% grades 1–4, < 1% grades 3 and 4; skin disorders: 4% grades 1–4, 0% grades 3 and 4 Panitumumab (Vectibix®) (Amgen Inc., 2006)—pruritus: 57% all grades, 2% grades 3 and 4; skin exfoliation: 25% all grades, 2% grades 3 and 4 Erlotinib (Tarceva®) (Genentech, Inc., 2007)—pruritus: 13% any grade, < 1% grade 3, 0% grade 4 Gefitinib (Iressa®) (AstraZeneca, 2004)—pruritus: 8% all grades, 7% grade 1, 1% grade 2, 0% grades 3 and 4

EGFR—epidermal growth factor receptor; EGFRI—epidermal growth factor receptor inhibitor; 5-FU—5-fluorouracil; GVHD—graft-versus-host disease; IFN—interferon; IL—interleukin; IV—intravenous; SPF—sun protection factor

Figure 27. Rash and Epidermal Growth Factor Receptor Targeted Therapy*

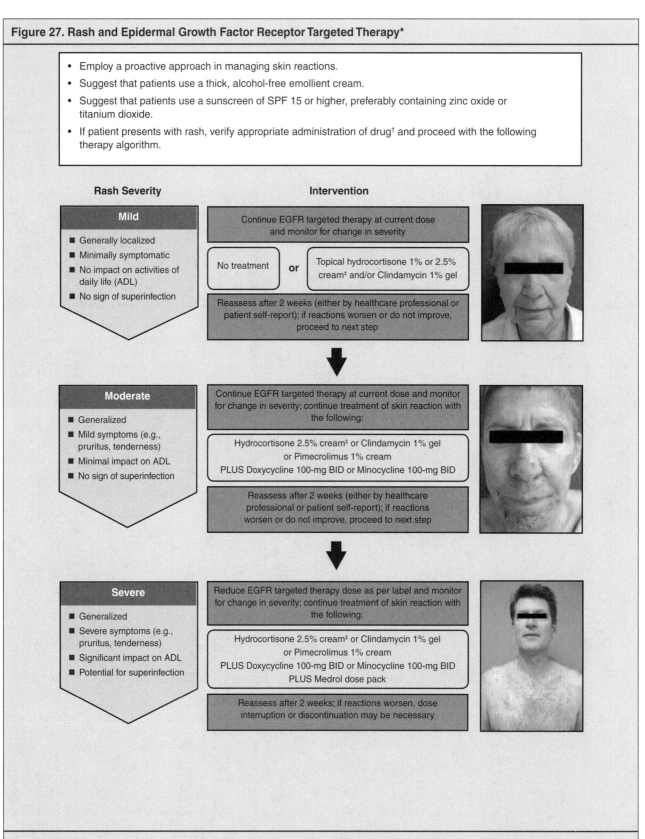

* erlotinib (Tarceva®); cetuximab (Erbitux®); panitumumab (Vectibix®); lapatinib (Tykerb®)
† Please refer to accompanying prescription information.
‡ The use of topical steroids should be employed in a pulse manner based on your institution's guidelines.

Note. From "Epidermal Growth Factor Receptor Inhibitor-Associated Cutaneous Toxicities: An Evolving Paradigm in Clinical Management," by T. Lynch, E.S. Kim, B. Eaby, J. Garey, D.P. West, and M.E. Lacouture, 2007, *Oncologist, 12*(5), pp. 617–618. Copyright 2007 by AlphaMed Press. Reprinted with permission.

Figure 28. Trichomegaly

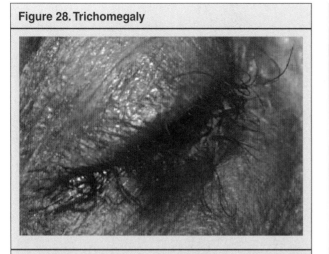

Note. From "Clinical Signs, Pathophysiology and Management of Skin Toxicity During Therapy With Epidermal Growth Factor Inhibitors," by S. Segaert and E. Van Cutsem, 2005, *Annals of Oncology, 16*(9), p. 1428. Copyright 2005 by Oxford University Press. Reprinted with permission.

Figure 29. Paronychia of the Nail

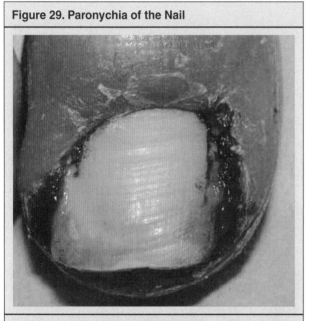

Note. From "Clinical Signs, Pathophysiology and Management of Skin Toxicity During Therapy With Epidermal Growth Factor Inhibitors," by S. Segaert and E. Van Cutsem, 2005, *Annals of Oncology, 16*(9), p. 1428. Copyright 2005 by Oxford University Press. Reprinted with permission.

Figure 30. Hyperpigmentation

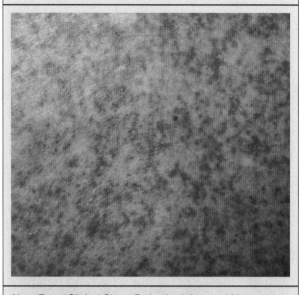

Note. From "Clinical Signs, Pathophysiology and Management of Skin Toxicity During Therapy With Epidermal Growth Factor Inhibitors," by S. Segaert and E. Van Cutsem, 2005, *Annals of Oncology, 16*(9), p. 1428. Copyright 2005 by Oxford University Press. Reprinted with permission.

Figure 31. Acral Erythema

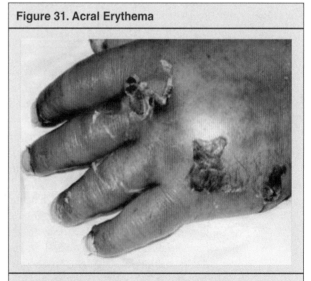

Note. From "Painful Blistered Hands and Feet," by C. Coyle and V. Wenhold, 2001, *Clinical Journal of Oncology Nursing, 5*(5), p. 230. Copyright 2001 by Oncology Nursing Society. Reprinted with permission.

(7) If there is a clinical diagnosis of impetigo, or if secondary infection with *S.
aureus* is confirmed, consider topical
mupirocin (Bactroban®) (Perez-Soler
et al., 2005).
9. Treatment of a secondarily infected rash
   a) If agents are used outside a trial setting, their
effectiveness should be evaluated after one

week and treatment continued for another
week.
   b) If there is no improvement after two weeks,
the treatment should be considered ineffective
and discontinued (Perez-Soler et al., 2005).
   c) Consider intranasal mupirocin (Bactroban
Nasal®) applied once daily to each nostril
(Perez-Soler et al., 2005).

Figure 32. Fissure

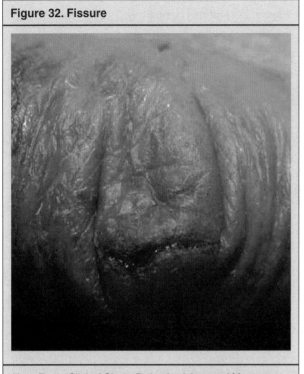

Note. From "Clinical Signs, Pathophysiology and Management of Skin Toxicity During Therapy With Epidermal Growth Factor Inhibitors," by S. Segaert and E. Van Cutsem, 2005, *Annals of Oncology, 16*(9), p. 1428. Copyright 2005 by Oxford University Press. Reprinted with permission.

d) Secondarily infected rash should be treated with a short course of oral antibiotics. Tetracyclines such as minocycline (Minocin®) have reasonably good activity against *S. aureus*, but many different antibiotics may be effective based on empirical, nonvalidated data (Perez-Soler et al., 2005).

e) Weak anecdotal evidence suggests that topical antibiotics may be effective (e.g., topical clindamycin [Cleocin®, Clindaderm®]). No clinical trials have been conducted, and no cases have shown clear benefit (Perez-Soler et al., 2005).

10. Rash and response/survival
    a) Data from several clinical trials with HER1/EGFR-targeted agents show a positive correlation between rash and patient response and/or survival (Perez-Soler et al., 2005; Perez-Soler & Van Cutsem, 2007).
    b) Findings suggest that rash might be a surrogate marker of efficacy and may be used as a tool to predict response. However, it is essential to analyze the correlation between the grade of rash and response/survival (Perez-Soler et al., 2005; Perez-Soler & Van Cutsem, 2007).

11. Psychosocial issues
    a) Skin toxicities from EGFRIs can have a significant impact on patients' physical, emotional, and social function and may interfere with treatment adherence (Wagner & Lacouture, 2007).
    b) In the majority of cases, there is no clinical need to withdraw EGFRI treatment; suspension of EGFRI treatment should only be temporary, simply allowing for diminution of the rash (Lynch et al., 2007).
    c) The most significant skin toxicities and health-related QOL factors are (Wagner & Lacouture, 2007)
        (1) Inability to work
        (2) Sleep disturbances
        (3) Interference with ADLs
        (4) Disruption of hobbies
        (5) Skin pain, burning, itching, and irritation
        (6) Increased facial hair
        (7) Depression, frustration, anxiety, and worry
        (8) Disruption of social life.
    d) More research is needed to develop effective treatments that can alleviate the physical and emotional discomfort experienced by patients, particularly those with advanced-stage cancer and a poor prognosis (Perez-Soler et al., 2005).
    e) Nursing interventions
        (1) Ensure that family and other support systems (friends, religious leader, visiting nurse, homecare personnel) can provide encouragement to patients to help to rebuild their self-esteem and self-belief.
        (2) Help patients to overcome their functional limitations with proactive management of the rash.
        (3) Refer patients to support groups, individual counseling, or a psychiatrist.
        (4) Listen actively and be supportive to patients.

12. Other cutaneous toxicities (Meniscus Ltd., 2006)
    a) Paronychia
    b) Hair alterations
    c) Xerosis
    d) Telangiectasia
    e) Nasal mucositis
    f) Ocular irritation
    g) Hyperpigmentation (see Table 23)

13. EGFRIs currently in clinical development: See Table 24.

Figure 33. Palmar-Plantar Erythrodysesthesia (Hand-Foot Syndrome)*

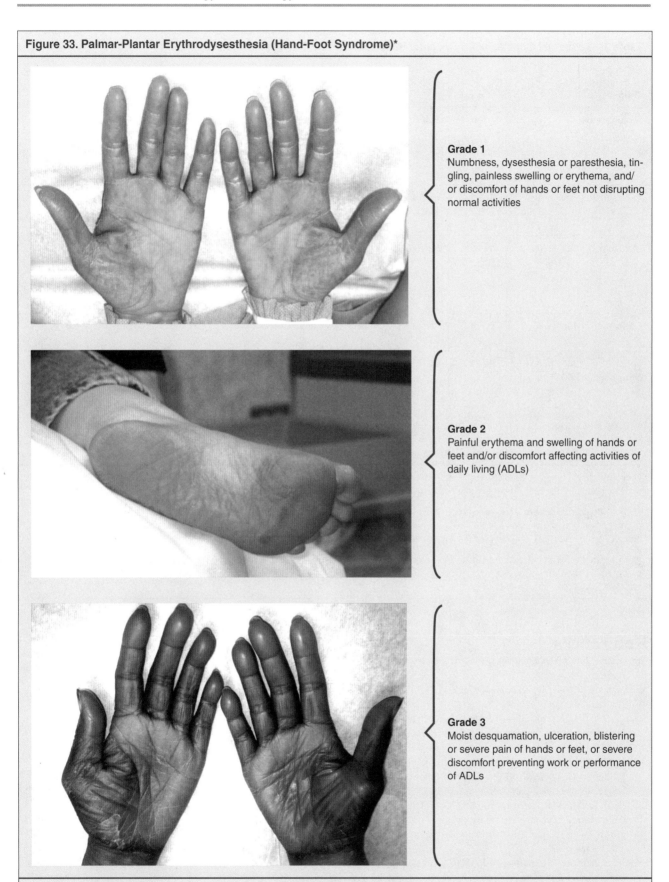

Grade 1
Numbness, dysesthesia or paresthesia, tingling, painless swelling or erythema, and/or discomfort of hands or feet not disrupting normal activities

Grade 2
Painful erythema and swelling of hands or feet and/or discomfort affecting activities of daily living (ADLs)

Grade 3
Moist desquamation, ulceration, blistering or severe pain of hands or feet, or severe discomfort preventing work or performance of ADLs

*Grading criteria from National Cancer Institute Cancer Therapy Evaluation Program. (2006). *Common terminology criteria for adverse events* (version 3.0). Bethesda, MD: National Cancer Institute.

Note. Photos courtesy of Susan Moore. Used with permission.

Table 24. Epidermal Growth Factor Receptor Inhibitors Currently in Clinical Development

Drug	Class	Target	Proposed Indications	Highest Development Phase US	EU
Nimotuzumab	MoAb	EGFR	NSCLC4 HNSCC Breast cancer Glioma Pancreatic cancer	Discovery	III
Pertuzumab (Omnitarg™)	MoAb	HER-2 (dimerization with EGFR)	NSCLC Ovarian cancer Breast cancer	II	N/A
Matuzumab/EMD 72000	MoAb	Pan-HER	NSCLC Ovarian cancer Uterine/cervical cancer Pancreatic cancer Stomach cancer	II	II
Canertinib/CI-1033	TKI	Pan-HER	Ovarian cancer	II	N/A
Lapatinib (Tykerb®) (Glaxo-SmithKline, 2007)	TKI	EGFR, HER-2	Breast cancer NSCLC HNSCC Renal cell carcinoma	III	III

Note: Lapatinib (Tykerb®) (GlaxoSmithKline, 2007) was approved by the U.S. Food and Drug Administration on 3/13/2007 for HER-2 positive metastatic breast cancer in conjunction with capecitabine.

EGFR—epidermal growth factor receptor; EGFRI—epidermal growth factor receptor inhibitor; EU—European Union; HER—human epidermal growth factor receptor; HNSCC—head and neck squamous cell carcinoma; MoAb—monoclonal antibody; N/A—not applicable; NSCLC—non-small cell lung cancer; TKI—tyrosine kinase inhibitor; US—United States

Note. From "Epidermal Growth Factor Receptor Inhibitor-Associated Cutaneous Toxicities: An Evolving Paradigm in Clinical Management," by T. Lynch, E.S. Kim, B. Eaby, J. Garey, D.P. West, and M.E. Lacouture, 2007, *Oncologist, 12*(5), p. 613. Copyright 2007 by AlphaMed Press. Reprinted with permission.

References

Amgen Inc. (2006). Vectibix [Package insert]. Thousand Oaks, CA: Author.

AstraZeneca. (2004). Iressa [Package insert]. Wilmington, DE: Author.

Basti, S. (2007). Ocular toxicities of epidermal growth factor receptor inhibitors and their management. *Cancer Nursing, 30*(Suppl. 4), S10–S16.

Bouche, O., Brixi-Benmansour, H., Bertin, A., Perceau, G., & Lagarde, S. (2005). Trichomegaly of the eyelashes following treatment with cetuximab. *Annals of Oncology, 16*(10), 1711–1712.

Braiteh, F., Kurzrock, R., & Johnson, F.M. (2008). Trichomegaly of the eyelashes after lung cancer treatment with the epidermal growth factor receptor erlotinib. *Journal of Clinical Oncology, 38*(7), 3460–3462.

Eaby, B., Culkin, A., & Lacouture, M.E. (2008). An interdisciplinary consensus on managing skin reactions associated with human epidermal growth factor receptor inhibitors. *Clinical Journal of Oncology Nursing, 12*(2), 283–290.

Esper, P., Gale, D., & Muehlbauer, P. (2007). What kind of rash is it? Deciphering the dermatologic toxicities of biologic and targeted therapies. *Clinical Journal of Oncology Nursing, 11*(5), 659–666.

Genentech, Inc. (2000). Herceptin [Package insert]. South San Francisco, CA: Author.

Genentech, Inc. (2007). Tarceva [Package insert]. South San Francisco, CA: Author.

GlaxoSmithKline. (2007). Tykerb [Package insert]. Research Triangle Park, NC: Author.

Goodman, M. (2004). Skin and nail bed changes. In C.H. Yarbro, M.H. Frogge, & M. Goodman (Eds.), *Cancer symptom management* (3rd ed., pp. 319–330). Sudbury, MA: Jones and Bartlett.

Hetherington, J., Andrews, C., Vaynshteyn, Y., & Fishel, R. (2007). Managing follicular rash related to chemotherapy and monoclonal antibodies. *Community Oncology, 4*(3), 157–162.

ImClone Systems & Bristol-Myers Squibb. (2006). Erbitux [Package insert]. Branchburg, NJ: Author.

Lacouture, M., Basti, S., Patel, J., & Benson, A. (2006). The SERIES Clinic: An interdisciplinary approach to the management of toxicities of EGFR inhibitors. *Journal of Supportive Oncology, 4*(5), 236–238.

Lacouture, M.E. (2007). *Tips to help with EGFR targeted therapy skin changes.* Durham, NC: AlphaMed Press.

Ligand Pharmaceuticals. (1999). Targretin [Package insert]. San Diego, CA: Author.

Luu, M., Lai, S.E., Patel, J., Guitart, J., & Lacouture, M.E. (2007). Photosensitive rash due to the epidermal growth factor receptor inhibitor erlotinib. *Photodermatology, Photoimmunology, and Photomedicine, 23*(1), 42–45.

Lynch, T., Kim, E.S., Eaby, B., Garey, J., West, D.P., & Lacouture, M.E. (2007). Epidermal growth factor receptor inhibitor-associated cutaneous toxicities: An evolving paradigm in clinical management. *Oncologist, 12*(5), 610–621.

Meniscus Ltd. (2006, October). *Cutaneous side effects associated with targeted therapy.* Retrieved October 7, 2008, from http://www.managecrc.com/html/side-effect-cutaneous-side-effects.asp

National Cancer Institute. (2008). *Pruritus (PDQ®).* Retrieved October 23, 2008, from http://www.cancer.gov/cancertopics/pdq/supportivecare/pruritus/HealthProfessional

National Cancer Institute Cancer Therapy Evaluation Program. (2006). *Common terminology criteria for adverse events* (version 3.0). Bethesda, MD: National Cancer Institute. Retrieved December 11, 2007, from http://ctep.cancer.gov/reporting/ctc_v30.html

Omoti, A.E., & Omoti, C.E. (2006). Ocular toxicity of systemic anti-cancer chemotherapy. *Pharmacy Practice, 4*(2), 55–59.

OncoLink. (2001). *Coping with cancer: Hair loss/alopecia.* Retrieved January 10, 2008, from http://www.oncolink.com/experts/article.cfm?c=1&s=5&ss=6&id=1057

Perez-Soler, R., Delord, J.P., Halpern, A., Kelly, K., Krueger, J., Sureda, B.M., et al. (2005). HER1/EGFR inhibitor-associated rash: Future directions for management and investigation outcomes from the HER1/EGFR Inhibitor Rash Management Forum. *Oncologist, 10*(5), 345–356.

Perez-Soler, R., & Van Cutsem, E. (2007). Clinical research of EGFR inhibitors and related dermatologic toxicities. *Oncology (Williston Park), 21*(11, Suppl. 5), 10–16.

Pfizer Labs. (2007). Sutent [Package insert]. New York: Author.

Rhee, J., Oishi, K., Garey, J., & Kim, E. (2005). Management of rash and other toxicities in patients treated with epidermal growth factor receptor-targeted agents. *Clinical Colorectal Cancer, 5*(Suppl. 2), S101–S106.

Roche Laboratories. (2008). *Xeloda product information.* Retrieved January 8, 2008, from http://www.xeloda.com

Segaert, S., & Van Cutsem, E. (2005). Clinical signs, pathophysiology and management of skin toxicity during therapy with epidermal growth factor inhibitors. *Annals of Oncology, 16*(9), 1425–1433.

Segaert, S., & Van Cutsem, E. (2007). Clinical management of EGFRI dermatologic toxicities: The European perspective. *Oncology (Williston Park), 21*(11, Suppl. 5), 22–26.

Vassallo, C., Brazzelli, V., Ardigo, M., & Borroni, G. (2001). The irreplaceable image: Nails changes in onco-hematologic patients. *Haematologica, 86*(3), 334–336. Retrieved January 11, 2008, from http://www.haematologica.it/2001_03/0334.htm

Wagner, L., & Lacouture, M. (2007). Dermatologic toxicities associated with EGFR inhibitors: The clinical psychologist's perspective. *Oncology (Williston Park), 21*(11, Suppl. 5), 34–36.

White, G., & Cox, N. (2006). *Diseases of the skin* (2nd ed.). St. Louis, MO: Elsevier Mosby. Retrieved January 10, 2008, from http://www.merckmedicus.com/ppdocs/us/hcp/contect/white/chapters/white-ch-018-s002.htm

Wyeth Pharmaceuticals. (2007). Torisel [Package insert]. Philadelphia: Author.

D. Alopecia
1. Pathophysiology: Alopecia is one of the most common and distressing side effects of chemotherapy. Men and women both report negative feelings about hair loss related to chemotherapy (Hilton, Hunt, Emslie, Salinas, & Ziebland, 2008). Chemotherapy-induced alopecia includes loss of hair anywhere on the body. In addition, this type of hair loss has a negative impact on body image, sexuality, and self-confidence. The pathobiology of the response of human hair follicles to chemotherapy remains largely unknown. Cells responsible for hair growth have high mitotic and metabolic rates. Certain cytotoxic agents disrupt the proliferative phase of hair growth. Most hair follicles on the scalp are in the anagen (growth) phase of the hair cycle (Hesketh et al., 2004). Recent investigations involve the role of *TP53* and its target genes, which mediate responses of hair follicle cells. It is suggested that pharmacologic inhibition of *TP53* may serve as an effective treatment in the prevention of chemotherapy-induced hair loss (Botchkarev, 2003). Other mechanisms of alopecia and potential targets for prevention are being investigated (Wang, Lu, & Au, 2006). Hair damage occurs either to the shaft or the root.
   a) Hair shaft damage results in partial atrophy or necrosis of the bulb, which causes constriction. Hair breaks off at the damaged area. The result of such damage is a head of hair that looks patchy and thin.
   b) Root damage is associated with complete alopecia. Hair falls out spontaneously or during washing or combing. The more potent epilators (e.g., cyclophosphamide, daunorubicin, doxorubicin, etoposide, ifosfamide, paclitaxel) are associated with root damage.
2. Incidence
   a) As many as 65% of patients undergoing chemotherapy will experience alopecia to some degree (Wang et al., 2006).
   b) The extent of alopecia depends on the mechanism of action of the drug, drug dose, serum half-life, infusion technique (e.g., bolus versus continuous infusion), the use of combination chemotherapy, and the condition of the hair prior to treatment (Batchelor, 2001).
3. Risk factors
   a) Type of cytotoxic drug(s) administered
      (1) The drugs that present the highest risk of alopecia are cyclophosphamide, daunorubicin, doxorubicin, etopo-

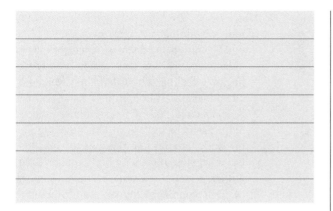

side, and ifosfamide (Hesketh et al., 2004).

   (2) Taxanes, camptothecins, and vinca alkaloids also are associated with significant hair loss (Batchelor, 2001).

  b) Certain noncytotoxic medications (e.g., propranolol hydrochloride, heparin sodium, lithium carbonate, prednisone, vitamin A, androgen preparations)

  c) High-dose chemotherapy: Busulfan-containing regimens used for blood or marrow transplantation have rarely been linked to permanent hair loss (Machado, Moreb, & Khan, 2007; Tosti, Piraccini, Vincenzi, & Misciali, 2005; Vowels, Chan, Giri, Russell, & Lam-Po-Tang, 1993).

  d) Certain medical conditions (e.g., hypothyroidism, aging)

  e) Poor hair condition before cytotoxic treatment

  f) Concomitant or previous radiotherapy to head (local effect)

4. Clinical manifestations: Scalp dryness, soreness, and rashes can occur before, during, or after hair loss.

  a) Degrees of alopecia (NCI CTEP, 2006)

   (1) Grade 0—No hair loss

   (2) Grade 1—Thinning or patchy

   (3) Grade 2—Complete

  b) Expected time frame (Freitas, 2005)

   (1) Hair loss begins approximately two to three weeks after administration of the drug and may last one to two months after completion of therapy.

   (2) Hair regrowth may take three to five months after cytotoxic therapy is complete.

5. Collaborative management: Alopecia can be so emotionally traumatic for patients that they may consider refusing therapy. Furthermore, alopecia is a constant reminder of patients' disease and greatly affects their sense of self. There is currently no known strategy for prevention of alopecia caused by cytotoxic therapy. Multiple pharmacologic and biologic therapies are being studied, such as growth factors, cytokines, antioxidants, and apoptosis inhibitors (Wang et al., 2006).

  a) Scalp hypothermia, although used in the past with mixed results, is not currently recommended.

   (1) There is long-standing concern that reducing circulation to the scalp through vasoconstriction may create a sanctuary site for malignant cells (Christodoulou, Tsakalos, Galani, & Skarlos, 2006).

   (2) Studies have explored the clinical benefit of using a digitized scalp cooling system in anthracycline-treated patients (Ridderheim, Bjurberg, & Gustavsson, 2003) and in patients receiving epirubicin and docetaxel (Macduff, Mackenzie, Hutcheon, Melville, & Archibald, 2003). Randomized clinical trials are needed to determine the proper technique for application, efficacy, and safety of scalp cooling in preventing chemotherapy-induced alopecia (Grevelman & Breed, 2005).

  b) Minoxidil has been studied for chemotherapy-induced alopecia. It appears to be most effective if used while hair still exists. Minoxidil has been associated with decreased severity or duration but does not eliminate chemotherapy-induced alopecia (Duvic et al., 1996; Wang et al., 2006).

6. Patient and family education: Advise patients and significant others about the following (Batchelor, 2001; Hesketh et al., 2004).

  a) The cause of alopecia and the time frame of hair loss and regrowth

  b) Strategies to manage hair loss and regrowth

   (1) Most strategies are literature-based and have not been tested in RCCTs.

   (2) Use shampoos without detergents, menthol, salicylic acid, alcohol, or heavy perfumes.

   (3) Avoid using permanent waves, bleach, and coloring agents on hair, as well as vigorous brushing, hot rollers, and hair dryer use.

   (4) Avoid excessive brushing or combing.

   (5) Consider shaving the head, as this may decrease itching and allow for wig application if warranted.

   (6) Protect the scalp from cold and sun with hats, scarves, wigs, and sunscreen.

(7) Protect the eyes with sunglasses or clear-glass glasses if lashes become thin or fall out completely; dust or particles can enter the eye more easily and cause irritation.

(8) Instruct patients that new hair that grows after completion of therapy may be different from the original hair (e.g., color, texture).

c) Local resources for support (e.g., wig salons, scarf and turban catalogs, support groups); refer interested patients to "Look Good . . . Feel Better," a program offered by the Personal Care Products Council Foundation through community organizations such as the American Cancer Society, to provide guidance and support regarding wigs and other head coverings, makeup, and skin care (Personal Care Products Council Foundation, 2004). A wig may be covered by the patient's insurance, which will help to defray costs. A prescription written for "hair prosthesis" may be required.

(1) Wigs can be synthetic or made of actual human hair, with the latter being the more costly choice. Salons or stores that specialize in wigs can provide a discussion of the pros and cons of each type of wig with the client.

(2) Wig specialists may have an easier time matching a wig to the patient's usual style if the patient consults the stylist before hair loss begins. It may be helpful to preserve a portion of normal hair prior to complete hair loss to allow for color and texture matching.

(3) If a wig is purchased prior to hair loss, it should be adjustable so that the size can be decreased as the hair loss occurs (Personal Care Products Council Foundation, 2004).

(4) A variety of scarves and turbans are available and assist with protection of the scalp and prevention of heat loss.

References

Batchelor, D. (2001). Hair and cancer chemotherapy: Consequences and nursing care—A literature study. *European Journal of Cancer Care, 10*(3), 147–163.

Botchkarev, V.A. (2003). Molecular mechanisms of chemotherapy-induced hair loss. *Journal of Investigative Dermatology Symposium Proceedings, 8*(1), 72–75.

Christodoulou, C., Tsakalos, G., Galani, E., & Skarlos, D.V. (2006). Scalp metastases and scalp cooling for chemotherapy-induced alopecia prevention. *Annals of Oncology, 17*(2), 350.

Duvic, M., Lemak, N.A., Valero, V., Hymes, S.R., Farmer, K.L., Hortobagyi, G.N., et al. (1996). A randomized trial of minoxidil

in chemotherapy-induced alopecia. *Journal of the American Academy of Dermatology, 35*(1), 74–78.

Freitas, B.A. (2005). Coping: Altered body image and alopecia. In J.K. Itano & K.N. Taoka (Eds.), *Core curriculum for oncology nursing* (4th ed., pp. 55–58). St. Louis, MO: Elsevier Saunders.

Grevelman, E.G., & Breed, W.P. (2005). Prevention of chemotherapy-induced hair loss by scalp cooling. *Annals of Oncology, 16*(3), 352–358.

Hesketh, P.J., Batchelor, D., Golant, M., Lyman, G.H., Rhodes, N., & Yardley, D. (2004). Chemotherapy-induced alopecia: Psychosocial impact and therapeutic approaches. *Supportive Care in Cancer, 12*(8), 543–549.

Hilton, S., Hunt, K., Emslie, C., Salinas, M., & Ziebland, S. (2008). Have men been overlooked? A comparison of young men and women's experiences of chemotherapy-induced alopecia. *Psycho-Oncology, 17*(6), 577–583.

Macduff, C., Mackenzie, T., Hutcheon, A., Melville, L., & Archibald, H. (2003). The effectiveness of scalp cooling in preventing alopecia for patients receiving epirubicin and docetaxel. *European Journal of Cancer Care, 12*(2), 154–161.

Machado, M., Moreb, J.S., & Khan, S.A. (2007). Six cases of permanent alopecia after various conditioning regimens commonly used in hematopoietic stem cell transplantation. *Bone Marrow Transplantation, 40*(10), 979–982.

National Cancer Institute Cancer Therapy Evaluation Program. (2006). *Common terminology criteria for adverse events* (version 3.0). Bethesda, MD: National Cancer Institute. Retrieved October 4, 2008, from http://ctep.cancer.gov/reporting/ctc_v30.html

Personal Care Products Council Foundation. (2004). *Look good . . . feel better.* Retrieved August 19, 2008, from http://www.lookgoodfeelbetter.org/general/facts.htm

Ridderheim, M., Bjurberg, M., & Gustavsson, A. (2003). Scalp hypothermia to prevent chemotherapy-induced alopecia is effective and safe: A pilot study of a new digitized scalp-cooling system used in 74 patients. *Supportive Care in Cancer, 11*(6), 371–377.

Tosti, A., Piraccini, B.M., Vincenzi, C., & Misciali, C. (2005). Permanent alopecia after busulfan chemotherapy. *British Journal of Dermatology, 152*(5), 1056–1058.

Vowels, M., Chan, L.L., Giri, N., Russell, S., & Lam-Po-Tang, R. (1993). Factors affecting hair regrowth after bone marrow transplantation. *Bone Marrow Transplantation, 12*(4), 347–350.

Wang, J., Lu, Z., & Au, J.L. (2006). Protection against chemotherapy-induced alopecia. *Pharmaceutical Research, 23*(11), 2505–2514.

E. Cardiovascular toxicity
1. Cardiovascular toxicity includes changes in conduction pathways (dysrhythmias), vasculature (hypotension, hypertension, Raynaud phenomenon), coronary arteries (unstable angina, acute myocardial infarction), cardiac myocytes (cardiomyopathy), and pericardial fluid accumulation (Sereno et al., 2008; Speyer, Ewer, & Freedberg, 2004). In some cases, the identification of cardiac dysfunction cannot be linked to a specific therapeutic agent (Chung et al., 2008). These cardiovascular toxicities are described in greater detail by chemotherapeutic drug category in Table 25.
2. Conduction pathway disorders
    a) Pathophysiology
        (1) Conduction disturbances are classified according to their origin (e.g., atrial, ventricular, heart blocks) or their degree of life-threatening symptoms.
        (2) Life-threatening dysrhythmias such as ventricular tachycardia, ventricular fibrillation, or advanced heart blocks are less common but may warrant permanent discontinuation of therapy. Other exacerbating factors often are involved and make it difficult to differentiate whether the disorder is truly triggered by the chemotherapeutic or biologic agent (Shelton, 2006a).
            (a) Electrolyte disturbances (e.g., hypokalemia, hyperkalemia, hypocalcemia, hypomagnesemia) (Bashir et al., 2007; Richardson, 2004)
            (b) Comorbid health conditions (e.g., chronic obstructive lung disease, heart disease) (Yusuf, Razeghi, & Yeh, 2008)
        (3) Mechanisms of arrhythmogenesis include (Shelton, 2006a)
            (a) Fluid volume loss through capillary leak, diarrhea, or profuse sweating can cause tachydysrhythmias, which usually respond to fluids and medications.
            (b) Oxygen free radicals released by ischemic cardiomyocytes lead to irritability with ectopic beats such as premature beats, atrial flutter, and ventricular tachycardia.
            (c) Inflammatory capillary permeability within the myocytes causes irritability and dysrhythmias.
            (d) Prolongation of the refractory period and interference with the action potential of myocytes leads to a risk of ventricular escape beats followed by irritable foci. This usually results in premature ventricular beats or an unusual type of ventricular tachycardia termed *torsades de pointes* (Roden, 2004; Wong & Rautaharju, 1998; Yap & Camm, 2003).
    b) Incidence
        (1) The prevalence of dysrhythmias specifically associated with cancer treatments is largely underestimated because of the probable attribution to other causes (Sereno et al., 2008).
        (2) In well-defined cases, the incidence can still only be imperfectly quantified because preventive measures are always employed when possible.
        (3) Incidence rates
            (a) Of patients with ovarian cancer who were treated with paclitaxel, 30% developed asymptomatic bradycardia. More profound cardiac events (i.e., ventricular tachycardia, left-bundle branch block) have been observed in 5% of patients (Rowinsky et al., 1991; Soe, Berkman, & Mardelli, 1996).
            (b) 10%–20% of dysrhythmias associated with cytokine therapies such as IL-2 are linked to fluid and electrolyte imbalances (Lee et al., 1989; Quesada, Talpaz, Rios, Kurzrock, & Gutterman, 1986; Sandstrom, 1996).
            (c) Lower incidence rates of less than 5% occur with agents that cause myocarditis or QT prolongation (Greenberg, 2003; Yap & Camm, 2003).
    c) Risk factors
        (1) Specific chemobiotherapeutic agents have been associated with dysrhythmias because of defined pathophysiologic mechanisms such as oxidative stress or QT prolongation (Shelton, 2006a).
        (2) All patients with reported "capillary permeability syndrome" are at risk for secondary tachydysrhythmias related to vascular depletion (Shelton, 2009).

Table 25. Cardiotoxicity of Chemotherapeutic Drugs

Classification	Drug	Incidence	Characteristic Effects	Nursing Considerations
Antitumor antibiotic	Bleomycin	Maximum lifetime dose is 400 units. Its more common dose-limiting toxicity is pulmonary fibrosis. Cardiomyopathy has been reported at similar doses (Bristol-Myers Squibb, 2006). Little is known about the incidence or risk factors for Raynaud phenomenon. It is believed that oxygen radical release causes localized ischemia in poorly perfused areas (Gayraud, 2007). Gangrenous digits have been reported. This seems to be idiosyncratic, not dose-related, and related to rate of infusion (Grunwald et al., 2005).	Raynaud phenomenon is infusion related and will resolve with discontinuation or completion of the agent. Raynaud phenomenon presents initially as pain and heaviness of the digits. Cardiomyopathy presents as progressive decline in ejection fraction with dyspnea as the usual first presenting symptom.	Perform routine monitoring of echocardiogram once close to maximum tolerated dose.
Anthracycline antitumor antibiotics	Daunorubicin	If total dose < 600 mg/m², incidence is 0%–41% (Kaszyk, 1986). If total dose is 1,000 mg/m², incidence is 12% (Kaszyk, 1986).	Nonspecific arrhythmia, tachycardia, cardiomyopathy, and/or CHF. Acute left ventricular failure can occur with high doses. CHF may be unresponsive to treatment (Bedford Laboratories, 2007b). Acute toxicity unrelated to dose may occur within hours. Although rare, myocarditis-pericarditis syndrome may be fatal (Wilkes & Barton-Burke, 2007). Pericardial effusion	Chronic effects are similar to those of doxorubicin, but higher cumulative doses may be tolerated (Bottomley, 2004; Von Hoff et al., 1977). Periodic monitoring with echocardiogram or MUGA scan is recommended.
	Daunorubicin citrate liposomal	Chronic therapy > 300 mg/m² has increased the incidence of cardiomyopathy and CHF. In a phase III study, 13.8% of patients reported a triad of back pain, flushing, and chest tightness (Gilead Sciences, Inc., 2006).	Cardiomyopathy associated with a decrease in LVEF, especially in patients with prior anthracycline experience or preexisting cardiac disease (Gilead Science, Inc., 2006)	Ensure that the patient undergoes a physical examination and cardiac evaluation with MUGA scan or echocardiogram before each course and at total cumulative doses of 300 mg/m² (160 mg/m² for higher risk patients) and at every 160 mg/m² thereafter. Periodic monitoring with echocardiogram or MUGA scans is recommended. Triad usually occurs during the first five minutes of infusion, subsides with infusion interruption, and generally does not recur if the infusion is resumed at a slower rate (Gilead Sciences, Inc., 2006).
	Doxorubicin	If total dose < 550 mg/m², incidence is 0.1%–1.2% (Kaszyk, 1986; Von Hoff et al., 1979). If total dose > 550 mg/m², incidence rises exponentially (Von Hoff et al., 1979). If total dose is 1,000 mg/m², incidence is nearly 50% (Carlson, 1992; Von Hoff et al., 1979).	ECG changes; nonspecific ST-T wave changes; premature ventricular and atrial contraction; low-voltage QRS changes; sinus tachycardia may occur acutely during administration (Kaszyk, 1986).	Chronic effects seen with cumulative doses may result in CHF. Concomitant administration of other antineoplastics (e.g., cyclophosphamide, taxanes, trastuzumab) has been implicated as a risk factor, although exact synergism is unclear (Rahman et al., 2007).

(Continued on next page)

Table 25. Cardiotoxicity of Chemotherapeutic Drugs *(Continued)*

Classification	Drug	Incidence	Characteristic Effects	Nursing Considerations
Anthracycline antitumor antibiotics *(cont.)*	Doxorubicin *(cont.)*	Incidence may manifest during therapy and last for months to years afterward (Pfizer Inc., 2006a). Late effects for pediatric patients: In one study, some relevant cardiac impairments (12% of 129 patients) occurred, 3 of which required cardiac drug therapy (Bryant et al., 2007; Langer et al., 2004).	Decreased ejection fraction, sinus tachycardia, and cardiomyopathy with symptoms of CHF occur later, with peak incidence 7 years after exposure (Barry et al., 2007; Carlson, 1992). It was once believed that continuous infusion caused more cardiotoxicity than intermittent delivery, but this has not been supported by systematic review (van Dalen et al., 2008). Pericardial effusion may be small and asymptomatic or may be hemorrhagic and produce acute symptoms.	Cardiotoxicity at lower doses may occur in mediastinally irradiated patients and/or patients with preexisting heart disease (Adams et al., 2003; Barry et al., 2007). Perform periodic monitoring of cardiac function with echocardiogram or MUGA scan throughout therapy and at least yearly after completion of treatment. Monitoring of troponin or BNP may be used to monitor for early changes (Anderson, 2008; Lenihan et al., 2007). Protection against cardiac toxicity with dexrazoxane in 10:1 ratio of dexrazoxane to doxorubicin. Protective agent administered by IV push or rapid infusion 30 minutes prior to doxorubicin (Ng & Green, 2007; Pfizer Inc., 2005; Swain & Vici, 2003). Coadministration of coenzyme 10 has shown some potential benefit in minimizing cardiotoxicity (Bryant et al., 2007; van Dalen et al., 2008).
	Mitoxantrone	Estimated risk is approximately 2.6% in doses of 140 mg/m². Risk increases with cumulative dose (OSI Pharmaceuticals, 2008).	Rare, but potentially fatal, CHF may occur during therapy or up to years after therapy completion.	Establish baseline cardiac function. Monitor for cardiac toxicity beyond doses of 100 mg/m². Risk is increased by other cardiotoxic medications, mediastinal radiation, or concomitant cardiovascular disease.
	Doxorubicin liposomal; pegylated liposomal doxorubicin	Effects on the myocardium have not been confirmed. In studies of patients with AIDS-related Kaposi sarcoma, 4.3% experienced cardiac-related adverse effects possibly related to the drug (Ortho Biotech, 2008). Irreversible toxicity may occur as the total dose nears 550 mg/m²; patients receiving mediastinal radiotherapy or previous or concomitant cardiotoxic therapy may experience heart failure at 400 mg/m² (Ortho Biotech, 2008).	Nonspecific arrhythmia, tachycardia, cardiomyopathy, and/or CHF Acute cardiac toxicity in the form of self-limiting atrial or ventricular dysrhythmias may occur with any dose and at any time during the treatment cycle. Second-degree atrioventricular heart block has also been reported (Kilickap et al., 2005; Safra, 2003). Acute left ventricular failure also can occur with isolated high doses. Delayed-onset, dose-related cardiomyopathy is the most common and well-known cardiotoxicity and is likely to be irreversible and unresponsive to treatment. Ten patients treated with pegylated doxorubicin developed protocol-defined cardiac events, compared with 48 doxorubicin-treated patients (O'Brien et al., 2004; Ortho Biotech, 2008). Pericardial effusion (Ortho Biotech, 2008)	Pegylated liposomal doxorubicin is believed to be associated with less risk of cardiotoxicity than the other anthracyclines (Escobar et al., 2003; Rivera et al., 2003). Experience with large cumulative doses is limited; consider the cardiac risk to be comparable to that of conventional doxorubicin formulation. Irreversible cardiac damage is dose-limiting. Long-term cardiac safety is unknown (Safra, 2003). Periodic monitoring with echocardiogram or MUGA scans is recommended.

(Continued on next page)

Table 25. Cardiotoxicity of Chemotherapeutic Drugs *(Continued)*

Classification	Drug	Incidence	Characteristic Effects	Nursing Considerations
Anthracycline antitumor antibiotics *(cont.)*	Epirubicin hydrochloride	The probability of developing clinically evident CHF is estimated as approximately 0.9% at a cumulative dose of 550 mg/m², 1.6% at 700 mg/m², and 3.3% at 900 mg/m² (Ryberg et al., 1998). The total cumulative dose has been established at 400 mg/m². The risk of developing CHF increases rapidly with increasing total cumulative doses in excess of 900 mg/m²; cumulative dose only should be exceeded with extreme caution (Berchem et al., 1996; OTN Generics, Inc., 2008).	Myocardial toxicity, manifested in its most severe form by potentially fatal CHF, may occur either during therapy with epirubicin or months to years after termination of therapy (OTN Generics, Inc., 2008).	Active or dormant cardiovascular disease, prior or concomitant radiotherapy to the mediastinal/pericardial area, previous therapy with other anthracyclines or anthracenediones, or concomitant use of other cardiotoxic drugs may increase the risk of cardiac toxicity. In the adjuvant treatment of breast cancer, the maximum cumulative dose used in clinical trials was 720 mg/m². Cardiac toxicity may occur at lower cumulative doses whether or not cardiac risk factors are present (OTN Generics, Inc., 2008).
	Idarubicin	Is reported to have less CHF than other anthracyclines, but its incidence rate is 1.2% at 150 mg/m² (Anderlini et al., 1995)	Myocardial toxicity, manifested in its most severe form by potentially fatal CHF, may occur either during therapy with idarubicin or months to years after termination of therapy (Pfizer Inc., 2006b)	Drug is approved for use with children (Pfizer Inc., 2006b).
Alkylating agents	Cisplatin	Oxygen radicals released with antineoplastic activity can produce acidosis, ischemia, and arterial vasospasm. It is cumulative, worsening with long-term exposure, but reversible as long as neuropathies also resolve.	Raynaud phenomenon has been reported, but no coronary artery disease (Bristol-Myers Squibb, 2007b). Hypomagnesemia induced by cisplatin has been associated with QT prolongation that subsequently results in bradycardia, and atrial or ventricular dysrhythmias (Slovacek et al., 2008).	Maintain magnesium levels > 2.0 mEq/L (Slovacek et al., 2008).
	Cyclophosphamide (high dose)	Toxicity is rare with cumulative or standard doses. There have been some reports of increased frequency with high-dose therapy > 180–200 mg/kg/day for 4 days (Bristol-Myers Squibb, 2005). Pediatric patients with thalassemia have been shown to have a potential for cardiac tamponade when cyclophosphamide is given with busulfan (Bristol-Myers Squibb, 2005).	ECG: Diminished QRS complex Cardiomegaly; pulmonary congestion; cardiac tamponade in children often is preceded by complaints of abdominal pain and vomiting (Bristol-Myers Squibb, 2005).	May result in acute lethal pericarditis, pericardial effusion, cardiac tamponade, and hemorrhagic myocardial necrosis in rare circumstances (Mills & Roberts, 1979; Wujcik & Downs, 1992) Cardiotoxicity usually is related to high doses for short intervals prior to BMT. Cases of cardiomyopathy with subsequent death have been reported following experimental high-dose therapy with cytarabine in combination with cyclophosphamide when used for BMT preparation (Bristol-Myers Squibb, 2005).

(Continued on next page)

Table 25. Cardiotoxicity of Chemotherapeutic Drugs (Continued)

Classification	Drug	Incidence	Characteristic Effects	Nursing Considerations
Alkylating agents (cont.)	Estramustine (estradiol and nitrogen mustard)	CHF in 3% of patients; MI in 3% of patients (Pfizer Inc., 2008a)	General fluid retention; exacerbation of pre-existing or incipient peripheral edema or CHF has been seen in some patients. Men receiving estrogens for prostatic cancer are at increased risk for thrombosis, including fatal and nonfatal MI (Pfizer Inc., 2008a).	Estramustine should be used with caution in patients with a history of cerebral vascular or coronary artery disease. Because hypertension may occur, blood pressure should be monitored periodically (Pfizer Inc., 2008a).
	Melphalan	Dose-related adverse effects are seen in < 5% of cases (GlaxoSmithKline, 2007a).	Raynaud phenomenon is dose-dependent, occurring only during active therapy, and resolving after completion of the cycle.	Teach patient to avoid cold exposure and quit smoking, which will exacerbate pain.
Antimetabolites	5-azacitidine	Capillary permeability is dose-related. Rare hypotension and dysrhythmias have been reported (Celgene Corporation, 2008b).	Pericardial effusion Dysrhythmias may be related to compensatory response to hypotension. Hypotension	Usually self-limiting and responds to a drug holiday
	5-FU	Incidence of 5-FU cardiotoxicity is dependent upon both dose and schedule. Incidence of 10% has been associated with doses > 800 mg/m²/day (Yusuf et al., 2008). The addition of other antineoplastic agents such as irinotecan or cisplatin may also influence the incidence of cardiotoxicity. Incidence is 1.6%–3% with bolus regimens (Labianca et al., 1982; Tsibiribi et al., 2006) but 7.6%–18% with prolonged infusion (4–5 days) regimens (Eskilsson et al., 1988; Meydan et al., 2005). One report with two-day infusional 5-FU (de Gramont's regimen) was 3.9% (Meydan et al.). One death was reported from myocardial ischemia (Soe et al., 1996), and other severe coronary artery events have been noted (Akhtar et al., 1996; Becker et al., 1999). Literature suggests the incidence is highest in the first and second cycles of therapy. In de Gramont's regimen, symptoms onset at night, a few hours after the bolus part of the infusion (Meydan et al., 2005).	Angina, palpitations, sweating, and/or syncope (Akhtar et al., 1993; Kleiman et al., 1987) Angina-like chest pain with or without MI, dysrhythmias, cardiogenic shock occurs due to coronary vasospasm. Sudden death also has been reported and is presumed to be due to acute myocardial ischemia or infarction (Akhtar et al., 1996; Gradishar & Vokes, 1990; Kleiman et al., 1987; Meydan et al., 2005). ECG changes without symptoms are unusual but have been reported. Transient symptomatic bradycardia was reported in a small group of patients receiving infusional 5-FU (Talapatra et al., 2007).	Patients at higher risk for development of cardiotoxicity include those with heart disease, electrolyte disturbances, and radiation exposure to the heart (Singh et al., 2004; Yusuf et al., 2008). It may be treated prophylactically or therapeutically with long-acting nitrates or calcium channel blockers (Eskilsson et al., 1988). 5-FU most commonly is discontinued in the face of cardiotoxicity, but careful rechallenge with the agent has been successfully achieved without exacerbation of previous cardiotoxicity (Weidmann et al., 1994).

(Continued on next page)

Table 25. Cardiotoxicity of Chemotherapeutic Drugs (Continued)

Classification	Drug	Incidence	Characteristic Effects	Nursing Considerations
Antimetabolites (cont.)	Capecitabine	Cardiotoxicity is rare; associated with fluorinated pyrimidine therapy is 1%–18% (Bertolini et al., 2001; Roche Pharmaceuticals, 2008; Van Cutsem et al., 2002). In a retrospective analysis of two randomized phase III clinical trials of capecitabine as a single agent administered at 1,250 mg/m² twice daily for days 1–14, followed by 7 days of rest, the incidence was noted in 3% of patients (Van Cutsem et al.). In two additional studies of patients receiving capecitabine previously treated with taxanes, the incidence also was 3% (Van Cutsem et al.).	Angina-like chest pain with or without MI, dysrhythmias, cardiogenic shock occurs because of coronary vasospasm. Sudden death also has been reported and is presumed to be associated with acute myocardial ischemia or infarction. ECG changes without symptoms are unusual but have been reported (Meydan et al., 2005). At least one case report of Raynaud phenomenon has been published (Coward et al., 2005).	These adverse events may be more common in patients with a prior history of coronary artery disease. Interrupt drug if grade 2 or 3 adverse reactions occur; discontinue drug for grade 4 toxicity (Roche Pharmaceuticals, 2008).
	Cladribine	Incidence of edema and tachycardia is 6%. Chest pain has been reported (Bedford Laboratories, 2007; Bryson & Sorkin, 1993; Wilkes & Barton-Burke, 2007).	Tachycardia Edema, generalized and not dependent Chest pain not associated with ischemic ECG changes	Most events occurred in patients with a history of cardiovascular disease or chest tumors (Bryson & Sorkin, 1993).
	Gemcitabine hydrochloride	CHF and MI have been reported rarely with the use of gemcitabine. Arrhythmias, predominantly supraventricular in nature, have been reported very rarely. Incidence of hypotension is 11% when given with cisplatin. A study of doses above 1,000 mg/m² on a daily x 5 dose schedule showed that patients developed significant hypotension (Eli Lilly & Co., 2007).	Hypotension, MI, arrhythmia, hypotension (Eli Lilly & Co., 2007)	Age, gender, and infusion time factors: Lower clearance in women and older adults results in higher concentrations of gemcitabine for any given dose. Toxicity is increased when administered more frequently than once weekly or with infusions longer than 60 minutes (Eli Lilly & Co., 2007).
Plant alkaloids	Vinorelbine tartrate	There have been rare reports of MI (Mayne Pharma, 2006). Chest pain was reported in 5% of patients (Mayne Pharma, 2006). Hypertension, hypotension, vasodilation, tachycardia, and pulmonary edema have been reported (GlaxoSmithKline, 2007b).	Rare incidence with variable symptoms that may be mistaken for evolving acute cardiac event	Most reports of chest pain were in patients who had either a history of cardiovascular disease or tumor within the chest (Mayne Pharma, 2006). There is a high level of suspicion for an acute cardiac event with symptoms. Temporarily discontinue vinorelbine and perform cardiac diagnostic tests when patients report cardiac symptoms (Mayne Pharma, 2006). Therapy may be resumed after resolution of symptoms (Mayne Pharma, 2006).
	Vinblastine	Idiosyncratic response to medication that is not dose-related but does not resolve until the medication is discontinued (Bedford Laboratories, 2007c)	Raynaud phenomenon	Teach patient to avoid cold exposure and quit smoking, which will exacerbate pain.

(Continued on next page)

Table 25. Cardiotoxicity of Chemotherapeutic Drugs *(Continued)*

Classification	Drug	Incidence	Characteristic Effects	Nursing Considerations
Plant alkaloids *(cont.)*	Vincristine	There have been isolated reports of Raynaud phenomenon with vincristine in adults and adolescents. It seems to be dose-related and does not resolve until the medication is discontinued (Gottschling et al., 2004; Mayne Pharma, 2007). One study of children associated symptomatic respiratory-phase heart-rate variation with use of vincristine (Steinherz & Steinherz, 1995).	Raynaud phenomenon has occurred even with single doses.	Advise patients to avoid cold exposure and quit smoking, which will exacerbate pain.
Miscellaneous	Arsenic trioxide	Dysrhythmias related to prolongation of the QT have occurred in approximately 10% of cases. It is usually asymptomatic but can induce ventricular tachycardia. Drug should not be administered unless the QTc is < 500 msec. Once held, therapy can be resumed once the QTc returns to < 460 msec (Cephalon Oncology, 2006).	Dysrhythmias	Check 12-lead ECG prior to therapy and hold if QTc is > 500 msec (Cephalon Oncology, 2006). Check all electrolytes prior to administration of medication and replenish prior to therapy. Potassium should be kept > 4.0 mEq/L, and magnesium > 1.8 mEq/L (Cephalon Oncology, 2006). Assess for other causes of dysrhythmias prior to administering drug.
Hormone	Tamoxifen	Rare cases of QT prolongation with dysrhythmia or heart failure (Barr Laboratories, 2007)	QT prolongation with bradycardia or ventricular dysrhythmias occurs infrequently and without clear risk factors such as dose or longevity of therapy (Slovacek et al., 2008).	Monitor ECG for QT prolongation. Avoid other medications known to prolong the QT interval.
Taxanes	Paclitaxel	Asymptomatic bradycardia occurred in almost 30% of patients with ovarian cancer; cardiac ischemia occurred in 5% (Rowinsky et al., 1991). Significant cardiac events occurred in 3% of all cases (Bristol-Myers Squibb, 2007c). Rare reports of cardiac ischemia or MI (Soe et al., 1996; Yusuf et al., 2008) CHF has been reported in cases of patients receiving other chemotherapy agents (Bristol-Myers Squibb, 2007c; D'Incalci et al., 1998; Platel et al., 2000).	Asymptomatic bradycardia (40–60 bpm), hypotension, asymptomatic ventricular tachycardia have been reported at all doses (Rowinsky et al., 1991). Atypical chest pain with and without cardiac ischemia occur occasionally and originally was thought to be related to agent's diluent Cremophor®, but this is now less clear (Salvatorelli et al., 2006; Soe et al., 1996). Pericardial effusion	Obtain a baseline ECG, H&P, and cardiac assessment before treatment; however, routine cardiac monitoring during infusion is not recommended (Arbuck et al., 1992; Rowinsky et al., 1991).
	Docetaxel	Hypotension is 2.8% (1.8% required treatment). Incidence related to high-dose treatment is unknown (Sanofi-Aventis Pharmaceuticals, 2008). Cardiac adverse effects similar to other microtubule inhibiting agents (Salvatorelli et al., 2006)	Hypotension during infusion that resolves with slowing of infusion rate CHF occurred in patients also treated with doxorubicin (> 360 mg/m^2) (Sparano, 1999). Sinus tachycardia, atrial flutter, dysrhythmia, unstable angina, and/or hypertension (Sanofi-Aventis Pharmaceuticals, 2008)	Drug is well-tolerated in older adult patients with NSCLC (Hainsworth et al., 2000).

(Continued on next page)

Table 25. Cardiotoxicity of Chemotherapeutic Drugs *(Continued)*

Classification	Drug	Incidence	Characteristic Effects	Nursing Considerations
Multikinase inhibitors	Lapatinib	Grade 4 heart failure with systolic dysfunction occurred in 1.6% of patients pooled from multiple studies (Perez et al., 2008). In pooled patients, 88% developed reversible disease (Perez et al., 2008). The QT interval may be prolonged and increase the risk for dysrhythmias (GlaxoSmithKline, 2008).	Most often occurred in individuals who received prior anthracyclines Onset averages 13 weeks after start of therapy and lasts approximately 7 weeks (Perez et al., 2008). QT prolongation most often leads to bradycardia but can cause life-threatening torsades de pointe (Shelton, 2006a).	Obtain baseline cardiac evaluation with echocardiogram or MUGA scan (GlaxoSmithKline, 2008). If the ejection fraction drops below the lower limit of normal, medication is stopped for at least 2 weeks, and when returned to normal and the patient remains asymptomatic, the dose is reduced and resumed at 1,000 mg/day (GlaxoSmithKline, 2008). Monitor for subtle signs of heart failure.
	Sorafenib	Cardiac failure or asymptomatic left ventricular end-diastolic dysfunction with reduced ejection fraction is infrequently (< 1%) reported (Force et al., 2007). No clear incidence rate has been identified (Kamba & McDonald, 2007; Patel et al., 2008; Porta et al., 2007). Cardiac ischemia with MI (< 1%) has been reported rarely (Bayer Healthcare Pharmaceuticals, 2008).	Cardiac failure Asymptomatic decreased left ventricular end-diastolic function with reduced ejection fraction Vasculitis with hypertension Asymptomatic myocardial ischemia and acute MI have been reported (Bayer Healthcare Pharmaceuticals, 2008). Chest pain with myocardial ischemia may occur.	Monitor blood pressure weekly throughout therapy. Standard antihypertensive agents are recommended for management of hypertension. Therapy breaks have been effective for resolution of hypertension. Hypertension seems to be related to presence of proteinuria, and both are usually present prior to cardiac failure (Force et al., 2007; Porta et al., 2007). Halt all therapy if symptomatic myocardial ischemia occurs temporally related to drug administration (Bayer Healthcare Pharmaceuticals, 2008).
	Sunitinib	Phase I and II studies evaluated for incidence of cardiac toxicities. Hypertension was reported in 35 of 75 patients with an incidence rate of 47% (Chu et al., 2007; Pfizer Inc., 2008b). This frequency has persisted through registration trials and existing clinical practice. There are well-established reports of both asymptomatic left ventricular end-diastolic dysfunction (> 15% reduction in ejection fraction) and cardiac failure, but incidence is 28% and 8%, respectively (Chu et al., 2007). Class effect (symptom occurring in most drugs in same category) involves mitochondrial injury and cardiomyocyte apoptosis, suggesting that there is risk for cardiac toxicities, but incidence rate is unclear (Chu et al.; Force et al., 2007). No clear incidence rate has been identified (Kamba & McDonald, 2007; Patel et al., 2008; Porta et al., 2007).	Hypertension Asymptomatic decreased left ventricular end-diastolic function with reduced ejection fraction Cardiac failure	See sorafenib.

(Continued on next page)

Table 25. Cardiotoxicity of Chemotherapeutic Drugs (Continued)

Classification	Drug	Incidence	Characteristic Effects	Nursing Considerations
mTOR inhibitor	Temsirolimus	Registration trials suggested prolongation of the QT interval with resultant dysrhythmias, particularly ventricular origin (Wyeth Pharmaceuticals, 2008b). Contingent upon approval, the FDA's licensing mandated follow-up studies of this effect, and they are currently under way (Micromedex, 2008).	Dysrhythmias	This is the first licensed drug in this class. Cardiac toxicities have not been identified but are possible given the targeted mechanism of action (Rubio-Viqueira & Hidalgo, 2006).
Monoclonal antibodies	Alemtuzumab	Cardiac toxicities are uncommon, although incidence is higher when this agent is used in lymphoproliferative malignancies, especially Sézary syndrome (Lenihan et al., 2004). In an 8-patient case series, 4 developed new-onset CHF caused by left ventricular dysfunction (Lenihan et al., 2004).	CHF may present even after one dose, but most symptoms present 6–11 weeks after starting therapy at doses of 30 mg 3 times a week (Bayer Healthcare Pharmaceuticals, 2007; Lenihan et al., 2004). No clear cardiac pathology was detectable on endomyocardial biopsy despite permanent reduction in ejection fraction. Dysrhythmias: Atrial fibrillation has been reported, but it is unclear if this is related to capillary leak and hypotension (Lenihan et al., 2004). The proposed mechanism of all cardiotoxicity associated with alemtuzumab is that of cytokine release (Lenihan et al., 2004).	Use with caution in patients who have received prior antitumor antibiotics (Bayer Healthcare Pharmaceuticals, 2007; Lenihan et al., 2004).
	Bevacizumab	Significant hypertension occurs in 15%–18% of patients receiving bevacizumab. It can occur as early as two weeks after start of therapy, and peak incidence is the second month of therapy (Genentech, Inc., 2007a). CHF was reported in 1.7% of patients overall, but the incidence was as high as 14% in patients who received prior anthracyclines (Genentech, Inc., 2007a).	Hypertension Thrombosis or hemorrhage CHF occurs more frequently in patients who have received prior anthracyclines or left chest wall radiation (Genentech, Inc., 2007a).	Check baseline vital signs and monitor with each clinic visit or establish home routine of twice daily while adjusting medications to treat hypertension. Temporarily suspend treatment if the urine has positive 3+ proteinuria, particularly if accompanied by hypertension. No clear antihypertensive treatment has been identified.
	Cetuximab	Unknown	Cardiac arrest of unclear etiology, but clear hypomagnesemia with this agent that could cause dysrhythmias related to QT prolongation	Maintain magnesium level 2.0 mEq/L. Monitor magnesium level throughout treatment and up to 8 weeks after conclusion of therapy (Bristol-Myers Squibb, 2007a).
	Gemtuzumab ozogamicin	Effects are infrequent and acute infusion-related at 9 mg/m² (all grade incidents): hypertension, 16% of participants; hypotension, 20%; and tachycardia, 11% (often in the first 24 hr of infusion) (Wyeth Pharmaceuticals, 2008a).	Hypertension, tachycardia, hypotension	Monitor vital signs before, during, and four hours after infusion. Assessment is complicated by concomitant combination chemotherapy.

(Continued on next page)

Table 25. Cardiotoxicity of Chemotherapeutic Drugs *(Continued)*

Classification	Drug	Incidence	Characteristic Effects	Nursing Considerations
Monoclonal antibodies *(cont.)*	Rituximab	Cardiac toxicity when used as a single agent is unknown. Infusion-related deaths within 24 hrs: 0.04%–0.07% (Genentech, Inc., 2007b) Incidence of mild to moderate hypotension requiring treatment interruption: 10% (Genentech, Inc., 2007b) Case reports of dysrhythmias	Hypotension and angioedema Infusion-related complex includes these cardiac events: MI, ventricular fibrillation, or cardiogenic shock (Genentech, Inc., 2008b). Although tachydysrhythmias are more common, case reports of bradycardia and heart block exist and may be related to prolongation of the QTc (Cervera Grau et al., 2008).	Nearly all fatalities have occurred on first infusion. Discontinue and medically treat patients who develop clinically significant cardiopulmonary reactions. After symptoms resolve, resume treatment by reducing the infusion rate by 50% (Genentech, Inc., 2007b).
	Trastuzumab	Incidence of cardiac dysfunction as a single agent: 7% Incidence with paclitaxel: 11% When combined with anthracycline and cyclophosphamide: 28% Advanced age may increase the probability of cardiac dysfunction (Bird & Swain, 2008; Genentech, Inc., 2008).	Signs and symptoms of cardiac dysfunction observed in patients treated with trastuzumab include dyspnea, increased cough, paroxysmal nocturnal dyspnea, peripheral edema, S3 gallop, or reduced ejection fraction (Genentech, Inc., 2008). Reducing the rate decreased infusion-related events for first infusion by 80%; 40% for subsequent infusions (Genentech, Inc., 2008).	CHF has been associated with disabling cardiac failure, death, and mural thrombosis leading to stroke. Discontinuing therapy is strongly suggested for those with significant CHF or asymptomatic ejection fraction decreases. Exercise extreme caution in treating patients with preexisting cardiac dysfunction. Patients should undergo frequent monitoring for deteriorating cardiac function (Genentech, Inc., 2008).
Cytokine	IFN alfa	Raynaud symptoms are rare but potentially severe. Peak incidence is 3 weeks–3 years after beginning therapy of 3,000,000 units daily. Concomitant administration of hydroxyurea may increase risk of this complication in some patients (Al-Zahrani et al., 2003; Schering Corp., 2008).	Raynaud phenomenon with superficial skin ulceration or gangrene (Al-Zahrani et al., 2003)	Teach patients to report Raynaud symptoms. Resolves with discontinuation of medication
Interleukin	IL-2	Side effects appear to be dose-related (Shelton, 2009). Risk increases with doses > 100,000 IU/kg (Wilkes & Barton-Burke, 2007). Average dose is 600,000 IU/kg (Novartis Oncology, 2007). Most adverse reactions are self-limiting and usually, but not invariably, reverse or improve within 2–3 days of discontinuing therapy. Hypotension of all grades occurs in as many as 71% of patients, but severe grade 4 toxicity occurs in only approximately 3% (Novartis Oncology, 2007). The rate of drug-related deaths in 255 patients with metastatic renal cell carcinoma who received single-agent IL-2 was 4% (11/255); the rate of drug-related deaths in 270 patients with metastatic melanoma who received single-agent IL-2 was 2% (6/270).	Alteration in cardiac output resulting from CLS. CLS results in hypotension and reduced organ perfusion, which may be severe and can result in death. CLS may be associated with cardiac arrhythmias (supraventricular and ventricular), CHF, angina, pleural and pericardial effusion, myocarditis, chest pain, and (rarely) MI (Novartis Oncology, 2007; Wilkes & Barton-Burke, 2007). CLS begins immediately after aldesleukin treatment starts. In most patients, this results in a concomitant drop in mean arterial blood pressure within 2–12 hr after the start of treatment.	IL-2 should be withheld in patients developing ventricular dysrhythmias until cardiac ischemia and wall motion can be assessed. Should adverse events occur, dosage should be withheld rather than reduced. Patients should have normal cardiac, pulmonary, hepatic, and CNS function at the start of therapy. Cardiac toxicities are worse when administered in conjunction with IFN alfa (Novartis Oncology, 2007). Medical management of CLS begins with careful monitoring of the patient's fluid and organ perfusion status; this is achieved by frequent determination of blood pressure and pulse and by monitoring organ function, which includes assessment of mental status and urine output.

(Continued on next page)

Table 25. Cardiotoxicity of Chemotherapeutic Drugs (Continued)

Classification	Drug	Incidence	Characteristic Effects	Nursing Considerations
Interleukin (cont.)	IL-2 (cont.)		With continued therapy, clinically significant hypotension (systolic blood pressure 90 mmHg or a 20 mmHg drop from baseline systolic pressure) and hypoperfusion will occur (Novartis Oncology, 2007). Electrical changes caused by cytokine biotherapy usually relate to cellular swelling or inflammatory cytokine release causing disruption of conduction pathways. Capillary permeability and hypovolemia enhance the risk of supraventricular tachycardia.	Hypovolemia is assessed by catheterization and central pressure monitoring. Electrical changes associated with biotherapeutic agents generally necessitate temporary discontinuation of the drug. Once inflammatory effects have resolved, rechallenge is possible (Shelton, 2009).
Immune modulator	Thalidomide	In a small phase I study, grade 3 dysrhythmias were experienced by 2% of patients (Sharma et al., 2006). Registration trial reported dysrhythmias, most commonly bradycardia not requiring clinical intervention (Celgene Corporation, 2007). Increased incidence (up to 23%) of thromboembolism, but it is unclear whether this is related to this agent or the cancer (Celgene Corporation, 2007).	Bradycardia is the most common dysrhythmia reported. Thromboembolism displays no established pattern of lower or upper extremities or a specific timing during treatment. It is associated with patients who are also receiving high-dose corticosteroids (Elice et al., 2008).	Assess patients for dizziness, palpitations, or other symptoms of dysrhythmias. Initiate thromboprophylaxis when not contraindicated. Lenalidomide is an additional immune modulator with similar actions and cardiotoxicities (Celgene Corporation, 2008a; Menon et al., 2008).
Immune conjugates	Denileukin diftitox	Vascular leak syndrome, also known as CLS, with vasodilation, hypotension, and compensatory tachycardia occurred in 27% of patients on registration trials, with 6% requiring hospitalization and rare deaths reported. Onset may be delayed up to 2 weeks after infusion and may persist or worsen after discontinuing the agent (Ligand Pharmaceuticals, 2006).	Hypotension, likely related to capillary permeability and vasodilation from immediate inflammatory responses of the vasculature (Ligand Pharmaceuticals, 2006) Dysrhythmias may occur but seem to be more often related to vasodilation and volume status.	Accurate intake and output, weight measurements, and central venous pressure readings may help to determine total fluid volume and vascular space volume status.

AIDS—acquired immunodeficiency syndrome; BMT—bone marrow transplant; BNP—brain natriuretic peptide; bpm—beats per minute; CHF—congestive heart failure; CLS—capillary leak syndrome; CNS—central nervous system; ECG—electrocardiogram; FDA—U.S. Food and Drug Administration; 5-FU—5-fluorouracil; H&P—history and physical; hr—hour; IFN—interferon; IL—interleukin; IU—international units; kg—kilogram; LVEF—left ventricular ejection fraction; mEq/L—milliequivalent per liter; MI—myocardial infarction; mmHg—millimeters of mercury; msec—millisecond; mTOR—mammalian target of rapamycin; MUGA—multigated acquisition; NSCLC—non-small cell lung cancer; QTc—QT interval corrected

(3) Patients with myocarditis, pericarditis, or pericardial effusion also are at risk for dysrhythmias because of their primary clinical complication (Shelton, 2006c).

(4) Dysrhythmias caused by poorly defined toxins, direct cardiotoxicity, or altered action potential are less predictable and, hence, potentially more dangerous (Floyd & Perry, 2008; Gianni, Salvatorelli, & Minotti, 2007; Loerzel & Dow, 2003).

(5) Individuals who have a personal history of heart disease, diabetes mellitus, hypertension, pulmonary hypertension, or electrolyte disturbances are more prone to dysrhythmias in conjunction with cancer therapy (Viale & Yamamoto, 2008; Yahalom & Portlock, 2005).

d) Clinical manifestations

(1) Most patients with dysrhythmias report subjective symptoms such as palpitations, chest discomfort, dyspnea, or dizziness.

(2) Syncope as the first presenting symptom is more common with ventricular dysrhythmias (Field & ACLS Subcommittee, 2006).

(3) Most patients report diminished functional capacity with atrial fibrillation. Dyspnea and fatigue are common, and loss of atrial contribution to cardiac output (approximately one-third of cardiac output) leads to worsening of all other cardiac disease symptoms (Kellen, 2004).

e) Assessment

(1) The first assessment to perform in patients with suspected dysrhythmias is a comparison of apical and peripheral heart rate. Not only does this provide an accurate heart rate, but it also demonstrates a pulse deficit that can occur with ventricular dysrhythmias or heart failure (Shelton, 2006a).

(2) While checking the heart rate by auscultation, abnormal heart sounds demonstrating pericardial effusion (muffled) or heart failure (gallops or murmurs) can be detected (Shelton, 2006a).

(3) Follow-up assessments of vital signs and associated symptoms such as dyspnea, hypoxemia (shown as low oxygen saturation), hypotension, or chest discomfort determine the sever-

ity of the rhythm disturbance (Field & ACLS Subcommittee, 2006).

(4) These abnormalities usually are followed by 12-lead electrocardiogram (ECG) for definitive assessment of the rhythm disturbance.

(5) Ongoing monitoring (continuous or intermittent) for rhythm assessment and interval measurement is implemented. Prolonged QT segment, even in the absence of dysrhythmias, warrants active assessment for potential etiologies (Roden, 2004; Shelton, 2006a; Yap & Camm, 2003).

(a) Chemobiotherapeutic agents associated with QT prolongation-induced dysrhythmias include 5-FU and its derivatives, tamoxifen, temsirolimus, and arsenic trioxide. Common contributing causes of QT prolongation that may require discontinuation include amphetamines, antidepressants, antiemetics, azole antifungals, fluoroquinolones, macrolides, calcium channel blockers, butyrophenones, histamine receptor antagonists, methadone, and proton pump inhibitors (Cephalon Oncology, 2006; Macdonald & Struthers, 2004; Roden, 2004; Slovacek, Ansorgova, Macingova, Haman, & Petera, 2008; Yap & Camm, 2003).

f) Collaborative management

(1) Correction of contributing factors such as hypoxemia, anemia, fluid imbalance, and electrolyte abnormalities is always initiated while determining if antidysrhythmic agents are warranted (Field & ACLS Subcommittee, 2006; Kellen, 2004).

(a) The major determinant of whether correction of etiologies precedes

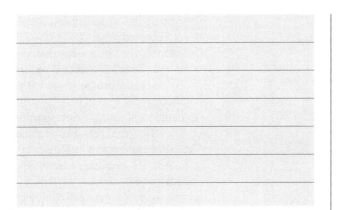

definitive treatment is the degree of clinical symptoms and cardiovascular decompensation at presentation (Field & ACLS Subcommittee, 2006).

(b) Spontaneous conversion of acute-onset atrial fibrillation may be as high as 71%, but it is unclear whether conversion represents treatment of potential underlying causes or is evidence that this dysrhythmia is commonly intermittent in nature (Ergene et al., 1999; Kellen, 2004).

(2) If correction of causes can be accomplished easily, no antidysrhythmic therapy may be necessary.

(a) Patients with dysrhythmias, or at high risk for their development, usually are monitored frequently and supported with electrolyte replacement to a goal potassium value of > 4.0 mEq/L and magnesium value > 2.0 mEq/L (Macdonald & Struthers, 2004; Shelton 2006a).

(b) Optimal calcium levels have not been established, but ionized calcium levels > 1.1 mEq/L are the usual goal.

(3) Symptomatic dysrhythmias should be treated with electricity in the form of synchronous cardioversion or pacing (Field & ACLS Subcommittee, 2006).

4) Antidysrhythmic medications are administered for immediate resolution of rhythm disturbances (Field & ACLS Subcommittee, 2006; Shelton, 2006a).

(a) Supraventricular tachycardia is treated with vagal maneuvers or adenosine as first-line measures

and amiodarone, beta-blockers, or calcium channel blockers for refractory rhythms. Dysrhythmia ablation through cardiac electrophysiology may be required with re-entrant rhythms.

(b) Atrial fibrillation has been managed in two different ways: rate control and conversion to sinus rhythm. Meta-analysis of various trials on these therapy options shows that rhythm control (conversion to normal) is associated with more hospitalizations and adverse effects, and stroke incidence is similar in both treatment groups (Cordina & Mead, 2005; Sherman, 2007). Rate control is achieved with beta-blockers, digoxin, and some calcium channel blockers. Rhythm control requires amiodarone, higher-dose calcium channel blockers, or electrical therapies (Field & ACLS Subcommittee, 2006).

(c) Abnormal ventricular rhythms are treated with amiodarone, lidocaine, or other agents to prolong the refractory period. These agents may also be proarrhythmic (Field & ACLS Subcommittee, 2006; Humphreys, 2002).

(d) Refractory dysrhythmias may require direct electrophysiology specialist-delivered electrical treatment, implantable defibrillator-pacers, synchronous cardioversion, atrial pacing, or ablation (Dunbar, Funk, Wood, & Valderama, 2004; Field & ACLS Subcommittee, 2006).

g) Patient and family education

(1) Patients and family are taught the symptoms of dysrhythmia and the potential urgency of treatment.

(2) They are advised when to call or come to the clinic and, more importantly, to call emergency medical services when they feel short of breath or dizzy.

(3) Once dysrhythmias have been identified for a patient, preventive strategies such as hydration or electrolyte replacement are taught.

(4) If supraventricular tachycardia has occurred, patients should be taught to induce vagal maneuvers via coughing or bearing down as if defecating (Field & ACLS Subcommittee, 2006).

(5) Patients with ventricular dysrhythmias are at risk for sudden death, and if indicated, family members may be advised to learn basic life support skills.

3. Vascular abnormalities

a) Capillary leak syndrome, a condition associated with the use of IL-2, involves extravasation of fluids and albumin into body issues. The results are decreased peripheral vascular resistance, hypotension, and decreased intravascular volume (Battiato & Wheeler, 2005; Newton, Jackowski, & Marrs, 2002).

b) Vasculitis: This syndrome may occur with high-dose cytarabine arabinoside, docetaxel, oprelvekin, suramin, and temsirolimus (Camp-Sorrell, 2005). Noncardiac arterial vasospasm and insufficiency may present as Raynaud phenomenon, whereby small distal arterial vessels constrict and prevent digit circulation (Lisse & Oberto-Medina, 2006; Viale & Yamamoto, 2008).

c) Hypertension: May be caused by a nonspecific vasospastic inflammation (Kamba & McDonald, 2007) or vasoconstriction.

(1) Pathophysiology

(a) Raynaud phenomenon is a temporary condition of vascular spasm of the arterial microvasculature of the digits, most commonly the fingers. Vasospasm causes immediate circulatory compromise that leads to local symptoms of pain and discoloration of the digits (Boin & Wigley, 2005).

(b) Abnormal nerve conduction and vascular diameter contribute to the pathophysiology of this disorder (Boin & Wigley, 2005).

(c) Increased protein tyrosine kinase activity and tyrosine phosphorylation within vascular smooth muscle cells respond to cooling by stimulating excessive alpha-2-adrenergic responses and vasospasm.

(d) The presence of anti-SS-A antibody and high levels of IL-6 are common findings in patients experiencing Raynaud phenomenon (Mitnick, 2000).

(e) In some agents, endothelial injury with inflammatory mediators can explain this process (e.g., taxanes, antiangiogenesis agents), but this mechanism does not provide a satisfactory explanation for the existence of Raynaud phenomenon with bleomycin, vincristine, or IFN (Gayraud, 2007; Gottschling, Meyer, Reinhard, Krenn, & Graf, 2004).

(f) Multikinase inhibition results in antiangiogenesis by blocking the BCR-ABL receptor and the actions of VEGF, which decreases cellular nitric oxide (NO) (Yusuf, Razeghi, & Yeh, 2008).

(g) Significant hypertension is highly associated with antiangiogenic VEGF inhibitors such as bevacizumab, sunitinib, and sorafenib. It has been reported that 11%–16% of patients receiving bevacizumab have significant enough hypertension to require addition or adjustment of antihypertensive medications (Yusuf et al., 2008).

(h) The pathophysiologic mechanism causing hypertension is thought to be related to the effect of loss of VEGF on the vascular endothelial wall, leading to diminished NO synthase and loss of vasodilatory effects of NO (Albert, 2005; Kamba & McDonald, 2007; Yusuf et al., 2008).

(i) Vasoconstriction subsequently leads to hypertension (Brunner et al., 2005; Mourad, des Guetz, Debbabi, & Levy, 2008; Zeb, Ali, & Rohra, 2007).

(j) Endothelial wall damage is thought to have a direct relationship to atherosclerotic events such as venous thromboembolism (VTE), supported by the fact that VTE occurs with higher incidence in patients treated with VEGF inhibi-

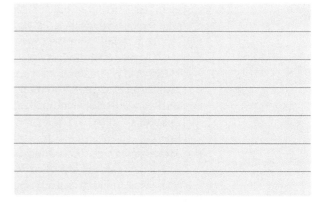

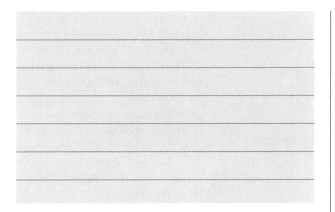

tors (Force, Krause, & Van Etten, 2007; Kamba & McDonald, 2007; Rosiak & Sadowski, 2005). The risk of VTE in patients with cancer ranges from 1.9% to 11% based upon a variety of risk factors. The addition of thalidomide increases this risk to as high as 30%, and antiangiogenic agents increase the risk up to 30%, even in lower-risk individuals (Yusuf et al., 2008).

(k) Lower NO levels have been associated with sodium and water retention that can exacerbate hypertension (Kamba & McDonald, 2007).

(2) Incidence

(a) Raynaud phenomenon is infrequent with most therapies, with few cases reported in registration trials and package insert materials. Only case reports are evident with any given therapy regimen (Al-Zahrani et al., 2003; Coward, Maisey, & Cunningham, 2005; Gayraud, 2007; Gottschling et al., 2004; Grunwald, Bolte, Wiebe, Ganser, & Schoffski, 2005; Story, 2005).

(b) Hypertension associated with antiangiogenic therapies and multikinase inhibitors occurs with high frequency (Albert, 2005; Chu et al., 2007; Floyd & Perry, 2008; Kamba & McDonald, 2007; Martel et al., 2006; Mourad et al., 2008; Patel et al., 2008; Porta et al., 2007; Viale & Yamamoto, 2008; Yusuf et al., 2008).

(c) Reports of hypertension with bevacizumab may be as high as 67% of all patients identified by analysis of clinical trial data (Chu

et al., 2007; Martel et al., 2006; Mourad et al., 2008; Rosiak & Sadowski, 2005).

(d) Hypertension with other multikinase inhibitors such as sunitinib is approximately 11%–18% (Ewer, Lenihan, & Khakoo, 2007; Patel et al., 2008; Porta et al., 2007).

d) Risk factors

(1) Increased incidence of Raynaud phenomenon has been noted with tyrosine kinase inhibitors, IFN, and bleomycin (Al-Zahrani et al., 2003; Boin & Wigley, 2005; Coward et al., 2005; Grunwald et al., 2005).

(2) Preexisting vascular insufficiency or hypertension are the most significant risk factors for development of Raynaud phenomenon related to drug therapy (Boin & Wigley, 2005; Lisse & Oberto-Medina, 2006).

(3) Drug-induced Raynaud phenomenon is a distinctly different entity from hereditary Raynaud disease (Boin & Wigley, 2005).

(4) It is also a secondary condition associated with certain malignancies (lymphoma, sarcoma), autoimmune disorders (rheumatoid arthritis, scleroderma, systemic lupus erythematosus), hormone imbalance (hypothyroidism, estrogen therapy), or specific medications (bleomycin) (Lisse & Oberto-Medina, 2006).

(5) Vasospasm is exacerbated by extreme hot or cold temperatures or emotional stress (Boin & Wigley, 2005; Gayraud, 2007).

(6) Patients who develop cancer therapy–related hypertension are more likely to have preexisting hypertension or cardiovascular disease than any other predisposing factors (Rosiak & Sadowski, 2005; Sharp, 2006).

(7) With bevacizumab therapy, proteinuria usually precedes hypertension, supporting the possibility that this toxicity is related to endothelial wall inflammation (Gerber, 2008; Patel et al., 2008).

e) Clinical manifestations

(1) Raynaud phenomenon is characterized by the classic cool, pale, and painful digits with an area of demarcation between perfused and nonperfused tissue (Boin & Wigley, 2005; Gayraud, 2007; Lisse & Oberto-Medina, 2006).

(a) The onset of symptoms is usually rapid, lasting a few minutes to several hours.

(b) It most often involves the fingers and often is unilateral, although different patterns have been observed.

(c) Vascular spasm with low blood flow first leads to pale-white and painful digits. This is followed by cyanosis and reduced pain, and lastly, flushing with return of circulation accompanied by pain.

(2) Hypertension is defined as blood pressure ≥ a systolic blood pressure of 140 mmHg or a diastolic blood pressure of 90 mmHg (Cushman, 2007; DHHS, NIH, & National Heart, Lung, and Blood Institute, 2004).

(a) Blood pressure rises with multikinase inhibitors and antiangiogenic agents and may be asymptomatic or accompanied by headache, visual disturbances, fatigue, tachycardia, or heart failure.

(b) There does not seem to be a specific pattern of primary systolic or diastolic hypertension; it appears to be reversible with a therapy break.

(c) Because the antiangiogenic agents are commonly used in patients who already have a propensity for hypertension (e.g., renal cell carcinoma, gastric cancer, colorectal cancer), it may be difficult to easily differentiate from other etiologic mechanisms.

(d) Refractoriness to traditional therapy is an important indicator that it is caused by anticancer therapies (Force et al., 2007).

f) Assessment

(1) Patients at risk for Raynaud phenomenon or hypertension should have a health history, blood pressure measurement, and examination of distal extremities at every clinic or hospital visit.

(2) Raynaud phenomenon is diagnosed by signs and symptoms in conjunction with a known risk factor.

(a) Raynaud phenomenon is visible and easily confirmed.

(b) Patient report is highly reliable because of the visibility of the condition and associated pain.

(3) Nailfold capillaroscopy and immunologic tests are useful in determining the etiology of Raynaud phenomenon (Gayraud, 2007; Pope, 2007).

(4) Hypertension may be a more subtle finding, requiring assessment of blood pressure at every clinic visit.

(5) The onset of treatment-related hypertension may occur as early as two weeks into therapy but peaks by the second month of treatment (Mourad et al., 2008; Rosiak & Sadowski, 2005).

g) Collaborative management

(1) Prevention of triggering factors will best alleviate symptoms of Raynaud phenomenon.

(a) Advise patients to avoid exposure to cold and to quit smoking (Pope, 2007).

(b) When it occurs in its mild form, Raynaud phenomenon may be managed with supportive interventions such as wearing gloves for tasks (removing items from the refrigerator) or placing hand warmers in gloves or pockets in cold weather.

(c) When severe, initial treatment is calcium channel blockers (Pope, 2007).

(d) Angiotensin-converting enzyme (ACE) inhibitors and angiotensin receptor blockers (ARBs) also may effectively treat Raynaud phenomenon by inhibiting activation of endothelin (Pope, 2007; Yusuf et al., 2008).

(e) Other treatments for refractory symptoms include phosphodiesterase-5 inhibitors (e.g., sudenafil), nitrates, endothelin receptor blockade (e.g., bosentan), and prostacyclin (Boin & Wigley, 2005; Gayraud, 2007; Lisse & Oberto-Medina, 2006; Pope, 2007).

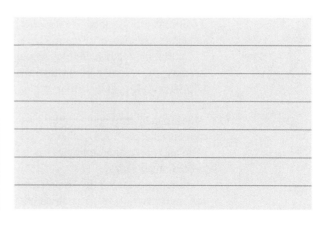

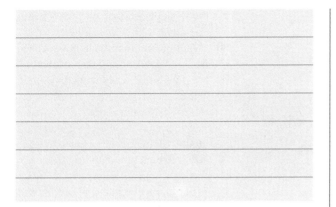

(2) Vascular constriction–induced hypertension is best treated with inducing vasodilation through inhibiting angiotensin II with ACE inhibitors or ARBs, or direct vasodilators (e.g., calcium channel blockers) (Higgins, Williams, & Guideline Development Group, 2007; Jurcut et al., 2008; Kolasinka-Malkowska, Filipiak, Gwizdala, & Tykarski, 2008).

    (a) Diuretics also reduce VEGF inhibitor-associated hypertension by reducing circulating blood volume (Mourad et al., 2008).

    (b) Nationally accepted guidelines for management of hypertension recommend thiazide diuretics as a first-line measure, although ACE inhibitors also are strongly encouraged if heart failure is a possible risk (Cushman, 2007; Higgins et al., 2007; Kolasinka-Malkowska et al., 2008).

    (c) Beta receptor blockers also are an important therapy option for some patients (London, 2008).

h) Patient and family education (Sharp, 2006; Viale & Yamamoto, 2008)

  (1) Teach patients the signs and symptoms of vascular complications.

  (2) Teach patients lifestyle changes, such as smoking cessation, low-fat diet, moderate exercise, or stress management, that may reduce incidence and severity of vascular complications (Appel et al, 2003; Elmer et al., 2006).

  (3) Advise patients to report complications to their care provider so that assessment and preventive strategies can be implemented early.

  (4) Hypertension can be life-threatening and cause stroke, so patients should be prepared to recognize signs of a hypertensive crisis or stroke.

    (a) Memory lapses

    (b) Blackouts or near syncope

    (c) Visual abnormalities

    (d) Persistent headache

    (e) Slurred words

    (f) Numbness or tingling of an extremity

    (g) Facial droop

  (5) Patients may require guidance with self-administration of antihypertensive agents.

  (6) Many agents can cause immediate orthostasis, dizziness, nausea, and risk of falling.

4. Coronary artery disease

  a) With the use of some drugs in high doses (e.g., 5-FU), coronary artery spasm leads to ischemia and possibly infarction (Anand, 1994; Becker, Erckenbrecht, Haussinger, & Frieling, 1999; Ewer & Yeh, 2006; Floyd & Perry, 2008; Gradishar & Vokes, 1990; Kleiman, Lehane, Geyer, Pratt, & Young, 1987; Labianca, Beretta, Clerici, Fraschini, & Luporini, 1982; Pottage, Holt, Ludgate, & Langlands, 1978; Tsibiribi et al., 2006; Yusuf et al., 2008).

  b) Increased incidence of ischemic myocardial disease and myocardial infarction occured with registration trials of cetuximab for locally advanced squamous cell head and neck cancer, although its association with the drug is unclear (Bristol-Myers Squibb, 2007a). Similar events did not occur with cetuximab when used for treatment of metastatic colorectal cancer.

  c) Capillary permeability with myocarditis, increased automaticity, and "myocardial stress" have been linked to myocardial infarction in patients receiving IL-2 (Jones & Ewer, 2006; Lee et al., 1989; Siegel & Puri, 1991).

  d) A rare instance of death resulting from myocardial ischemia and infarction has been documented with taxane therapy (Soe, Berkman, & Mardelli, 1996). Follow-up of dysrhythmia or other symptoms with serum cardiac enzymes or troponin levels can detect early myocardial infarction prior to definitive ECG changes (Field & ACLS Subcommittee, 2006; Shelton, 2006b). Few patients suffer this adverse effect with now-established drug monitoring and dose attenuation plans.

  e) Thrombotic heart disease may occur with agents enhancing hypercoagulability, although no relationship to any specific chemotherapy or biotherapy agent has been demonstrated (Ewer & Yeh, 2006; Floyd & Perry, 2008; Ng, Better, & Green, 2006; Yusuf et al., 2008).

f) Kleiman et al. (1987) and Soe et al. (2004) reported a type of vasospastic angina similar to Prinzmetal angina that is associated with high-dose chemotherapy. Unexplained chest pain with ischemic ECG changes that spontaneously resolve (Prinzmetal-like) continue to be reported on rare occasions (Ewer & Yeh, 2006; Yusuf et al., 2008).

g) Aromatase inhibitors are associated with an increased incidence of coronary artery disease. The mechanism of coronary artery disease is unclear (Bird & Swain, 2008; Towns, Bedard, & Verma, 2008). Myocardial infarction clearly associated with any chemotherapeutic or biologic agents warrants permanent discontinuation of therapy (Jones & Ewer, 2006).

5. Cardiac failure/cardiomyopathy

a) Cardiac failure is defined as inadequate contractile force to eject the required amount of blood for perfusion of the body (Heart Failure Society of America, 2006; Hunt et al., 2005).

b) Pathophysiology (Barry, Alvarez, Scully, Miller, & Lipshulta, 2007; Ewer & Ewer, 2008; Ewer & Yeh, 2006; Jones & Ewer, 2006; Jones, Swanton, & Ewer, 2006; Ng et al., 2006; Slordal & Spiget, 2006; University of Florida Shands Cancer Center, 2006; Yusuf et al., 2008)

(1) Physiologic mechanisms that contribute to heart failure include available oxygen content (e.g., reduced RBC count with decreased oxygen carrying capacity), myocyte strength, ventricular hypertrophy, ventricular dilation, and circulating blood volume (Yusuf et al., 2008).

(2) Anemia indirectly results in decreased available oxygen. Reduced oxygen saturation with decreased oxygen delivery causes the heart to contract stronger and more frequently to deliver the desired oxygen to tissues. With extended increased workload, the heart will fail. This is called "high-output failure." The consequences are the same as other etiologic mechanisms.

(3) Capillary permeability with interstitial fluid collection around the myocytes and eosinophilic infiltration of the heart muscle are the etiology of IL-2 cardiac failure (Jones & Ewer, 2006; Viale & Yamamoto, 2008).

(4) Renal retention of sodium associated with IL-11 leads to fluid retention and functional cardiomyositis (Smith, 2000).

(5) Anthracycline-induced cardiomyopathy is caused by drugs such as the antitumor antibiotics doxorubicin, daunorubicin, epirubicin, and idarubicin, which are known as DNA intercalators or anthracyclines. This is the most well-documented etiology of chemotherapy-induced cardiomyopathy associated with myocyte atrophy (Barry et al., 2007; Doroshow, 1991; Grenier & Lipshultz, 1998; Jones et al., 2006; Singal & Iliskovic, 1998).

(6) Oxidative stress in the presence of increased free radicals and decreased antioxidants results in myocyte injury and/or death (Santos, Moreno, Leino, Froberg, & Wallace, 2002; Singal & Iliskovic, 1998; Speyer & Wasserheit, 1998; Viale & Yamamoto, 2008; Yusuf et al., 2008).

(7) Irreversible damage already may occur prior to changes in ejection fraction or left ventricular wall thickness (Ewer & Lenihan, 2008).

c) Types of anthracycline toxicity (Barry et al., 2007; Jones et al., 2006; Yusuf et al., 2008)

(1) Early-onset anthracycline toxicity (type I)

(a) Occurs during or within one year of completion of anthracycline therapy (Gianni et al., 2007; Krischer et al., 1997)

i) Cases vary in severity.

ii) Some cases involve stable, asymptomatic abnormalities in left ventricular function.

iii) Other cases are progressive and involve ECG changes, associated signs of cardiomyopathy, changes in exercise-stress capacity, and overt CHF (Grenier & Lipshultz, 1998).
   (b) Is dose-related; toxicity increases with higher cumulative doses and higher maximal doses (Floyd & Perry, 2008; Grenier & Lipshultz, 1998; Yusuf et al., 2008).
(2) Late-onset anthracycline toxicity (type II) (Barry et al., 2007; Ganz et al., 2008)
   (a) Occurs one year or more after completion of anthracycline therapy
   (b) Presumably is caused by decreased left ventricular contractility and inappropriately thin left ventricular wall, elevated wall stress, and progressive ventricular dysfunction (Ewer & Lenihan, 2008; Grenier & Lipshultz, 1998)
   (c) Is dose-related; incidence increases with higher cumulative doses as well as higher maximal dose (Speyer & Wasserheit, 1998; Swain, Whaley, & Ewer, 2003).
   (d) Is more common than early-onset anthracycline toxicity (Jones & Ewer, 2006).
d) Types of nonanthracycline cardiomyopathy (Ewer & Ewer, 2008; Ewer & Lenihan, 2008; Ewer & Yeh, 2006; Ng et al., 2006; Slordal & Spigot, 2006; Yusuf et al., 2008)
   (1) Acute (Loerzel & Dow, 2003)
      (a) Occurs within 24 hours of drug administration
      (b) Is self-limiting
      (c) Is not dose-related (Camp-Sorrell, 2005)

   (d) May cause electrical changes in the heart that an ECG may reflect
   (e) Electrical changes caused by chemotherapy: The most frequent electrical change is decreased voltage (Steinherz & Yahalom, 1997).
   (f) Chemotherapy has led to cardiac decompensation and collapse (Kaszyk, 1986); however, transient changes usually do not call for discontinuation of therapy (Ewer & Ewer, 2008; Ewer & Lenihan, 2008; Ewer & Tan-Chiu, 2007).
   (g) The following call for discontinuation of therapy (Ewer & Lenihan, 2008).
      i) Acute changes associated with 5-FU (Akhtar, Salim, & Bano, 1993; Georgieva et al., 2007)
      ii) Endothelial damage leading to myocardial necrosis with use of high-dose cyclophosphamide (Chung et al., 2008; Mills & Roberts, 1979)
      iii) Serious arrhythmias resulting from a drug
(2) Subacute (Story, 2005)
   (a) Symptoms appear four to five weeks following therapy.
   (b) Fibrinous pericarditis and myocardial dysfunction, which may be diagnosed with a radionuclide cardiac multigated acquisition (MUGA) scan (Kaszyk, 1986)
   (c) Usually is reversible
   (d) Chemotherapy may or may not be stopped, depending on the patient's condition.
   (e) Biotherapy usually is discontinued if symptoms of subacute cardiac toxicity appear (Sandstrom, 1996; Siegel & Puri, 1991).
(3) Chronic (Story, 2005)
   (a) Nonreversible cardiomyopathy may occur weeks or months after drug administration (Camp-Sorrell, 2005; Floyd & Perry, 2008; Yusuf et al., 2008).
   (b) Seen with cumulative doses of cardiotoxic drugs that cause myocardial weakening because of direct damage to myocytes (Yahalom & Portlock, 2005)
   (c) Enhanced if radiation therapy has been given to the left chest, thorax, and/or mediastinum (Carlson,

1992; Jones & Ewer, 2006; Loerzel & Dow, 2003; Yusuf et al., 2008)

(d) Cardiotoxic chemotherapy is stopped if chronic toxicity occurs (Yahalom & Portlock, 2005).

(e) Erb-2 receptor blockers such as trastuzumab and lapatinib may cause cardiomyopathy via inhibition of mitochondrial function and the tyrosine kinase pathway (a major metabolic pathway) shared by cardiac myocytes (Ewer & Ewer, 2008; Ewer & O'Shaughnessy, 2007; Ewer & Tan-Chiu, 2007; Perez et al., 2008; Suter et al., 2007). When tumor cell tyrosine kinase is targeted, cancer cells die, but if cardiac tyrosine kinase also is inhibited, atrophy and death of myocytes occur.

(f) Probably reversible (Telli, Hunt, Carlson, & Guardino, 2007)

(g) Timing: As few as 48 hours after administration, but as late as 89 days (Perez et al., 2008; Suter et al., 2007)

(h) Newer multikinase inhibitors (e.g., sunitinib) and antiangiogenic agents (e.g., bevacizumab) are less direct in inhibiting tyrosine kinase with similar potential myocyte dysfunction (Chu et al., 2007; Force et al., 2007; Gerber, 2008).

(i) Longevity ranges from two to eight weeks (Perez et al., 2008).

(j) Average left ventricular ejection fraction (LVEF) decrease is 10%–15%, mean value is 40%–43% (Ewer et al., 2007; Perez et al., 2008).

e) Incidence

(1) Krischer et al. (1997) reported an incidence of early-onset anthracycline toxicity in 1.6% of 6,000 children with cancer who had been treated with anthracycline chemotherapy according to Pediatric Oncology Group protocols. This has been supported by more recent data (Bryant et al., 2007).

(2) Acute and subacute toxicity occur infrequently (Story, 2005); approximately 10% of acute toxicities consist of transient electrical changes in the heart (Camp-Sorrell, 2005).

(3) Chronic toxicity is related to cumulative dose (Loerzel & Dow, 2003).

(4) Studies show that some drugs (e.g., epirubicin, idarubicin, mitoxantrone) produce less cardiac toxicity than do other anthracyclines (Hurteloup & Ganzina, 1986; Loerzel & Dow, 2003; Shenkenberg & Von Hoff, 1986).

(5) More recent data suggest that even lower levels of anthracyclines that do not alter ejection fraction may compromise the heart's ability to handle other stressors, thereby increasing the risk of adverse cardiac events (Ewer & Lenihan, 2008).

(6) Escalating cardiotoxicity incidence with anthracyclines, taxanes, and trastuzumab in adjuvant and therapeutic breast cancer treatment is leading to more studies to assess best drug order and combinations (Barry et al., 2007; D'Incalci, Schuller, Colombo, Zucchetti, & Riva, 1998; Ewer & O'Shaughnessy, 2007; Ganz et al., 2008; Gianni et al., 2007; Jones et al., 2006; Perez et al., 2008; Suter et al., 2007).

f) Risk factors

(1) Direct insult of myofibrils by drugs such as the antitumor antibiotics doxorubicin, daunorubicin, epirubicin, and idarubicin

(2) Cardiac toxicity can be potentiated when taxanes are given with other cardiotoxic drugs such as doxorubicin. Paclitaxel (but not docetaxel) appears to interfere with the pharmacokinetic elimination of doxorubicin (Bird & Swain, 2008; D'Incalci et al., 1998; Ewer & O'Shaughnessy, 2007; Mackey et al., 2008; Perez et al., 2008; Sparano, 1999; Towns et al., 2008).

(3) Occasional cases of hemorrhagic myocarditis have been reported in adults who received very high doses

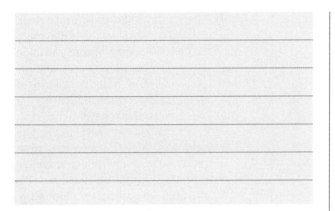

of cyclophosphamide, such as patients who are being prepared for BMT (Mills & Roberts, 1979; Satti et al., 2007). High-dose cyclophosphamide is considered potentially cardiotoxic for children (Bryant et al., 2007; van Dalen, Caron, Dickinson, & Kremer, 2008). The effects may be additive with those of anthracyclines.

(4) Anthracycline-induced cardiotoxicity (Rahman, Yusuf, & Ewer, 2007)

(a) Chemotherapy-induced cardiac toxicity in pediatric patients is almost always attributable to anthracyclines (Bottomley, 2004; Iarussi et al., 2001).

(b) In children and adults, cardiac toxicity has been associated with all anthracyclines in clinical use (Floyd & Perry, 2008; Grenier & Lipshultz, 1998; Jones & Ewer, 2006; van Dalen et al., 2008).

(c) The cumulative dose at which cardiac toxicity occurs varies from drug to drug.

(d) Doxorubicin is the most widely used anthracycline and the most extensively studied (Loerzel & Dow, 2003; Speyer & Wasserheit, 1998). It serves as a model for identifying anthracycline-related cardiomyopathies (Jones & Ewer, 2006; Yusuf et al., 2008).

(5) Exposure to other agents may potentiate anthracycline-induced cardiac toxicity.

(a) Mitoxantrone: This agent is known to be cardiotoxic; reports indicate that it potentiates cardiotoxicity when administered following anthracyclines or radiation to the mediastinal area (Kaszyk, 1986).

(b) Dactinomycin

(c) Mitomycin C

(d) Bleomycin

(e) Amsacrine: Krischer et al. (1997) reported that administration of amsacrine after anthracycline therapy resulted in a risk of cardiac toxicity that was 2.5 times higher than the risk associated with an anthracycline alone.

(f) Very high-dose cyclophosphamide (usually > 100 mg/kg)

(g) Dacarbazine

(h) Vincristine

(i) Diethylstilbestrol diphosphate: Cardiac toxicity has been reported 10 times more frequently with combined therapy than with doxorubicin alone (6.75% compared to 0.7%) (Leaf et al., 2003).

(j) Tamoxifen has been rarely associated with reduced left ventricular function (Barr Laboratories, 2007).

(k) Taxanes (e.g., paclitaxel, docetaxel) added to standard anthracycline regimens have proved effective in adjuvant and therapeutic breast cancer treatment regimens but provide added cardiotoxicity (Gianni et al., 2007).

(l) Trastuzumab is administered to patients with HER2-positive breast tumors. It has been shown to escalate severity when given simultaneously with anthracyclines or taxanes (Ewer & Ewer, 2008; Ewer & O'Shaughnessy, 2007; Gianni et al., 2007; Suter et al., 2007).

  i) Does not cause structural myocyte damage like anthracyclines

  ii) Average reduction in ejection fraction is 10%–15%, with overt heart failure symptoms occurring in 0%–3.9% of patients.

  iii) Reversible in 88% of cases, not requiring permanent drug discontinuation

(m) Cardiomyopathy has a reported incidence of approximately 6% with anthracyclines alone, 11% with anthracyclines and taxanes, and up to 28% with all three agents (Ganz et al., 2008; Gianni et al., 2007; Suter et al., 2007).

(6) High-dose therapy

(a) Administration schedule: Higher doses of cardiotoxic drugs given over a shorter period demonstrate increased toxicity (Hortobagyi et al., 1989; Iarussi et al., 2001). Dividing doses into smaller boluses has been shown to decrease toxicity (Von Hoff et al., 1979).

(b) Thoracic irradiation to the lungs or mediastinum (Adams, Hardenbergh, Constine, & Lipshultz, 2003; Bottomley, 2004; Carlson, 1992): Cardiac toxicity may occur at lower radiation doses when patients receive anthracyclines and mediastinal radiation (Chronowski et al., 2003).

(c) High-dose chemotherapy associated with HSCT may cause a spectrum of subacute to life-threatening cardiomyopathy peaking in incidence between the 6th and 16th day after administration of the preparative regimen (Chung et al., 2008).

(7) Age

(a) Malnutrition may increase cardiotoxicity. In cases of preexisting malnutrition, children are at higher risk than adults because of biologic and metabolic differences, the high tissue sensitivity of children, and the intensity of pediatric chemotherapy regimens (Carlson, 1992; Kaszyk, 1986).

(b) Conflicting evidence regarding older adults

i) Some researchers maintain that older adults are at higher risk than other adults because of the inability of an older person's body to self-repair and the greater likelihood of preexisting cardiac disease (Carlson, 1992; Kaszyk, 1986; Von Hoff, Rozencweig, Layard, Slavik, & Muggia, 1977).

ii) Other studies indicate that older adults can tolerate aggressive treatment and that, in regard to treatment for solid tumors, geriatric patients tolerate chemotherapy as well as young people do (Damon, 1992). Advanced age may increase the chances of cardiac

dysfunction with selected drugs (e.g., trastuzumab). Studies of older women receiving adjuvant chemotherapy with anthracyclines showed an increased risk for cardiomyopathy (Gianni et al., 2007).

(8) Preexisting cardiac disease (Kaszyk, 1986), such as cardiac abnormalities, or tumors in the chest, increases risk of cardiomyopathy (Bottomley, 2004; Jones & Ewer, 2006; Yusuf et al., 2008).

(9) Smoking also is associated with cardiac changes such as vasoconstriction, hypertension, and atherosclerosis (Kaszyk, 1986).

(10) Mediastinal radiotherapy increases risk of cardiomyopathy.

g) Clinical manifestations (Fares, 2008; Heart Failure Society of America, 2006; Hunt et al., 2005; Ng et al., 2006)

(1) The most common clinical finding is dyspnea.

(2) Heart failure usually presents with symptoms of increased work of the heart, such as tachycardia, full bounding pulses, gallops, or murmurs.

(3) Compensatory symptoms that reflect the body's attempt to improve tissue perfusion of the major organs in the face of inadequate contractile force include tachypnea, distended neck veins, cool and pale or cyanotic extremities, decreased bowel sounds with nausea or poor digestion, and decreased urine output.

(4) When the blood cannot enter the heart for a prolonged period of time, venous congestion occurs. Peripheral and dependent edema is accompanied by hepatosplenomegaly; crackles are de-

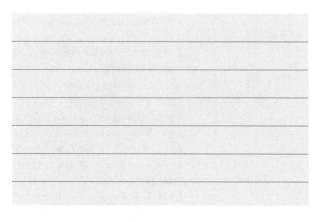

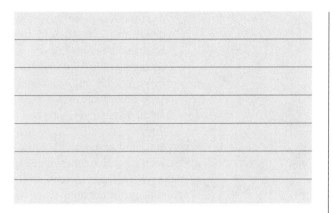

tected on lung auscultation; and pleural or pericardial effusions may occur.

(5) Late effects of compromised peripheral circulation may be detected by poor distal extremity wound healing.

h) Assessment

(1) Assess daily weights in high-risk patients when inpatient or at home. The heart failure literature validates that patient weight gain is a highly sensitive and specific predictor for decompensating heart failure (Hunt et al., 2005).

(2) When patients call with symptoms, the ability to determine the degree of heart failure is dependent upon the patient's report of dyspnea, weight gain, or edema.

(3) Assess breath sounds and heart sounds of patients at risk for cardiomyopathy at every hospital or home health visit.

(4) Anthracycline-toxicity diagnosis (Jannazzo, 2007; Jurcut et al., 2008; Shelton, 2009)

(a) Cardiac toxicity associated with anthracycline therapy is best diagnosed by serial endocardial biopsy (Ewer & Lenihan, 2008; Loerzel & Dow, 2003). The means for doing such a biopsy are not available in all institutions, however, and obtaining the tissue needed for the biopsy is an invasive procedure. Serial endocardial biopsy seldom is used in pediatric patients.

(b) MUGA scans are widely used as a means of detecting early-onset anthracycline cardiac toxicity. They are reliable indicators of cardiac damage but may not reflect early reversible changes (Ewer & Lenihan, 2008; Speyer & Wasserheit, 1998; Yusuf et al., 2008).

(5) Three-dimensional color Doppler echocardiography is widely used to diagnose all types of cardiomyopathy. It has the advantage of being noninvasive and can measure LVEF, fractional shortening, and left ventricular wall thickness (Ewer & Lenihan, 2008; Jurcut et al., 2008; Speyer & Wasserheit, 1998; Yusuf et al., 2008).

(6) Blood levels of cardiac troponin can detect early myocardiocyte injury (Speyer & Wasserheit, 1998) caused by anthracycline toxicity (Anderson, 2008; Ewer & Lenihan, 2008; Jurcut et al., 2008).

(7) Brain natriuretic peptide levels are used to monitor left ventricular heart failure. They may be inappropriately elevated postoperatively or in patients with anemia, atrial fibrillation, cor pulmonale, ventricular hypertrophy, pulmonary embolism, or lung cancer (Anderson, 2008).

(8) ECG can detect abnormalities in cardiac electrophysiology caused by cardiotoxicity. The most common abnormal findings are low QRS voltage or tachycardia. Ischemic ST changes may be present or accompanied by left ventricular strain seen as ischemia on anterior chest leads 4, 5, and 6.

(9) Assessment before biotherapy (Loerzel & Dow, 2003; Novartis Oncology, 2007; Shelton, 2009)

(a) Before treatment with IL-2: Ensure that patients have a baseline cardiac evaluation of left ventricular function to determine eligibility for treatment with IL-2.

(b) Before treatment with certain MoAbs (e.g., trastuzumab) and chemotherapy agents: Ensure that patients have a MUGA scan and ECG to establish baseline cardiac function.

(10) Assessment throughout therapy, especially for high-risk patients (Loerzel & Dow, 2003)

(a) Check the results of baseline cardiac studies (e.g., ejection fraction) before administering the drug. Ejection fraction may not be the most sensitive indicator and should not be the only parameter used to assess cardiotoxicity (Ewer & Lenihan, 2008). Other clinical assessments may include

ventricular dilatation, ventricular wall thickness, or wall motion abnormalities.

(b) Observe for clinical manifestations of CHF (e.g., tachycardia, shortness of breath, nonproductive cough, neck-vein distention, ankle edema, displaced point of maximal impulse crackles, hepatomegaly).

(11) Calculate and assess the cumulative dose of the applicable drug (e.g., doxorubicin) and document it in the patient's records. Cardiotoxic levels of common anthracyclines are

(a) Doxorubicin 400–450 mg/m^2 (Swain et al., 2003)

(b) Daunorubicin 400 mg/m^2 (Jannazzo, 2007)

(c) Epirubicin 900 mg/m^2 (Ryberg et al., 1998)

(d) Idarubicin 150 mg/m^2 (Anderlini et al., 1995).

(12) Assess heart rate, rhythm, and regularity, including murmurs, split sounds, and extra sounds (a gallop or third heart sound may indicate insufficiency).

(13) Assess electrolytes (e.g., potassium, calcium); abnormal electrolyte levels can interfere with cardiac function.

i) Collaborative management (Fares, 2008; Yusuf et al., 2008)

(1) Administer, if part of the protocol in your institution, the cardioprotective iron-chelating agent dexrazoxane during or prior to the administration of doxorubicin to prevent cardiotoxicity in some patients (e.g., patients with metastatic breast cancer who have received > 300 mg/m^2 doxorubicin) (Barry et al., 2007; Carlson, 1992; Safra, 2003; Speyer et al., 1992; Swain & Vici, 2003; van Dalen et al., 2008). Iron-chelating agents inhibit the generation of free radicals. Speyer and Wasserheit (1998) reported that dexrazoxane significantly decreased cardiac toxicity in children when the drug was administered in pediatric trials. Additional trials involving pediatric patients are ongoing (Bryant et al., 2007; Swain & Vici, 2003). Dexrazoxane is FDA approved to reduce cardiac toxicity in adults (Pfizer Inc., 2005).

(2) Administer liposomal formulation of anthracyclines (liposomal doxorubicin [Doxil®] or liposomal daunorubicin [DaunoXome®]) when indicated. They have demonstrated less cardiotoxicity, permitting higher dose delivery (Escobar, Markman, Zanotti, Webster, & Belinson, 2003; Rahman et al., 2007).

(3) Administer medications as prescribed to treat CHF and support cardiac output (e.g., diuretics, inotropic cardiac medications, vasodilators, oxygen).

(a) ACE inhibitors have been administered to prevent cardiomyopathy in patients receiving irradiation to the left breast and children receiving TBI (Cardinale et al., 2006; Nakamae et al., 2005).

(b) Metoprolol tartrate, a beta-blocker, has been used effectively to treat pediatric patients who have severe CHF following doxorubicin therapy (Shaddy et al., 1995).

(c) Develop an activity or exercise plan.

(d) Institute dietary modifications (e.g., a low-salt diet) as necessary for patients with CHF. Omega-3 fatty acids have been reported to both enhance and abrogate doxorubicin toxicities, but no clinical effects have been proven (Germain et al., 2003).

(4) Expect to discontinue or reduce the dose of the cardiotoxic agent if the patient's ejection fraction is less than 40%–45% (Ewer & Lenihan, 2008; Ewer & Tan-Chiu, 2007; Loerzel & Dow, 2003; Ng et al., 2006).

(5) Monitor results of ECGs; for patients receiving chemotherapy, an ECG is recommended at three months, six months, and one year post–anthracycline therapy (Barry et al., 2007; Ng & Green, 2007).

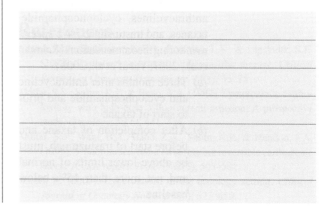

Al-Zahrani, H., Gupta, V., Minden, M.D., Messner, M.A., & Lipton, J.H. (2003). Vascular events associated with alfa-interferon therapy. *Leukemia and Lymphoma, 44*(3), 471–475.

Anand, A.J. (1994). Fluorouracil cardiotoxicity. *Annals of Pharmacotherapy, 28*(3), 374–378.

Anderlini, P., Benjamin, R.S., Wong, F.C., Kantarjian, H.M., Andreeff, M., Kornblau, S.M., et al. (1995). Idarubicin cardiotoxicity: A retrospective study in acute myeloid leukemia and myelodysplasia. *Journal of Clinical Oncology, 13*(11), 2827–2834.

Anderson, K.M. (2008). Clinical uses of brain natriuretic peptide in diagnosing and managing heart failure. *Journal of the American Academy of Nurse Practitioners, 20*(6), 305–310.

Appel, L.J., Champagne, C.M., Harsha, D.W., Cooper, L.S., Obarzanek, E., Elmer, P.J., et al. (2003). Effects of comprehensive lifestyle modification on blood pressure control: Main results of the PREMIER clinical trial. *JAMA, 289*(16), 2083–2093.

Arbuck, S.G., Adams, J., & Strauss, H. (1992, September). *A reassessment of cardiac toxicity associated with Taxol.* Abstract presented at the Second National Cancer Institute Workshop on Taxol and Taxus, Alexandria, VA.

Barr Laboratories. (2007). Tamoxifen [Package insert]. Pomona, NY: Author.

Barry, E., Alvarez, J.A., Scully, R.E., Miller, T.L., & Lipshultz, S.E. (2007). Anthracycline-induced cardiotoxicity: Course, pathophysiology, prevention, and management. *Expert Opinion on Pharmacotherapy, 8*(8), 1039–1058.

Bashir, H., Crom, D., Metzger, M., Mulcahey, J., Jones, D., & Hudson, M.M. (2007). Cisplatin-induced hypomagnesemia and cardiac dysrhythmia. *Pediatric Blood and Cancer, 49*(6), 867–869.

Battiato, L.A., & Wheeler, V.S. (2005). Biotherapy. In C.H. Yarbro, M.H. Frogge, & M. Goodman (Eds.), *Cancer nursing: Principles and practice* (6th ed., pp. 543–558). Sudbury, MA: Jones and Bartlett.

Bayer Healthcare Pharmaceuticals. (2008). Nexavar [Package insert]. West Haven, CT: Author.

Becker, K., Erckenbrecht, J.F., Haussinger, D., & Frieling, T. (1999). Cardiotoxicity of antiproliferative compound fluorouracil. *Drugs, 57*(4), 475–484.

Bedford Laboratories. (2007a). Cladribine [Package insert]. Bedford, OH: Author.

Bedford Laboratories. (2007b). Daunorubicin hydrochloride [Package insert]. Bedford, OH: Author.

Bedford Laboratories. (2007c). Vinblastine [Package insert]. Bedford, OH: Author.

Berchem, G.J., Ries, F., Hanfelt, J., Duhem, C., Keipes, M., Delagardelle, C., et al. (1996). Epirubicin cardiotoxicity: A study comparing low with high-dose–intensity weekly schedules. *Supportive Care in Cancer, 4*(4), 308–312.

Bertolini, A., Flumano, M., Fusco, O., Muffatti, A., Scarinici, A., Pontiggia, G., et al. (2001). Acute cardiotoxicity during capecitabine treatment: A case report. *Tumori, 87*(3), 200–206.

Bird, B.R., & Swain, S.M. (2008). Cardiac toxicity in breast cancer survivors. Review of potential cardiac problems. *Clinical Cancer Research, 14*(1), 14–24.

Boin, F., & Wigley, F.M. (2005). Understanding, assessing, and treating Raynaud's phenomenon. *Current Opinions in Rheumatology, 17*(6), 752–760.

Bottomley, S.J. (2004). Late effects of childhood cancer: Cardiovascular system. In N.E. Kline (Ed.), *Essentials of pediatric oncology nursing: A core curriculum* (pp. 273–274). Glenview, IL: Association of Pediatric Oncology Nurses.

Bristol-Myers Squibb. (2005). Cytoxan [Package insert]. Princeton, NJ: Author.

Bristol-Myers Squibb. (2006). Blenoxane [Package insert]. Princeton, NJ: Author.

Bristol-Myers Squibb. (2007a). Erbitux [Package insert]. Princeton, NJ: Author.

Bristol-Myers Squibb. (2007b). Platinol [Package insert]. Princeton, NJ: Author.

Bristol-Myers Squibb. (2007c). Taxol [Package insert]. Princeton, NJ: Author.

Brunner, H., Cockcroft, J.R., Deanfield, J., Donald, A., Ferrannini, E., Halcox, J., et al. (2005). Endothelial function and dysfunction Part II: Association with cardiovascular risk factors and diseases. A statement by The Working Group on Endothelins and Endothelial Factors of the European Society of Hypertension. *Journal of Hypertension, 23*(2), 233–246.

Bryant, J., Picot, J., Levitt, G., Sullivan, I., Baxter, L., & Clegg, A. (2007). Radioprotection against the toxic effects of anthracyclines given to children with cancer: A systematic review. *Health Technology Assessment, 11*(27), iii, ix–x, 1–84.

Bryson, H.M., & Sorkin, E.M. (1993). Cladribine: A review of its pharmacodynamic and pharmacokinetic properties and therapeutic potential in hematological malignancies. *Drugs, 46*(5), 872–894.

Camp-Sorrell, D. (2005). Chemotherapy: Toxicity management. In C.H. Yarbro, M.H. Frogge, & M. Goodman (Eds.), *Cancer nursing: Principles and practice* (6th ed., pp. 412–457). Sudbury, MA: Jones and Bartlett.

Cardinale, D., Colombo, A., Sandri, M.T., Lamantia, G., Colombo, N., Civelli, M., et al. (2006). Prevention of high-dose chemotherapy-induced cardiotoxicity in high-risk patients by angiotensin-converting enzyme inhibition. *Circulation, 114*(23), 2474–2481.

Carlson, R.W. (1992). Reducing the cardiotoxicity of the anthracyclines. *Oncology, 6*(6), 95–108.

Celgene Corporation. (2007). Thalomid [Package insert]. Summit, NJ: Author.

Celgene Corporation. (2008a). Revlimid [Package insert]. Summit, NJ: Author.

Celgene Corporation. (2008b). Vidaza [Package insert]. Summit, NJ: Author.

Cephalon Oncology. (2006). Trisenox [Package insert]. Frazer, PA: Author.

Cervera Grau, J.M., Esquerdo Galiana, G., Belso Candela, A., Llorca Ferrandiz, C., Juarez Marroqui, A., & Macia Escalante, S. (2008). Complete atrioventricular block induced by rituximab in monotherapy in an aged patient with non-Hodgkin's diffuse large B-cell lymphoma. *Clinical and Translational Oncology, 10*(5), 298–299.

Chronowski, G.M., Wilder, R.B., Tucker, S.L., Ha, C.S., Younes, A., Fayad, L., et al. (2003). Analysis of in-field control and late toxicity for adults with early-stage Hodgkin's disease treated with chemotherapy followed by radiotherapy. *International Journal of Radiation Oncology, Biology, Physics, 55*(1), 36–43.

Chu, T.F., Rupnick, M.A., Kerkela, R., Dallabrida, S.M., Zurakowski, D., Nguyen, L., et al. (2007). Cardiotoxicity associated with tyrosine kinase inhibitor sunitinib. *Lancet, 370*(9604), 2011–2019.

Chung, T., Lim, W.C., Sy, R., Cunningham, I., Trotman, J., & Kritharides, L. (2008). Subacute cardiac toxicity following autologous hematopoietic stem-cell transplantation in patients with normal cardiac function. *Heart, 94*(7), 911–918.

Cordina, J., & Mead, G. (2005). Pharmacological cardioversion for atrial fibrillation and flutter. *Cochrane Database of Systematic Reviews* 2005, Issue 2. Art. No.: CD003713. DOI: 10.1002/14651858.CD003713.pub2.

Coward, J., Maisey, N., & Cunningham, D. (2005). The effects of capecitabine in Raynaud's disease: A case report. *Annals of Oncology, 16*(5), 835–836.

Cushman, W.C. (2007). JNC-7 guidelines: Are they still relevant? *Current Hypertension Reports, 9*(5), 380–386.

Damon, L.E. (1992). Anemia of chronic disease in the aged: Diagnosis and treatment. *Geriatrics, 47*(4), 47–54, 57.

D'Incalci, M., Schuller, J., Colombo, T., Zucchetti, M., & Riva, A. (1998). Taxoids in combination with anthracyclines and other agents: Pharmacokinetic considerations. *Seminars in Oncology, 25*(Suppl. 13), 16–20.

Doroshow, J.H. (1991). Doxorubicin-induced cardiac toxicity. *New England Journal of Medicine, 324*(12), 343–345.

Dunbar, S.B., Funk, M., Wood, K., & Valderama, A.L. (2004). Ventricular dysrhythmias: Nursing approaches to health outcomes. *Journal of Cardiovascular Nursing, 19*(5), 316–328.

Eli Lilly & Co. (2007). Gemzar [Package insert]. Indianapolis, IN: Author.

Elice, F., Jacoub, J., Rickles, F.R., Falanga, A., & Rodeghiero, F. (2008). Hemostatic complications of angiogenesis inhibitors in cancer patients. *American Journal of Hematology, 83*(11), 862–870.

Elmer, P.J., Obarzanek, E., Vollmer, W.M., Simons-Morton, D., Stevens, V.J., Young, D.R., et al. (2006). Effects of comprehensive lifestyle modification on diet, weight, physical fitness, and blood pressure control: 18-month results of a randomized trial. *Annals of Internal Medicine, 144*(7), 485–495.

Ergene, U., Ergene, O., Fowler, J., Kinay, O., Cete, Y., Oktay, C., et al. (1999). Must antidysrhythmic agents be given to all patients with new-onset atrial fibrillation? *American Journal of Emergency Medicine, 17*(7), 659–662.

Escobar, P.F., Markman, M., Zanotti, K., Webster, K., & Belinson, J. (2003). Phase 2 trial of pegylated liposomal doxorubicin in advanced endometrial cancer. *Journal of Cancer Research and Clinical Oncology, 129*(11), 651–654.

Eskilsson, J., Albertsson, M., & Mercke, C. (1988). Adverse cardiac effects during induction chemotherapy treatment with cisplatin and 5-fluorouracil. *Radiotherapy and Oncology, 13*(1), 41–46.

Ewer, M.S., & Lenihan, D.J. (2008). Left ventricular ejection fraction and cardiotoxicity: Is our ear really to the ground? *Journal of Clinical Oncology, 26*(8), 1201–1203.

Ewer, M.S., Lenihan, D.J., & Khakoo, A.Y. (2007). Sunitinib-related cardiotoxicity: An interdisciplinary issue. *Lancet, 370*(9604), 2011–2019.

Ewer, M.S., & O'Shaughnessy, J.A. (2007). Cardiac toxicity of trastuzumab-related regimens in HER2-overexpressing breast cancer. *Clinical Breast Cancer, 7*(8), 600–607.

Ewer, M.S., & Tan-Chiu, E. (2007). Reversibility of trastuzumab cardiotoxicity: Is the concept alive and well? *Journal of Clinical Oncology, 25*(34), 5532–5533.

Ewer, M.S., & Yeh, E. (2006). *Cancer and the heart.* Hamilton, Ontario, Canada: BC Decker.

Ewer, S.M., & Ewer, M.S. (2008). Cardiotoxicity profile of trastuzumab. *Drug Safety, 31*(6), 459–467.

Fares, W.H. (2008). Management of acute decompensated heart failure in an evidence-based era: What is the evidence behind the current standard of care? *Heart and Lung, 37*(3), 173–178.

Field, J.M., & ACLS Subcommittee. (2006). *Advanced cardiovascular life support provider manual.* Dallas, TX: American Heart Association.

Floyd, J.D., & Perry, M.C. (2008). Cardiotoxicity of cancer therapy. In M.C. Perry (Ed.), *The chemotherapy source book* (4th ed., pp. 179–190). Philadelphia: Lippincott Williams & Wilkins.

Force, T., Krause, D.S., & Van Etten, R.A. (2007). Molecular mechanisms of cardiotoxicity of tyrosine kinase inhibition. *National Review of Cancer, 7*(5), 332–344.

Ganz, P.A., Hussey, M.A., Moinpour, C.M., Unger, J.M., Hutchins, L.F., Dakhil, S.R., et al. (2008). Late cardiac effects of adjuvant chemotherapy in breast cancer survivors treated on Southwest Oncology Group Protocol S8897. *Journal of Clinical Oncology, 26*(8), 1223–1230.

Gayraud, M. (2007). Raynaud's phenomenon. *Joint, Bone, Spine, 74*(1), e1–e8.

Genentech, Inc. (2007a). Avastin [Package insert]. South San Francisco, CA: Author.

Genentech, Inc. (2007b). Rituxan [Package insert]. South San Francisco, CA: Author.

Genentech, Inc. (2008). Herceptin [Package insert]. South San Francisco, CA: Author.

Georgieva, S., Kinova, E., Iordanov, V., Gudev, A., Tzekova, V., & Velikova, M. (2007). Acute heart failure after treatment with 5-fluorouracil. *Journal of B.U.ON., 12*(1), 113–116.

Gerber, D.E. (2008). Targeted therapies: A new generation of cancer treatments. *American Family Physician, 77*(3), 311–319.

Germain, E., Bonnet, P., Aubourg, L., Grangepont, M.C., Chajes, V., & Bougnoux, P. (2003). Anthracycline-induced cardiac toxicity is not increased by dietary omega-3 fatty acids. *Pharmacological Research, 47*(2), 111–117.

Gianni, L., Salvatorelli, E., & Minotti, G. (2007). Anthracycline cardiotoxicity in breast cancer patients: Synergism with trastuzumab and taxanes. *Cardiovascular Toxicology, 7*(2), 67–71.

Gilead Sciences, Inc. (2006). Daunoxome [Package insert]. San Dimas, CA: Author.

GlaxoSmithKline. (2007a). Alkeran [Package insert]. Research Triangle Park, NC: Author.

GlaxoSmithKline. (2007b). Navelbine [Package insert]. Retrieved April 30, 2004, from http://www.gsk.com

GlaxoSmithKline. (2008). Tykerb [Package insert]. Research Triangle Park, NC: Author.

Gottschling, S., Meyer, S., Reinhard, H., Krenn, T., & Graf, N. (2004). First report of a vincristine dose-related Raynaud's phenomenon in an adolescent with malignant brain tumor. *Journal of Pediatric Hematology and Oncology, 26*(11), 768–769.

Gradishar, W.J., & Vokes, E.E. (1990). 5-fluorouracil cardiotoxicity: A critical review. *Annals of Oncology, 1*(6), 409–414.

Greenberg, M.I. (2003). The dose makes the poison: Arsenic trioxide. *Emergency Medicine News, 25*(7), 23–25.

Grenier, M.A., & Lipshultz, S.E. (1998). Epidemiology of anthracycline cardiotoxicity in children and adults. *Seminars in Oncology, 25*(Suppl. 10), 72–85.

Grunwald, V., Bolte, O., Wiebe, S., Ganser, A., & Schoffski, P. (2005). Acral necrosis after inadequate excessive administration of bleomycin in a testicular cancer patient. *Onkologie, 28*(1), 41–43.

Hainsworth, J.D., Burris, H.A., III, Litchy, S., Morrissey, L.H., Barton, J.H., Bradhof, J.E., et al. (2000). Weekly docetaxel in the treatment of elderly patients with advanced nonsmall cell lung carcinoma: A Minnie Pearl Cancer Research Network phase II trial. *Cancer, 89*(2), 328–333.

Heart Failure Society of America. (2006). HFSA 2006 comprehensive heart failure practice guidelines: Executive summary. *Journal of Cardiac Failure, 12*(1), 10–38.

Higgins, B., Williams, B., & Guideline Development Group. (2007). Pharmacologic management of hypertension. *Clinical Medicine, 7*(6), 612–616.

Hortobagyi, G.N., Frye, D., Buzdar, A.U., Ewer, M.S., Fraschini, G., Hug, V., et al. (1989). Decreased cardiac toxicity of doxorubicin administered by continuous intravenous infusion in combination chemotherapy for metastatic breast carcinoma. *Cancer, 63*(1), 37–45.

Humphreys, M. (2002). Ventricular tachycardia: A life-threatening dysrhythmia. *CONNECT: The World Journal of Critical Care Nursing, 2*(2), 48–50, 52.

Hunt, S.A., Abraham, W.T., Chin, M.H., Feldman, A.M., Francis, G.S., Ganiats, T.G., et al. (2005). ACC/AHA 2005 guideline update for the diagnosis and management of chronic heart failure in the adult. A report of the American College of Cardiology/American Heart Association Task Force on Practice Guidelines (Writing Committee to Update the 2001 Guidelines for the Evaluation and Management of Heart Failure): Developed in collaboration with American College of Chest Physicians and the International Society for Heart and Lung Transplantation: Endorsed by the Heart Rhythm Society. *Circulation, 112*(12), e154–e235.

Hurteloup, P., & Ganzina, F. (1986). Clinical studies with new anthracyclines: Epirubicin, idarubicin, esorubicin [Abstract]. *Drugs Under Experimental and Clinical Research, 12*(1–3), 233–246.

Iarussi, D., Indolfi, P., Casale, F., Coppolino, P., Tedesco, M.A., & Di Tullio, M.T. (2001). Recent advances in the prevention of anthracycline cardiotoxicity in childhood. *Current Medicinal Chemistry, 8*(13), 1649–1660.

Jannazzo, A. (2007). Monitoring of anthracycline-induced cardiotoxicity. *Annals of Pharmacotherapy, 42*(1), 99–104.

Jones, R.L., & Ewer, M.S. (2006). Cardiac and cardiovascular toxicity of nonanthracycline anticancer drugs. *Expert Review of Anticancer Therapy, 6*(9), 1249–1269.

Jones, R.L., Swanton, C., & Ewer, M.S. (2006). Anthracycline cardiotoxicity. *Expert Opinions on Drug Safety, 5*(6), 791–809.

Jurcut, R., Wildiers, H., Ganame, J., D'Hooge, J., Paridaens, R., & Voigt, J.U. (2008). Detection and monitoring of cardiotoxicity—What does modern cardiology offer? *Supportive Care in Cancer, 16*(5), 437–445.

Kamba, T., & McDonald, D.M. (2007). Mechanisms of adverse effects of anti-VEGF therapy for cancer. *British Journal of Cancer, 96*(12), 1788–1795.

Kaszyk, L.K. (1986). Cardiac toxicity associated with cancer therapy. *Oncology Nursing Forum, 13*(4), 81–88.

Kellen, J.C. (2004). Implications for nursing care of patients with atrial fibrillation: Lessons learned from the AFFIRM and RACE studies. *Journal of Cardiovascular Nursing, 19*(2), 128–137.

Kilickap, S., Barista, I., Akgul, E., Aytemir, K., Aksoyek, S., Aksoy, S., et al. (2005). cTnT can be a useful marker for early detection of anthracycline cardiotoxicity. *Annals of Oncology, 16*(5), 798–804.

Kleiman, N.S., Lehane, D.E., Geyer, C.E., Jr., Pratt, C.M., & Young, J.G. (1987). Prinzmetal's angina during 5-fluorouracil chemotherapy. *American Journal of Medicine, 82*(3), 566–568.

Kolasinska-Malkowska, K., Filipiak, K.J., Gwizdala, A., & Tykarski, A. (2008). Current possibilities of ACE inhibitor and ARB combination in arterial hypertension and its complications. *Expert Review of Cardiovascular Therapy, 6*(5), 759–771.

Krischer, J.P., Epstein, S., Cuthbertson, D.D., Goorin, A.M., Epstein, M.L., & Lipshultz, S.E. (1997). Clinical cardiotoxicity following anthracycline treatment for childhood cancer: The Pediatric Oncology Group experience. *Journal of Clinical Oncology, 15*(4), 1544–1552.

Labianca, R., Beretta, G., Clerici, M., Fraschini, P., & Luporini, G. (1982). Cardiac toxicity of 5-fluorouracil: A study of 1083 patients. *Tumori, 68*(6), 505–510.

Langer, T., Stohr, W., Bielack, S., Paulussen, M., Treuner, J., & Beck, J.D. (2004). Late effects surveillance system for sarcoma patients. *Pediatric Blood and Cancer, 42*(4), 373–379.

Leaf, A.N., Propert, K., Corcoran, C., Catalano, P.J., Trump, D.L., Harris, J.E., et al. (2003). Phase III study of combined chemohormonal therapy in metastatic prostate cancer (ECOG 3882): An Eastern Cooperative Oncology Group study. *Medical Oncology, 20*(2), 137–146.

Lee, R., Lotze, M., Skibber, J., Tucker, E., Bonow, R., Ognibene, F., et al. (1989). Cardiorespiratory effects of immunotherapy with interleukins. *Journal of Clinical Oncology, 7*(1), 7–20.

Lenihan, D.J., Alencar, A.J., Yang, D., Kurzrock, R., Keating, M.J., & Duvic, M. (2004). Cardiac toxicity of alemtuzumab in patients with mycosis fungoides/Sezary syndrome. *Blood, 104*(3), 655–658.

Lenihan, D.J., Massey, M.R., Baysinger, K.B., Adorno, C., Warneke, D., Steinert, L., et al. (2007). Superior detection of cardiotoxicity during chemotherapy using biomarkers [Abstract]. *Journal of Cardiac Failure, 13*(6, Suppl. 2), S151.

Ligand Pharmaceuticals. (2006). Ontak [Package insert]. San Diego, CA: Author.

Lisse, J.R., & Oberto-Medina, M. (2006). *Raynaud phenomenon.* Retrieved January 26, 2008, from http://www.emedicine.com/MED/topic1993.htm

Loerzel, V.W., & Dow, K.H. (2003). Cardiac toxicity related to cancer treatment. *Clinical Journal of Oncology Nursing, 7*(5), 557–562.

London, M.J. (2008). Beta blockers and alpha2 agonists for cardioprotection. *Best Practice and Research in Clinical Anaesthesiology, 22*(1), 95–110.

Macdonald, J.E., & Struthers, A.D. (2004). What is the optimal serum potassium level in cardiovascular patients? *Journal of the American College of Cardiology, 43*(2), 156–161.

Mackey, J.R., Clemons, M., Cole, M.A., Delgato, D., Dent, S., Paterson, A., et al. (2008). Cardiac management during adjuvant trastuzumab therapy: Recommendations of the Canadian Trastuzumab Working Group. *Current Oncology, 15*(1), 24–35.

Martel, C.L., Presant, C.A., Ebrahimi, B., Upadhyaya, G., Vakil, M., Yeon, C., et al. (2006). Bevacizumab-related toxicities: Association of hypertension and proteinuria. *Community Oncology, 3*(2), 90–99.

Mayne Pharma. (2006). Navelbine [Package insert]. Paramus, NJ: Author.

Mayne Pharma. (2007). Vincristine [Package insert]. Paramus, NJ: Author.

Meydan, N., Kundak, I., Yavuzsen, T., Oztop, I., Barutca, S., Yilmaz, U., et al. (2005). Cardiotoxicity of de Gramont's regimen: Incidence, clinical characteristics and long-term follow-up. *Japanese Journal of Clinical Oncology, 35*(5), 265–270.

Menon, S.P., Rajkumar, S.V., Lacy, M., Falco, P., & Palumbo, A. (2008). Thromboembolic events with lenalidomide-based therapy for multiple myeloma. *Cancer, 112*(7), 1522–1528.

Micromedex. (2008). *Temsirolimus.* Retrieved November 28, 2008, from http://www.thomsonhc.com

Mills, B.A., & Roberts, R.W. (1979). Cyclophosphamide-induced cardiomyopathy: A report of two cases and review of the English literature. *Cancer, 43*(6), 2223–2226.

Mitnick, H.J. (2000). Paraneoplastic rheumatic syndromes. *Current Rheumatology Reports, 2*(2), 163–170.

Mourad, J.J., des Guetz, G., Debbabi, H., & Levy, B.I. (2008). Blood pressure rise following angiogenesis inhibition by bevacizumab. A crucial role for microcirculation. *Annals of Oncology, 19*(5), 927–934.

Nakamae, H., Tsumura, K., Terada, Y., Nakane, T., Nakamae, M., Ohta, K., et al. (2005). Notable effects of angiotensin II receptor blockade, valsarten, on acute cardiotoxic changes after standard chemotherapy with cyclophosphamide, doxorubicin, vincristine, and prednisone. *Cancer, 104*(11), 2492–2498.

Newton, S., Jackowski, C., & Marrs, J. (2002). Biotherapy skin reaction. *Clinical Journal of Oncology Nursing, 6*(3), 181–182.

Ng, R., Better, N., & Green, M.D. (2006). Anticancer agents and cardiotoxicity. *Seminars in Oncology, 33*(1), 2–14.

Ng, R., & Green, M.D. (2007). Managing cardiotoxicity in anthracycline-treated breast cancers. *Expert Opinion on Drug Safety, 6*(3), 315–312.

Novartis Oncology. (2007). Proleukin [Package insert]. East Hanover, NJ: Author.

O'Brien, M.E.R., Wigler, N., Inbar, M., Rosso, R., Grischke, E., Santoro, A., et al. (2004). Reduced cardiotoxicity and comparable efficacy in a phase 3 trial of pegylated liposomal doxorubicin HCl (CAELYX/DOXIL) versus conventional doxorubicin for first-line treatment of metastatic breast cancer. *Annals of Oncology, 15*(3), 440–449.

Ortho Biotech. (2008). Doxil [Package insert]. Raritan, NJ: Author.

OSI Pharmaceuticals. (2008). Novantrone [Package insert]. Melville, NY: Author.

OTN Generics, Inc. (2008). Epirubicin hydrochloride [Package insert]. San Francisco: Author.

Patel, T.V., Morgan, J.A., Demetri, G.D., George, S., Maki, R.G., Quigley, M., et al. (2008). A preeclampsia-like syndrome characterized by reversible hypertension and proteinuria induced by the multitargeted kinase inhibitors sunitinib and sorafenib. *Journal of the National Cancer Institute, 100*(4), 282–284.

Perez, E.A., Suman, V.J., Davidson, N.E., Sledge, G.W., Kaufman, P.A., Hudis, C.A., et al. (2008). Cardiac safety analysis of doxorubicin and cyclophosphamide followed by paclitaxel with or without trastuzumab in the North Central Cancer Treatment Group N9531 adjuvant breast cancer trial. *Journal of Clinical Oncology, 26*(8), 1231–1238.

Pfizer Inc. (2005). Zinecard [Package insert]. New York: Author.

Pfizer Inc. (2006a). Adriamycin [Package insert]. New York: Author.

Pfizer Inc. (2006b). Idamycin [Package insert]. New York: Author

Pfizer Inc. (2008a). Emcyt [Package insert]. New York: Author.

Pfizer Inc. (2008b). Sutent [Package insert]. New York: Author

Platel, D., Pouna, P., Bonoron-Adele, S., & Robert, J. (2000, March 1). Preclinical evaluation of the cardiotoxicity of taxane-anthracycline combinations using the model of isolated perfused rat heart [Abstract]. *Toxicology and Applied Pharmacology, 163*(2), 135–140.

Pope, J.E. (2007). The diagnosis and treatment of Raynaud's phenomenon: A practical approach. *Drugs, 67*(4), 517–525.

Porta, C., Paglino, C., Imarisio, I., & Bonomi, L. (2007). Uncovering Pandora's vase: The growing problem of new toxicities from novel anticancer agents. The case of sorafenib and sunitinib. *Clinical and Experimental Medicine, 7*(4), 127–134.

Pottage, A., Holt, S., Ludgate, S., & Langlands, A.O. (1978). Fluorouracil cardiotoxicity. *BMJ, 1*(6112), 547.

Quesada, J.R., Talpaz, M., Rios, A., Kurzrock, R., & Gutterman, J.U. (1986). Clinical toxicity of interferons in cancer patients: A review. *Journal of Clinical Oncology, 4*(2), 234–243.

Rahman, A.M., Yusuf, S.W., & Ewer, M.S. (2007). Anthracycline-induced cardiotoxicity and the cardiac sparing effect of liposomal formulation. *International Journal of Nanomedicine, 2*(4), 567–583.

Richardson, M.T. (2004). Electrolyte imbalances. In C.H. Yarbro, M.H. Frogge, & M. Goodman (Eds.), *Cancer symptom management* (3rd ed., pp. 440–460). Sudbury, MA: Jones and Bartlett.

Rivera, E., Valero, V., Arun, B., Royce, M., Adinin, R., Hoelzer, K., et al. (2003). Phase II study of pegylated liposomal doxorubicin in combination with gemcitabine in patients with metastatic breast cancer. *Journal of Clinical Oncology, 21*(17), 3249–3254.

Roche Pharmaceuticals. (2008). Xeloda [Package insert]. Nutley, NJ: Author.

Roden, D.M. (2004). Drug-induced prolongation of the QT interval. *New England Journal of Medicine, 350*(10), 1013–1022.

Rosiak, J., & Sadowski, L. (2005). Hypertension associated with bevacizumab. *Clinical Journal of Oncology Nursing, 9*(4), 407–411.

Rowinsky, E.K., McGuire, W.P., Guarnieri, T., Fisherman, J.S., Christian, M.C., & Donehower, R.C. (1991). Cardiac disturbances during the administration of Taxol. *Journal of Clinical Oncology, 9*(9), 1704–1712.

Rubio-Viqueira, B., & Hidalgo, M. (2006). Targeting mTOR for cancer treatment. *Current Opinion in Investigational Drugs, 7*(6), 501–512.

Ryberg, M., Nielsen, D., Skovsgaard, T., Hansen, J., Jensen, B.V., & Dombernowsky, T. (1998). Epirubicin cardiotoxicity: An analysis of 469 patients with metastatic breast cancer. *Journal of Clinical Oncology, 16*(11), 3502–3508.

Safra, T. (2003). Cardiac safety of liposomal anthracyclines. *Oncologist, 8*(Suppl. 2), 17–24.

Salvatorelli, E., Menna, P., Cascegna, S., Liberi, G., Calafiore, A.M., Gianni, L., et al. (2006). Paclitaxel and docetaxel stimulation of doxorubicinol formation in the human heart: Implications for cardiotoxicity of doxorubicin-taxane chemotherapies. *Journal of Pharmacology and Experimental Therapy, 318*(1), 424–433.

Sandstrom, S.K. (1996). Nursing management of patients receiving biological therapy. *Seminars in Oncology Nursing, 12*(2), 152–162.

Sanofi-Aventis Pharmaceuticals. (2008). Taxotere [Package insert]. Bridgewater, NJ: Author.

Santos, D.L., Moreno, A.J., Leino, R.L., Froberg, M.K., & Wallace, K.B. (2002). Carvedilol protects against doxorubicin-induced mitochondrial cardiomyopathy. *Toxicology and Applied Pharmacology, 185*(3), 218–227.

Satti, T.M., Ullah, K., Ahmed, P., Raza, S., Chaudry, Q.U., Ikram, A., et al. (2007). Cardiac complications after stem cell transplantation. *Journal of the College of Physicians and Surgeons—Pakistan, 17*(7), 420–422.

Schering Corp. (2008). Intron [Package insert]. Kenilworth, NJ: Author.

Sereno, M., Brunello, A., Chiappori, A., Barriuso, J., Casado, E., Belda, C., et al. (2008). Cardiac toxicity: Old and new issues in anti-cancer drugs. *Clinical Translational Oncology, 10*(1), 35–46.

Shaddy, R.E., Olsen, S.L., Bristow, M.R., Taylor, D.O., Bullock, E.A., Tani, L.Y., et al. (1995). Efficacy and safety of metoprolol in the treatment of doxorubicin-induced cardiomyopathy in pediatric patients. *American Heart Journal, 129*(1), 197–199.

Sharma, R.A., Steward, W.P., Daines, C.A., Knight, R.D., O'Byme, K.J., & Dalgeish, A.G. (2006). Toxicity of the immunomodulatory thalidomide analogue, lenalidomide: Phase I clinical trial of three dosing schedules in patients with solid malignancies. *European Journal of Cancer, 42*(14), 2318–2325.

Sharp, K. (2006). Hypertension: Just the facts. *Clinical Journal of Oncology Nursing, 10*(6), 727–729.

Shelton, B.K. (2006a). Dysrhythmias. In D. Camp-Sorrell & R. Hawkins (Eds.), *Clinical manual for the oncology advanced practice nurse* (2nd ed., pp. 299–319). Pittsburgh, PA: Oncology Nursing Society.

Shelton, B.K. (2006b). Myocardial infarction. In D. Camp-Sorrell & R. Hawkins (Eds.), *Clinical manual for the oncology advanced practice nurse* (2nd ed., pp. 349–368). Pittsburgh, PA: Oncology Nursing Society.

Shelton, B.K. (2006c). Pericarditis, pericardial effusion, and pericardial tamponade. In D. Camp-Sorrell & R. Hawkins (Eds.), *Clinical manual for the oncology advanced practice nurse* (2nd ed., pp. 369–384). Pittsburgh, PA: Oncology Nursing Society.

Shelton, B.K. (2009). Biological agents. In D. Ashenbrenner & S. Venable (Eds.), *Drug therapy in nursing* (3rd ed., pp. 644–668). Philadelphia: Lippincott Williams & Wilkins.

Shenkenberg, T.D., & Von Hoff, D.D. (1986). Mitoxantrone: A new anticancer drug with significant clinical activity. *Annals of Internal Medicine, 105*(1), 67–81.

Sherman, D.G. (2007). Stroke prevention in atrial fibrillation: Pharmacologic rate versus rhythm control. *Stroke, 38*(2), 615–617.

Siegel, J.P., & Puri, R.K. (1991). Interleukin-2 toxicity. *Journal of Clinical Oncology, 9*(4), 694–704.

Singal, P.K., & Iliskovic, N. (1998). Doxorubicin-induced cardiomyopathy. *New England Journal of Medicine, 339*(13), 900–904.

Singh, R., Sagar, T., & Ramanan, S. (2004). 5-fluorouracil cardio toxicity—Revisited. *Indian Journal of Medical and Paediatric Oncology, 25*(4), 35–38.

Slordal, L., & Spiget, O. (2006). Heart failure induced by noncardiac drugs. *Drug Safety, 29*(7), 567–586.

Slovacek, L., Ansorgova, V., Macingova, Z., Haman, L., & Petera, J. (2008). Tamoxifen-induced QT interval prolongation. *Journal of Clinical Pharmacy and Therapeutics, 33*(4), 453–455.

Smith, J.W. (2000). Tolerability and side effect profile of rhIL-11. *Oncology, 14*(9, Suppl. 8), 41–47.

Soe, M.S., Berkman, A., & Mardelli, J. (1996). Case report: Paclitaxel induced myocardial ischemia. *Maryland Medical Journal, 45*(1), 41–43.

Sparano, J.A. (1999, June). Doxorubicin/taxane combinations: Cardiac toxicity and pharmacokinetics. *Seminars in Oncology, 26*(Suppl. 9), 14–19.

Speyer, J., & Wasserheit, C. (1998). Strategies for reduction of anthracycline cardiac toxicity. *Seminars in Oncology, 25*(5), 525–537.

Speyer, J.L., Ewer, M.S., & Freedberg, R.S. (2004). Cardiac effects of cancer therapy. In M.D. Abeloff, J.D. Armitage, J.E. Niederhuber, M. Kaston, & W. McKenna (Eds.), *Abeloff's clinical oncology* (4th ed., pp. 1251–1268). New York: Churchill Livingstone.

Speyer, J.L., Green, M.D., Zeleninch-Jacquotte, A., Wernz, J.C., Rey, M., Sanger, J., et al. (1992). ICRF-187 permits longer treatment with doxorubicin in women with breast cancer. *Journal of Clinical Oncology, 10*(1), 117–127.

Steinherz, L.J., & Steinherz, P.G. (1995). Cardiac failure and dysrhythmias 6–19 years after anthracycline therapy: A series of 15 patients. *Medical and Pediatric Oncology, 24*(6), 352–361.

Steinherz, L.J., & Yahalom, J. (1997). Adverse effects of treatment. In V.T. DeVita Jr., S. Hellman, & S.A. Rosenberg (Eds.), *Cancer: Principles and practice of oncology* (5th ed., pp. 2739–2747). Philadelphia: Lippincott-Raven.

Story, K.T. (2005). Alterations in circulation. In J.K. Itano & K.N. Taoka (Eds.), *Core curriculum for oncology nursing* (4th ed., pp. 364–379). St. Louis, MO: Elsevier Saunders.

Suter, T.M., Procter, M., van Veldhusen, D.J., Muscholl, M., Bergh, J., Carlomagno, C., et al. (2007). Trastuzumab-associated cardiac

adverse effects in the Herceptin adjuvant trial. *Journal of Clinical Oncology, 25*(25), 3859–3865.

Swain, S., Whaley, F.S., & Ewer, M.S. (2003). Congestive heart failure in patients treated with doxorubicin: A retrospective analysis of three trials. *Cancer, 97*(11), 2869–2879.

Swain, S.M., & Vici, P. (2003). The current and future role of dexrazoxane as a cardioprotectant in anthracycline treatment: Expert panel review. *Journal of Cancer Research and Clinical Oncology, 130*(1), 1–7.

Talapatra, K., Rajesh, I., Rajesh, B., Selivamani, B., & Subhashini, J. (2007). Transient asymptomatic bradycardia in patients on infusional 5-fluorouracil. *Journal of Cancer Research and Therapeutics, 3*(3), 169–171.

Telli, M.L., Hunt, S.A., Carlson, R.W., & Guardino, A.E. (2007). Trastuzumab-related cardiotoxicity: Calling into question the concept of reversibility. *Journal of Clinical Oncology, 25*(23), 3525–3533.

Towns, K., Bedard, P.L., & Verma, S. (2008). Matters of the heart: Cardiac toxicity of adjuvant systemic therapy for early-stage breast cancer. *Current Oncology, 15*(Suppl. 1), 516–529.

Tsibiribi, P., Descotes, J., Lombard-Bohas, C., Barel, C., Bui-Xuan, B., Belkhiria, M., et al. (2006). Cardiotoxicity of 5-fluorouracil in 1350 patients with no history of heart disease. *Bulletins in Cancer, 93*(3), E27–E30.

University of Florida Shands Cancer Center. (2006). *Cardiac toxicity.* Retrieved November 11, 2008, from http://www.ufscc.ufl.edu/Patient/content.aspx?section=UFSCC&id=23159

Urbanova, D., Urban, L., Danova, K., & Simkova, I. (2008). Natriuretic peptides: Biochemical markers of anthracycline cardiac toxicity. *Oncology Research, 17*(2), 51–58.

U.S. Department of Health and Human Services, National Institutes of Health, & National Heart, Lung, and Blood Institute. (2004). *The seventh report of the Joint National Committee on Prevention, Detection, Evaluation, and Treatment of High Blood Pressure (JNC-7)* [NIH Pub # 04-5230, August 2004]. Retrieved November 28, 2008, from http://www.nhlbi.nih.gov/guideline/hypertension/jnc7full.pdf

Van Cutsem, E., Hoff, P.M., Blum, J.L., Abt, M., & Osterwalder, B. (2002). Incidence of cardiotoxicity with the oral fluoropyrimidine capecitabine is typical of that reported with 5-fluorouracil. *Annals of Oncology, 13*(3), 484–485.

van Dalen, E.C., Caron, H.N., Dickinson, H.O., & Kremer, L.C. (2008). Cardioprotective interventions for cancer patients receiving anthracyclines. *Cochrane Database of Systematic Reviews* 2008, Issue 2. Art. No.: CD003917. DOI: 10.1002/14651858.CD003917.pub3.

Viale, P.H., & Yamamoto, D.S. (2008). Cardiovascular toxicity associated with cancer treatment. *Clinical Journal of Oncology Nursing, 12*(4), 627–638.

Von Hoff, D.D., Layard, M.W., Basa, P., Davis, H.L., Von Hoff, A.L., Rozencweig, M., et al. (1979). Risk factors for doxorubicin-induced congestive heart failure. *Annals of Internal Medicine, 91*(5), 710–717.

Von Hoff, D.D., Rozencweig, M., Layard, M., Slavik, M., & Muggia, F.M. (1977). Daunomycin-induced cardiotoxicity in children and adults: A review of 110 cases. *American Journal of Medicine, 62*(2), 200–208.

Weidmann, B., Teipel, A., & Niederle, N. (1994). The syndrome of 5-fluorouracil cardiotoxicity: An elusive cardiopathy. *Cancer, 73*(7), 2001–2002.

Wilkes, G.M., & Barton-Burke, M.B. (2007). *2007 oncology nursing drug handbook.* Sudbury, MA: Jones and Bartlett.

Wong, S., & Rautaharju, F.M. (1998). The QT interval: Physiological determinants, pathophysiological changes and significance for clinical practice. *Canadian Journal of Cardiovascular Nursing, 9*(1), 23–28.

Wujcik, D., & Downs, S. (1992). Bone marrow transplantation. *Critical Care Clinics of North America, 4*(1), 149–166.

Wyeth Pharmaceuticals. (2008a). Mylotarg [Package insert]. Philadelphia: Author.

Wyeth Pharmaceuticals. (2008b). Torisel [Package insert]. Philadelphia: Author.

Yahalom, J., & Portlock, C.S. (2005). Cardiac toxicity. In V.T. DeVita Jr., S. Hellman, & S.A. Rosenberg (Eds.), *Cancer: Principles and practice of oncology* (7th ed., pp. 2545–2555). Philadelphia: Lippincott Williams & Wilkins.

Yap, Y.G., & Camm, A.J. (2003). Drug induced QT prolongation and torsades de pointes. *Heart, 89*(11), 1363–1372.

Yusuf, S.W., Razeghi, P., & Yeh, E.T. (2008). The diagnosis and management of cardiovascular disease in cancer patients. *Current Problems in Cardiology, 33*(4), 163–196.

Zeb, A., Ali, S.R., & Rohra, D.K. (2007). Mechanism underlying hypertension and proteinuria caused by bevacizumab. *Journal of the College of Physicians and Surgeons—Pakistan, 17*(7), 448–449.

F. Pulmonary toxicity

Pulmonary toxicity ranges from reversible short-term reactive airway disease to diffuse permanent fibrosis and structural destruction. Most are rare, occurring in < 1% of low-risk patients and up to 8% in high-risk groups (Chernecky, 2008). On rare occasions, these toxicities have been fatal (Boeck, Hausman, Reibke, Schultz, & Heinemann, 2007; Giusti, Shastri, Cohen, Keegan, & Pazdur, 2007; Gupta & Mahipal, 2007; Keijzer & Kuenen, 2007; Leimgruber et al., 2006; Makris et al., 2007). As patients survive increasingly aggressive and multimodal therapy, and use of multitargeted therapies becomes more commonplace, additional pulmonary toxicities are emerging. As in the case of acute promyelocytic leukemia differentiation syndrome or pulmonary veno-occlusive disease (VOD), it may be unclear whether defined pulmonary changes are related to the disease, rejection phenomena, chemotherapy agents, or the combined effects of chemoradiotherapy. Chemotherapy-induced pulmonary toxicities are divided into acute, undefined, and chronic disorders. Diagnosing the etiology of pulmonary signs and symptoms in patients with cancer can be challenging because toxicity can mimic a broad spectrum of pathogenic causes, including infectious agents and neoplastic lung disorders (Chernecky & Shelton, 2001; Meadors, Floyd, & Perry, 2006; Tietjen & Stover, 2002). Consequently, it is imperative to detect evidence of pulmonary toxicity as early as possible and have a clear understanding of potential for toxicity.

1. Interstitial lung disease (ILD): Pneumonitis—acute chemotherapy-induced/pulmonary capillary permeability syndrome/chemotherapy-related adult respiratory distress syndrome and pulmonary fibrosis (NCI CTEP, 2006).
   a) Pathophysiology (Vahid & Marik, 2008)
      (1) A heterogeneous group of lung disorders involving damage to the alveoli and surrounding interstitium (King, 2007a)
      (2) Postulated pathologic changes include (Daba, El-Tahir, Al-Arifi, & Gubara, 2004; Kachel & Martin, 1994; King, 2007a; Koh & Castro, 1996; Specks, 2008)
         (a) Injury to lung parenchyma
         (b) Inflammation of alveoli, alveolar cell walls, interstitial spaces, and terminal bronchioles
         (c) Release of ILs and transforming growth factors (Daba et al., 2004)
         (d) Destruction of the alveolar-capillary endothelium leading to changes in interstitial fibroblasts (Kachel & Martin, 1994; Koh & Castro, 1996)
         (e) Activation of fibroblasts and microfibroblasts, which cause collagen deposition in the alveolar interstitium (Chernecky, 2008).
      (3) Disease results predominantly from inflammatory features (Chernecky, 2008; Chernecky & Shelton, 2001; Meadors et al., 2006).
         (a) Fluid or bloody exudates in alveoli
         (b) Fluid between alveoli (interstitial spaces) resulting from degradation of alveolar wall (Budinger & Sznajder, 2006)
         (c) Fibrosis and stiffening of vascular, airway, and/or alveolar walls

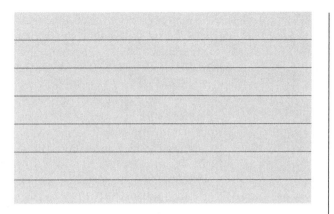

(4) Resolution of disorder results in scarring and fibrosis of tissue, beginning in the interstitium and later involving the alveolar sacs.

(5) Stiff, noncompliant lungs cause poor elasticity and increased work of breathing (Chernecky, 2008).

(6) Chronic exposure to chemotherapy agents resulting in extensive alteration of pulmonary parenchyma such as changes in the connective tissue, obliteration of alveoli, and dilatation of air spaces lead to "honeycombing" appearance of x-rays and scans (Daba et al., 2004; King, 2007a; Koh & Castro, 1996).

(7) Increased pulmonary pressure leads to pulmonary hypertension, cor pulmonale, and heart failure (Chernecky, 2008; Segura et al., 2001).

(8) Cellular mechanisms of injury (Meadors et al., 2006)

(a) Direct damage: Some chemotherapy agents cause direct damage to the alveoli and capillary endothelium, such as high-dose cytarabine or mitomycin-C (Chan & King, 2007; Forghieri, Luppi, Morselli, & Potenza, 2007; Morgensztern & Govidan, 2008; Wickham, 1986).

(b) Metabolic damage: Cyclophosphamide metabolism in the lung leads to the formation of alkylating metabolites and acrolein (a reactive aldehyde), which may cause toxicity (Gupta & Mahipal, 2007; Hamada et al., 2003; Kachel & Martin, 1994; Malik, Myers, DeRemee, & Specks, 1996; Specks, 2008; Vahid & Marik, 2008; Wilkes & Barton-Burke, 2008).

(c) Multi-kinase inhibitors, including tyrosine kinase inhibitors (e.g., imatinib, dasatinib), and EGFR inhibitors (e.g., cetuximab, panitumumab) (Vahid & Marik, 2008)

i) Act upon the transmembrane receptors regulating the enzyme tyrosine kinase.

ii) Inhibition of this pathway has effects upon multiple cell structures in the body, including the alveoli and lung pneumocytes (Vahid & Marik, 2008).

(d) Pulmonary edema (noncardiogenic)

i) Acute onset is related to capillary leak syndrome.

ii) It is clinically indistinguishable from other causes of pulmonary edema, but high-resolution CT may be helpful in distinguishing the etiology (Forghieri et al., 2007; LeChiong & Matthay, 2004).

(e) Hemorrhagic pneumonitis is parenchymal injury and microvascular bleeding similar to alveolar hemorrhage but occurring in both alveolar and interstitial spaces (Balk, 2007).

(f) Acute hypersensitivity reactions cause an immunologic reaction with rapid onset of capillary permeability. This may be a combined effect of direct injury, pulmonary edema, and small airway hemorrhage (Balk, 2007).

b) Incidence is variable based upon host and medication-related factors. Most pneumonitis syndromes are infrequent.

c) Risk factors

(1) The chemotherapy drugs most commonly associated with pulmonary toxicity are bleomycin, busulfan, carmustine, cyclophosphamide, cytosine arabinoside, gemcitabine, methotrexate, mitomycin, and tamoxifen (Boeck et al., 2007; Daba et al., 2004; Tietjen & Stover, 2002).

(2) Other agents associated with dyspnea include azathioprine, chlorambucil, chlorozotocin, docetaxel, erlotinib, etoposide, gemcitabine, lomustine, melphalan, mercaptopurine, procarbazine, semustine, teniposide, trans-retinoic acid, vinblastine, vindesine, and teni-

poside (Camp, Gilmore, Gullatte, & Hutcherson, 2007; Tietjen & Stover, 2002).

(3) General host risk factors for ILD

(a) Age: A normal physiologic phenomenon that has been observed with aging is a decrease in the effectiveness of the antioxidant defense system. Therefore, susceptibility to pulmonary toxicity from certain cytotoxic drugs increases significantly after age 70 (Hydzik, 1990; Wagner, Mehta, & Laber, 2007; Wickham, 1986).

(b) Smoking (Chernecky, 2008)

(c) Deteriorating CrCl can be an important parameter in predicting drug clearance and has been implicated with increased risk for pneumonitis and pulmonary fibrosis (McLeod, Lawrence, Smith, Vogt, & Gandara, 1987; Ngan, Liang, Lam, & Chan, 1993; Patel, 1990; Van Barneveld et al., 1984; Yahalom & Portlock, 2008).

(d) High oxygen concentrations (about 60% FiO_2), such as those used during administration of general anesthesia, can enhance the pulmonary toxicity of bleomycin (Ginsberg & Comis, 1984).

(e) Prior lung disease (e.g., chronic obstructive lung disease) or reduced lung reserve (Chernecky, 2008; Segura et al., 2001; Wickham, 1986)

(f) Autoimmune disease enhances release of inflammatory mediators that increase propensity for drug-related pulmonary toxicity (Chernecky, 2008; King, 2007a; Lake, 2007; Varga, 2007).

(4) Treatment-related factors (see Table 26)

(a) ILD increases with thoracic radiation therapy (Chernecky, 2008; Comis, 1992; Segura et al., 2001; Senan, Paul, Thompson, & Kay, 1992).

(b) Multidrug regimens may increase the incidence and severity of pulmonary toxicity, but this is not clearly defined. Typically, these chemotherapy regimens include bleomycin, mitomycin, cyclophosphamide, methotrexate, or

carmustine (Boeck et al., 2007; Czarnecki & Voss, 2006; Segura et al., 2001).

(c) It has not been determined whether any single drug is the causative agent or if the interaction of these antineoplastics results in enhanced toxicity (Boeck et al., 2007).

(d) Concurrent chemotherapy and radiation therapy, especially employing agents such as bleomycin, carmustine, cyclophosphamide, or doxorubicin, has been associated with interstitial pulmonary pneumonitis (Chernecky, 2008; Chernecky & Shelton, 2001; Hydzik, 1990; Segura et al., 2001; Wickham, 1986).

(e) Cumulative dose: Cytotoxic agents that are directly toxic to the lungs generally exhibit increasing toxicity with increasing dose. This is believed to be a result of drug accumulation in the lung itself. Two patterns of dose-related pulmonary toxicity are clinically observed.

i) A definite increase in risk for development of pulmonary toxicity occurs once a threshold effect has been reached (e.g., total lifetime dose of bleomycin exceeds 450–500 units). Pulmonary toxicity secondary to busulfan, in the absence of other predisposing factors, only has been noted with total doses > 500 mg (GlaxoSmithKline, 2008b).

ii) Maximum recommended dose of mitomycin is 30 mg/m^2 (Chan & King, 2007).

iii) With linear effect, there is a constantly increasing risk for

Table 26. Pulmonary Toxicity of Chemotherapeutic Drugs

Classification	Drug	Incidence	Characteristic Effects	Comments
Alkylating agents	Busulfan	Incidence is rare but serious. Busulfan is associated with pulmonary damage and pneumonitis. It occurs in 2.5%–11.5% of patients, usually those on long-term treatment, although it can occur more acutely. A progressive and often untreatable pneumonitis is an important complication of therapy. Bronchopulmonary dysplasia with pulmonary fibrosis occurs with chronic therapy (GlaxoSmithKline, 2008b).	Insidious onset cough, dyspnea, and low-grade fever; bronchodysplasia progressing to interstitial pulmonary fibrosis ("busulfan lung") (Barton-Burke et al., 2007) Bronchopulmonary dysplasia with pulmonary fibrosis is a rare but serious complication following chronic busulfan therapy. The average onset of symptoms is 4 years after therapy; delayed onsets have occurred (range = 4 months–10 years) (GlaxoSmithKline, 2008b). Chest x-rays show diffuse linear densities, sometimes with reticular nodular or nodular infiltrates or consolidation. Pleural effusions have occurred (GlaxoSmithKline, 2008b; Smalley & Wall, 1966).	Establish baseline pulmonary function. Assess x-rays, PFTs, or CT scans as indicated
	Chlorambucil	Incidence is low. Respiratory dysfunction is reported at high doses (GlaxoSmithKline, 2006).	Pulmonary fibrosis; bronchopulmonary dysplasia in patients receiving long-term therapy (GlaxoSmithKline, 2006)	Establish baseline pulmonary function.
	Cyclophosphamide	Incidence is rare. Diffuse alveolar damage is the most common manifestation of cyclophosphamide-induced lung disease (Rossi et al., 2000). In early-onset toxicity occurring within the first 48 days, there is no relationship among development of lung injury, dose, and duration of administration (Erasmus, 2000; Hamada et al., 2003; Patel, 1990; Specks, 2008). Incidence of pulmonary toxicity has been reportedly increased in patients who have received concomitant methotrexate or amiodarone and in chronic graft-versus-host disease (Bhagat et al., 2001; Gupta & Mahipal, 2007; Hamada et al., 2003; Specks, 2008).	Edema, fibrosis, alveolar hemorrhage, and fibrin deposition are thought to be due to accumulation of the alkylating agent metabolite acrolein (Patel, 1990; Twohig & Matthay, 1990). The metabolite causes lipid peroxidation normally cleared by pulmonary antioxidant mechanisms, but when accumulated, erode the lipid layer and cause microvascular damage (Patel; Specks, 2008). Onset of chronic fibrosis can be 15 weeks–6 years after medication administration (Hamada et al., 2003). Interstitial pulmonary fibrosis has been reported in patients receiving high doses of cyclophosphamide over a prolonged period (Gupta & Mahipal, 2007). Anaphylactic reactions are associated with death. Possible cross-sensitivity with other alkylating agents has been reported (Bristol-Myers Squibb, 2005). One clinical change in PFTs that has proven significantly predictive for cyclophosphamide pulmonary toxicity is reduction of the diffusing lung capacity for carbon monoxide (DLCO) (Hamada et al., 2003; Malik et al., 1996).	Incidence and severity may be exacerbated by concomitant oxygen delivery > 60% FiO_2 (Specks, 2008). Treatment involves discontinuing the agent and steroids, which has good to variable response in early-onset toxicity (Bristol-Myers Squibb, 2005; Specks, 2008). Delayed-onset interstitial fibrosis with pleural thickening is less responsive to corticosteroids (Hamada et al., 2003).
	Ifosfamide	Interstitial pneumonitis with pulmonary fibrosis occurs with variable incidence, with the highest incidence of 6% in non-small cell lung cancer (Vahid & Marik, 2008). Acute dyspnea with hypoxemia may occur in some patients due to transient methemoglobinemia (Vahid & Marik, 2008).	Dyspnea, tachypnea, and cough warrant investigation of possible pulmonary toxicity (Bristol-Myers Squibb, 2008a).	Methemoglobinemia occurs due to reactions between 4-thioifosfamide and glutathione to deplete antioxidant reserves (Vahid & Marik, 2008).

(Continued on next page)

Table 26. Pulmonary Toxicity of Chemotherapeutic Drugs *(Continued)*

Classification	Drug	Incidence	Characteristic Effects	Comments
Alkylating agents *(cont.)*	Melphalan	Reports of bronchopulmonary dysplasia (Glaxo-SmithKline, 2007) Acute hypersensitivity reactions including anaphylaxis were reported in 2.4% of 425 patients receiving the injected drug for myeloma (GlaxoSmithKline, 2007).	Pulmonary fibrosis, interstitial pneumonia, bronchospasm, and dyspnea also may be a sign of rare hypersensitivity, not pulmonary toxicity. These patients appeared to respond to antihistamine and corticosteroid therapy (GlaxoSmithKline, 2007).	If a hypersensitivity reaction occurs, IV or PO melphalan should not be readministered because hypersensitivity reactions also have been reported with PO melphalan (GlaxoSmithKline, 2007).
	Oxaliplatin	Associated with pulmonary fibrosis (< 1% of study patients), which may be fatal (Pasetto & Monfardini, 2006). Incidence of events increases with combined therapy (Ruiz-Casado et al., 2006). An acute syndrome of pharyngolaryngeal dysesthesia is seen in 1%–2% (grade 3 or 4) of patients previously untreated for advanced colorectal cancer. The combined incidence of cough, dyspnea, and hypoxia was 43% (any grade) and 7% (grades 3 and 4) in the oxaliplatin plus 5-FU/LV arm compared to 32% (any grade) and 5% (grades 3 and 4) in the irinotecan plus 5-FU/LV arm for patients with previously untreated colorectal cancer (Sanofi-Aventis Pharmaceuticals, 2007).	Anaphylactic-like reactions, thought to be related to eosinophilic infiltration of the lungs, are treatable with epinephrine, corticosteroids, and antihistamines (Vahid & Marik, 2008). Previously treated patients experienced subjective sensations of dysphagia or dyspnea, without laryngospasm or bronchospasm (no stridor or wheezing) (Sanofi-Aventis Pharmaceuticals, 2007).	In cases of unexplained respiratory symptoms such as nonproductive cough, dyspnea, crackles, or radiologic pulmonary infiltrates, oxaliplatin should be discontinued until further pulmonary investigation excludes ILD or pulmonary fibrosis (Sanofi-Aventis Pharmaceuticals, 2007).
	Temozolomide	Dyspnea 5%–8% Sinusitis: 6% Coughing: 5% (Schering Corporation, 2007) Interstitial pneumonitis in up to 4.8% of patients receiving doses exceeding 150–200 mg/m² (Maldonado et al., 2007; Vahid & Marik, 2008)	Allergic reactions, including rare cases of anaphylaxis; when used with nitrosoureas and procarbazine (Maldonado et al., 2007; Schering Corporation, 2007) Pneumonitis with high doses	Establish baseline pulmonary function.
Anticancer cytokines	Aldesleukin (IL-2)	Life-threatening grade 4 respiratory disorders: 3% (ARDS, respiratory failure, intubation); 1% (apnea) Adverse events occurring in 10% of patients (N = 525) (Chiron Corporation, 2002) Dyspnea: 43% Lung disorder: 24% (physical findings associated with pulmonary congestion, rales, rhonchi) Respiratory disorder: 11% (ARDS, chest x-ray infiltrates, unspecified pulmonary changes) Increased cough: 11%	Pulmonary congestion, dyspnea, pulmonary edema, respiratory failure, tachypnea, pleural effusion, wheezing, apnea, pneumothorax, hemoptysis (Chiron Corporation, 2002)	Establish baseline pulmonary function, and assess eligibility for high-dose aldesleukin. Consider fluid limitations with respiratory symptoms if blood pressure tolerates. Consider dose holding or discontinuation with refractory symptoms.

(Continued on next page)

Table 26. Pulmonary Toxicity of Chemotherapeutic Drugs *(Continued)*

Classification	Drug	Incidence	Characteristic Effects	Comments
Anticancer cytokines *(cont.)*	IFN alfa-2b	Rare (Schering Corporation, 2008)	Fever, cough, dyspnea, pulmonary infiltrates, pneumonitis, pneumonia	Consider holding drug while evaluating symptoms.
	Oprelvekin (IL-11)	Dyspnea: 48% Increased cough: 29% Pleural effusions: 10% (Wyeth Pharmaceuticals, 2008b)	Peripheral edema, dyspnea; preexisting fluid collections, including pericardial effusions or ascites, should be monitored. Patients should be advised to immediately seek medical attention if any of the following signs or symptoms develop: swelling of the face, tongue, or throat; difficulty breathing, swallowing, or talking; shortness of breath; wheezing (Wyeth Pharmaceuticals, 2008b).	Fluid retention is reversible within several days following discontinuation of the oprelvekin. Fluid balance should be monitored, and appropriate medical management is advised. Closely monitor for fluid and electrolyte status in patients receiving chronic diuretic therapy (Wyeth Pharmaceuticals, 2008b).
Antimetabolites	Capecitabine	Dyspnea: 14% (Roche Pharmaceuticals, 2006) Not considered a major toxicity but has demonstrated these side effects: 0.1% cough; 0.1% epistaxis and hemoptysis and respiratory distress; 0.2% asthma (Roche Pharmaceuticals, 2006)	Dyspnea, cough, respiratory distress; manage toxicities with symptomatic treatment, dose interruptions, and dose adjustment.	Once dose has been adjusted, it should not be increased at a later time (Roche Pharmaceuticals, 2006).
	Cytarabine	"Cytarabine syndrome" in doses > 5 g/m^2 (6–12 hours after dose) (Castleberry et al., 1981; Haupt et al., 1981; Mayne Pharma, 2006a; Spratto & Woods, 2004) Cytarabine liposomal: No pulmonary data (Enzon Pharmaceuticals, 2007)	A syndrome of sudden respiratory distress, rapidly progressing to pulmonary edema, capillary leak syndrome, respiratory failure, and adult respiratory disease (Haupt et al., 1981)	High-resolution CT will show diffuse bilateral patchy infiltrates (Forghieri et al., 2007). May be reduced with fluid restrictions.
	Fludarabine phosphate	Cough: 10%*; 44%** Pneumonia: 16%*; 22%** Dyspnea: 9%*; 22%** Allergic pneumonitis: 0%*; 6%** *N = 101; **N = 32 (Berlex Laboratories, 2006)	Pulmonary hypersensitivity reactions such as dyspnea, cough, and interstitial pulmonary infiltrate have been observed. In a clinical investigation using fludarabine phosphate injection in combination with pentostatin for the treatment of refractory chronic lymphocytic leukemia in adults, there was an unacceptably high incidence of fatal pulmonary toxicity. Therefore, this combination is not recommended (Berlex Laboratories, 2006).	—

(Continued on next page)

Table 26. Pulmonary Toxicity of Chemotherapeutic Drugs (Continued)

Classification	Drug	Incidence	Characteristic Effects	Comments
Antimetabo-lites (cont.)	Gemcitabine hydrochloride	Some kind of pulmonary toxicity is reported in 0.2%–13% of patients (Roychowdhury et al., 2000; Vahid & Marik, 2008). Dyspnea: 23% (severe dyspnea in 3%) (Eli Lilly & Co., 2007). Parenchymal lung toxicity, including interstitial pneumonitis, pulmonary fibrosis, pulmonary edema, and adult respiratory distress syndrome, has been reported rarely (Eli Lilly & Co., 2007). Severe pulmonary toxicities likely to be related to bronchospastic events, capillary permeability-induced pulmonary edema, or diffuse alveolar hemorrhage have been reported (Vahid & Marik, 2008). These have led to death in rare circumstances (Boeck et al., 2007; Vahid & Marik). Late pulmonary fibrosis has also been reported in < 1% of patients. Pulmonary hemorrhage has been associated with a 20% mortality rate (Vahid & Marik, 2008).	Dyspnea, cough, bronchospasm, and parenchymal lung toxicity (rare) may occur. If such effects develop, gemcitabine should be discontinued. Early use of supportive care measures may help to ameliorate these conditions (Eli Lilly & Co., 2007). Respiratory failure and death occurred very rarely in some patients despite discontinuation of therapy (Pavlakis et al., 1997). Some patients experienced the onset of pulmonary symptoms up to two weeks after the last dose (Eli Lilly & Co., 2007).	Prolonged infusion time beyond 60 minutes and doses more than once weekly increase toxicities (Castleberry et al., 1981; Spratto & Woods, 2004). Risk is increased when administered with other pulmonary toxic medications (Boeck et al., 2007; Vahid & Marik, 2008). Bronchospasm can be treated and resolved with corticosteroids. Rechallenge may require premedication with corticosteroids (Vahid & Marik, 2008).
	Methotrexate	Pulmonary edema: 1%–2% (Hospira, Inc., 2007) The incidence of allergic pneumonitis is 5%–10% (Rossi et al., 2000). The toxicity is not dose related, but patients who receive treatment more frequently may be more susceptible to lung injury (Aronchick & Gefter, 1991; Kohli et al., 2004; Lateef et al., 2005).	Fever, dyspnea, cough (especially dry nonproductive), nonspecific pneumonitis, or a chronic interstitial obstructive pulmonary disease (deaths have been reported); pulmonary infiltrates (Hospira, Inc., 2007; Kohli et al., 2004; Lateef et al., 2005).	Readministration with a desensitization protocol has been successfully implemented (Davis et al., 2003; Kohli et al., 2004).
Antitumor antibiotics	Bleomycin sulfate	10% of treated patients (Bristol-Myers Squibb, 2006a) Nonspecific pneumonitis in approximately 1% progresses to pulmonary fibrosis and death (Keijzer & Kuenen, 2007). More common in patients older than 70 years of age receiving > 400 units total dose. Toxicity is unpredictable and has been seen occasionally in young patients receiving low doses (Bristol-Myers Squibb, 2006a). Possible lower toxicity if not given as IV bolus (Bristol-Myers Squibb, 2006a; Chisholm et al., 1992)	The characteristics of bleomycin-induced pneumonitis include dyspnea and fine rales. Bleomycin-induced pneumonitis produces patchy x-ray opacities usually of the lower lung fields that look the same as infectious bronchopneumonia or even lung metastases in some patients. Carbon monoxide diffusion capacity may be abnormal before other symptoms appear (Sleijfer et al., 1995).	Early toxicity may be self-resolving. Monitor for early warning signs of toxicity to avoid irreversible pulmonary damage. Chest x-rays should be taken every one to two weeks. If pulmonary changes are noted, treatment should be discontinued. Conflicting studies regarding exposure to increasing concentrations of oxygen-increasing toxicity warrants prudently maintaining oxygen levels at room air (25%) (Bristol-Myers Squibb, 2006a).

(Continued on next page)

Table 26. Pulmonary Toxicity of Chemotherapeutic Drugs *(Continued)*

Classification	Drug	Incidence	Characteristic Effects	Comments
Antitumor antibiotics *(cont.)*	Mitomycin	Pulmonary toxicity has been reported with both single-agent therapy and combination chemotherapy, 3%–36%, 6–12 months after therapy. Prior treatment with mitomycin, cumulative doses > 30 mg/m², and other anticancer drugs may increase risk of toxicity (Bristol-Myers Squibb, 2000).	Dyspnea, nonproductive cough, diffuse alveolar damage, capillary leak, and pulmonary edema; severe bronchospasm has been reported following administration of vinca alkaloids in patients who previously or simultaneously received mitomycin. Acute respiratory distress occurred within minutes to hours after the vinca alkaloid injection. The total doses for each drug varied considerably (Bristol-Myers Squibb, 2000).	Signs and symptoms of pneumonitis may be reversed if therapy is instituted early. Drug may be discontinued if dyspnea occurs even with normal chest radiograph (Luedke et al., 1985). Caution should be exercised when using oxygen because oxygen itself is toxic to the lungs. Pay careful attention to fluid balance, and avoid overhydration (Bristol-Myers Squibb, 2000).
Miscellaneous	Mitoxantrone	Hypersensitivity-like acute pneumonitis occurs variably when given in combination with other chemotherapeutic agents (Vahid & Marik, 2008).	Sudden-onset dyspnea and tachypnea with hypoxemia. Patchy infiltrates on x-ray or CT scan	Organizing pneumonia detectable on bronchial biopsy or open lung biopsy usually is responsive to corticosteroid treatment (Vahid & Marik, 2008).
Miscellaneous	Arsenic trioxide	Respiratory events (all grades, N = 40): • Cough: 65% • Dyspnea: 53% • Hypoxia: 23% • Pleural effusion: 20% • Wheezing: 13% Grades 3 and 4: • Dyspnea: 10% • Hypoxia: 10% • Pleural effusion: 3% (Cephalon, 2006)	These adverse effects have not been observed to be permanent or irreversible, nor do they usually require interruption of therapy (Cephalon, 2006).	Establish baseline pulmonary function.
Miscellaneous: Antiangiogenesis agent	Bevacizumab	Pulmonary hemorrhage occurs rarely (< 1%) (Vahid & Marik, 2008).	More common in patients with squamous cell carcinoma of the lung (Vahid & Marik, 2008). Most common clinical presentation is hemoptysis (Vahid & Marik, 2008).	This medication is always discontinued when this toxicity occurs (Genentech, Inc., 2007a).
Miscellaneous: Proteasome inhibitor	Bortezomib	Acute pneumonitis syndrome reported rarely as case reports from Japanese patients treated after hematopoietic stem cell transplant and an African American without history of transplant (Ohri & Arena, 2006)	Sudden respiratory distress with accompanying pulmonary infiltrates. Proposed pathophysiology is acute vasculitis (Pitini et al., 2007).	Immediate discontinuation of this drug is recommended when pulmonary symptoms occur (Millennium Pharmaceuticals, Inc., 2008).
Miscellaneous	Lenalidomide	Hypersensitivity reactions	Hypersensitivity pneumonitis-like syndrome (Thornburg et al., 2007)	Immediate discontinuation of medication is indicated if pulmonary toxicity is suspected (Celgene Corporation, 2008).

(Continued on next page)

Table 26. Pulmonary Toxicity of Chemotherapeutic Drugs (Continued)

Classification	Drug	Incidence	Characteristic Effects	Comments
Miscellaneous (cont.)	Thalidomide	Acute pulmonary toxicity is rare and has no reported incidence rate (Celgene Corporation, 2007). Case reports of suspected but not verified alveolar hemorrhage exist.	Sudden onset ground glass opacities have been noted with thalidomide. It is unclear whether they represent infection, interstitial lung toxicity, or alveolar hemorrhage. It is believed that antiangiogenic properties have been temporally associated with alveolar hemorrhage in patients receiving thalidomide; however, hemorrhagic pathogens have not been ruled out (Khalsa et al., 2007).	Consider infectious etiology as higher risk for pulmonary symptoms than drug toxicity. Other bleeding symptoms may support suspicion for alveolar hemorrhage in patients with respiratory distress temporally related to thalidomide administration (Khalsa et al., 2007).
Monoclonal antibodies	Alemtuzumab	Infusion-rate–related dyspnea: 17%. Acute infusion-related events were most common during the first week of therapy. Incidence (N = 149): • Dyspnea: 26% • Cough: 25% • Bronchitis/pneumonitis: 21% • Pneumonia: 16% • Bronchospasm: 9% (Bayer Healthcare Pharmaceuticals, 2007)	Alemtuzumab has been associated with infusion-related events, including hypotension, rigors, fever, shortness of breath, bronchospasm, chills, and/or rash. Side effects include asthma, bronchitis, chronic obstructive pulmonary disease, hemoptysis, hypoxia, pleural effusion, pleurisy, pneumothorax, pulmonary edema, pulmonary fibrosis, pulmonary infiltration, respiratory depression, respiratory insufficiency, sinusitis, stridor, and throat tightness (Bayer Healthcare Pharmaceuticals, 2002).	To ameliorate or avoid infusion-related events, patients should be premedicated with an oral antihistamine and acetaminophen prior to dosing and monitored closely for infusion-related adverse events.
	Cetuximab	ILD < 1% is idiosyncratic in nature (Bristol-Myers Squibb/ImClone, 2007).	Serious but potentially fatal. May worsen after discontinuation of medication. Characterized by dyspnea, tachypnea, and activity intolerance. Progressive worsening of symptoms even after initial discontinuation of medication	All dyspnea noted between cycles warrants evaluation of PFTs. Hold medication until ILD is ruled out. If drug is resumed, administer at 50% previous rate (Bristol-Myers Squibb/ImClone, 2007).
	Gemtuzumab ozogamicin	Hypoxia: 5%. Pneumonia: 13%. Increased cough: 17%. Dyspnea: 32% (often during the first 24 hours). Severe pulmonary events leading to death have been reported infrequently (Wyeth Pharmaceuticals, 2008a).	Signs, symptoms, and clinical findings include dyspnea, pulmonary infiltrates, pleural effusions, noncardiogenic pulmonary edema, pulmonary insufficiency and hypoxia, and ARDS. These events occur as sequelae of infusion reactions. Monitor for increased cough, dyspnea, pharyngitis, and pneumonia, and check vital signs before, during, and after infusion.	Do not administer as an IV push or bolus (Wyeth Pharmaceuticals, 2008a). Patients with white blood cell counts > 30,000 µl may be at increased risk; also, patients with symptomatic intrinsic lung disease may have more severe pulmonary reactions.
	Panitumumab	ILD: 1% (Amgen Inc., 2008; Giusti et al., 2007)	Monitor for infusion reactions (Giusti et al., 2007). ILD characterized by dyspnea, cough, and pulmonary infiltrates that occur 2–4 months into therapy and worsen even after drug discontinuation (Amgen Inc., 2008; Cohenuram & Saif, 2007).	Evidence of interstitial pneumonitis via PFTs and high resolution CT scan prompt permanent discontinuation of the drug (Cohenuram & Saif, 2007).

(Continued on next page)

Table 26. Pulmonary Toxicity of Chemotherapeutic Drugs *(Continued)*

Classification	Drug	Incidence	Characteristic Effects	Comments
Monoclonal antibodies *(cont.)*	Rituximab	38% (N = 135) experienced pulmonary events in clinical trials. Infusion-related deaths involving pulmonary function: 0.04%–0.07% Bronchospasm: 8% (Genentech, Inc., 2007b)	Most common adverse events were increased cough, rhinitis, bronchospasm, dyspnea, and sinusitis. Infusion-related symptom complex includes pulmonary effects: hypoxia, bronchospasm, dyspnea, pulmonary infiltrates, and ARDS (Genentech, Inc., 2007b). There have been reports of bronchiolitis obliterans presenting up to 6 months postinfusion and a limited number of reports of pneumonitis (including interstitial pneumonitis) presenting up to 3 months postinfusion, some of which resulted in fatal outcomes (Wagner et al., 2007).	Treatment should be interrupted for severe reactions and resumed at 50% reduced infusion rate when symptoms resolve. The safety of resuming or continuing administration of rituximab in patients with pneumonitis or bronchiolitis obliterans is unknown (Genentech, Inc., 2007b).
	Trastuzumab	As a single agent: • Increased cough: 26% • Dyspnea: 22% In the postmarketing setting, severe hypersensitivity reactions (including anaphylaxis), infusion reactions, and pulmonary adverse events have been reported. Severe pulmonary events leading to death have been reported rarely (Genentech, Inc., 2008).	Increased cough, dyspnea, rhinitis, pharyngitis, pulmonary infiltrates, pleural effusions, noncardiac edema, pulmonary insufficiency, hypoxia, and ARDS (Genentech, Inc., 2008) Other severe events reported rarely in the postmarketing setting include pneumonitis and pulmonary fibrosis (Genentech, Inc., 2008).	Patients with symptomatic intrinsic lung disease or extensive tumor involvement of the lungs, resulting in dyspnea at rest, may be at greater risk for severe reactions. Adverse effects increase with combined drug therapy (Genentech, Inc., 2008).
Nitrosoureas	Carmustine	Although rare, cases of fatal pulmonary toxicity have been reported. Most of these patients were receiving prolonged therapy with total doses of carmustine greater than 1,400 mg/m². However, there have been reports of pulmonary fibrosis in patients receiving lower total doses (Bristol-Myers Squibb Oncology, 2007a). In a long-term study of carmustine, all those initially treated at younger than 5 years of age died of delayed pulmonary fibrosis (Bristol-Myers Squibb, 2007a).	Pulmonary infiltrates and/or fibrosis have been reported to occur from 9 days to 43 months after treatment and appear to be dose-related. Fibrosis may be slowly progressive (Bristol-Myers Squibb, 2007a). When used in high doses (300–600 mg/m²) prior to bone marrow transplantation, pulmonary toxicity may occur and may be dose limiting. The pulmonary toxicity of high-dose carmustine may manifest as severe interstitial pneumonitis, which occurs most frequently in patients who have had recent radiation to the mediastinum. There is a linear relationship between total dose and pulmonary toxicity at doses > 1,000 mg/m², with 50% of patients developing pulmonary toxicity at total cumulative doses of 1,500 mg/m². Risk factors include preexisting lung disease, smoking, cyclophosphamide therapy, and recent (within months) thoracic radiation. Patients with baseline forced vital capacity and/or pulmonary diffusion capacity for carbon monoxide that are less than 70% of the predicted value are at high risk (Bristol-Myers Squibb, 2007a).	Perform baseline and regular PFTs tests, especially in patients with risk factors or who have received > 800 mg/m².

(Continued on next page)

Table 26. Pulmonary Toxicity of Chemotherapeutic Drugs *(Continued)*

Classification	Drug	Incidence	Characteristic Effects	Comments
Nitrosoureas *(cont.)*	Lomustine	Rare, usually in doses > 1,100 mg/m^2 (one reported case at a dose of 600 mg/m^2) (Bristol-Myers Squibb, 2006b) There appeared to be some late reduction of pulmonary function of all long-term survivors. This form of lung fibrosis may be slowly progressive and has resulted in death in some cases (Bristol-Myers Squibb, 2006b).	Pulmonary toxicity characterized by pulmonary infiltrates and/or fibrosis has been reported rarely with lomustine. Onset of toxicity has occurred after an interval of 6 months or longer from the start of therapy with cumulative doses of lomustine usually > 1,100 mg/m^2 (Bristol-Myers Squibb, 2006b). Delayed-onset pulmonary fibrosis occurring up to 17 years after treatment has been reported in patients who received nitrosoureas in childhood and early adolescence (1–16 years) combined with cranial radiotherapy for intracranial tumors (Bristol-Myers Squibb, 2006b).	Establish baseline pulmonary function. Monitor high-risk patients with PFTs.
Plant alkaloids	Docetaxel	Non-dose-related interstitial pneumonitis with pulmonary fibrosis occurs in approximately 3%–5% of cases, most often manifesting 4–8 weeks after exposure (Leimgruber et al., 2006; Sanofi-Aventis Pharmaceuticals, 2008).	Pulmonary infiltrates, pleural effusion, pulmonary edema	Pleural effusions may be reversible with diuretics (Sanofi-Aventis Pharmaceuticals, 2008). Pulmonary fibrosis is not consistently responsive to corticosteroids (Sanofi-Aventis Pharmaceuticals, 2008).
	Etoposide	Reported cases of pulmonary events have been reported infrequently: interstitial pneumonitis/pulmonary fibrosis; anaphylactic-like reactions characterized by chills, fever, tachycardia, bronchospasm, dyspnea, and/or hypotension have been reported to occur in 0.7%–2% of patients receiving IV etoposide and in less than 1% of patients treated with the oral capsules (Bristol-Myers Squibb, 2007b; Post et al., 2007).	Anaphylactic-like reactions have occurred during the initial infusion of etoposide. Facial/tongue swelling, coughing, diaphoresis, cyanosis, tightness in throat, laryngospasm, back pain, and/or loss of consciousness have sometimes occurred in association with aforementioned reactions. In addition, an apparent hypersensitivity-associated apnea has been reported rarely.	Higher rates of anaphylactic-like reactions have been reported in children who received infusions at concentrations higher than those recommended. The role that concentration of infusion (or rate of infusion) plays in the development of anaphylactic-like reactions is uncertain. Treatment is symptomatic (Bristol-Myers Squibb, 2007b). PET scintigraphy may demonstrate clear ventilation abnormalities with etoposide pulmonary toxicity (Post et al., 2007).
	Paclitaxel	Rare for single agent: 2% dyspnea Rare reports of interstitial pneumonia, lung fibrosis, and pulmonary embolism (Bristol-Myers Squibb, 2007c) 8.5%–9% combined therapy Events usually occur with high doses or in combined therapy (Bristol-Myers Squibb, 2007c; Dunsford et al., 1999).	Hypersensitivity pneumonitis (Dunsford et al., 1999) Rare reports of radiation pneumonitis have been received in patients receiving concurrent radiotherapy (Bristol-Myers Squibb, 2007c).	Rarely severe or fatal, often responsive to corticosteroids (Ostoros et al., 2006)

(Continued on next page)

Table 26. Pulmonary Toxicity of Chemotherapeutic Drugs (Continued)

Classification	Drug	Incidence	Characteristic Effects	Comments
Plant alkaloids (cont.)	Vinorelbine tartrate	Shortness of breath was reported in 3% of patients; it was severe in 2% receiving vinorelbine. Rare but severe: Reported cases of interstitial pulmonary changes and ARDS, most of which were fatal, occurred in patients treated with single-agent vinorelbine (Mayne Pharma, 2006b).	Acute shortness of breath and severe bronchospasm, most commonly when vinorelbine was used in combination with mitomycin; these adverse events may require treatment with supplemental oxygen, bronchodilators, and/or corticosteroids, particularly when there is preexisting pulmonary dysfunction. The mean time to onset of these symptoms after vinorelbine administration was 1 week (range = 3–8 days).	Patients with alterations in their baseline pulmonary symptoms or with new onset of dyspnea, cough, hypoxia, or other symptoms should be evaluated promptly (Mayne Pharma, 2006b).
Targeted therapies: mTOR inhibitors	Temsirolimus	Incidence is 1%–36% of patients treated for renal cell cancer (Duran et al., 2006; Vahid & Marik, 2008).	Unclear mechanism of non-dose-dependent interstitial pneumonitis (Vahid & Marik, 2008)	Because clinical features are ill-defined, discontinuation of the medication is recommended when signs of interstitial pneumonitis are evident (Vahid & Marik, 2008).
Targeted therapies: Tyrosine kinase inhibitors	Dasatinib	Pleural effusion occured in approximately 35% of patients across multiple studies (Bristol-Myers Squibb, 2008b; Quintas-Cardama et al., 2007).	Most effusions are exudative and are characterized by lymphocytic infiltration of the pleura (Bergeron et al., 2007). Most patients who develop grades 3 and 4 pleural effusions have accelerated or blast phase chronic myeloid leukemia (Quintas-Cardama et al., 2007). Pleural effusion is more prevalent in twice-daily dosing (Quintas-Cardama et al., 2007). Symptoms include dyspnea, cough, and chest pain (Bergeron et al., 2007; Bristol-Myers Squibb, 2008b).	Most pleural effusions are reversible but may recur with future treatment (Bergeron et al., 2007). Treatment may include interruption of medication, diuretics, or corticosteroids (Bergeron et al., 2007; Quintas-Cardama et al., 2007).
	Erlotinib	Incidence is rare (< 1%) except when given in combination with gemcitabine, where incidence is approximately 2.5% (Genentech, Inc. & OSI Pharmaceuticals, 2007; Vahid & Marik, 2008).	Fatal ILD has been associated with oral erlotinib therapy for lung cancer (Liu et al., 2007; Vahid & Marik, 2008). Can occur days to months after exposure. Occasional pleural effusion has been reported (Toh et al., 2007).	Some patients have shown clinical improvement with corticosteroid treatment (Vahid & Marik, 2008). Strongly suspicious erlotinib-induced lung injury warrants discontinuation of the drug (Genentech, Inc. & OSI Pharmaceuticals, 2007).
	Gefitinib	Cases of ILD have been observed in patients at an overall incidence of about 1%. Approximately one-third of the cases have been fatal. Reports indicated that ILD has occurred in patients who have received prior radiation therapy (31%), prior chemotherapy (57%), and no previous therapy (12%) (AstraZeneca Pharmaceuticals, 2005).	Interstitial pneumonia, pneumonitis, and alveolitis. Patients often present with acute-onset dyspnea, sometimes associated with cough or low-grade fever, often becoming severe within a short time and requiring hospitalization. Increased mortality has been observed in patients with concurrent idiopathic pulmonary fibrosis whose condition worsens while receiving gefitinib (AstraZeneca Pharmaceuticals, 2005).	If acute onset or worsening of pulmonary symptoms (dyspnea, cough, fever) occurs, therapy should be interrupted and promptly investigated. If ILD is confirmed, discontinue.

(Continued on next page)

Table 26. Pulmonary Toxicity of Chemotherapeutic Drugs (Continued)

Classification	Drug	Incidence	Characteristic Effects	Comments
Targeted therapies: Tyrosine kinase inhibitors (cont.)	Imatinib mesylate	Severe superficial edema and severe fluid retention (pleural effusion, pulmonary edema, and ascites) were reported in 1%–6% of patients taking imatinib for gastrointestinal stromal tumors (Vahid & Marik, 2008). Dyspnea was reported in 14%–15% of patients. Interstitial pneumonitis and pulmonary fibrosis are rare (Novartis Pharmaceuticals, 2007).	In two studies, 54%–74% of patients had fluid retention, making pulmonary events difficult to identify. Fluid retention events include pleural effusion, ascites, pulmonary edema, pericardial effusion, and anasarca (Ishii et al., 2006). Fluid extravasation and pleural effusions appear to be dose-related, were more common in the blast crisis and accelerated phase studies (where the dose was 600 mg/day), and were more common in older adults (Vahid & Marik, 2008). However, a few of these events may be serious or life-threatening, and one patient with blast crisis died with pleural effusion, congestive heart failure, and renal failure (Deininger et al., 2003; Novartis Pharmaceuticals, 2007).	These events usually were managed by interrupting imatinib mesylate treatment and using diuretics or other appropriate supportive care measures. The symptoms often resurface when rechallenging with this agent (Vahid & Marik, 2008). The overall safety profile of pediatric patients (39 children studied) was similar to that found in studies with adult patients treated with imatinib; however, no peripheral edema has been reported (Novartis Pharmaceuticals, 2007).
	Topotecan hydrochloride	The incidence of grades 3 and/or 4 dyspnea was 4% in patients with ovarian cancer and 12% in patients with small cell lung cancer (GlaxoSmithKline, 2008a). Pulmonary fibrosis may occur, but there is only one documented pathologic confirmation of this complication (Maitland et al., 2006). All grades, dyspnea: 22% (GlaxoSmithKline, 2008a)	Dyspnea, coughing, and pneumonia are the main pulmonary side effects (GlaxoSmithKline, 2008a).	Establish baseline pulmonary function.

ARDS—adult respiratory distress syndrome; CT—computed tomography; 5-FU/LV—5-fluorouracil/leucovorin; IFN—interferon; IL—interleukin; ILD—interstitial lung disease; IV—intravenous; mTOR—mammalian target of rapamycin; PET—positron-emission tomography; PFT—pulmonary function test; PO—oral

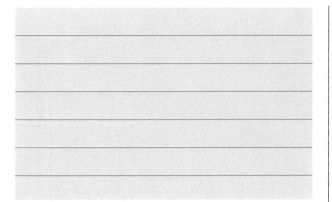

the development of pulmonary toxicity as more drug is administered (e.g., carmustine) (Bristol-Myers Squibb, 2007a).

(f) Long-term treatment (e.g., busulfan treatment) (Barton-Burke et al., 2007)

(5) Risk factors of direct injury

(a) Use of hydroxyurea has resulted in rare reports of interstitial pulmonary infiltrates and acute alveolitis (Hennemann, Bross, Reichle, & Andreesen, 1993; Kavuru, Gadsden, Lichtin, & Gephardt, 1994).

(b) Metabolic injury

i) Metabolites of cyclophosphamide cause acute pneumonitis that may be hemorrhagic in nature. The mortality rate associated with this syndrome is approximately 50% (Kachel & Martin, 1994; Malik et al., 1996; Specks, 2008; Twohig & Matthay, 1990).

ii) Renal dysfunction may cause delayed drug excretion and increased pulmonary toxicity of cyclophosphamide and bleomycin (Kachel & Martin, 1994; McLeod et al., 1987; Specks, 2008).

(c) Disruption of intracellular kinases

i) Tyrosine kinase inhibitors (e.g., gefitinib, erlotinib) (Endo, Johkoh, Kimura, & Yamamoto, 2006; Ieki, Saitoh, & Shibuya, 2003)

ii) EGFRIs (e.g., cetuximab)

iii) mTOR inhibitors (e.g., temsirolimus) (Duran et al., 2006; Klastersky, 2006)

- An intracellular kinase that directs protein production
- When activated, mTOR fosters cancer cell growth and proliferation, and angiogenesis (Novartis Oncology U.S., 2008).

(d) Pulmonary edema

i) Biologic agents are key offending agents that cause this toxicity (Antoniou, Ferdoutsis, & Bouros, 2003; Schwartzentruber, 2005).

- A high incidence of capillary leak syndrome is associated with IL-2, but it resolves quickly after therapy ends and diuresis begins.
- Pulmonary edema is a dose-limiting toxicity of high-dose IL-2 therapy (NCI CTEP, 2006; Siegel & Puri, 1991).
- Severity depends on the route, dose, and administration schedule (Conant, Fox, & Miller, 1989; Schwartzentruber, 2005).

ii) Docetaxel is associated with fluid retention and associated alveolar permeability and pulmonary infiltrates that may be prevented with corticosteroid premedication and is treatable with diuretics (King, 2007c; Leimgruber et al., 2006; Pronk, Stoter, & Verweij, 1995).

iii) Cytosine arabinoside (Forghieri et al., 2007; Haupt, Hutchins, & Moore, 1981)

iv) Leuprolide acetate (Ferrari, Pezzuto, & Coppola, 2007)

v) Tyrosine kinase inhibitors, such as bortezomib, gefitinib, dasatinib, and imatinib mesylate, cause capillary permeability, pulmonary edema, and effusions (Miyakoshi et al., 2006; Vahid & Marik, 2008).

(e) Hemorrhagic pneumonitis

i) Cyclophosphamide

ii) Gemcitabine (Carron et al., 2001)

iii) Rituximab (Alexandrescu et al., 2004)

iv) Thalidomide

(f) Hypersensitivity pneumonitis
  i) Paclitaxel can cause acute pneumonitis, which appears to be a hypersensitivity reaction to Cremophor® EL emulsifier (Camp et al., 2007; Goldberg & Vannice, 1995; Ramanathan, Belani, & Reddy, 1996; Read, Mortimer, & Picus, 2002).
  ii) Docetaxel: Occurs in 7%–47%; factors affecting variability of occurrence include total dose, chemotherapy schedule, and concurrent administration with gemcitabine or radiotherapy (Grande, Villanueva, Huidobro, & Casal, 2007).
  iii) Acute methotrexate reaction is likely allergic in origin (Davis, Williams, & Walker, 2003; Lateef, Shakoor, & Balk, 2005).

d) Clinical manifestations
  (1) May be difficult to detect when clinical manifestations are subtle
  (2) Signs and symptoms
    (a) Dyspnea
    (b) Tachypnea
    (c) Increased work of breathing
    (d) Dry nonproductive cough
    (e) Hypoxemia: Cyanosis, low oxygen saturation
    (f) Demonstrated anxiety, uneasiness
  (3) Timing of signs and symptoms
    (a) Hypersensitivity reactions may occur as early as hours after exposure (Kohli, Ferencz, & Calderon, 2004).
    (b) Average timing of hypersensitivity pneumonitis is 7–10 days after exposure.
    (c) Methotrexate hypersensitivity reactions occur 12–18 hours after first dose (Balk, 2007).
    (d) Delayed toxicity may occur 8 months–10 years after therapy initiation (Tenenbaum, 1994).

e) Assessment
  (1) Past medical history
    (a) Key chemobiotherapy drug exposure
    (b) Other medications known to cause pulmonary toxicity: These may include but are not limited to amiodarone, nitrofurantoin, penicillamine, phenytoin, and procainamide (Bhagat, Spor, Long, & Folz, 2001; Chernecky, 2008; Vahid & Marek, 2008).
    (c) Other pulmonary conditions—recent or chronic (Klastersky, 2006)
    (d) Recent viral illnesses that predispose to hemorrhagic airway disease
    (e) Autoimmune or connective tissue disease (Chernecky, 2008; King, 2007a; Lake, 2007; Varga, 2007)
    (f) Occupational exposures: Can help to rule out similar lung disorders and unexpected exposures such as exposure to silica, dusts, coal, and cotton (Chernecky, 2008; Daba et al., 2004)
    (g) Environmental exposures such as asbestos, gases, and dusts (Chernecky, 2008; Daba et al., 2004)
  (2) Physical examination
    (a) Vital signs—tachypnea, tachycardia
    (b) Crackles on auscultation
    (c) Cough and sputum production, hemoptysis
    (d) Pleuritic pain—may accompany some disorders (e.g., erlotinib)
    (e) Accessory muscle use for breathing
    (f) Evidence of poor tissue oxygenation—cyanosis, oliguria, decreased bowel sounds, altered mentation
  (3) Diagnostic tests
    (a) Arterial blood gases usually show hypoxemia with respiratory alkalosis.
    (b) Changes suggesting pulmonary edema are observed in approxi-

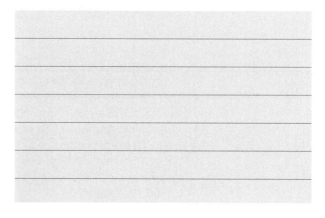

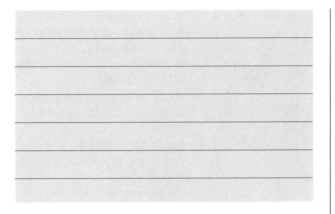

mately 20% of radiographs of patients receiving high-dose IL-2 (Berthiaume et al., 1995; Siegel & Puri, 1991).

(c) Chest x-ray shows ground glass opacities/infiltrates and interstitial or alveolar thickening of interlobular septum (Endo et al., 2006; Stark, 2007). Nodular patterns indicate fibrosis (Stark).

(d) Chest CT is highly sensitive and able to differentiate pneumonitis from pulmonary embolism or fibrosis that may also occur in patients with cancer experiencing respiratory distress (Endo et al., 2006; Forghieri et al., 2007).

(e) A sensitive test of pulmonary function is the carbon monoxide diffusing capacity that is reduced prior to symptoms in many patients (Bahhady & Unterborn, 2003; Ngan et al., 1993; Segura et al., 2001).

(f) Serum markers KL-6, SP-A, and SP-D have been used as indicators of ILD for some agents (e.g., gefitinib) (Kitajima et al., 2006).

(g) Positron-emission tomography scintigraphy has been helpful for early diagnosis of pulmonary fibrosis related to etoposide (Post et al., 2007).

(h) Open lung biopsy provides definitive diagnosis (King, 2007b).

f) Collaborative management

(1) Pulmonary function testing is a prerequisite for the following patients being evaluated for biotherapy (particularly for treatment with IL-2) (Chiron Corporation, 2002; Letizia & Conway, 1996).

(a) Heavy smokers (> 10 cigarettes/day) (Fernander, Schumacher, Wei, Crooks, & Wedlund, 2008)

(b) Patients with extensive pulmonary disease

(c) Patients with symptoms suggesting decreased pulmonary reserve such as exercise intolerance, new cough, or tachypnea (Chernecky & Shelton, 2001; Ngan et al., 1993)

(2) Avoid exceeding maximum doses.

(a) Bleomycin: 400 units/m^2 (Lasky & Ortiz, 2007)

(b) Mitomycin-C: 30 mg/m^2 (Chan & King, 2007)

(3) If pulmonary toxicity is suspected, hold chemotherapy and notify prescriber.

(4) Administer oxygen cautiously and only if patient is hypoxemic.

(a) Some lung-toxic medications have increased toxicity with oxygen therapy (e.g., bleomycin).

(b) Oxygen can cause absorption atelectasis and loss of surfactant that may exacerbate toxicity risk.

(5) Establish fluid balance goals.

(a) Carefully record intake and output.

(b) Determine if fluid boluses or fluid restrictions are warranted.

(c) Consider using goal "dry" weight to target diuretic therapy. Weigh patient on a regular basis.

(d) Diuretics work to decrease parenchymal edema by filtering fluid from the vascular space, thereby causing the body to replenish vascular fluid by drawing fluid from interstitial spaces. This is not always effective when capillary permeability is impaired and cell and vessel boundaries have been compromised.

(6) Supportive care

(a) Oxygen therapy: When using bleomycin, be aware of reports of oxygen-induced lung damage (Bristol-Myers Squibb, 2004).

(b) Bronchodilators: Metered dose inhaler provides better delivery than nebulizer.

(c) Position for best breathing: Head of bed elevated, tripod position (arms elevated and extended with knees separated while leaning forward), legs over side of bed

(7) Treatment of possible etiologies of ILD

(a) Administer corticosteroids as ordered. Corticosteroids usually are contraindicated for patients receiving biotherapy that acts by enhancing immunostimulatory activity.

(b) Antimicrobial therapy may be considered when it is unclear if there is an infection superimposed upon other lung toxicities.

(c) Oral carnosine to abrogate bleomycin pulmonary toxicity has anecdotal reports of success (Cuzzocrea et al., 2007).

(8) Follow-up evaluation of patients at risk

(a) Monitor x-rays and CT scans routinely.

i) Targeted therapies are recommend at least monthly.

ii) Frequency is based upon perceived risk for ILD and may increase in frequency with cumulative dose or added risk factors.

iii) A chest radiograph may be recommended every one to two weeks to monitor for bleomycin toxicity (Bristol-Myers Squibb, 2004).

(b) Periodic monitoring of pulmonary function tests (average of every three months) (Chernecky, 2008)

i) Forced vital capacity and forced expiratory volume in one minute are sensitive for fibrotic changes

ii) Used more frequently to detect pulmonary fibrosis.

g) Patient and family education (Camp-Sorrell, 2005; Hood & Harwood, 2004)

(1) Provide education regarding symptoms associated with pulmonary toxicity (e.g., cough, dyspnea, chest pain, shallow breathing, chest wall discomfort). Make sure all patients, including outpatients receiving SC IL-2, know to seek medical assistance immediately if symptoms begin.

(2) Make sure that patients receiving therapy know that agent may be delayed or held until pulmonary symptoms resolve.

(3) Explore with patients their wishes regarding intubation and resuscitation status; establish advance directives.

(4) Teach patients that raising the head of the bed may facilitate breathing.

(5) Instruct patients to conserve energy by performing daily activities when their energy level is highest.

(6) Teach patients and significant others methods to decrease symptoms of dyspnea by exercising to tolerance, practicing pursed-lip breathing, refraining from smoking, and using a small fan.

(7) Teach patients to take an opioid (in most cases, morphine) as prescribed by a physician; opioids may relieve the discomfort caused by air hunger.

(8) Review the safety issues (e.g., flammability) related to oxygen administration.

2. Alveolar hemorrhage

a) Pathophysiology

(1) Bleeding into the alveolar spaces has long been associated with viral infection and certain toxic injuries.

(2) Vascular endothelial wall destruction by chemotherapy or chemoradiotherapy causes microcapillary bleeding. Why the alveolus is the target organ rather than GI system or uroendothelium is unclear, and pulmonary hemorrhage often occurs in isolation rather than linked to GI bleeding or hematuria.

b) Incidence

(1) Alveolar hemorrhage incidence rates are 1.9% in nonmyeloablative transplant regimens (Wanko, Broadwater, Foltz, & Chao, 2006) and as high as 10.3% in myeloablative HSCT (Lewis, DeFor, & Weisdorf, 2000; Majhail, Parks, DeFor, & Weisdorf, 2006; Wanko et al., 2006).

(2) Pediatric transplant sources suggest an incidence rate of about 5% (Heggen et al., 2002).

c) Risk factors

(1) Alveolar hemorrhage is most well-documented in the setting of HSCT,

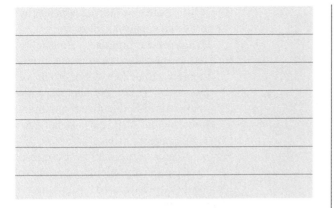

although some acute pneumonitis syndromes also may be hemorrhagic in nature (Alexandrescu et al., 2004; Carron et al., 2001; Lin et al., 2005).

(2) Alveolar hemorrhage has been rarely associated with normal doses of gemcitabine, bevacizumab, and cyclophosphamide (Vahid & Marik, 2008).

(3) Concomitant pulmonary infection is documented with cytomegalovirus, adenovirus, and strongloides (parasite).

(4) Unlike other bleeding syndromes, pulmonary hemorrhage is not always related to platelet counts or coagulation values.

d) Clinical manifestations

(1) The onset of bleeding is usually within the first two weeks after the preparative regimen.

(2) Symptoms include dyspnea, cough, chest discomfort, and profound hypoxemia.

(3) Hemoptysis is rare, although pink, frothy sputum may occur, and bronchoalveolar specimens may be bloody.

e) Assessment

(1) Breath sounds

(2) Sputum quantity and quality

(3) Hgb, platelet count, coagulation parameters

(a) Hgb may not fall until bleeding is life-threatening.

(b) Platelet goal is > 50,000/mm^3.

(4) Diagnosis may be suspected with bilateral interstitial infiltrates on x-ray or CT scan.

(5) Bronchoalveolar lavage with bloody returns, higher yield than instilled, and positive hemosiderin-laden macrophages in the sputum is considered diagnostic (Vahid & Marik, 2008).

f) Collaborative management

(1) Corticosteroids are standard treatment although not proven effective

(Grigoriyan, Rishi, Molina, Homer, & Manthous, 2007).

(2) Coagulation factors are the standard treatments, although no one therapy is proven effective (Grigoriyan et al., 2007).

(3) Consider mechanical ventilation with positive pressure to tamponade bleeding.

3. Acute promyelocytic leukemia differentiation syndrome/retinoic acid syndrome (NCI CTEP, 2006)

a) Pathophysiology

(1) Created by rapid proliferation and differentiation of WBCs causing immunologic stimulation with inflammatory capillary permeability of the lungs and rash (Ahmed et al., 2007; Bi & Jiang, 2006)

(2) First named retinoic acid syndrome because of its propensity to occur when patients with acute progranulocytic leukemia (M3 leukemia) received all-trans-retinoic acid (Au & Kwong, 2008; Fenaux, Wang, & Degos, 2007)

(3) More a condition of tumor responsiveness to therapy than an actual toxicity of the therapy

b) Incidence

(1) Also associated with administration of arsenic trioxide in the same population of patients (Au & Kwong, 2008; Fenaux et al., 2007; Jin, Hou, Liu, & Yu, 2006)

(2) Also has occurred in other settings of retinoid administration, even with non-M3 leukemia, emphasizing the need for monitoring when administering any retinoid or differentiating agent (DiNardo et al., 2008)

(3) Reported to occur in 10%–15% of patients receiving combination retinoid and chemotherapy and is more prevalent in patients with high WBC counts (Fenaux et al., 2007)

c) Risk factors

(1) High WBC count

(2) Acute leukemia, M3 subtype

(3) All-trans-retinoic acid treatment

(4) Arsenic trioxide

d) Clinical manifestations

(1) Fever, rash, dyspnea, cough, crackles, and hypoxemia

(2) Occurs 7–20 days after initiation of treatment (Bi & Jiang, 2006)

e) Assessment

(1) WBC count daily

(2) Periodic evaluation of coagulation parameters, platelet count

(3) Intake and output; monitor for over-hydration.

(4) Breath sounds

f) Collaborative management

(1) Prevention

(a) Immediate administration of chemotherapy when WBC count rises

(b) Platelet goal 50,000/mm³

(c) Fluid management (strict intake and output)

(2) Immediate treatment with corticosteroids (Cupitt, 2000) and conventional chemotherapy may improve outcomes, but the syndrome still carries an approximate 10% mortality rate (Ahmed et al., 2007; Fenaux et al., 2007).

4. Pleural effusions

a) Pathophysiology

(1) Pleural effusions are defined as accumulation of excess fluid in the pleural space that impairs lung expansion.

(2) As excess fluid is retained in the pleural space, there is resistance to full alveolar expansion (Allibone, 2006).

(3) Four to six liters of pleural fluid usually pass daily through the potential space between the visceral and parietal pleura.

b) Incidence of drug-related pleural effusions

(1) Incidence varies and is dependent upon agent, dose, schedule, and comorbid conditions.

(2) Pleural effusions can be detected radiographically in 42%–52% of patients receiving IL-2. In general, no intervention is required; effusions resolve after IL-2 is discontinued (Shelton, 2009).

(3) Incidence can be as high as 35% with some agents (Quintas-Cardama et al., 2007).

c) Risk factors

(1) Major causes of pleural effusion

(a) Obstruction to fluid outflow (Allibone, 2006)

(b) Pleural irritation leading to exudative capillary permeability into the space (Allibone, 2006)

(2) Pleural effusions are a common complication of cancer and other medical disorders such as CHF, renal failure, or hypothyroidism.

(3) When associated with chemotherapy and biologic therapies, pleural effusions are the result of capillary permeability that is temporally related to administration of the offending agent.

(4) Chemotherapy and biotherapy agents that have been associated with development of pleural effusions include

(a) Bortezomib (Pitini, Arrigio, Altavilla, & Naro, 2007)

(b) Cytosine arabinoside

(c) Cyclophosphamide (high-dose)

(d) Dasatinib (Bergeron et al., 2007; Hochhaus, 2007; Ishii, Shoji, Kimura, & Ohyashiki, 2006; Quintas-Cardama et al., 2007)

(e) Docetaxel (Toh et al., 2007)

(f) Erlotinib (Toh et al., 2007)

(g) Imatinib (2%–6%) (Bergeron et al., 2007; Ishii et al., 2006)

(h) Oprelvekin (Wyeth Laboratories, 2008b)

(i) Pemetrexed (Brandes, Grossman, & Ahmad, 2006).

d) Clinical manifestations/assessment

(1) Patients present with tachypnea, dyspnea, increased work of breathing, abnormal chest excursion, and fatigue.

(2) Large pleural effusions are easily documented by obtaining an upright chest x-ray.

(3) Smaller effusions are seen on chest CT.

(4) Tyrosine kinase inhibitor–induced pleural effusions are characterized by exudative features and lymphocytic infiltration of the pleura.

e) Collaborative management

(1) In most cases, pleural effusions are uncomplicated, and discontinuing the causative agents results in spontaneous resolution of the pleural effusion (Quintas-Cardama et al., 2007).

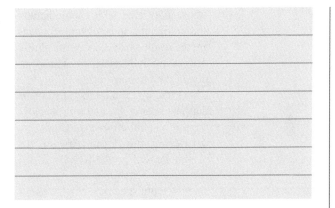

(2) Dose reduction has been success-ful at eliminating pleural effusion related to dasatinib (Bergeron et al., 2007).

(3) Other treatment strategies have includ-ed diuretics and corticosteroids, but neither intervention has a large body of evidence to support use (Bergeron et al., 2007; Quintas-Cardama et al., 2007).

5. Pulmonary alveolar proteinosis
   a) Pathophysiology
      (1) Condition is characterized by intra-alveolar accumulation of surfactant components and cell fragments.
      (2) The thick proteinacious exudate causes bronchiolar occlusion, poor respiratory compliance, and hypoxemia (Pedroso et al., 2007).
   b) Incidence: Disorder is rare.
   c) Risk factors (Inaba et al., 2007; Miyoshi, Daibata, Takemoto, Machida, & Taguchi, 2005; Pamuk et al., 2003; Shoji et al., 2002)
      (1) Hematologic malignancies
      (2) MDS
      (3) Profound neutropenia at the onset of the disorder
      (4) It is unclear whether this disorder is caused by antineoplastic agents such as alkylating agents (Inaba et al., 2007) or imatinib (Wagner et al., 2003) or the underlying disease itself.
      (5) It has also been linked to the infection with *Acinetobacter* (Goldschmidt et al., 2003), *Pneumocystis* (Akin & Nguyen, 2004), or *Mycobacterium* (Goldschmidt et al.).
   d) Clinical manifestations
      (1) Dyspnea, tachypnea, cough, and in-creased work of breathing
      (2) Tend to occur over a few days, with progressive worsening

(3) CT scans show widespread air-space consolidation with "crazy-paving" patterns (Akin & Nguyen, 2004).
(4) Diagnosed by bronchoscopy or lung biopsy specimens that stain positive for periodic acid-Schiff
(5) Usually corrects itself when patients go into remission or recover normal WBC counts (Pamuk et al., 2003)
(6) May be fatal in patients with persistent disease or those who failed to recover counts (Goldschmidt et al., 2003; Inaba et al., 2007)
   e) Collaborative management (Inaba et al., 2007; Kim, Kim, & Kim, 2004; Pamuk et al., 2003)
      (1) Antibiotics
      (2) Corticosteroids
      (3) Lung lavage
6. Pulmonary VOD
   a) Pathophysiology
      (1) VOD of the liver is a common reported complication of high-dose alkylating agents, TBI, and gemtuzumab (Bunte, Patnaik, Pritzker, & Burns, 2008; McKoy et al., 2007).
      (2) Fibrotic changes in the hepatic venules lead to stiff and fibrotic vessels with portal hypertension. This pathophysi-ology is likely the same in the lungs.
      (3) Post-capillary pulmonary venular obstruc-tion has been documented in the lungs and is called pulmonary VOD (Bunte et al., 2008; Hackman, Madtes, Petersen, & Clark, 1989; Salzman, Adkins, Craig, Freytes, & LeMaistre, 1996).
      (4) Endothelial wall damage is the pro-posed mechanism of injury (Bunte et al., 2008).
      (5) The clinical result of this process is pulmonary hypertension, with right heart failure.
      (6) Pulmonary VOD presents 40–60 days post-HSCT as hypoxemia, volume dependent hypotension, atrial arrhyth-mias, right bundle branch block, or he-patic congestion (Bunte et al., 2008).
   b) Incidence
      (1) Infrequent manifestation of endothelial injury in < 2% of transplant recipients
      (2) Likely underestimated because of symptoms mimicking other similar adverse effects
   c) Risk factors
      (1) Matched unrelated transplant
      (2) High-dose alkylating agents
      (3) Prior lung injury

d) Clinical manifestations and assessment
  (1) Definitive diagnosis requires a right heart catheterization, but elevated right heart pressures on echocardiogram also may be suggestive of this disorder.
  (2) CT demonstrates perihilar infiltrates, and thickening of major pulmonary veins that are unique to pulmonary VOD differentiate pulmonary hypertension from other causes (Bunte et al., 2008; Dufour et al., 1998).
e) Collaborative management
  (1) No clear treatment has been identified.
  (2) Most documented cases have been fatal (Bunte et al., 2008).

References

Ahmed, Z., Shaikh, M.A., Raval, A., Mehta, J.B., Byrd, R.P. Jr., & Roy, T.M. (2007). All-trans retinoic acid syndrome: Another cause of drug-induced respiratory failure. *Southern Medical Journal, 100*(9), 899–902.

Akin, M.R., & Nguyen, G.K. (2004). Pulmonary alveolar proteinosis. *Pathology, Research and Practice, 200*(10), 693–698.

Alexandrescu, D.T., Dutcher, J.P., O'Boyle, K., Albulak, M., Oiseth, S., & Wiernik, P.H. (2004). Fatal intra-alveolar hemorrhage after rituximab in a patient with non-Hodgkin lymphoma. *Leukemia and Lymphoma, 45*(11), 2321–2325.

Allibone, L. (2006). Assessment and management of patients with pleural effusions. *Nursing Standard, 20*(37), 59.

Amgen Inc. (2008). Vectibix [Package insert]. Thousand Oaks, CA: Author.

Antoniou, K.M., Ferdoutsis, E., & Bouros, D. (2003). Interferons and their application in the diseases of the lung. *Chest, 123*(1), 209–216.

Aronchick, J.M., & Gefter, W.B. (1991). Drug-induced pulmonary disease: An update. *Journal of Thoracic Imaging, 6*(1), 19–29.

AstraZeneca Pharmaceuticals. (2005). Iressa [Package insert]. Wilmington, DE: Author.

Au, W.Y., & Kwong, Y.L. (2008). Arsenic trioxide: Safety issues and their management. *Acta Pharmacologica Sinica, 29*(3), 296–304.

Bahhady, I.J., & Unterborn, J. (2003). What pulmonary function tests can and cannot tell you: Results help assess disease severity in ILD and COPD. *Journal of Respiratory Diseases, 24*(4), 170–176.

Balk, R.A. (2007). *Methotrexate-induced lung injury* [Up-To-Date Version 15.3, current as of August 2007]. Retrieved March 21, 2008, from http://www.uptodate.com/home/index.html

Bayer Healthcare Pharmaceuticals. (2007). Campath-1h [Package insert]. Wayne, NJ: Author.

Bergeron, A., Rea, D., Levy, V., Picard, C., Meignin, V., Tamburini, J., et al. (2007). Lung abnormalities after dasatinib treatment for chronic leukemia: A case series. *American Journal of Respiratory and Critical Care Medicine, 176*(8), 814–818.

Berlex Laboratories. (2006). Fludara [Package insert]. Richmond, CA: Author.

Berthiaume, Y., Boiteau, P., Fick, G., Kloiber, R., Sinclair, G.D., Fong, C., et al. (1995). Pulmonary edema during IL-2 therapy: Combined effect of increased permeability and hydrostatic pressure. *American Journal of Respiratory and Critical Care Medicine, 152*(1), 329–335.

Bhagat, R., Spor, T.A., Long, G.D., & Folz, R.J. (2001). Amiodarone and cyclophosphamide enhanced lung toxicity. *Bone Marrow Transplantation, 27*(10), 1109–1111.

Bi, K.H., & Jiang, G.S. (2006). Relationship between cytokines and leukocytosis in patients with APL induced by all-trans retinoic acid or arsenic trioxide. *Cellular and Molecular Immunology, 3*(6), 421–427.

Boeck, S., Hausmann, A., Reibke, R., Schultz, C., & Heinemann, V. (2007). Severe lung and skin toxicity during treatment with gemcitabine and erlotinib for metastatic pancreatic cancer. *Anticancer Drugs, 18*(9), 1109–1111.

Brandes, J.C., Grossman, S.A., & Ahmad, H. (2006). Alteration of pemetrexed excretion in the presence of acute renal failure and effusions: Presentation of a case and review of the literature. *Cancer Investigation, 24*(3), 283–287.

Bristol-Myers Squibb. (2000). Mutamycin [Package insert]. Princeton, NJ: Author.

Bristol-Myers Squibb. (2005). Cytoxan [Package insert]. Princeton, NJ: Author.

Bristol-Myers Squibb. (2006a). Blenoxane [Package insert]. Princeton, NJ: Author.

Bristol-Myers Squibb. (2006b). Lomustine [Package insert]. Princeton, NJ: Author.

Bristol-Myers Squibb. (2007a). BiCNU [Package insert]. Princeton, NJ: Author.

Bristol-Myers Squibb. (2007b). Etophos [Package insert]. Princeton, NJ: Author.

Bristol-Myers Squibb. (2007c). Taxol [Package insert]. Princeton, NJ: Author.

Bristol-Myers Squibb. (2008a). Ifex [Package insert]. Princeton, NJ: Author.

Bristol-Myers Squibb. (2008b). Sprycel [Package insert]. Princeton, NJ: Author.

Bristol-Myers Squibb/ImClone Systems. (2007). Erbitux [Package insert]. Princeton, NJ: Author.

Budinger, G.R., & Sznajder, J.I. (2006). The alveolar-epithelial barrier: A target for potential therapy. *Clinics in Chest Medicine, 27*(4), 655–669.

Bunte, M.C., Patnaik, M.M., Pritzker, M.R., & Burns, L.J. (2008). Pulmonary veno-occlusive disease following hematopoietic stem cell transplantation: A rare model of endothelial dysfunction. *Bone Marrow Transplantation, 41*(8), 677–686.

Camp, M.J., Gilmore, J.W., Gullatte, M.M., & Hutcherson, D.A. (2007). Antineoplastic agents. In M.M. Gullatte (Ed.), *Clinical guide to antineoplastic therapy: A chemotherapy handbook* (2nd ed., pp. 77–362). Pittsburgh, PA: Oncology Nursing Society.

Camp-Sorrell, D. (2005). Chemotherapy: Toxicity management. In C.H. Yarbro, M.H. Frogge, & M. Goodman (Eds.), *Cancer nursing: Principles and practice* (6th ed., pp. 412–457). Sudbury, MA: Jones and Bartlett.

Carron, P.L., Cousin, L., Caps, T., Belle, E., Pernet, D., Neidhardt, A., et al. (2001). Gemcitabine-associated diffuse alveolar hemorrhage. *Intensive Care Medicine, 27*(9), 1554.

Castleberry, R.P., Grist, W.M., Holbrook, T., Malluh, A., & Gaddy, D. (1981). The cytosine arabinoside (Ara-C) syndrome. *Medical and Pediatric Oncology, 9*(3), 257–264.

Celgene Corporation. (2007). Thalomid [Package insert]. Summit, NJ: Author.

Celgene Corporation. (2008). Revlimid [Package insert]. Summit, NJ: Author.

Cephalon. (2006). Trisenox [Package insert]. Frazer, PA: Author.

Chan, E.D., & King, Jr., T. (2007). *Mitomycin-C pulmonary toxicity* [Up-To-Date Version 15.3, current as of August 2007]. Retrieved March 21, 2008, from http://www.uptodate.com/home/index .html

Chernecky, C. (2008). Pulmonary fibrosis. In C.C. Chernecky & K. Murphy-Ende (Eds.), *Acute care oncology nursing* (2nd ed., pp. 442–454). Philadelphia: Elsevier Saunders.

Chernecky, C., & Shelton, B.K. (2001). Pulmonary complications in patients with cancer. *American Journal of Nursing, 101*(5), 24A–24H.

Chiron Corporation. (2002). Proleukin [Package insert]. Emeryville, CA: Author.

Chisholm, R.A., Dixon, A.K., Williams, M.V., & Oliver, R.T. (1992). Bleomycin lung: The effect of different chemotherapeutic regimens. *Cancer Chemotherapy and Pharmacology, 30*(2), 158–160.

Cohenuram, M., & Saif, M.W. (2007). Panitumumab: The first fully humanized monoclonal antibody, from bench to the clinic. *Anticancer Drugs, 18*(1), 7–15.

Comis, R.L. (1992). Bleomycin pulmonary toxicity: Current status and future directions. *Seminars in Oncology, 19*(2, Suppl. 5), 64–70.

Conant, E.F., Fox, K.R., & Miller, W.T. (1989). Pulmonary edema as a complication of interleukin-2 therapy. *American Journal of Roentgenology, 152*(4), 749–752.

Cupitt, J.M. (2000). A case for steroids in acute lung injury associated with the retinoic acid syndrome. *Anaesthesia and Intensive Care, 28*(2), 202–204.

Cuzzocrea, S., Genovese, T., Failla, M., Vecchio, G., Fruciano, M., Mazzon, E., et al. (2007). Protective effect of orally administered carnosine on bleomycin-induced lung injury. *American Journal of Physiology—and Lung Cellular Molecular Physiology, 292*(5), 1095–1104.

Czarnecki, A., & Voss, S. (2006). Pulmonary toxicity in patients treated with gemcitabine and a combination of gemcitabine and a taxane: Investigation of a signal using postmarketing data. *British Journal of Cancer, 94*(11), 1759–1760.

Daba, M.H., El-Tahir, K.E., Al-Arifi, M.N., & Gubara, O.A. (2004). Drug-induced pulmonary fibrosis. *Saudi Medical Journal, 25*(6), 700–706.

Davis, K.A., Williams, P., & Walker, J.C. (2003). Successful desensitization to high-dose methotrexate after systemic anaphylaxis. *Annals of Allergy, Asthma and Immunology, 90*(1), 87–89.

Deininger, M., O'Brien, S.G., Ford, J.M., & Druker, B.J. (2003). Practical management of patients with chronic myeloid leukemia receiving imatinib. *Journal of Clinical Oncology, 21*(8), 1637–1647.

DiNardo, C.D., Ky, B., Vogl, D.T., Forfia, P., Loren, A., Luger, S., et al. (2008). Differentiation syndrome in non-M3 acute myeloid leukemia treated with retinoid X receptor agonist bexarotene. *Medical Oncology, 25*(3), 299–302.

Dufour, B., Maitre, S., Humbert, M., Capron, F., Simmoneau, G., & Musset, D. (1998). High-resolution CT of the chest in four patients with pulmonary capillary hemangiomatosis or pulmonary venoocclusive disease. *American Journal of Roentgenology, 171*(5), 1321–1324.

Dunsford, M.L., Mead, G.M., Bateman, A.C., Cook, T., & Tung, K. (1999). Severe pulmonary toxicity in patients treated with a combination of docetaxel and gemcitabine for metastatic transitional cell carcinoma. *Annals of Oncology, 10*(8), 943–947.

Duran, I., Siu, L.L., Oza, A.M., Chung, T.B., Sturgeon, J., Townsley, C.A., et al. (2006). Characterization of the lung toxicity of the cell cycle inhibitor temsirolimus. *European Journal of Cancer, 42*(12), 1875–1880.

Eli Lilly & Co. (2007). Gemzar [Package insert]. Indianapolis, IN: Author.

Endo, M., Johkoh, T., Kimura, K., & Yamamoto, N. (2006). Imaging of gefitinib-related interstitial lung disease: Multi-institutional analysis by the West Japan Thoracic Oncology Group. *Lung Cancer, 52*(2), 135–140.

Enzon Pharmaceuticals. (2007). DepoCyt [Package insert]. Bridgewater, NJ: Author.

Erasmus, J.J. (2000). *Pulmonary drug toxicity: Pathogenesis and radiologic manifestations. Society of Thoracic Radiology Annual Meeting 2000* [Course syllabus]. Retrieved June 5, 2004, from http://www.thoracicrad.org/str99/TI2000/sundaypm.htm

Fenaux, P., Wang, Z.Z., & Degos, L. (2007). Treatment of acute promyelocytic leukemia by retinoids. *Current Topics in Microbiology and Immunology, 313,* 101–128.

Fernander, A., Schumacher, M., Wei, X., Crooks, P., & Wedlund, P. (2008). Smoking risk and the likelihood of quitting among African-American female light and heavy smokers. *JAMA, 100*(10), 1199–206.

Ferrari, B., Pezzuto, A., & Coppola, F. (2007). Massive ascites and hydrothorax after leuprolide acetate administration in a down-regulated woman undergoing assisted reproduction. *Fertility and Sterility, 88*(4), 9–11.

Forghieri, F., Luppi, M., Morselli, M., & Potenza, L. (2007). Cytarabine-related lung infiltrates on high resolution computerized tomography: A possible complication with benign outcome in leukemic patients. *Haematologica, 92*(9), e85–e90.

Genentech, Inc. (2007a). Avastin [Package insert]. South San Francisco, CA: Author.

Genentech, Inc. (2007b). Rituxan [Package insert]. South San Francisco, CA: Author.

Genentech, Inc. (2008). Herceptin [Package insert]. South San Francisco, CA: Author.

Genentech, Inc. & OSI Oncology. (2007). Tarceva [Package insert]. Melville, NY: Author.

Ginsberg, S.J., & Comis, R.L. (1984). The pulmonary toxicity of antineoplastic agents. In M.C. Perry & J.W. Yarbro (Eds.), *Toxicity of chemotherapy* (pp. 227–268). New York: Grune and Stratton.

Giusti, R.M., Shastri, K.A., Cohen, M.H., Keegan, P., & Pazdur, R. (2007). FDA drug approval summary: Panitumumab (Vectibix). *Oncologist, 12*(5), 577–583.

GlaxoSmithKline. (2006). Leukeran [Package insert]. Research Triangle Park, NC: Author.

GlaxoSmithKline. (2007). Alkeran [Package insert]. Research Triangle Park, NC: Author.

GlaxoSmithKline. (2008a). Hycamtin [Package insert]. Research Triangle Park, NC: Author.

GlaxoSmithKline. (2008b). Myleran [Package insert]. Research Triangle Park, NC: Author.

Goldberg, H.L., & Vannice, S.B. (1995). Pneumonitis related to treatment with paclitaxel. *Clinical Journal of Oncology, 13*(2), 534–535.

Goldschmidt, N., Nusair, S., Gural, A., Amir, G., Izhar, U., & Laxer, U. (2003). Disseminated *Mycobacterium kansasii* infection with pulmonary alveolar proteinosis in a patient with chronic myelogenous leukemia. *American Journal of Hematology, 74*(3), 221–223.

Grande, C., Villanueva, M.J., Huidobro, G., & Casal, J. (2007). Docetaxel-induced interstitial pneumonitis following non-small-cell lung cancer treatment. *Clinical and Translational Oncology, 9*(9), 578–581.

Grigoriyan, A., Rishi, A., Molina, J., Homer, R., & Manthous, C.A. (2007). Diffuse alveolar damage and hemorrhage in acute myelogenous leukemia treated with corticosteroids. *Connecticut Medicine, 71*(4), 201–204.

Gupta, S., & Mahipal, A. (2007). Fatal pulmonary toxicity after a single dose of cyclophosphamide. *Pharmacotherapy, 27*(4), 616–618.

Hackman, R.C., Madtes, D.K., Petersen, F.B., & Clark, J.G. (1989). Pulmonary venoocclusive disease following bone marrow transplantation. *Transplantation, 47*(6), 989–992.

Hamada, K., Nagal, S., Kitaichi, M., Jin, G., Shigermatsu, M., Nagao, T., et al. (2003). Cyclophosphamide-induced late-onset lung disease. *Internal Medicine, 42*(1), 82–87.

Haupt, H.M., Hutchins, G.M., & Moore, G.W. (1981). Ara-C lung: Noncardiogenic pulmonary edema complicating cytosine arabinoside therapy of leukemia. *American Journal of Medicine, 70*(2), 256–261.

Heggen, J., West, C., Olson, E., Olson, T., Teague, G., Fortenberry, J., et al. (2002). Diffuse alveolar hemorrhage in pediatric hematopoietic cell transplant patients. *Pediatrics, 109*(5), 965–967.

Hennemann, B., Bross, K.J., Reichle, A., & Andreesen, R. (1993). Acute alveolitis induced by hydroxyurea in a patient with chronic myeloproliferative syndrome. *Annals of Hematology, 67*(3), 133–134.

Hochhaus, A. (2007). Management of Bcr-Abl-positive leukemias with dasatinib. *Expert Review of Anticancer Therapy, 7*(11), 1529–1536.

Hood, L.E., & Harwood, K.V. (2004). Dyspnea. In C.H. Yarbro, M.H. Frogge, & M. Goodman (Eds.), *Cancer symptom management* (3rd ed., pp. 29–46). Sudbury, MA: Jones and Bartlett.

Hospira, Inc. (2007). Methotrexate [Package insert]. Lake Forest, IL: Author.

Hydzik, C.A. (1990). Late effects of chemotherapy: Implications for patient management and rehabilitation. *Nursing Clinics of North America, 25*(2), 423–446.

Ieki, R., Saitoh, E., & Shibuya, M. (2003). Acute lung injury as a possible adverse drug reaction related to gefitinib. *European Respiratory Journal, 22*(1), 179–181.

Inaba, H., Jenkins, J.J., McCarville, M.B., Morrison, R.R., Howard, S.C., Pui, C.H., et al. (2007). Pulmonary alveolar proteinosis in pediatric leukemia. *Pediatric Blood and Cancer, 51*(1), 66–70.

Ishii, Y., Shoji, N., Kimura, Y., & Ohyashiki, K. (2006). Prominent pleural effusion possibly due to imatinib mesylate in adult Philadelphia chromosome-positive acute lymphoblastic leukemia. *Internal Medicine, 45*(5), 339–340.

Jin, B., Hou, K.Z., Liu, Y.P., & Yu, P. (2006). Leukocytosis and retinoic acid syndrome in patients with acute promyelocytic leukemia treated with arsenic trioxide. *Chinese Medical Sciences Journal, 21*(3), 171–174.

Kachel, D.L., & Martin, W.J., II. (1994). Cyclophosphamide-induced lung toxicity: Mechanism of endothelial cell injury. *Journal of Pharmacology and Experimental Therapeutics, 268*(1), 42–46.

Kavuru, M.S., Gadsden, T., Lichtin, A., & Gephardt, G. (1994). Hydroxyurea-induced acute interstitial lung disease. *Southern Medical Journal, 87*(7), 767–769.

Keijzer, A., & Kuenen, B. (2007). Fatal pulmonary toxicity in testis cancer with bleomycin-containing chemotherapy. *Journal of Clinical Oncology, 25*(23), 3543–3544.

Khalsa, S.K., Roberts, C.C., & Underhill, M.S. (2007). Acute pulmonary toxicity from thalidomide in a patient with multiple myeloma. *Radiology Case Reports, 2*(2), 254.

Kim, K.H., Kim, J.H., & Kim, Y.W. (2004). Use of extracorporeal membrane oxygenation (ECMO) during whole lung lavage in pulmonary alveolar proteinosis associated with lung cancer. *European Journal of Cardiothoracic Surgery, 26*(5), 1050–1051.

King, T., Jr. (2007a). *Approach to the adult with interstitial lung disease* [Up-To-Date Version 15.3, current as of August 2007]. Retrieved March 21, 2008, from http://www.uptodate.com/home/index.html

King, T., Jr. (2007b). *Role of the lung biopsy in diagnosis of interstitial lung disease* [Up-To-Date Version 15.3, current as of August 2007]. Retrieved March 21, 2008, from http://www.uptodate.com/home/index.html

King, T., Jr. (2007c). *Taxane-induced pulmonary toxicity* [Up-To-Date Version 15.3, current as of August 2007]. Retrieved March 21, 2008, from http://www.uptodate.com/home/index.html

Kitajima, H., Takahashi, H., Harada, K., Kanai, A., Inomata, S., Taniguchi, H., et al. (2006). Gefitinib-induced interstitial lung disease showing improvement after cessation: Dissociation of serum markers. *Respirology, 11*(2), 217–220.

Klastersky, J. (2006). Adverse effects of the humanized antibodies used as cancer therapeutics. *Current Opinion in Oncology, 18*(4), 316–320.

Koh, D.W., & Castro, M. (1996). Pulmonary toxicity of chemotherapy drugs. In M.C. Perry (Ed.), *The chemotherapy source book* (3rd ed., pp. 665–695). Baltimore: Williams & Wilkins.

Kohli, A., Ferencz, T.M., & Calderon, J.G. (2004). Readministration of high-dose methotrexate in a patient with suspected immediate hypersensitivity and T-cell acute lymphoblastic lymphoma. *Allergy and Asthma Proceedings, 25*(4), 249–252.

Lake, F.R. (2007). *Interstitial lung disease in rheumatoid arthritis* [Up-To-Date Version 15.3, current as of August 2007]. Retrieved March 21, 2008, from http://www.uptodate.com/home/index.html

Lasky, J.A., & Ortiz, L. (2007). *Bleomycin-induced lung injury* [Up-To-Date Version 15.3, current as of August 2007]. Retrieved March 21, 2008, from http://www.uptodate.com/home/index.html

Lateef, O., Shakoor, N., & Balk, R.A. (2005). Methotrexate pulmonary toxicity. *Expert Opinion on Drug Safety, 4*(4), 723–730.

Le-Chiong, T., Jr., & Matthay, R.A. (2004). Drug-induced pulmonary edema and acute respiratory distress syndrome. *Clinics in Chest Medicine, 25*(1), 95–104.

Leimgruber, K., Negro, R., Baier, S., Moser, B., Resch, G., Sansone, S., et al. (2006). Fatal interstitial pneumonitis associated with docetaxel administration in a patient with hormone-refractory prostate cancer. *Tumori, 92*(6), 542–544.

Letizia, M., & Conway, A.M. (1996). Interleukin-2 therapy for renal cell cancer: Indications, effects, and nursing implications. *Critical Care Nurse, 16*(5), 20–35.

Lewis, I.D., DeFor, T., & Weisdorf, D.J. (2000). Increasing incidence of diffuse alveolar hemorrhage following allogeneic bone marrow transplantation: Cryptic etiology and uncertain therapy. *Bone Marrow Transplantation, 26*(5), 539–543.

Lin, T.S., Penza, S.L., Avalos, B.R., Lucarelli, M.R., Farag, S.S., Byrd, J.C., et al. (2005). Diffuse alveolar hemorrhage following gemtuzumab ozogamicin. *Bone Marrow Transplantation, 35*(8), 823–824.

Liu, V., White, D.A., Zakowski, M.F., Travis, W., Kris, M.G., Ginserberg, M.S., et al. (2007). Pulmonary toxicity associated with erlotinib. *Chest, 132*(3), 1042–1044.

Luedke, D., McLaughlin, T.T., Daughaday, C., Luedke, S., Harrison, B., Reed, G., et al. (1985). Mitomycin C and vindesine associated pulmonary toxicity with variable clinical expression. *Cancer, 55*(3), 542–545.

Maitland, M.L., Wilcox, R., Hogarth, D.K., Desai, A.A., Caligiuri, P., Abrahams, C., et al. (2006). Diffuse alveolar damage after a single dose of topotecan in a patient with pulmonary fibrosis and small cell lung cancer. *Lung Cancer, 54*(2), 243–245.

Majhail, N.S., Parks, K., DeFor, T.E., & Weisdorf, D.J. (2006). Alveolar hemorrhage following hematopoietic cell transplantation using reduced-intensity conditioning. *Bone Marrow Transplantation, 38*(11), 765–768.

Makris, D., Scherpereel, A., Copin, M.C., Colin, G., Brun, L., Lafitte, J.J., et al. (2007). Fatal interstitial lung disease associated with oral erlotinib therapy for lung cancer. *BMC Cancer, 7,* 150.

Maldonado, F., Limper, A.H., Lim, K.G., & Aubrey, M.C. (2007). Temozolomide-associated organizing pneumonitis. *Mayo Clinic Proceedings, 82*(6), 771–773.

Malik, S.W., Myers, J.L., DeRemee, R.A., & Specks, U. (1996). Lung toxicity associated with cyclophosphamide use. Two distinct patterns. *American Journal of Respiratory and Critical Care Medicine, 154*(6, Pt. 1), 1851–1856.

Mayne Pharma. (2006a). Cytarabine [Package insert]. Paramus, NJ: Author.

Mayne Pharma. (2006b). Navelbine [Package insert]. Paramus, NJ: Author.

McKoy, J.M., Angelotta, C., Bennett, C.L., Tallman, M.S., Wadleigh, M., Evens, A.M., et al. (2007). Gemtuzumab ozogamicin-associated sinusoid obstructive syndrome (SOS): An overview from the research on adverse drug events and reports (RADAR) project. *Leukemia Research, 31*(5), 599–604.

McLeod, B.F., Lawrence, H.J., Smith, D.W., Vogt, P.J., & Gandara, D.R. (1987). Fatal bleomycin toxicity from a low cumulative dose in a patient with renal insufficiency. *Cancer, 60*(11), 2617–2620.

Meadors, M., Floyd, J., & Perry, M.C. (2006). Pulmonary toxicity of chemotherapy. *Seminars in Oncology, 33*(1), 98–105.

Millennium Pharmaceuticals, Inc. (2008). Velcade [Package insert]. Cambridge, MA: Author.

Miyakoshi, S., Kami, M., Yuji, K., Matsumara, T., Takatoku, M., Sasaki, M., et al. (2006). Severe pulmonary complications in Japanese patients after bortezomib treatment for refractory multiple myeloma. *Blood, 107*(9), 3492–3494.

Miyoshi, I., Daibata, M., Takemoto, S., Machida, H., & Taguchi, H. (2005). Pulmonary alveolar proteinosis complicating acute myeloid leukaemia, *British Journal of Haematology, 131*(1), 1.

Morgensztern, D., & Govidan, R. (2008). Pulmonary toxicity of antineoplastic therapy. In M.C. Perry (Ed.), *The chemotherapy source book* (4th ed., pp. 191–196). Philadelphia: Williams & Wilkins.

National Cancer Institute Cancer Therapy Evaluation Program. (2006). *Common terminology criteria for adverse events* (version 3.0). Retrieved March 18, 2008, from http://ctep.cancer.gov/forms/CTCAEv3.pdf

Ngan, H.Y., Liang, R.H., Lam, W.K., & Chan, T.K. (1993). Pulmonary toxicity in patients with non-Hodgkin's lymphoma treated with bleomycin-containing combination chemotherapy. *Cancer Chemotherapy and Pharmacology, 32*(5), 407–409.

Novartis Oncology U.S. (2008). *mTOR pathway.* Retrieved September 17, 2008, from http://www.novartisoncology.us/research/mtor-pathway.jsp?source=01030&irmasrc=OUSWB0004&campaign=ONC-90088&site=msn&HBX_PK=mtor_inhibitor&HBX_OU=52

Novartis Pharmaceuticals. (2007). Gleevec [Package insert]. East Hanover, NJ: Author.

Ohri, A., & Arena, F.P. (2006). Severe pulmonary complications in African-American patient after bortezomib therapy. *American Journal of Therapeutics, 13*(6), 553–555.

Ostoros, G., Pretz, A., Fillinger, J., Soltesz, I., & Dome, B. (2006). Fatal pulmonary fibrosis induced by paclitaxel: A case report and review of the literature. *International Journal of Gynecologic Cancer, 16*(Suppl. 1), 391–393.

Pamuk, G.E., Turgut, B., Vural, O., Demir, M., Hatipoglu, O., & Unlu, E. (2003). Pulmonary alveolar proteinosis in a patient with acute lymphoid leukemia regression after G-CSF therapy. *Leukemia and Lymphoma, 44*(5), 871–874.

Pasetto, L.M., & Monfardini, S. (2006). Is acute dyspnea related to oxaliplatin administration? *World Journal of Gastroenterology, 12*(36), 5907–5908.

Patel, J.M. (1990). Metabolism and pulmonary toxicity of cyclophosphamide. *Pharmacologic Therapy, 47*(1), 137–146.

Pavlakis, N., Bell, D.R., Millward, M.J., & Levi, J.A. (1997). Fatal pulmonary toxicity resulting from treatment with gemcitabine. *Cancer, 80*(2), 286–291.

Pedroso, S.L., Martins, L.S., Sousa, S., Reis, A., Dias, L., Henriques, A.C., et al. (2007). Pulmonary alveolar proteinosis: A rare pulmonary complication of sirolimus. *Transplant International, 20*(3), 291–296.

Pitini, V., Arrigo, C., Altavilla, G., & Naro, C. (2007). Severe pulmonary complications after bortezomib treatment for multiple myeloma: An unrecognized pulmonary vasculitis? *Leukemia Research, 31*(7), 1027–1028.

Post, M.C., Grutters, J.C., Verzijlbergen, J.F., & Biesma, D.H. (2007). PET scintigraphy of etoposide-induced pulmonary toxicity. *Clinical Nuclear Medicine, 32*(9), 683–684.

Pronk, L.C., Stoter, G., & Verweij, J. (1995). Docetaxel (Taxotere®): Single agent activity, development of combination treatment and reducing side effects. *Cancer Treatment Reviews, 21*(5), 463–478.

Quintas-Cardama, A., Kantarjian, H., O'Brien, S., Borthakur, G., Brussi, J., & Munden, R. (2007). Pleural effusion in patients with chronic myelogenous leukemia treated with dasatinib after imatinib failure. *Journal of Clinical Oncology, 25*(25), 3908–3914.

Ramanathan, R.K., Belani, C.P., & Reddy, V.V. (1996). Transient pulmonary infiltrates: A hypersensitivity reaction to paclitaxel. *Annals of Internal Medicine, 124*(2), 278.

Read, W.L., Mortimer, J.E., & Picus, J. (2002). Severe interstitial pneumonitis associated with docetaxel administration. *Cancer, 94*(3), 847–853.

Roche Pharmaceuticals. (2006). Xeloda [Package insert]. Nutley, NJ: Author.

Rossi, S.E., Erasmus, J.J., McAdams, H.P., Sporn, T.A., & Goodman, P.C. (2000). Pulmonary drug toxicity: Radiologic and pathologic manifestations. *Radiographics, 20*(5), 1245–1259.

Roychowdhury, D., Smith, C., Peterson, A., Pedersen, C., Schep, C., Kilgour-Christie, J., et al. (2000). Infrequency of serious pulmonary toxicity (SPT) with Gemzar (G): Analysis of a large database. *Proceedings of the American Society of Clinical Oncology, 19,* Abstract 762.

Ruiz-Casado, A., Garcia, M.D., & Racionero, M.A. (2006). Pulmonary toxicity of 5-fluorouracil and oxaliplatin. *Clinical and Translational Oncology, 8*(8), 624.

Salzman, D., Adkins, D.R., Craig, F., Freytes, C., & LeMaistre, C.F. (1996). Malignancy-associated pulmonary veno-occlusive disease: Report of a case following autologous bone marrow transplantation and review. *Bone Marrow Transplantation, 18*(4), 755–760.

Sanofi-Aventis Pharmaceuticals. (2007). Eloxatin [Package insert]. Bridgewater, NJ: Author.

Sanofi-Aventis Pharmaceuticals. (2008). Taxotere [Package insert]. Bridgewater, NJ: Author.

Schering Corporation. (2007). Temodar [Package insert]. Kenilworth, NJ: Author.

Schering Corporation. (2008). Intron-A [Package insert]. Kenilworth, NJ: Author.

Schwartzentruber, D.J. (2005). Interleukin-2: Clinical applications: Principles of administration and management of side effects. In S.A. Rosenberg (Ed.), *Principles and practice of the biologic therapy of cancer* (4th ed., pp. 36–56). Philadelphia: Lippincott Williams & Wilkins.

Segura, A., Yuste, A., Cercos, A., Lopez-Tendero, P., Girones, R., Perez-Fidalgo, J.A., et al. (2001). Pulmonary fibrosis induced by cyclophosphamide. *Annals of Pharmacotherapy, 35*(7–8), 894–897.

Senan, S., Paul, J., Thompson, N., & Kay, S.B. (1992). Cigarette smoking is a risk factor for bleomycin-induced pulmonary toxicity. *European Journal of Cancer, 28*A(12), 2084.

Shelton, B.K. (2009). Biological agents. In D. Ashenbrenner & S. Venable (Eds.), *Drug therapy in nursing* (3rd ed., pp. 644–668). Philadelphia: Lippincott Williams & Wilkins.

Shoji, N., Ito, Y., Kimura, Y., Nishimaki, J., Kuriyama, Y., Tauchi, T., et al. (2002). Pulmonary alveolar proteinosis as a terminal complication in myelodysplastic syndromes: Report of four cases detected on autopsy. *Leukemia Research, 26*(6), 591–595.

Siegel, J.P., & Puri, R.K. (1991). Interleukin-2 toxicity. *Journal of Clinical Oncology, 9*(4), 694–704.

Sleijfer, S., van der Mark, T.W., Schraffordt Koops, K., & Mulder, N.H. (1995). Decrease in pulmonary function during bleomycin-containing combination chemotherapy for testicular cancer: Not only a bleomycin effect. *British Journal of Cancer, 71*(1), 120–123.

Smalley, R.V., & Wall, R.L. (1966). Two cases of busulfan toxicity. *Annals of Internal Medicine, 64*(1), 154–164.

Specks, U. (2008). *Cyclophosphamide pulmonary toxicity.* Retrieved July 26, 2008, from http://www.uptodate.com/patients/content/topic.do?topicKey=int_lung/24001

Spratto, G.R., & Woods, A.L. (2004). *PDR nurse's drug handbook.* Clifton Park, NY: Delmar Learning.

Stark, P. (2007). *Evaluation of diffuse lung disease by plain chest radiograph* [Up-To-Date Version 15.3, current as of August 2007]. Retrieved March 21, 2008, from http://www.uptodate.com/home/index.html

Tenenbaum, L. (1994). *Cancer chemotherapy and biotherapy: A reference guide.* Philadelphia: Saunders.

Thornburg, A., Abonour, R., Smith, P., Knox, K., & Twigg, H.L., III. (2007). Hypersensitivity pneumonitis-like syndrome associated with the use of lenalidomide. *Chest, 131*(5), 1572–1574.

Tietjen, P.E., & Stover, D.E. (2002). Lung injury associated with cancer treatment. *Pulmonary and Critical Care Update, 17*(Lesson 10). Retrieved November 24, 2008, from http://www.chestnet.org/education/online/pccu/vol17/lessons9_10/lesson10.php

Toh, C.K., Lee, P., Chowbay, B., Goh, J.W., Mancer, K., & Tan, P.H. (2007). An inflammatory response with worsening of pleural effusion on treatment with erlotinib in non-small cell lung cancer. *Acta Oncologica, 46*(2), 256–258.

Twohig, K.J., & Matthay, R.A. (1990). Pulmonary effects of cytotoxic agents other than bleomycin. *Clinics in Chest Medicine, 11*(1), 31–54.

Vahid, B., & Marik, P.E. (2008). Pulmonary complications of novel antineoplastic agents for solid tumors. *Chest, 133*(2), 528–538.

Van Barneveld, P.W., van der Mark, T.W., Sleijfer, D.T., Mulder, N.H., Koops, H.S., Sluiter, H.J., et al. (1984). Predictive factors for bleomycin-induced pneumonitis. *American Review of Respiratory Disease, 130*(6), 1078–1081.

Varga, J. (2007). *Prognosis and treatment of interstitial lung disease in systemic sclerosis* [Up-To-Date Version 15.3, current as of August 2007]. Retrieved March 21, 2008, from http://www.uptodate.com/home/index.html

Wagner, S.A., Mehta, A.C., & Laber, D.A. (2007). Rituximab-induced interstitial lung disease. *American Journal of Hematology, 82*(10), 916–919.

Wagner, U., Staats, P., Moll, R., Feek, U., Vogelmeier, C., & Groneberg, D.A. (2003). Imatinib-associated pulmonary alveolar proteinosis. *American Journal of Medicine, 115*(8), 674.

Wanko, S.O., Broadwater, G., Foltz, R.J., & Chao, N.J. (2006). Diffuse alveolar hemorrhage: Retrospective review of clinical outcome in allogeneic transplant recipients treated with aminocaproic acid. *Biology of Blood and Marrow Transplantation, 12*(9), 949–953.

Wickham, R. (1986). Pulmonary toxicity secondary to cancer treatment. *Oncology Nursing Forum, 13*(5), 69–76.

Wilkes, G.M., & Barton-Burke, M. (2008). *2008 oncology nursing drug handbook.* Sudbury, MA: Jones and Bartlett.

Wyeth Pharmaceuticals. (2008a). Mylotarg [Package insert]. Philadelphia: Author.

Wyeth Pharmaceuticals. (2008b). Neumega [Package insert]. Philadelphia: Author.

Yahalom, J., & Portlock, C.S. (2008). Long-term cardiac and pulmonary complications of cancer therapy. *Hematology/Oncology Clinics of North America, 22*(2), 305–318.

G. Hemorrhagic cystitis: An irritation of the bladder that ranges from microscopic hematuria to acute exsanguinating hematuria (Strohl & Camp-Sorrell, 2006)
   1. Pathophysiology: Irritation, inflammation, and ulceration occur as a result of the binding of drug metabolites or byproducts to the bladder mucosa primarily related to cyclophosphamide and ifosfamide therapy (Strohl & Camp-Sorrell, 2006).
      a) Acrolein is a drug metabolite of cyclophosphamide.
      b) Acrolein and chloroacetaldehyde are metabolites of ifosfamide.
   2. Incidence (ASCO, 2002; Hogle, 2007)
      a) Toxicity occurs in rare instances with bortezomib and with repeated cycles of gemcitabine and irinotecan.
      b) Toxicity primarily is associated with cyclophosphamide and ifosfamide.
         (1) In adults
            (a) Standard- or low-dose cyclophosphamide (< 1,000 mg): Associated with a 6%–10% incidence of toxicity usually manifested as microscopic hematuria that may or may not be symptomatic (Choudhury & Ahmed, 1997; Shahab & Patterson, 2007)
            (b) High-dose cyclophosphamide (at least 120 mg/kg): Associated with

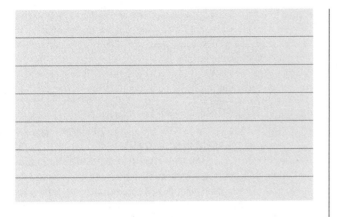

up to a 40% incidence of toxicity ranging from microscopic to frank hematuria with clotting (ASCO, 2002; Hogle, 2007; Shahab & Patterson, 2007)

(c) Ifosfamide: Associated with 18%–40% incidence of frank hematuria. Incidence of combined microscopic and frank hematuria is up to 50%. Mortality with severe hemorrhage is 2%–4% (ASCO, 2002).

(2) In children: Symptoms occur as early as a few weeks following chemotherapy or as late as several years after treatment and can be long-term in duration (Adamson, Balis, Berg, & Blaney, 2005; McCarville, Hoffer, Gingrich, & Jenkins, 2000).

(a) Mild dysuria to severe hemorrhage occurs in 5%–10% of children receiving low-dose cyclophosphamide (Adamson et al., 2005).

(b) Mild dysuria to severe hemorrhage occurs in 20%–40% of children receiving ifosfamide (Adamson et al., 2005).

3. Risk factors

a) Immunosuppression can cause increased risk for bladder damage as a result of increased susceptibility to toxins, bacteria, and viruses (Perez-Brayfield, 2007).

b) Cyclophosphamide therapy (Stillwell & Benson, 1988)

(1) IV administration presents a greater risk than does cyclophosphamide administered orally.

(2) High-dose administration presents a greater risk than does low-dose administration.

(3) Toxicity can occur with a single dose of IV cyclophosphamide or with up to

57 mg/kg administered cumulatively over two years.

c) Cumulative doses of ifosfamide 45 g/m^2 or greater, especially for children younger than age three, have been associated with increased incidence and severity of renal toxicity (Loebstein et al., 1999).

d) Prior radiation therapy to the pelvis or bladder increases risk (ASCO, 2002; Hogle, 2007; McCarville et al., 2000; Stillwell & Benson, 1988).

e) Smoking, because of bladder wall friability, increases risk.

4. Clinical manifestations (Shahab & Patterson, 2007; Stillwell & Benson, 1988; Strohl & Camp-Sorrell, 2006)

a) Dysuria

b) Frequency

c) Burning during urination

d) Nocturia or oliguria

e) Microscopic or frank hematuria

5. Assessment: Obtain a baseline urinalysis before therapy, and regularly monitor subsequent urinalysis results and subjective reports.

6. Preventive strategies

a) Preventive measures for hemorrhagic cystitis focus on assessment and monitoring, forced hydration and diuresis, and frequent voiding or continuous bladder irrigation (Friend & Pruett, 2004; Strohl & Camp-Sorrell, 2006; Sylvanus, 2007; West, 1997).

(1) Assess baseline blood urea nitrogen (BUN), serum creatinine (SCr), and the results of routine urinalysis and urine cultures as needed to rule out renal pathology and infection.

(2) Maintain and monitor intake and output; instruct patient and caregiver in this process.

(3) Instruct patients to increase oral fluid intake (adults: two to three liters/day); provide parenteral hydration if the patient is unable to drink and retain oral fluids. Encourage hydration to begin 12–24 hours prior to scheduled chemotherapy. Urinary output should be > 100 cc/hr/m^2 (Amerinet Choice, 2006; West, 1997). Prevention includes forced diuresis and administration of chemoprotectants (e.g., mesna).

(4) Administer final daily dose of oral cyclophosphamide prior to 4 pm to allow the drug to pass through the bladder prior to bedtime.

(5) Encourage frequent voiding, around the clock, day and night.

(6) Instruct the patient on visual observation of urine and to call if pink, red, dark, or cloudy.

(7) Administer forced NS hydration and forced diuresis with ifosfamide and high-dose cyclophosphamide.

b) Administer the bladder protectant mesna with high-dose cyclophosphamide and any dose of ifosfamide. Mesna binds to drug metabolite, inactivating and detoxifying it, then allowing it to be flushed from the bladder (ASCO, 2002; Hogle, 2007).

(1) For adults receiving standard-dose ifosfamide via short infusion, the total daily mesna dose should be equal to 60% of the total daily ifosfamide dose and administered 15 minutes before (0 hours) and at four and eight hours after each infusion dose of ifosfamide. Therefore, each bolus mesna dose is approximately 20% of the total daily dose of ifosfamide to equal 60% when three bolus mesna doses are complete (ASCO, 2002). Oral mesna is given in a dosage equal to 40% of the ifosfamide dose two and six hours after each dose of ifosfamide (Amerinet Choice, 2006).

(2) For adults receiving standard-dose ifosfamide via continuous infusion, mesna can be administered with ifosfamide, as a continuous infusion at 60%–100% of the ifosfamide dose, following a loading dose of 20% of the total daily ifosfamide dose.

(3) Another recommendation for adults receiving standard-dose ifosfamide by continuous infusion is to include one bolus loading dose of mesna equal to 20% of the total daily ifosfamide dose followed by a continuous infusion of mesna at a dose of up to 40% of the total daily ifosfamide dose and continuing the mesna infusion for 12–24 hours following completion of the ifosfamide. Note: No relevant clinical data are available to support a mesna dose of > 60% of the ifosfamide dose, and doses above 60% have been associated with increased GI toxicity (Amerinet Choice, 2006; ASCO, 2002; Fischer, Knobf, Durivage, & Beaulieu, 2003).

(4) For adults with high-dose ifosfamide (> 2.5 g/m²/day), no guidelines have yet been established regarding the concomitant mesna dosing. Some studies indicate that more frequent and prolonged mesna dosing is needed for maximum uroprotection with high-dose ifosfamide (ASCO, 2002).

(5) For adults receiving high-dose cyclophosphamide therapy, mesna dosing should be at 40% of the total cyclophosphamide dose. Doses of up to 60%–120% of the cyclophosphamide dose have been administered, but the efficacy of higher mesna dosing has not yet been established. Administer mesna 15 minutes before and at four and eight hours after the cyclophosphamide dose (ASCO, 2002; Hogle, 2007; Shepherd et al., 1991).

(6) For children, an IV mesna dose is typically 60% of the ifosfamide or cyclophosphamide dose; some studies recommend a 1:1 ratio. The most common pediatric administration schedule consists of IV mesna 15 minutes prior to chemotherapy and at four and eight hours after chemotherapy (Amerinet Choice, 2006; Katz et al., 1995; Links & Lewis, 1999).

(7) The initial loading bolus dose of mesna should be administered via IV, but subsequent doses can be administered intravenously or orally. SC dosing also has been utilized. Oral dosing may be higher, and the dose can be mixed with juices or beverages to mask the taste (ASCO, 2002; Hogle, 2007).

(8) Adverse effects of mesna include nausea, vomiting, diarrhea, abdominal pain, altered taste, rash, urticaria, headache, and hypotension (Amerinet Choice, 2006).

7. Collaborative management

a) Discontinue ifosfamide or cyclophosphamide administration if evidence of gross hematuria or cystitis is noted.

b) Insert a urinary catheter.

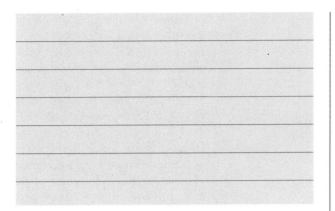

(1) In adult patients, place a three-way Foley catheter to provide continuous irrigation with saline or acetylcysteine (Shahab & Patterson, 2007).

(2) In patients who have clots obstructing their ability to void, place a large-bore urethral catheter to provide irrigation with a saline solution (Kunkle, Hirshberg, & Greenberg, 2006; West, 1997).

c) Administer an antifibrinolytic agent, such as aminocaproic acid, to promote clotting. Other agents aiding in the formation of a protein precipitate over bleeding surfaces include saline, potassium aluminum sulfate, silver nitrate, and formalin (Choudhury & Ahmed, 1997; Kunkle et al., 2006; West, 1997).

d) Obtain a urology consultation. Cystoscopy with electrocautery or cryosurgery may be used to control bleeding. Cystectomy may be necessary for last-resort cases.

e) Follow-up is needed because prolonged mucosal irritation, inflammation, and bleeding can lead to persistent cystitis, irreversible bladder fibrosis, and an increased risk for bladder cancer (ASCO, 2002; Hogle, 2007). Follow-up recommendations include the following (Kunkle et al., 2006; Stillwell & Benson, 1988).

(1) Periodic and at least annual urinalysis, urine cytology, and cystoscopy

(2) Periodic excretory urograms for patients with gross hematuria, new microhematuria, abnormal cytologic findings regarding the urine, or persistent irritative voiding

8. Patient and family education (Kunkle et al., 2006)

a) Tell patients about the possibility of hemorrhagic cystitis with ifosfamide and cyclophosphamide regimens.

b) Ensure that patients know the signs and symptoms to report.

c) Encourage patients to void at least every two hours while awake and just prior to bedtime and to take oral cyclophosphamide early in the day, with the last dose before 4 pm.

d) Instruct patients to increase fluid intake daily as able.

References

Adamson, P.C., Balis, F.M., Berg, S., & Blaney, S.M. (2005). General principles of chemotherapy. In P.A. Pizzo & D.G. Poplack (Eds.), *Principles and practice of pediatric oncology* (5th ed., pp. 290–365). Philadelphia: Lippincott Williams & Wilkins.

American Society of Clinical Oncology. (2002). *2002 update of recommendations for the use of chemotherapy and radiotherapy protectants: Clinical practice guidelines of the American Society of Clinical Oncology.* Retrieved November 10, 2007, from http://jco.ascopubs.org/cgi/content/full/20/12/2895

Amerinet Choice. (2006). Mesnex [Package insert]. Retrieved October 27, 2008, from http://dailymed.nlm.nih.gov/dailymed

Choudhury, D., & Ahmed, Z. (1997). Drug-induced nephrotoxicity. *Medical Clinics of North America, 81*(3), 705–717.

Fischer, D.S., Knobf, M.T., Durivage, H.J., & Beaulieu, N.J. (Eds.). (2003). *The cancer chemotherapy handbook* (6th ed.). St. Louis, MO: Mosby.

Friend, P.H., & Pruett, J. (2004). Bleeding and thrombotic complications. In C.H. Yarbro, M.H. Frogge, & M. Goodman (Eds.), *Cancer symptom management* (3rd ed., pp. 240–241). Sudbury, MA: Jones and Bartlett.

Hogle, W.P. (2007). Cytoprotective agents used in the treatment of patients with cancer. *Seminars in Oncology Nursing, 23*(3), 213–224.

Katz, A., Epelman, S., Anelli, A., Gorender, E.F., Cruz, S.M., Oliveira, R.M., et al. (1995). A prospective randomized evaluation of three schedules of mesna administration in patients receiving an ifosfamide-containing chemotherapy regimen: Sustained efficiency and simplified administration. *Journal of Cancer Research in Clinical Oncology, 121*(2), 128–131.

Kunkle, D.A., Hirshberg, S.J., & Greenberg, R.E. (2006). Urologic issues in palliative and supportive care. In A.M. Berger, J.L. Shuster, & J.H. Von Roehn (Eds.), *Principles and practice of palliative care and supportive oncology* (3rd ed., pp. 357–371). Philadelphia: Lippincott Williams & Wilkins.

Links, M., & Lewis, C. (1999). Chemoprotectants: A review of their clinical pharmacology and therapeutic efficacy. *Drugs, 57*(3), 293–306.

Loebstein, R., Atanackovic, G., Bishai, R., Wolpin, J., Khattak, S., Hashemi, G., et al. (1999). Risk factors for long-term outcome of ifosfamide-induced nephrotoxicity in children. *Journal of Clinical Pharmacology, 39*(5), 454–461.

McCarville, M.B., Hoffer, F.A., Gingrich, J.R., & Jenkins, J.J. (2000). Imaging findings of hemorrhagic cystitis in pediatric oncology patients. *Pediatric Radiology, 30*(3), 131–138.

Perez-Brayfield, M.R. (2007). *Hemorrhagic cystitis.* Retrieved November 11, 2007, from http://www.emedicine.com/ped/topic3081.htm

Shahab, I., & Patterson, W.P. (2007). Renal and electrolyte abnormalities due to chemotherapy. In M.C. Perry (Ed.), *The chemotherapy source book* (4th ed., pp. 223–231). Philadelphia: Lippincott Williams & Wilkins.

Shepherd, J.D., Pringle, L.E., Barnett, M.J., Klingemann, H.G., Reece, D.E., & Phillips, G.L. (1991). Mesna versus hyperhydration for the prevention of cyclophosphamide-induced hemorrhagic cystitis in bone marrow transplantation. *Journal of Clinical Oncology, 9*(11), 2016–2020.

Stillwell, T.J., & Benson, R.C. (1988). Cyclophosphamide-induced hemorrhagic cystitis: A review of 100 patients. *Cancer, 61*(3), 451–457.

Strohl, R.A., & Camp-Sorrell, D. (2006). Hemorrhagic cystitis. In D. Camp-Sorrell & R.A. Hawkins (Eds.), *Clinical manual for the oncology advanced practice nurse* (2nd ed., pp. 661–663). Pittsburgh, PA: Oncology Nursing Society.

Sylvanus, T. (2007). Prevention of hemorrhagic cystitis: The evidence says what?! [Abstract 2433]. *Oncology Nursing Forum, 34*(2), 574.

West, N.J. (1997). Prevention and treatment of hemorrhagic cystitis. *Pharmacotherapy, 17*(4), 696–706.

H. Hepatotoxicity
1. Pathophysiology (Andrade, Salmeron, & Lucena, 2006)
   a) Hepatotoxicity can occur through the following mechanisms.
      (1) Direct toxic effect to the hepatocyte
      (2) Elicitation of antibody-mediated cytotoxicity
      (3) Activation of apoptotic cascade through intracellular stress
      (4) Alternation of transporter proteins by the drug, preventing bile flow and leading to cholestasis
   b) Pediatric considerations
      (1) The organ systems of preterm and term infants and children are immature, causing many drugs, including antineoplastics, to have a different disposition from that seen in adults.
      (2) The clearance rates of adolescents may be lower than the high rates typical of toddlers and higher than typical adult rates. Toxicity alters drug clearance (Grochow & Baker, 1998).
      (3) Liver injury may manifest as fatty changes, hepatocellular necrosis, cholestasis, peliosis hepatitis, VOD (McDonald et al., 1993), nodular regenerative hyperplasia, hepatic neoplasms, hepatic fibrosis, or parenchymal cell damages.
2. Incidence (see Table 27)
3. Risk factors (Aydinli & Bayraktar, 2007; Fregonese & Stolk, 2008; Kaler, 2007; Weiss, 2005)
   a) Prior liver infection, damage, or disorder (e.g., cirrhosis, hepatitis, Budd-Chiari syndrome)
   b) Hepatotoxic chemotherapeutic drugs (risk increases with higher dosing)
   c) Family history of hereditary liver diseases (e.g., alpha-1 antitrypsin deficiency, hemochromatosis, Wilson disease)
   d) Prior tumor involvement of the liver
   e) Past medical history of transplant (e.g., liver, kidney, bone marrow, peripheral blood stem cell): Cholestasis is present in 80% of patients with chronic GVHD; chronic hepatitis is seen in the majority of HSCT survivors who experienced hepatitis C infection; chronic cyclosporine therapy can lead to gallstones and biliary symptoms (Peffault de Latour et al., 2004; Strasser et al., 1999, 2000; Strasser & Shulman, 2000).
   f) Prior radiation therapy to the liver or right side of abdomen
   g) History of alcohol abuse, especially if liver is cirrhotic
   h) Use of illicit drugs
   i) Concurrent administration of noncytotoxic hepatotoxic drugs or herbal products
   j) Intrahepatic chemotherapy administration
   k) Advancing age
4. Clinical manifestations (Bryant, 2006)
   a) Varying degrees of jaundice, from mild seen in sclera to severe seen in tissue
   b) Hyperpigmentation of the skin
   c) Ascites
   d) Fatigue, malaise, and other flu-like symptoms
   e) Anorexia
   f) Mild to severe nausea with varying degree of emesis
   g) Diarrhea, weight loss, dehydration, cachectic appearance
   h) Right upper quadrant pain
   i) Hepatosplenomegaly
   j) Dark-orange urine, clay-colored stools
   k) Pruritus
   l) Elevated transaminases (aspartate aminotransferase, alanine aminotransaminase), prolonged PTT
   m) Bruising and/or bleeding
   n) Portal hypertension
   o) Encephalopathy: Mental status changes ranging from subtle changes, such as decrease in memory, mental fogginess, and mild confusion, to profound coma
   p) Arthralgia/myalgia

Table 27. Hepatotoxicity of Chemotherapeutic and Biotherapeutic Drugs

Classification	Medication Name(s)	Route of Administration	Indications	Side Effects	Nursing Considerations
Alkylating agent	Busulfan	PO, IV	CML, conditioning regimens for BMT	Increased ALT, hyperbilirubinemia, veno-occlusive disease: High busulfan AUC values (> 1,500 μM/min) are associated with increased risk of hepatic veno-occlusive disease during conditioning for allogeneic BMT.	Monitor LFTs, bilirubin, alkaline phosphatase.
	Cisplatin	IV, IM, SC, IT	Bladder, testicular, and ovarian cancers	Hepatic dysfunction, increased transaminases (acute); jaundice	Monitor LFTs.
	Melphalan	PO, IV	Palliative treatment of multiple myeloma; nonresectable epithelial ovarian carcinoma; part of an induction regimen for BMT and SCT	Although melphalan is not associated with hepatotoxicity at usual PO doses, transient LFT abnormalities have been reported with the higher doses used in the setting of hematopoietic SCT (Giralt et al., 2001).	Ensure adequate patient hydration. Monitor LFTs.
Alkylating agent (nitrosourea)	Carmustine	IV, wafer	Brain tumor, multiple myeloma, Hodgkin disease, non-Hodgkin lymphoma Wafer is adjuvant in patients with high-grade malignant glioma or recurrent glioblastoma multiforme.	Reversible increases in bilirubin, alkaline phosphatase, and AST occur in 20%–25% of patients; subacute hepatitis and hepatic coma occur in < 1% (UpToDate, 2008).	Monitor LFTs. May require dose adjustment in hepatic impairment, but no dosing guidelines are available.
Anthracenedione; antibiotic	Mitoxantrone	IV	Remission-induction therapy of ANLL and AML Mitoxantrone is also active against other leukemias, lymphomas, and breast cancer and moderately active against pediatric sarcoma; initial chemotherapy for patients with pain related to advanced hormone-refractory prostate cancer; reducing neurologic disability and/or frequency of clinical relapses in patients with worsening relapsing-remitting multiple sclerosis	Transient elevation of liver enzymes, jaundice	Consider dose adjustments in patients with severe hepatic dysfunction (bilirubin > 3.4 mg/dl). Not recommended for treatment of multiple sclerosis in patients with concurrent hepatic impairment. Monitor LFTs.
Antibiotic	Bleomycin	IM, IV, SC, intracavitary	Squamous cell carcinomas, melanomas, sarcomas, testicular cancer, Hodgkin lymphoma, and non-Hodgkin lymphoma; sclerosing agent for malignant pleural effusion	Hepatotoxicity < 1%	Monitor LFTs.

(Continued on next page)

Table 27. Hepatotoxicity of Chemotherapeutic and Biotherapeutic Drugs *(Continued)*

Classification	Medication Name(s)	Route of Administration	Indications	Side Effects	Nursing Considerations
Antibiotic *(cont.)*	Dactinomycin	IV	Testicular cancer, melanoma, gestational trophoblastic neoplasm, Wilms tumor, neuroblastoma, retinoblastoma, rhabdomyosarcoma, uterine sarcomas, Ewing sarcoma, Kaposi sarcoma, sarcoma botryoides, and soft-tissue sarcoma	Ascites, hepatic failure, hepatitis, hepatomegaly, hepatotoxicity, LFT abnormality. May cause veno-occlusive liver disease (increased risk in children < 4 years of age); use with caution in hepatobilliary dysfunction.	Avoid dactinomycin use within 2 months of radiation treatment for right-sided Wilms tumor, as it may increase the risk of hepatotoxicity.
	Doxorubicin	IV	Leukemias, lymphomas, multiple myeloma, osseous and nonosseous sarcomas, mesotheliomas, germ cell tumors of the ovary or testes, Wilms tumor, neuroblastoma, and carcinomas of the head and neck, thyroid, lung, breast, stomach, pancreas, liver, ovary, bladder, prostate, and uterus	Increased bilirubin levels, hepatitis	Hepatic impairment [U.S. Boxed Warning]: Use with caution in patients with hepatic impairment; dosage adjustment recommended. Use with caution in patients with hepatobilliary dysfunction. Extensively metabolized in liver; reduce dose for altered hepatic function (Sifton, 2002).
Antimetabolite	6-mercaptopurine	PO	Treatment (maintenance and induction) of ALL	Hepatic: Intrahepatic cholestasis and focal centralobular necrosis (40%), characterized by hyperbilirubinemia, increased alkaline phosphatase and AST, jaundice, ascites, encephalopathy; more common at doses > 2.5 mg/kg/day	Hepatic effects usually occur within 2 months of therapy; may occur within 1 week, or may be delayed up to 8 years.
	Clofarabine	IV	AML, CML, ALL, MDS	Elevated ALT, AST, bilirubin, hepatomegaly, jaundice	Monitor LFTs.
Antimetabolite (antifolate)	Methotrexate	IM, IV, IT, SC	Trophoblastic neoplasms; leukemias; psoriasis; RA, including polyarticular-course juvenile RA; osteosarcoma; soft-tissue sarcomas; lymphomas; and carcinomas of the breast, head and neck, lung, GI tract, esophagus, and testes	U.S. Boxed Warning: Methotrexate has been associated with acute (elevated transaminases) and potentially fatal chronic (fibrosis, cirrhosis) hepatotoxicity. Risk is related to cumulative dose and prolonged exposure. Ethanol abuse, obesity, advanced age, and diabetes may increase the risk of hepatotoxic reactions. Use caution with preexisting liver impairment; may require dosage reduction.	Monitor closely (with LFTs, including serum albumin) for liver toxicities. Use caution when used with other hepatotoxic agents (e.g., azathioprine, retinoids, sulfasalazine).

(Continued on next page)

Table 27. Hepatotoxicity of Chemotherapeutic and Biotherapeutic Drugs *(Continued)*

Classification	Medication Name(s)	Route of Administration	Indications	Side Effects	Nursing Considerations
Antimetabolite (purine antagonist)	Cytarabine	IV	Treatment of AML, ALL, CML (blast phase), and lymphomas; prophylaxis and treatment of meningeal leukemia	Transient elevations of liver enzymes, jaundice	Dose may need to be adjusted in patients with liver failure because cytarabine is partially detoxified in the liver. There is no FDA-approved hepatic dosing adjustment guideline; the following guideline has been used by some clinicians (dose level not specified): Bilirubin > 2 mg/dl Administer 50% of dose and elevate subsequent doses with lack of toxicity (Koren et al., 1992).
Antimetabolite (pyrimidine antagonist)	Capecitabine	PO	Metastatic colorectal cancer; adjuvant therapy of Dukes' C colon cancer; treatment of metastatic breast cancer	Increased bilirubin (22%–48%; grades 3 and 4: 11%–23%); hepatic failure, hepatic fibrosis, hepatitis < 5%	Use with caution in patients with hepatic impairment.
	Floxuridine	Intra-arterial, IV	Management of hepatic metastases of colorectal and gastric cancers	Hepatocellular injury with increased aminotransferases, alkaline phosphatase, and serum bilirubin (hepatitis pattern); stricture of the intrahepatic or extrahepatic bile ducts (sclerosing cholangitis) accompanied by elevated alkaline phosphatase and serum bilirubin (Chang et al., 1987; Hohn et al., 1989)	Hepatic impairment: Use with caution in patients with hepatic impairment.
	Gemcitabine	IV	Metastatic breast cancer; locally advanced or metastatic NSCLC or pancreatic cancer; advanced, relapsed ovarian cancer	Increased transaminases (67%–78%; grades 3 and 4: 1%–12%), increased alkaline phosphatase (55%–77%; grades 3 and 4: 2%–16%), increased bilirubin (13%–26%; grades 3 and 4: < 1%–6%)	Serious hepatotoxicity has been reported; use caution with hepatic impairment (history of cirrhosis, hepatitis, or alcoholism) or in patients with hepatic metastases; may lead to exacerbation of hepatic impairment; dose reduction recommended for patients with elevated bilirubin levels (Venook et al., 2000).

(Continued on next page)

Table 27. Hepatotoxicity of Chemotherapeutic and Biotherapeutic Drugs (Continued)

Classification	Medication Name(s)	Route of Administration	Indications	Side Effects	Nursing Considerations
Anthracycline	Epirubicin	IV	Breast cancer	—	U.S. Boxed Warning: Use with caution in patients with mid-to-moderate hepatic impairment. See FDA-approved labeling for dosing guidelines. Monitor LFTs.
Biologic response modulator	IL-2; aldesleukin	IV, SC	Metastatic renal cell cancer, melanoma	Increased transaminases and alkaline phosphatase; jaundice. The mechanism of hepatic damage appears to be impaired sinusoidal perfusion and hypoxic damage caused by activation of Kupffer cells, and leukocyte and platelet adhesion to hepatic sinusoidal endothelium (Nakagawa et al., 1996); patients receiving high-dose IV IL-2 experience jaundice with serum bilirubin levels in the range of 2–7 mg/dl, thought to be caused by intrahepatic cholestasis (Fisher et al., 1989).	Dosing guidelines are not available for patients with preexisting liver dysfunction; dosing is typically delayed until resolution of hepatic dysfunction.
Miscellaneous	Asparaginase	IM, IV, SC	ALL	Hepatic: Transaminases, bilirubin, and alkaline phosphatase increased (transient)	Hepatic impairment: Use with caution in patients with preexisting hepatic impairment; may alter function.
	Bexarotene	Topical, PO	Cutaneous lesions of T-cell lymphoma	Increased LDH; Hepatic failure (above with oral formulation)	Extensive hepatic elimination. Monitor LFTs; consider stopping if values are three times the upper limit of normal (UpToDate, 2008).
	Denileukin diftitox	IV	Persistent or recurrent cutaneous T-cell lymphoma whose malignant cells express the CD25 component of the IL-2 receptor	Increased transaminases (61%; grades 3 and 4: 15%)	Monitor LFTs.
Monoclonal antibody	Gemtuzumab ozogamicin	IV	Relapsed CD33-positive AML in patients 60 years of age and older who are not candidates for cytotoxic chemotherapy	Abnormal LFTs (20%; grades 3 and 4: 7%), increased LDH (18%), hyperbilirubinemia (11%); increased alkaline phosphatase (10%), increased PT/PTT, veno-occlusive disease (5%–10%; up to 20% in relapsed patients; higher frequency in patients with prior history of subsequent hematopoietic SCT) (Giles et al., 2001)	U.S. Boxed Warning: Has been associated with severe veno-occlusive disease or hepatotoxicity use; risk may be increased by combination chemotherapy, previous hepatic disease, or hematopoietic SCT.

(Continued on next page)

Table 27. Hepatotoxicity of Chemotherapeutic and Biotherapeutic Drugs (Continued)

Classification	Medication Name(s)	Route of Administration	Indications	Side Effects	Nursing Considerations
Natural source (plant) derivative	Irinotecan	IV	Metastatic carcinoma of the colon or rectum	Increased bilirubin (84%), increased alkaline phosphatase (13%); increased AST (10%), ascites and/or jaundice (grades 3 and 4: 9%)	Hepatic impairment: Use with caution in patients with hepatic impairment. Hyperbilirubinemia: Patients with even modest elevations in total serum bilirubin levels (1–2 mg/dl) have a significantly greater likelihood of experiencing first-course grade 3 or 4 neutropenia than those with bilirubin levels that were < 1 mg/dl. Patients with abnormal glucuronidation of bilirubin, such as those with Gilbert syndrome, may also be at greater risk of myelosuppression when receiving therapy with irinotecan. Use caution when treating patients with known hepatic dysfunction or hyperbilirubinemia; dosage adjustments should be considered (Venook et al., 2003).
Tyrosine kinase inhibitor	Imatinib mesylate	PO	GIST kit-positive (CD117); Ph+ CML; Ph+ ALL; hypereosinophilic syndrome and/or chronic eosinophilic leukemia	Elevations in serum AST and ALT levels in 1%–5% of patients with CML, most commonly during the first 12 months of treatment	Hepatic impairment: Use with caution in patients with hepatic impairment; may require dosage adjustment.
Vinca alkaloid; natural source (plant) derivative	Vincristine	IV	Leukemias, Hodgkin disease, non-Hodgkin lymphomas, Wilms tumor, neuroblastoma, rhabdomyosarcoma	Metabolized extensively in the liver	Hepatic impairment: Use with caution in patients with hepatic impairment; dosage modification required.

ALL—acute lymphocytic leukemia; ALT—alanine aminotransferase; AML—acute myeloid leukemia; ANLL—acute nonlymphocytic leukemia; AST—aspartate aminotransferase; AUC—area under the concentration versus time curve; BMT—bone marrow transplant; CML—chronic myeloid leukemia; FDA—U.S. Food and Drug Administration; GI—gastrointestinal; GIST—gastrointestinal stromal tumor; IL-2—interleukin-2; IM—intramuscular; IT—intrathecal; IV—intravenous; LDH—lactic dehydrogenase; LFT—liver function test; MDS—myelodysplastic syndrome; min—minute; NSCLC—non-small cell lung cancer; Ph+—Philadelphia chromosome-positive; PO—oral; PT/PTT—prothrombin time/partial thromboplastin time; RA—rheumatoid arthritis; SC—subcutaneous; SCT—stem cell transplant

5. Assessment (Bryant, 2006)
   a) Physical examination to find and document the preceding clinical manifestations
      (1) Integument: Assess for presence of jaundice, ecchymosis, petechiae.
      (2) Head, eyes, ears, nose, and throat examination: Assess for icteric sclera.
      (3) Neurologic examination: Assess level of orientation, mental status.
      (4) Abdominal examination: Assess bowel sounds, liver/spleen, ascites, venous distension, Charcot triad.
   b) Baseline liver function tests (LFTs) prior to initiation of therapy
   c) History of hepatotoxic drug and/or alcohol use
   d) Past medical history (organ transplant, hepatitis, exposure to infected individuals)
   e) Hereditary liver diseases
6. Collaborative management: Few guidelines exist for the dosing of drugs based on elevated LFTs.
   a) Avoid using hepatotoxic drugs other than chemotherapy agents if LFT results are abnormal.
   b) It may be necessary to adjust the dose of chemotherapy in the presence of impaired hepatic function (Wilkes & Barton-Burke, 2003).
   c) Monitor the full blood chemistry, CBC, and clotting factor results.
   d) Instruct and assist the patient in following a low-fat, high-glucose diet containing vitamin B and C additives.
   e) Assess the patient's level of consciousness.
   f) Evaluate for signs of bleeding.
   g) Monitor subsequent LFT results.
7. Patient and family education
   a) If appropriate, inform patients and significant others that hepatotoxicity is a possible side effect of the chemotherapy agent.
   b) Instruct patients to avoid all alcoholic beverages if hepatotoxicity is noted.
   c) Provide instruction about signs and symptoms of liver failure (e.g., jaundice, liver tenderness, and changes in color of urine or stool).
   d) Promote rest.
   e) Encourage use of soothing lotions and cool baths to promote skin comfort. Remind patients not to scratch.
   f) Suggest that patients wear lightweight, loose clothing.
   g) Encourage patients to continue eating a light, high-glucose diet.
   h) Reinforce the importance of having lifelong annual follow-up assessments performed by a healthcare provider familiar with their cancer history, treatment, and risk of developing late effects (Bottomley, 2004).
   i) Encourage patients to have periodic LFTs and to plan appropriate follow-up.

References

Andrade, R.J., Salmeron, J., & Lucena, M.I. (2006). Drug hepatotoxicity. In K.R. Reddy & T. Faust (Eds.), *The clinician's guide to liver disease* (pp. 321–344). Thorofare, NJ: SLACK, Inc.

Aydinli, M., & Bayraktar, Y. (2007). Budd-Chiari syndrome: Etiology, pathogenesis, and diagnosis. *World Journal of Gastroenterology, 13*(19), 2693–2696.

Bottomley, S.J. (2004). Late effects of childhood cancer: Promoting health after childhood cancer. In N.E. Kline (Ed.), *Essentials of pediatric oncology nursing: A core curriculum* (2nd ed., pp. 290–291). Glenview, IL: Association of Pediatric Oncology Nurses.

Bryant, G. (2006). Hepatotoxicity. In D. Camp-Sorrell & R.A. Hawkins (Eds.), *Clinical manual for the oncology advanced practice nurse* (2nd ed., pp. 553–557). Pittsburgh, PA: Oncology Nursing Society.

Chang, A.E., Schneider, P.D., Sugarbaker, P.H., Simpson, C., Culnane, M., & Steinberg, S.M. (1987). A prospective randomized trial of regional versus systemic continuous 5-fluorodeoxyuridine chemotherapy in the treatment of colorectal liver metastases. *Annals of Surgery, 206*(6), 685–693.

Fisher, B., Keenan, A.M., Garra, B.S., Steinberg, S.M., White, D.E., DiBisceglie, A.M., et al. (1989). Interleukin-2 induces profound reversible cholestasis: A detailed analysis in treated cancer patients. *Journal of Clinical Oncology, 7*(12), 1852–1862.

Fregonese, L., & Stolk, J. (2008). Hereditary alpha-1-antitrypsin deficiency and its clinical consequences. *Orphanet Journal of Rare Disease, 3*(16). Retrieved October 28, 2008, from http://www.ojrd.com/content/3/1/16

Giles, F.J., Kantarjian, H.M., Kornblau, S.M., Thomas, D.A., Garcia-Manero, G., Waddelow, T., et al. (2001). Mylotarg (gemtuzumab ozogamicin) therapy is associated with hepatic venoocclusive disease in patients who have not received stem cell transplantation. *Cancer, 92*(2), 406–413.

Giralt, S., Thall, P.F., Khouri, I., Wang, X., Braunschweig, I., Ippolitti, C., et al. (2001). Melphalan and purine analog-containing preparative regimens: Reduced-intensity conditioning for patients with hematologic malignancies undergoing allogeneic progenitor cell transplantation. *Blood, 97*(3), 631–637.

Grochow, L.B., & Baker, S.D. (1998). The relationship of age to the disposition and effects of anticancer drugs. In L.B. Grochow & M.M. Ames (Eds.), *A clinician's guide to chemotherapy pharmacokinetics and pharmacodynamics* (pp. 35–53). Baltimore: Williams & Wilkins.

Hohn, D.C., Stagg, R.J., Friedman, M.A., Hannigan, J.F., Jr., Rayner, A., Ignoffo, R.J., et al. (1989). A randomized trial of continuous intravenous versus hepatic intraarterial floxuridine in patients with colorectal cancer metastatic to the liver: The Northern California Oncology Group trial. *Journal of Clinical Oncology, 7*(11), 1646–1654.

Kaler, S.G. (2007). Wilson's disease. In L. Goldman & D. Ausiello (Eds.), *Goldman: Cecil medicine* (23rd ed.). Philadelphia: Elsevier Saunders. Retrieved October 28, 2008, from http://www.mdconsult.com/das/book/body/108871545-2/0/1492/0.html

Koren, G., Beatty, K., Seto, A., Einarson, T.R., & Lishner, M. (1992). The effects of impaired liver function on the elimination of antineoplastic agents. *Annals of Pharmacotherapy, 26*(3), 363–371.

McDonald, G.N., Hinds, M.S., Fisher, L.D., Schoch, H.G., Wolford, J.L., Banaji, M., et al. (1993). Veno-occlusive disease of the liver and multiorgan failure after bone marrow transplantation: A cohort study of 35 patients. *Annals of Internal Medicine, 118*(4), 255–267.

Nakagawa, K., Miller, F.N., Sims, D.E., Lentsch, A.B., Miyzazki, M., & Edwards, M.J. (1996). Mechanisms of interleukin-2–induced hepatic toxicity. *Cancer Research, 56*(3), 507–510.

Peffault de Latour, R., Levy, V., Asselah, T., Marcellin, P., Scieux, C., Aldes, L., et al. (2004). Long-term outcome of hepatitis C infection after bone marrow transplantation. *Blood, 103*(5), 1618–1624.

Sifton, D.W. (Ed.). (2002). *Physicians' desk reference* (56th ed.). Montvale, NJ: Medical Economics.

Strasser, S.I., Shulman, H.M., Flowers, M.E., Reddy, R., Margolis, D.A., Prumbaum, M., et al. (2000). Chronic graft-vs-host disease of the liver: Presentation as an acute hepatitis. *Hepatology, 32*(6), 1265–1271.

Strasser, S.I., Sullivan, K.M., Myerson, D., Spurgeon, C.L., Storer, B., Schoch, H.G., et al. (1999). Cirrhosis of the liver in long-term marrow transplant survivors. *Blood, 93*(10), 3259–3266.

UpToDate. (2008). *Carmustine: Drug information.* Retrieved October 29, 2008, from http://www.uptodate.com/home/index.html

Venook, A.P., Egorin, M.J., Rosner, G.L., Hollis, D., Mani, S., Hawkins, M., et al. (2000). Phase I and pharmacokinetic trial of gemcitabine in patients with hepatic or renal dysfunction: Cancer and Leukemia Group B 9565. *Journal of Clinical Oncology, 18*(14), 2780–2787.

Venook, A.P., Enders Klein, C., Fleming, G., Hollis, D., Leichman, C.G., Hohl, R., et al. (2003). A phase I and pharmacokinetic study of irinotecan in patients with hepatic or renal dysfunction or with prior pelvic radiation: CALGB 9863. *Annals of Oncology, 14*(12), 1783–1790.

Weiss, R.B. (2005). Miscellaneous toxicities. In V.T. DeVita Jr., S. Hellman, & S.A. Rosenberg (Eds.), *Cancer: Principles and practice of oncology* (7th ed., pp. 2602–2614). Philadelphia: Lippincott Williams & Wilkins.

Wilkes, G.M., & Barton-Burke, M. (2008). *2008 oncology nursing drug handbook.* Sudbury, MA: Jones and Bartlett.

I. Nephrotoxicity: Approximately one million nephrons are present in each child at birth. Not all become fully functional until adulthood. New nephrons are not formed after birth (Bergstein, 2000). Nephrotoxicity is a dose-limiting effect of some chemotherapy and biotherapy agents.
   1. Pathophysiology: The kidneys are responsible for approximately 20% of the cardiac output. The renal system filters and/or excretes chemotherapy drugs, leaving the kidneys and other renal organs susceptible to toxic effects (Flombaum, 2005). Damage to vasculature and/or structure of the kidneys is possible along with specific renal syndromes and agent-specific renal deficiencies (Kuck & Ricciardi, 2005). Nephrotoxicity can cause

the following (Lydon, 1986; Moracic & Van Nostrand, 2007).
   a) Direct renal cell damage (including potential damage to the glomerulus, renal blood vessels, and/or different parts of the nephron): Initial studies show that damage may be irreversible and lead to necrosis, especially with cisplatin and high-dose methotrexate therapy (Lydon, 1986). More recent studies show the chief dose-limiting side effect of cisplatin is nephrotoxicity due to the kidneys accumulating cisplatin at a higher rate than other organs, primarily as a result of mediated transport (Arany & Safirstein, 2003).
   b) Growth impairment and gradual reduction in GFR have been noted in pediatric patients experiencing ifosfamide-induced renal tubular dysfunction (Stohr, Patzer, et al., 2007; Stohr, Paulides, et al., 2007).
   c) Precipitation of metabolites in the acidic environment of the urine: As a result of rapid tumor-cell lysis, metabolite precipitation causes obstructive nephropathy, also known as tumor lysis syndrome (TLS) (Higdon & Higdon, 2006).
      (1) TLS is an oncologic emergency and a metabolic risk for patients with large tumor burdens or tumor cell loads that are very sensitive to antineoplastic treatment modalities (e.g., acute leukemia, high-grade lymphoma, small cell lung cancer, multiple myeloma).
      (2) Patients presenting with elevated lactic dehydrogenase levels are at higher risk for TLS.
      (3) Tumor cells rapidly lyse following treatment, sending intracellular components into peripheral circulation. The results are severe and potentially life-threatening metabolic electrolyte imbalances characterized by hyperuricemia, hyperkalemia, hyperphosphatemia, and hypocalcemia (Cope & Brant, 2004).
      (4) TLS can be life-threatening if not identified and treated early. Early and aggressive treatment is crucial for possible reversal of adverse effects. Clinical consequences include acute renal failure, cardiac arrhythmias and failure, multisystem organ failure, and death (Cope & Brant, 2004).
      (5) The goals of preventive and treatment measures for TLS include vigorous hydration, urinary alkalinization, reduction of uric acid production with

allopurinol or rasburicase, and forced diuresis (Brant, 2002; Sanofi-Aventis, 2007; Shahab & Patterson, 2007).

d) Impaired water excretion: Treatment with certain antineoplastic agents (e.g., cyclophosphamide, ifosfamide, vinca alkaloids, cisplatin, melphalan, bortezomib) can cause a potentially emergent clinical situation known as water intoxication or the syndrome of inappropriate antidiuretic hormone (SIADH) (Flounders, 2003; Higdon & Higdon, 2006; Millennium Pharmaceuticals, Inc., 2007).

(1) SIADH leads to water resorption and decreased water excretion, hypervolemia, hyponatremia, and hyposmolality. SIADH should be suspected with clinical presentation of normovolemic hyponatremia (Higdon & Higdon, 2006).

(2) SIADH can have a rapid onset with life-threatening outcomes if the sodium level is < 105 mEq/L.

(3) SIADH can occur in regimens requiring vigorous hydration to prevent nephrotoxicity because they create a potential for water retention and severe hyponatremia.

(4) A clinical consequence is cerebral edema with neurologic signs and excess thirst as common symptoms.

(5) Treatment for SIADH relates to the presenting symptomatology and includes fluid restriction, forced diuresis, demeclocycline, and administration of hypertonic 3% saline (Higdon & Higdon, 2006).

e) Decreased renal perfusion and prerenal azotemia (Strohl & Camp-Sorrell, 2007)

(1) In patients receiving IL-2, factors contributing to nephrotoxicity include hypotension, impaired cardiac function, and decreased intravascular volume.

(2) These lead to decreased renal perfusion and prerenal azotemia.

(3) Most nephrotoxic effects of IL-2 are prerenal and fully reversible.

f) Proteinuria: With IFN and bevacizumab, the most common renal presentation is proteinuria (Genentech, Inc., 2007a).

g) Nephrotic syndrome and interstitial nephritis are rare (Genentech, Inc., 2007a; Kirkwood, 2000; Skalla, 1996).

2. Incidence (see Table 28)

3. Risk factors

a) Age less than 12 months: Renal blood flow, glomerular filtration, and tubular function are not completely developed in children until they are 12 months old. These physiologic characteristics affect drug disposition as well as excretion and secretion rates, predisposing children to nephrotoxicity (Balis, Holcenberg, & Blaney, 2001).

b) Advancing age, during which the kidneys become slightly smaller and renal function decreases (Shahab & Patterson, 2007): Research focusing on the older adult receiving nephrotoxic chemotherapy indicates a potential need for consideration of dose reductions or extended time between doses (Sawhey, Sehl, & Naeim, 2005). NCCN has instituted guidelines for treating the older adult patient with cancer (NCCN, 2007).

c) Preexisting renal disease, which presents a direct risk (Bergstein, 2000; Cope & Brant, 2004; Davies, 2006; Shahab & Patterson, 2007)

d) Connective tissue, liver, or cardiac disease, which presents an indirect risk (Shahab & Patterson, 2007)

e) Poor nutrition and hydration status

f) Hypovolemia, which may increase the risk of acute renal failure (Davies, 2006; Flounders, 2003; Jenkins & Rieselbach, 1982)

g) Administration of other nephrotoxic drugs (e.g., NSAIDs, aminoglycoside antibiotics, amphotericin B, cyclosporine, ibandronic acid) (Balis et al., 2001; McCormack & Plosker, 2006; Raymond, 1984)

h) The use of unconventional herbal preparations used in some cultures during chemotherapy has been associated with renal dysfunction, including electrolyte imbalances, tubular necrosis, and nephritis (Bagnis, Deray, Baumelou, Le Quintrec, & Vanherweghem, 2004).

i) Extravascular fluid shifts

j) Nephrectomy

k) Pretherapy hypercalcemia or SCr levels > 1.5 mg/dl

Table 28. Nephrotoxicity of Chemotherapeutic and Biotherapeutic Drugs

Classification	Drug	Incidence of Nephrotoxicity	Comments
Alkylating agent	Cisplatin	Adults: 12%–36% Adults and children: Renal sodium wasting, 10%; hypomagnesium, 1%–10% (Rossi et al., 1999)	Toxicity increases significantly with high-dose therapy (> 85 mg/m²) (Marceau et al., 1999). Dose-limiting renal insufficiency may be cumulative (Wilkes & Barton-Burke, 2008). The most common pediatric toxicities are dose-limiting azotemia and electrolyte disturbances secondary to decreased renal blood flow, decreased glomerular filtration rate, and loss of tubular function (Balis et al., 2001).
	Eloxatin	Adults: Serum creatinine changes, 10%	Elevated serum creatinine levels are most common (FDA, 2007).
	Ifosfamide	Adults: Renal toxicity, 6% (Bristol-Myers Squibb, 2006a) Children: Fanconi syndrome, 5%; subclinical tubular dysfunction, 15% (Rossi et al., 1999)	May cause tubular damage. Incidence of damage may increase with existing renal dysfunction or prior cisplatin therapy (Vogelzang, 1991). Pediatric patients have a slightly higher incidence of tubular damage (Skinner et al., 1993). Children tend to develop proximal tubular damage as well as a condition similar to Fanconi syndrome (Balis et al., 2001; Grochow & Baker, 1998).
Antimetabolite	Fludarabine	Adults: < 1% Children: Rare	Acute uric acid nephropathy related to TLS can occur with acute leukemias, high-grade lymphomas, and small cell lung cancer, and in patients with large tumor burden who have not received prophylactic allopurinol (Cheson et al., 1998).
	Gemcitabine	Adults: Hemolytic uremic syndrome (rare), elevated BUN and SCr, proteinuria, hematuria	BUN (17%) and SCr (8%) changes; up to 50% in clinical trials developed mild proteinuria and hematuria. Potential to lead to hemolytic uremic syndrome is rare (Flombaum, 2005).
	Methotrexate	Adults: < 10% with high-dose therapy Children: Child-specific incidence is unavailable.	In high-dose therapy, methotrexate enters renal tubules, precipitating tubular injury (Balis et al., 2001; Crom, 1998; Vogelzang, 1991).
Antitumor antibiotic	Mitomycin-C	Adults: 2%–10% Children: Child-specific incidence is unavailable.	Cumulative doses > 60 mg/m² may cause hemolytic uremic syndrome, a serious complication that includes hemolytic anemia, thrombocytopenia, and irreversible renal failure (Bristol-Myers Squibb, 2006b; Flombaum, 2005; Hrozencik & Connaughton, 1988; Vogelzang, 1991). Mitomycin-C is not commonly used for children.
Cytokine	Interferon	Adults: Rare, dose-related, generally reversible upon treatment cessation	Direct renal toxicity and neurogenic bladder and renal effects related to dehydration and metabolic or hemodynamic instability (Kirkwood, 2000; Sandstrom, 1996; Schering-Plough, 2008)
	Interleukin-2	Adults: Common, dose-related, transient, quickly reversible upon treatment cessation Children: Unknown	Alterations include impaired renal function, including direct renal toxicity and neurogenic bladder and renal effects related to dehydration and metabolic or hemodynamic instability (Novartis, 2007; Siegel & Puri, 1991).
Miscellaneous	Bortezomib	Adults: Rare Children: Unknown	Rare toxicities include renal failure and signs of hyperuricemia, hypokalemia, hypocalcemia, and hyponatremia with possible TLS and SIADH. Also noted are rare occurrences of renal calculus, hydronephrosis, and glomerular nephritis (Millennium Pharmaceuticals, Inc., 2007).
Monoclonal antibody	Bevacizumab	Adults: Rare Children: Unknown	Rare toxicities include proteinuria and nephrotic syndrome (Genentech, Inc., 2007a).
	Gemtuzumab ozogamicin	Adults: Rare, related to TLS	Rapid reduction of tumor cells can result in renal insufficiency, acute renal failure, uric acid nephropathy, acute renal failure resulting from renal tubular obstruction, and nephrolithiasis. Patients with large tumor burden are at increased risk for TLS (Wyeth Pharmaceuticals, 2007).

(Continued on next page)

Table 28. Nephrotoxicity of Chemotherapeutic and Biotherapeutic Drugs *(Continued)*

Classification	Drug	Incidence of Nephrotoxicity	Comments
Monoclonal antibody *(cont.)*	Rituximab	Adults: Rare, related to TLS	Same as gemtuzumab ozogamicin (Genentech, Inc., 2007b)
Nitrosourea	Carmustine	Adults: Common with cumulative doses > 1,500 mg/m² Children: Child-specific incidence is unavailable.	Effects include interstitial fibrosis and glomerular sclerosis, progressive azotemia, decrease in kidney size, and renal failure even with lower doses (Bristol-Myers Squibb, 2007a; Vogelzang, 1991). The onset of renal toxicity may occur months to years after chemotherapy (Shahab & Patterson, 2007).
	Lomustine	Adults: Common with cumulative doses > 1,500 mg/m² (Shahab & Patterson, 2007) Children: Child-specific incidence is unavailable.	Effects include interstitial fibrosis and glomerular sclerosis as well as progressive azotemia, decrease in kidney size, and renal failure even with lower doses (Bristol-Myers Squibb, 2007b; Vogelzang, 1991). The onset of renal toxicity may occur months to years after chemotherapy (Shahab & Patterson, 2007). In children, high cumulative doses of lomustine (> 1,000 mg/m²), nitrosourea therapy longer than 15 months, and semustine therapy are associated with progressive renal atrophy (Balis et al., 2001).
	Streptozotocin	Adults: Variable Children: Child-specific incidence is unavailable.	Common dose-related, cumulative renal toxicities include azotemia, anuria, hypophosphatemia, glycosuria, and renal tubular acidosis. Adequate hydration can help to reduce the risk of these toxicities (Sicor Pharmaceuticals, 2006). May cause tubular interstitial nephritis and tubular atrophy (Myerowitz et al., 1976); however, nephrotoxicity is rarely reported if the weekly dose is < 1 g/m² (Sadoff, 1970; Vogelzang, 1991). Streptozotocin is not commonly used for children.

BUN—blood urea nitrogen; SCr—serum creatinine; SIADH—syndrome of inappropriate antidiuretic hormone; TLS—tumor lysis syndrome

l) Previous radiation to the kidneys or abdomen without renal protection, especially in BMT recipients (Cohen & Moulder, 2005)

4. Clinical manifestations (Davies, 2006; Shahab & Patterson, 2007): Although hypomagnesemia, hypocalcemia, hypophosphatemia, and decreased serum bicarbonate are common during IL-2 and IFN alfa therapy, the conditions are accompanied by hypoalbuminemia and are not attributable to altered renal function (Kirkwood, 2000; Schwartzentruber, 2000). Signs and symptoms are listed previously for specific syndromes of TLS and SIADH. Signs and symptoms associated with renal dysfunction that require attention include the following (Cohen & Moulder, 2005).

   a) Oliguria
   b) Increasing SCr
   c) Declining CrCl
   d) Elevated BUN
   e) Hypomagnesemia
   f) Proteinuria
   g) Hematuria
   h) Weight gain from fluid retention or edema

5. Affected laboratory values (Cohen & Moulder, 2005): For pediatric patients, reference ranges are age-specific. Reference ranges differ from institution to institution. Similarly, indications to hold or delay chemotherapy for pediatric patients are based on evidence of nephrotoxicity as defined by treatment protocol. Consult institutional guidelines in regard to specific pediatric cases (Nicholson & Pesce, 2000). Note: The values cited in this section apply to adults only.

   a) BUN (Cohen & Moulder, 2005)
      (1) Assess baseline and consecutive levels.
         (a) For patients not requiring vasopressors, monitor levels daily.
         (b) For inpatients requiring vasopressors, monitor levels twice daily.
         (c) For outpatients, monitor levels weekly or as clinically indicated.
         (d) Remember that BUN is very sensitive to hydration status and BUN levels increase as dehydration increases in severity.
      (2) Make a rough estimate of renal function.
      (3) Hold or reduce dose of chemotherapy per physician order or protocol guidelines with evidence of renal impairment.

 b) SCr (Cohen & Moulder, 2005)
  (1) Assess baseline and consecutive levels. If the patient is on a research protocol, refer to protocol guidelines.
   (a) For patients not requiring vasopressors, monitor levels daily.
   (b) For inpatients requiring vasopressors, monitor levels twice daily.
   (c) For outpatients, monitor levels weekly or as clinically indicated.
  (2) SCr is a specific and sensitive indicator of renal function.
  (3) Consider holding or reducing dose of chemotherapy if SCr is ≥ grade 2 toxicity (> 1.5–3.0 × upper limit of normal) (NCI CTEP, 2006)
 c) 12-hour CrCl (Cohen & Moulder, 2005)
  (1) Assess baseline and consecutive levels. If the patient is on a research protocol, refer to protocol guidelines.
  (2) The 12-hour CrCl can be the most sensitive test of renal function. The 12-hour test is as effective as the 24-hour test and may be less costly. For pediatric patients, a test of nuclear GFR frequently is used.
  (3) Accuracy depends on collecting all urine in a specified time.
  (4) Consider holding or reducing dose of chemotherapy as indicated by the physician or treatment protocol if CrCl is decreasing.
 d) Urine cytology: Urine cytology is inaccurate if patients are cachectic because of various states of malnutrition and dehydration (Cohen & Moulder, 2005).
  (1) Assess changes in urine cytology (e.g., RBCs, WBCs, epithelial cells).
  (2) The presence of casts in urine can indicate renal tubular damage.
 e) Urine protein: Proteinuria indicates damage to the glomerular and tubular systems (Cohen & Moulder, 2005).

 f) Urine-specific gravity and osmolality (Cohen & Moulder, 2005)
  (1) A measure of renal ability to concentrate or dilute urine
  (2) Indicates presence or absence of tubular or medullary damage
  (3) Is often elevated in patients who are not adequately hydrated
 g) Urine pH (Cohen & Moulder, 2005)
  (1) A measure of the free hydrogen-ion concentration in urine
  (2) Expresses the strength of the urine as a dilute acid or a base solution
 h) Serum electrolytes, especially magnesium, uric acid, sodium, potassium, and calcium levels (Cohen & Moulder, 2005)
  (1) Measure serum electrolytes when giving cisplatin or high-dose chemotherapy and if the patient is at risk for TLS.
  (2) Monitor serum electrolytes during biotherapy, particularly IL-2, at the following frequencies (Wilkes & Barton-Burke, 2008).
   (a) For patients not requiring vasopressors, monitor levels daily.
   (b) For patients requiring vasopressors, monitor levels as clinically indicated.
  (3) Assess patient for fluid imbalance.
6. Objective physical assessment data (Strohl & Camp-Sorrell, 2007)
 a) Monitor intake and output.
 b) Monitor weight changes, especially weight gain and edema, daily or as clinically indicated.
 c) Monitor for changes in level of consciousness, mental status, or behavior.
7. Collaborative management
 a) General strategies
  (1) Monitor renal function tests regularly.
  (2) Institute hydration of approximately three liters per day to prevent or minimize renal damage, especially with cisplatin and high-dose methotrexate regimens (Rossi, Kleta, & Ehrich, 1999; Widemann, 2006). Hydration for pediatric patients is one-and-one-half to two times maintenance.
  (3) Confer with physician if BUN, creatinine, or electrolytes do not return to baseline.
  (4) Treat oliguria judiciously with fluid boluses.
  (5) Replace electrolytes as ordered.
 b) Follow-up recommendations (Strohl & Camp-Sorrell, 2007)

(1) Conduct periodic evaluation, including urinalysis, CrCl, and serum chemistries.

(2) If renal toxicity is severe, refer patients to a nephrologist to assess and possibly provide further workup and treatment, such as hemodialysis.

c) Drug-specific prevention strategies (Flombaum, 2005; Wilkes & Barton-Burke, 2008)

(1) Cisplatin regimens

(a) Assess BUN, SCr, and 24-hour CrCl to establish baseline prior to drug administration.

(b) Administer vigorous NS hydration to minimize toxicity.

(c) Strictly monitor intake and output and total body fluid balance.

(d) Assess for fluid overload.

(e) Induce diuresis with mannitol and/or a loop diuretic before or after administering cisplatin as a means of ensuring adequate urine flow to prevent fluid overload. Note that an increase in cisplatin toxicity has been shown with the use of furosemide for diuresis.

(f) Monitor renal function tests.

(g) Monitor serum sodium, potassium, magnesium, calcium, and phosphate.

(h) One study indicates selenium may provide some protection against cisplatin-induced nephrotoxicity (Conklin, 2000).

(i) Consider amifostine for reduction of nephrotoxicity associated with cisplatin-based regimens (ASCO, 2002; MedImmune Inc., 2007; Schrier, 2002; Shahab & Patterson, 2007).

i) Amifostine is a chemoprotectant and has been shown to decrease the harmful metabolites of cisplatin and some alkylating agents.

ii) Half-life (Wilkes & Barton-Burke, 2008)
  • Distribution less than one minute
  • Elimination in eight minutes

iii) The drug is administered intravenously over not more than 5–15 minutes and is given within 30 minutes of cisplatin after one liter of hydration has been administered.

iv) Side effects include hypotension, nausea and vomiting, flushing, and fever and chills.

v) Pretreat with antiemetics, administer hydration, monitor blood pressure every three to five minutes, keep patient in Trendelenburg position during and immediately after infusion, and interrupt the amifostine infusion if blood pressure drops below the threshold level.

vi) Hold antihypertensives 24 hours prior to amifostine administration.

(2) High-dose methotrexate regimens

(a) Alkalinize the urine by giving sodium bicarbonate PO or by IV. Assess urine pH for a minimum > 7.0 (Wilkes & Barton-Burke, 2008).

(b) It is essential to administer leucovorin at scheduled times (first dose usually 24 hours after methotrexate). Subsequent doses are given at six-hour intervals and continue until methotrexate level is within acceptable range. Leucovorin bypasses the folic acid antagonizing effect of methotrexate, decreasing the overall toxicities of methotrexate.

(c) Avoid taking folic acid, aspirin, penicillins, and sulfonylureas (e.g., glipizide) 48 hours before and after methotrexate (Wilkes & Barton-Burke, 2008).

(d) Discontinue treatment with NSAIDs, clotrimazole, and trimethoprim-sulfamethoxazole until the methotrexate level has decreased (Wilkes & Barton-Burke, 2008).

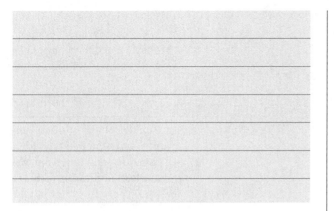

 (e) Reduce subsequent doses based on degree of toxicity.

 (3) For patients receiving IL-2 and IFN, know if doses are standard or one of the varying levels of high-dose, as toxicity increases with higher doses.

  (a) Encourage the patient to drink two to three liters of noncaffeinated fluid daily.

  (b) Monitor output.

 (4) Regimens for TLS: Allopurinol or rasburicase (Cheson, Frame, Vena, Quashu, & Sorensen, 1998)

  (a) Anticipate TLS in patients with tumors that have high growth fractions (e.g., Burkitt and other high-grade lymphomas, acute and chronic leukemias).

  (b) Administer allopurinol or rasburicase to decrease uric acid level, which can rapidly lead to acute uric acid nephropathy and renal failure if untreated.

8. Patient and family education (Lydon, 1986; Strohl & Camp-Sorrell, 2007)

 a) Ensure that patients understand the reasons for changes in urine output, electrolyte depletion, and increasing creatinine and BUN.

 b) Inform patients that nephrotoxicity is a risk associated with certain cytotoxic agents.

 c) Reinforce the importance of complying with preventive measures.

 d) Reinforce the importance of collecting all urine for 12 and 24 hours for CrCl.

 e) Encourage patients to increase fluid intake; intake should be two to three liters of noncaffeinated fluid daily.

 f) Ensure that patients understand the need to comply with instructions to alkalinize urine and complete leucovorin rescue, allopurinol therapy, and/or amifostine treatment.

 g) Explain the reason for weight gain during

specific therapies and the need for diuresis after therapy is completed.

 h) Instruct patients to avoid the use of drugs that potentiate renal dysfunction. Give them a list of those drugs.

 i) Ensure that patients know to notify the healthcare team if

  (1) They are unable to make urine for more than 12 hours.

  (2) Urine becomes very dark, concentrated, pink, bloody, or cloudy.

  (3) They produce only very small amounts of urine.

  (4) Weight gain or edema occur.

References

American Society of Clinical Oncology. (2002). *2002 update of recommendations for the use of chemotherapy and radiotherapy protectants: Clinical practice guidelines of the American Society of Clinical Oncology.* Retrieved November 10, 2007, from http://jco.ascopubs.org/cgi/content/full/20/12/2895

Arany, I., & Safirstein, R.L. (2003). Cisplatin nephrotoxicity. *Seminars in Nephrology, 23*(5), 460–464.

Bagnis, C.I, Deray, G., Baumelou, A., Le Quintrec, M., & Vanherweghem, J.L. (2004). Herbs and the kidney. *American Journal of Kidney Diseases, 44*(1), 1–11.

Balis, F.M., Holcenberg, J.S., & Blaney, S.M. (2001). General principles of chemotherapy. In P.A. Pizzo & D.G. Poplack (Eds.), *Principles and practice of pediatric oncology* (4th ed., pp. 237–308). Philadelphia: Lippincott Williams & Wilkins.

Bergstein, J.M. (2000). Glomerular disease and renal failure. In R.E. Berhman, R.M. Kliegman, & H.B. Jenson (Eds.), *Nelson textbook of pediatrics* (16th ed., pp. 1573–1576, 1604–1612). Philadelphia: Saunders.

Brant, J. (2002). Rasburicase: An innovative new treatment for hyperuricemia associated with tumor lysis syndrome. *Clinical Journal of Oncology Nursing, 6*(1), 12–16.

Bristol-Myers Squibb. (2006a). Ifex [Package insert]. Retrieved October 27, 2008, from http://dailymed.nlm.nih.gov/dailymed

Bristol-Myers Squibb. (2006b). Mutamycin [Package insert]. Retrieved October 27, 2008, from http://dailymed.nlm.nih.gov/dailymed

Bristol-Myers Squibb. (2007a). BiCNU [Package insert]. Retrieved October 27, 2008, from http://dailymed.nlm.nih.gov/dailymed

Bristol-Myers Squibb. (2007b). CeeNu [Package insert]. Retrieved October 27, 2008, from http://dailymed.nlm.nih.gov/dailymed

Cheson, D.D., Frame, J.N., Vena, D., Quashu, N., & Sorensen, J.M. (1998). Tumor lysis syndrome: An uncommon complication of fludarabine therapy of chronic lymphocytic leukemia. *Journal of Clinical Oncology, 16*(7), 2313–2320.

Cohen, E.P., & Moulder, J.E. (2005). Radiation nephropathy. In E.P. Cohen (Ed.), *Cancer and the kidney* (pp. 169–170). New York: Oxford University Press.

Conklin, K.A. (2000). Dietary antioxidants during chemotherapy: Impact on chemotherapeutic effectiveness and development of side effects. *Nutrition and Cancer, 37*(1), 1–18.

Cope, D., & Brant, J.M. (2004). Tumor lysis syndrome. *Clinical Journal of Oncology Nursing, 8*(4), 415–416.

Crom, W.R. (1998). Methotrexate. In L.B. Grochow & M.M. Ames (Eds.), *A clinician's guide to chemotherapy pharmacokinetics and pharmacodynamics* (pp. 311–330). Baltimore: Williams & Wilkins.

Davies, M.J. (2006). Acute renal failure. In D. Camp-Sorrell & R.A. Hawkins (Eds.), *Clinical manual for the oncology advanced practice nurse* (2nd ed., pp. 637–645). Pittsburgh, PA: Oncology Nursing Society.

Flombaum, C.D. (2005). Nephrotoxicity in chemotherapy agents. In E.P. Cohen (Ed.), *Cancer and the kidney* (pp. 127–130). New York: Oxford University Press.

Flounders, J. (2003). Syndrome of inappropriate antidiuretic hormone. *Oncology Nursing Forum, 30*(8), E63–E70. Retrieved October 14, 2008, from http://www.ons.org/publications/journals/ONF/Volume30/Issue3/3003381.asp

Genentech, Inc. (2007a). Avastin [Package insert]. Retrieved November 11, 2007, from http://www.gene.com/gene/products/information/oncology/avastin/index.jsp

Genentech, Inc. (2007b). Rituxan [Package insert]. Retrieved November 11, 2007, from http://www.gene.com/gene/products/information/oncology/rituxan/index.jsp

Grochow, L.B., & Baker, S.D. (1998). The relationship of age to the disposition and effects of anticancer drugs. In L.B. Grochow & M.M. Ames (Eds.), *A clinician's guide to chemotherapy pharmacokinetics and pharmacodynamics* (pp. 35–54). Baltimore: Williams & Wilkins.

Higdon, M.L., & Higdon, J.A. (2006). Treatment of oncologic emergencies. *American Family Physician, 74*(11), 1873–1880.

Hrozencik, S.P., & Connaughton, M.J. (1988). Cancer-associated hemolytic uremic syndrome. *Oncology Nursing Forum, 15*(6), 755–759.

Jenkins, P.G., & Rieselbach, R.E. (1982). Acute renal failure: Diagnosis, clinical spectrum, and management. In R.E. Rieselbach & M.B. Garnick (Eds.), *Cancer and the kidney* (pp. 103–179). Philadelphia: Lea & Febiger.

Kirkwood, J.M. (2000). Interferon-alpha and -beta: Clinical applications. In S.A. Rosenberg (Ed.), *Principles and practice of the biologic therapy of cancer* (pp. 224–251). Philadelphia: Lippincott Williams & Wilkins.

Kuck, A.W., & Ricciardi, E. (2005). Alterations in elimination. In J.K. Itano & K.N. Taoka (Eds.), *Core curriculum for oncology nursing* (4th ed., pp. 340–341). St. Louis, MO: Elsevier Saunders.

Lydon, J. (1986). Nephrotoxicity of cancer treatment. *Oncology Nursing Forum, 13*(2), 68–77.

Marceau, D., Poirer, M., Masson, E., & Beaulieu, E. (1999, May). *High incidence of nephrotoxicity with cisplatin therapy despite adequate hydration: Risk factor correlation.* Abstract presented at the Annual Meeting of the American Society of Clinical Oncology, Atlanta, GA.

McCormack, P.L., & Plosker, G.L. (2006). Ibandronic acid: A review of its use in the treatment of bone metastases of breast cancer. *Drugs, 66*(5), 711–728.

MedImmune Inc. (2007). Ethyol [Package insert]. Retrieved November 11, 2007, from http://www.medimmune.com/products/ethyol/index.asp

Millennium Pharmaceuticals, Inc. (2007). Velcade [Package insert]. Retrieved November 11, 2007, from http://www.mlnm.com/products/velcade/index.asp

Moracic, L., & Van Nostrand, J. (2007). Anesthetic implications for cancer chemotherapy. *AANA Journal, 75*(3), 218–226.

Myerowitz, R.L., Sartiano, G.P., & Cavallo, T. (1976). Nephrotoxic and cytoproliferative effects of streptozotocin. *Cancer, 38*(4), 1550–1555.

National Cancer Institute Cancer Therapy Evaluation Program. (2006). *Common terminology criteria for adverse events* (version 3.0). Bethesda, MD: National Cancer Institute. Retrieved October 27, 2008, from http://ctep.cancer.gov/forms/CTCAEv3.pdf

National Comprehensive Cancer Network. (2007). *NCCN Clinical Practice Guidelines in Oncology™: Senior adult oncology* [v.2.2007]. Retrieved October 14, 2008, from http://www.nccn.org/professionals/physician_gls/PDF/senior.pdf

Nicholson, J.F., & Pesce, M.A. (2000). Reference ranges for laboratory tests and procedures. In R.E. Berhman, R.M. Kliegman, & H.B. Jenson (Eds.), *Nelson textbook of pediatrics* (16th ed., pp. 2181–2234). Philadelphia: Saunders.

Novartis. (2007). Proleukin [Package insert]. Retrieved October 27, 2008, from http://dailymed.nlm.nih.gov/dailymed

Raymond, J.R. (1984). Nephrotoxicities and antineoplastic and immunosuppressive agents. *Current Problems in Cancer, 8*(16), 1–32.

Rossi, R., Kleta, R., & Ehrich, J.H.H. (1999). Renal involvement in children with malignancies. *Pediatric Nephrology, 13*(2), 153–162.

Sadoff, L. (1970). Nephrotoxicity of streptozotocin (NSC85998). *Cancer Chemotherapy Reports, 54*(6), 457–459.

Sandstrom, S.K. (1996). Nursing management of patients receiving biological therapy. *Seminars in Oncology Nursing, 12*(2), 152–162.

Sanofi-Aventis. (2007). Elitek [Package insert]. Retrieved November 11, 2007, from http://www.sanofi-aventis.us/live/us/en/layout.jsp?scat=8D52920D-5655-4CCB-A499-EE05C6172519

Sawhey, P., Sehl, M., & Naeim, A. (2005). Physiologic aspects of aging: Impact on cancer management and decision making: Part 1. *Cancer, 11*(6), 449–460.

Schering-Plough. (2008). Intron-A [Package insert]. Retrieved October 27, 2008, from http://dailymed.nlm.nih.gov/dailymed

Schrier, R.W. (2002). Cancer therapy and renal injury. *Journal of Clinical Investigation, 110*(6), 473.

Schwartzentruber, D.J. (2000). Interleukin-2: Clinical applications: Principles of administration and management of side effects. In S.A. Rosenberg (Ed.), *Principles and practice of the biologic therapy of cancer* (3rd ed., pp. 32–50). Philadelphia: Lippincott Williams & Wilkins.

Shahab, I., & Patterson, W.P. (2007). Renal and electrolyte abnormalities due to chemotherapy. In M.C. Perry (Ed.), *The chemotherapy source book* (4th ed., pp. 223–231). Philadelphia: Lippincott Williams & Wilkins.

Sicor Pharmaceuticals. (2006). Zanosar [Package insert]. Retrieved October 27, 2008, from http://dailymed.nlm.nih.gov/dailymed

Siegel, J.P., & Puri, R.K. (1991). Interleukin-2 toxicity. *Journal of Clinical Oncology, 9*(4), 694–704.

Skalla, K. (1996). The interferons. *Seminars in Oncology Nursing, 12*(2), 97–105.

Skinner, R., Sharkey, I.M., Pearson, A.D., & Craft, A.W. (1993). Ifosfamide, mesna, and nephrotoxicity in children. *Journal of Clinical Oncology, 11*(1), 173–190.

Stohr, W., Patzer, L., Paulides, M., Kretzer, A., Beck, J., Langer, T., et al. (2007). Growth impairment after ifosfamide-induced nephrotoxicity in children. *Pediatric Blood and Cancer, 48*(5), 571–576.

Stohr, W., Paulides, M., Bielack, S., Jürgens, H., Koscielniak, E., Rossi, R., et al. (2007). Nephrotoxicity of cisplatin and carboplatin in sarcoma patients: A report from the late effects surveillance system. *Pediatric Blood and Cancer, 48*(2), 140–147.

Strohl, R.A., & Camp-Sorrell, D. (2007). Hemorrhagic cystitis. In D. Camp-Sorrell & R.A. Hawkins (Eds.), *Clinical manual for the oncology advanced practice nurse* (2nd ed., pp. 661–663). Pittsburgh, PA: Oncology Nursing Society.

U.S. Food and Drug Administration. (2007). *Eloxatin prescribing information.* Retrieved November 12, 2007, from http://www.fda.gov/cder/drug/infopage/eloxatin

Vogelzang, N.J. (1991). Nephrotoxicity from chemotherapy: Prevention and management. *Oncology, 5*(10), 97–102.

Widemann, B.C. (2006). Understanding and managing methotrexate nephrotoxicity. *Oncologist, 11*(6), 694–703.

Wilkes, G.M., & Barton-Burke, M. (2008). *2008 oncology nursing drug handbook.* Sudbury, MA: Jones and Bartlett.

Wyeth Pharmaceuticals. (2007). Mylotarg [Package insert]. Retrieved November 11, 2007, from http://www.wyeth.com/products?product=/wyeth_html/home/products/prescription/Mylotarg%c2%ae%20(gemtuzumab%20ozogamicin%20for%20Injection)/prescribinginfo.html

J. Neurotoxicity: Neurotoxicity can arise as direct or indirect damage to the CNS, peripheral nervous system, cranial nerves (CNs), or any combination of the three (Gilbert, 2000). Many cancer treatments are neurotoxic. Some drugs cause neurotoxicity at low doses, whereas others cause neurotoxicity only during intensive therapy. Neurologic toxicity is a dose-limiting factor in several cancer treatments, such as radiation therapy, and patients suffer more from the toxicities than from the cancer itself (Keime-Guibert, Napolitano, & Delattre, 1998; Quasthoff & Hartung, 2002).
1. Pathophysiology
   a) CN deficits: These deficits result from damage to one of the 12 CNs arising from the brain stem. The result depends on which nerve is damaged (Barker, 2008; Cassidy & Misset, 2002). Examples of CN deficits include the following.
      (1) Olfactory (CN I): Loss or decrease of smell
      (2) Optic (CN II): Loss of visual acuity, optic atrophy, altered visual field
      (3) Oculomotor (CN III): Ptosis, dilated pupils, altered ocular muscle function, nystagmus
      (4) Trochlear (CN IV): Altered ocular muscle function causing nystagmus
      (5) Trigeminal (CN V): Numbness, poor blink reflex, weakened chewing
      (6) Abducens (CN VI): Altered ocular muscle function causing nystagmus
      (7) Facial (CN VII): Facial paralysis, drooping mouth, sagging lower eyelid, flat nasolabial fold
      (8) Acoustic (CN VIII): Sensory neuronal hearing loss, vertigo, ataxia, nausea and/or vomiting
      (9) Glossopharyngeal (CN IX): Altered sense of taste, altered throat sensation
      (10) Vagus (CN X): Hoarseness, altered gag reflex, altered swallowing function
      (11) Spinal accessory (CN XI): Tilting of head, weakness of shoulder muscles
      (12) Hypoglossal (CN XII): Abnormal tongue movement
   b) Peripheral nervous system deficits are a result of damage to sensory and motor nerves outside the CNS, including the autonomic nerves. Peripheral neuropathy is caused by chemotherapy injuring the sensory and motor axons. This results in demyelination, which reduces nerve conduction velocity leading to loss of deep tendon reflexes. Disorders of one or more peripheral nerves cause signs and symptoms that correspond to the anatomical distribution and normal function of the nerve. The signs and symptoms of a peripheral nerve disorder may include sensory, motor, or autonomic disturbances (Hickey, 2003). See NCI CTCAE in Table 29.
      (1) Sensory nerve fibers: Decrease or loss of light touch and pinprick sensation along the involved dermatome. Tingling, numbness, paresthesias and dysesthesias are common. Paresthesias are unusual sensations such as "pins and needles," whereas dysesthesias are unpleasant sensations such as burning (Hickey, 2003).
      (2) Motor nerve fibers: Symmetrical generalized motor weakness that may affect balance, strength, activity level, foot or wrist drop, myalgias, and muscle cramping (Armstrong, Almadrones, & Gilbert, 2005)
      (3) Decreased or absent deep-tendon reflexes
      (4) Autonomic nerves: Constipation, paralytic ileus (rare), urinary retention, incontinence, erectile dysfunction, orthostatic hypotension
   c) CNS deficits: These deficits have multiple causes (e.g., metabolic imbalances, intracranial hemorrhage, or infection related to chemotherapy-induced coagulopathy or myelosuppression, IT or intra-arterial chemotherapy, high-dose therapy). Deficits depend on the area of brain or brain stem affected (Armstrong, Rust, & Kohtz, 1997; Gilbert, 2000).

Table 29. Common Terminology Criteria for Adverse Events—Neuropathies

Adverse Event	Grade 1	Grade 2	Grade 3	Grade 4	Grade 5
Neuropathy—cranial	Asymptomatic, detected on exam/testing only	Symptomatic, not interfering with ADL	Symptomatic, interfering with ADL	Life-threatening; disabling	Death
Neuropathy—motor	Asymptomatic, weakness on exam/testing only	Symptomatic weakness interfering with function, but not interfering with ADL	Weakness interfering with ADL; bracing or assistance to walk (e.g., cane or walker) indicated	Life-threatening; disabling (e.g., paralysis)	Death
Neuropathy—sensory	Asymptomatic; loss of deep tendon reflexes or paresthesia (including tingling) but not interfering with function	Sensory alteration or paresthesia (including tingling), interfering with function, but not interfering with ADL	Sensory alteration or paresthesia interfering with ADL	Disabling	Death

ADL—activities of daily living

Note. From *Common Terminology Criteria for Adverse Events* (Version 3.0), by National Cancer Institute Cancer Therapy Evaluation Program, 2006, Bethesda, MD: National Cancer Institute.

(1) Acute or chronic encephalopathy: Somnolence and lethargy, confusion, disorientation, memory loss, cognitive dysfunction, seizures

(2) Cerebellar dysfunction: Truncal, limb, and gait ataxia; dysarthria (staggered gait and postural imbalance); difficulty speaking; slow or irregular speech; nystagmus

(3) The blood-brain barrier contributes to the immune privilege of the CNS; however, significant cross-talk and bidirectional communication occur between the CNS and the immune system (Maier & Watkins, 2003). In addition, the release of proinflammatory cytokines, including IL-1, IL-6, and TNF-α, in the peripheral blood leads to penetration of the blood-brain barrier as well as production of proinflammatory cytokines in the CNS (Myers, Pierce, & Pazdernik, 2008). The proinflammatory cytokines also are associated with a syndrome of behaviors and symptoms known as sickness behavior (Kronfol & Remick, 2000). Sickness behavior includes fever, fatigue, lethargy, muscle aches, decreased ability to concentrate, and decreased social interaction (Parnet, Kelley, Bluthe, & Dantzer, 2002; Pollmacher, Haack, Schuld, Reichenberg, & Yirmiya, 2002; Wilson, Finch, & Cohen, 2002).

(4) Ifosfamide and some of its metabolites can cross the blood-brain barrier (Verstappen, Heimans, Hockman, & Postma, 2003). Nitrosoureas are alkylating agents that can cross the blood-brain barrier and are used to treat brain tumors, melanoma, and lymphomas (Verstappen et al., 2003). Concomitant administration of dexamethasone or mannitol may be given to reduce side effects of cerebral edema as a result of penetration of the blood-brain barrier (Wilkes & Barton-Burke, 2007).

(5) Thalidomide's mechanism of action is unclear, but it is thought to possess immunomodularity, anti-inflammatory, and antiangiogenic properties. It was found to inhibit angiogenesis and is known to cause nerve damage that may

276 Chemotherapy and Biotherapy Guidelines and Recommendations for Practice, Third Edition

be permanent. Peripheral neuropathy is common (Celgene Corporation, 1998).

2. Incidence: Exact incidence is unknown, but incidence is increasing with greater use of high-dose chemotherapy, the use of more than one neurotoxic agent at a time or sequentially, and with increased detection because of objective and subjective assessment (Armstrong & Gilbert, 2002; Cavalletti & Zanna, 2002; Postma & Heimans, 2000) (see Table 30).

3. Risk factors
   a) Regimens that include high-dose chemotherapy are associated with blood-brain barrier penetration (Taxen & Hansen, 1994), and most chemotherapeutic agents have not been reported to cross the blood-brain barrier in standard doses (Saykin, Ahles, & McDonald,

2003), with the exception of methotrexate, cisplatin, cytarabine, ifosfamide, procarbazine, temozolomide, carmustine, lomustine (Wilkes & Barton-Burke, 2007), and topotecan (Wong & Berkenblit, 2004).
   b) Route of administration: IT methotrexate and cytarabine may be used to treat meningeal leukemia or lymphoma (Tuxen & Hansen, 1994). High peripheral doses can cause neurotoxicity (e.g., lethargy, somnolence) and cerebellar toxicity (e.g., nystagmus, dysarthria, ataxia, slurred speech, decreased ability to make fine coordinated movements) (Wilkes & Barton-Burke, 2007). IT doses may cause paraparesis or seizure (Tuxen & Hansen).
   c) Concomitant cranial radiation therapy causes the cells in the CNS to replicate

Table 30. Neurotoxicity of Chemotherapeutic and Biotherapeutic Drugs			
Classification	**Drug**	**Incidence of Neurotoxicity**	**Characteristic Effects and Comments**
Alkylating agents	Busulfan	Low at conventional dosing; high dosing can cause seizures (Ben Venue Labs, Inc., 2007).	Administer seizure prophylaxis—anticonvulsants (e.g., phenytoin) (Ben Venue Labs, Inc., 2007).
	Cisplatin	Occurs with cumulative doses beyond 400 mg/m² (Van der Hoop et al., 1990) Symptomatic hearing loss affects 15%–20% of patients, and hearing impairment can be found in more than three-fourths of the patients (Oldenburg et al., 2007). Lhermitte sign can occur in 20%–40% of patients after weeks or months of treatment (Forsyth & Cascino, 1995).	Numbness, paresthesia, and pain in toes and fingers spreading proximally to the arms and legs; proprioception is impaired and reflexes are lost, but power is almost always spared (Hilkens et al., 1995). Radiotherapy to the normal cochlea or cranial nerve VIII with concurrent administration of cisplatin results in ototoxicity (Low et al., 2006). Ototoxicity can be severe in children (Li et al., 2004). Lhermitte sign is a shock-like nonpainful paresthesia radiating from the back to the feet during neck flexion (Forsyth & Cascino, 1995).
	Ifosfamide	10%–20% of patients will develop an encephalopathy (David & Picus, 2005). Rare toxicities are seizures, ataxia, weakness, and neuropathies (Posner, 2001).	Symptoms can occur during drug administration and usually resolve within several days (David & Picus, 2005). Patients at risk for toxicities include those with a prior history of ifosfamide-related encephalopathy, renal dysfunction, or low serum albumin prior to treatment (Posner, 2001).
	Oxaliplatin	Acute symptoms are observed more frequently at doses > 130 mg/m² than at < 85 mg/m² and are infusion rate dependent (Gamelin et al., 2002).	Symptoms consist of striking paresthesias and dysesthesias of the hands, feet, and perioral region with jaw tightness. Symptoms are often induced or aggravated by the cold (Lehky et al., 2004).
Antimetabolites	Capecitabine	Paresthesias were common for fewer than 10% of patients treated (Renouf & Gill, 2006).	Paresthesias, headaches, dizziness, or insomnia can occur. Cerebellar toxicity has been reported (Renouf & Gill, 2006). Symptoms resolved after stopping the drug (Videnovic et al., 2005).

(Continued on next page)

Table 30. Neurotoxicity of Chemotherapeutic and Biotherapeutic Drugs *(Continued)*

Classification	Drug	Incidence of Neurotoxicity	Characteristic Effects and Comments
Antimetabo-lites *(cont.)*	Cytarabine	Conventional doses cause little toxicity. High-dose, 3 g/m^2, every 12 hours for 6 doses can cause an acute cerebellar syndrome in 10%–25% of patients (Smith et al., 1997). Patients over 50 years of age with abnormal liver or renal function or who received a total dose of > 30 g are likely to develop cerebellar toxicity (Smith et al., 1997).	Symptoms begin with somnolence and occasionally encephalopathy. Immediately thereafter, cerebellar signs are noted. Symptoms range from mild ataxia to an inability to sit or walk. No specific treatment, but cytarabine should be stopped immediately. In some, the syndrome resolves immediately, but it is permanent in others (Friedman & Shetty, 2001).
	5-fluoroura-cil (5-FU)	Rare side effects including encephalopathy, optic neuropathy, or seizures have been recorded (Pirzada et al., 2000).	Symptoms of an acute onset of ataxia, dysmetria, and dysarthria can develop weeks to months after beginning treatment. The 5-FU should be stopped in any patient with cerebellar toxicity; with time, symptoms will resolve (Pirzada et al., 2000).
	Gemcitabine	Up to 10% of patients experience mild par-esthesias during treatment, but severe peripheral and autonomic neuropathies can occur (Dormann et al., 1998).	An acute inflammatory myopathy and asymmetrical, painful, proximal muscle weakness can occur (Ardavanis et al., 2005). Myositis can occur when gemcitabine is given during or after radiation (radiation recall phenomenon) (Friedlander et al., 2004).
	Methotrexate (MTX)	Generalized or focal seizures have been reported among pediatric patients with acute lymphocytic leukemia treated with intermediate-dose IV MTX (Bedford Laboratories, 2000). Acute chemical arachnoiditis can occur after intrathecal MTX. Acute neurotoxicity is most frequently seen after high-dose MTX and may develop in the second or third week of therapy (Forsyth & Cascino, 1995).	Symptomatic patients were commonly noted to have leukoencephalopathy and/or microangiopathic calcifications on diagnostic imaging studies (Bedford Laboratories, 2000). Headache, back pain, nuchal rigidity, fever, and lethargy can begin 2–4 hours after drug is injected and may last 12–72 hours, self-limiting (Bedford Laboratories, 2000). Symptoms such as somnolence, confusion, transient blindness, seizures, and coma (Bedford Laboratories, 2000); leucovorin administration should begin as promptly as possible. Monitoring of the serum MTX concentration is essential in determining the optimal dose and duration of the treatment with leucovorin (Bedford Laboratories, 2000).
Interferon (IFN)	IFN alfa	Low-dose toxicity causes tremors. High-dose toxicity is rare and includes oculo-motor palsy and sensory motor neuropa-thies (Rutkove, 1997).	Neurotoxicity tends to be dose-related. High doses can cause confusion, lethargy, confusion, hallucinations, and seizures (Meyers et al., 1991).
	IFN alfa-2a IFN alfa-2b	Incidence of neuropsychiatric depression and suicidal behavior was > 15% (Hensley et al., 2000). Depression, anxiety, or emotional lability was seen in 4%–40% of patients (Hensley et al., 2000).	Motor weakness can be seen at high doses (> 100 million units) and reverses within days (Hensley et al., 2000). All patients recovered upon withdrawal of drug. Those with psychiatric history were more likely to develop neuropsychiatric toxicity (Hensley et al., 2000).
Interleukin	IL-2	Neuropsychiatric complications occur in 30%–50% of patients (Denicoff et al., 1987).	Toxicity is dose dependent. Confusion may be dose-limiting effect of high-dose IL-2 (Buzaid & Atkins, 2001).
Miscellaneous	Bortezomib	Peripheral neuropathy is the main dose-limiting toxicity, and grade 1 or 2 peripheral neuropathies affect 33% of patients (Richardson et al., 2003).	Peripheral neuropathy is length dependent, sensory rather than motor (Cata et al., 2007; Cavaletti & Zanna, 2007). Symptoms include reduced ankle reflexes, decreased vibration sensation, and impaired heel to toe gait (Gidal, 2006). Symptoms can improve or stabilize after patient stops or decreases the dose of the drug (Jagganath et al., 2004).

(Continued on next page)

Table 30. Neurotoxicity of Chemotherapeutic and Biotherapeutic Drugs *(Continued)*

Classification	Drug	Incidence of Neurotoxicity	Characteristic Effects and Comments
Miscellaneous *(cont.)*	Thalidomide	Peripheral neuropathy develops in approximately 75% of patients who receive a prolonged course of thalidomide (Cavaletti et al., 2004; Mileshkin et al., 2006; Tosi et al., 2005). Somnolence can occur and stops after a few weeks on therapy.	The neuropathy is partially reversible, and dose reduction or cessation of treatment is required in up to 60% of patients (Mileshkin et al., 2006; Tosi et al., 2005). Patients should be examined at monthly intervals for the first 3 months to detect early signs of neuropathy, which include numbness, tingling, and pain in hands and feet (Celgene Corporation, 1998).
Monoclonal antibody	Bevacizumab	Reversible posterior leukoencephalopathy syndrome (RPLS) occurs infrequently (Allen et al., 2006; Ozcan et al., 2006).	Headache, seizure, lethargy, confusion, and blindness can occur. RPLS associated with mild to moderate hypertension has been reported. Symptoms can occur up to 1 year after therapy. Symptoms usually resolve after stopping the bevacizumab and controlling hypertension (Allen et al., 2006; Ozcan et al., 2006).
Plant alkaloids	Docetaxel	Sensory and motor neuropathies can occur. Grade 3 or 4 (NCI CTEP, 2006) neuropathies occur in less than 5% of patients (Smith et al., 1997).	Treatment with docetaxel has been associated with the development of Lhermitte sign, a nonpainful electrical shock that shoots down the neck with flexion (Smith et al., 1997).
	Paclitaxel	Sensory and motor neuropathies are commonly seen with paclitaxel. The incidence of grade 3 or 4 neuropathy occurs in patients receiving 250 mg/m² every 3 weeks compared to 5%–12% with dosing < 200 mg/m² every 3 weeks (Lee & Swain, 2006).	Neuropathy with burning paresthesias of the hands and feet can occur (Lee & Swain, 2006). Paresthesias are dose-dependent and can be profound with numbness and a decrease in deep tendon reflexes (Postma & Heimans, 2000).
	Vincristine	Vincristine causes some degree of neuropathy. The toxicity is severe in adults, dose dependent, and more prominent with hepatic dysfunction (Donelli et al., 1998). Autonomic neuropathy such as colicky abdominal pain and constipation occur in almost 50% of patients; paralytic ileus may result (Legha, 1986).	Symptoms include paresthesias of the fingertips and feet. Can occur with first dose, and symptoms may appear after drug has been stopped; can progress before improving. Weakness can be mild—patients can lose ability to walk on heels, lose strength in wrists—and more severe—develop foot drop and slap feet when walking (Verstappen et al., 2005).

slowly or not at all. The brain and spinal cord and, to a lesser degree, peripheral nerves are susceptible to damage by ionizing radiation that usually causes symptoms months or years after radiation treatment has been completed (Belka, Budach, Kortmann, & Bamberg, 2001).

d) Age
   (1) Cerebellar neurotoxicity of cytarabine and vincristine increases with increasing age. However, both cytarabine and vincristine neurotoxicity varies with dose and route of administration (Voss & Wilkes, 1999).
   (2) Children are at higher risk for ototoxicity than are adults because children's inner ears are not fully developed.
   (3) Compared to adults, children are at higher risk for neurotoxicity resulting from cranial radiation. Children

younger than age three are particularly susceptible.
   (4) Older adults and pediatric patients receiving biologic agents are at increased risk for neurotoxicity (Battiato & Wheeler, 2005).
e) Cumulative doses of vinca alkaloids (especially vincristine), platinum analogs (especially cisplatin), and taxanes will cause peripheral neuropathies.
f) Renal failure or renal impairment
g) Concurrent or subsequent administration of diuretics or aminoglycoside antibiotics may increase cisplatin-induced sensory neuropathy and ototoxicity and may increase cerebellar damage from cytarabine administration (Gilbert, 2000).
h) Steroids cause neurotoxicity in the form of myopathy, alterations in mental status such as anxiety, and steroid psychosis

(Zochodone, 1998). Patients can develop symmetric proximal weakness in their arms and legs. Treatment is dose reduction or taper with discontinuation (La Pier, 1997).

i) Preexisting neuropathy caused by concomitant medical conditions (e.g., diabetes, vitamin B_{12} deficiency, thyroid dysfunction, cachexia, Charcot-Marie-Tooth disease, hearing loss) (Armstrong & Gilbert, 2002); peripheral neuropathy can have other etiologies, including alcoholism, HIV and other immunosuppressive illnesses, congenital neuropathy, other neurotoxic medications, and exposure to certain toxins and metals (du Bois et al., 1999; Hughes, 2002).

j) Standard-dose chemotherapy has been associated with cognitive impairment, also referred to as "chemo brain" (Ahles & Saykin, 2001). Cognitive impairment has been observed in patients receiving standard-dose chemotherapy for lymphoma and cancers of the breast, lung, and testes (Ahles & Saykin; Shapiro et al., 2005). The cognitive difficulties typically are subtle and most commonly include trouble with concentration, memory, ability to focus, organizational skills, and working with numbers (Ahles & Saykin). Executive function, which includes attention regulation, planning and initiating purposeful activity, anticipating consequences of one's actions, problem solving, and inhibition of inappropriate activity (Grigsby, Kay, Kowalsky, & Kramer, 2002) also has been affected (Saykin et al., 2003). The subtlety of cognitive impairment is reflected by patients' perceptions of difficulty as compared to scores within the normal range on standard neurocognitive testing (Tannock, Ahles, Ganz, & Van Dam, 2004). The potential to significantly affect an individual's QOL exists, regardless of the severity of the side effects.

4. Assessment
   a) The ability to determine changes in the CNS, peripheral nervous system, and CNs is through neurologic assessment. The hallmark for optimal care begins with assessment followed by documentation of findings (Barker, 2008).
   b) Identify patients who are at increased risk for neurotoxicity based on risk factors.
   c) Perform a neurologic examination prior to each chemotherapy/biotherapy treatment and subsequent medical visit that includes evaluation of level of consciousness, sensory and motor function, gait, range of motion, CN function, and reflexes (Brant,

1998; Seidel, Ball, Dains, & Benedict, 1999). Manifestations include
   (1) Peripheral neuropathy grading criteria scale (NCI CTEP, 2006)
   (2) CNS deficits as described in Section 1.c
   (3) CN assessment (see Table 31).

d) Assess pain management. Undertreated cancer pain is a particular problem in women, minority ethnic groups, and older patients (de Leon-Casasola & Lema, 2003). A pathophysiologic approach to pain management is required in patients with cancer. Such an approach includes a patient history, physical examination, and dedicated testing to determine whether pain is visceral, somatic, or neuropathic (de Leon-Casasola & Lema). Patients describe visceral pain as gnawing, cramping, aching, or sharp (NCCN, 2007). Visceral pain is diffuse, and many patients use a whole hand to describe where it hurts. Somatic pain is well localized (de Leon-Casasola & Lema; Payne, 1987). Patients can describe where it hurts with one finger. Neuropathic pain is usually described as sharp, tingling, burning, or shooting (NCCN). Patients often describe the pain as electric shock sensations (de Leon-Casasola, 2008).

e) Administer self-report questionnaires that assess neurologic function and QOL at baseline and subsequent visits (Almadrones, McGuire, Walczak, Florio, & Tian, 2004; Cella, Peterman, Hudgens, Webster, & Socinski, 2003; Greimel et al., 2003; Postma & Heimans, 2000).

f) Assess hearing with audiogram prior to ototoxic chemotherapy (e.g., cisplatin, carboplatin) to establish baseline.

g) Assess patient and family coping. Older adults require different examination considerations.
   (1) Use a quiet area; reduce background noise.

Table 31. Neurologic Assessment of the Cranial Nerves

Cranial Nerve	Test	Dysfunction
Olfactory I	Check first for obstruction, mucus, and inflammation. Test one nostril at a time.	Anosmia
Optic II	Determine if patient wears glasses. Have patient read held up fingers.	Blind eye
Oculomotor III	Test one eye at a time. Shine flashlight in eye, note brisk constriction. Lids should not dip below top of iris (ptosis). Ask patient to follow your finger/light as you move it up, down, and medially.	Nonreactive pupil, ptosis
Trochlear IV	Ability to move eyes down and in	Inability to move eyes down and in
Trigeminal V	Patient closes eyes. Stroke three zones of face, comparing right to left. If awake, stroke cornea gently with cotton. Normal response is lid closure.	Decreased or absent, no blink
Abducens VI	Ability to look out (abduct)	Inability to look out
Facial VII	Test all three zones; close eyelids, wrinkle brow, raise eyebrows, wiggle nose, pucker, show teeth, smile, puff out cheek.	Inability to close eyes
Acoustic VIII	Open lids, turn head side to side. Eyes will move to opposite direction. Have patient close eyes, and test for high frequency sounds (tick of watch, rubbing fingers, faint whisper).	Eyes will not move when turning head side to side.
Glossopharyngeal/ vagus IX and X	Gag, palate, swallow, and speech. Look for midline uvula. Note ability to give healthy cough.	Palate sags on weak side. Uvula swings to strong side. Decreased cough
Spinal accessory XI	Have patient turn chin against resisting examiner's hand. Push down on both shoulders as patient elevates them.	Weakness
Hypoglossal XII	Ask patient to stick out tongue; note position and symmetry. Ask patient to put his tongue in his cheek and push.	Tongue deviates to weak side. Weakness

Note. From *The Clinical Practice of Neurological and Neurosurgical Nursing* (5th ed., p. 170), by J.V. Hickey, 2003, Philadelphia: Lippincott Williams & Wilkins. Copyright 2003 by Lippincott Williams & Wilkins. Adapted with permission.

(2) Use low-pitched, soft voice; address by surnames.
(3) Review medicines at every encounter.
(4) Always ask about pain.
(5) Do not expect typical presentation of chronic or acute diseases (Barker, 2008).
h) Assess patients' environment to ensure safety with impaired function.
5. Collaborative management
   a) Use assessment guidelines for early detection and treatment.
   b) Reduce drug dose, discontinue drug, or switch to a less-neurotoxic drug as ordered when neurologic deficits occur (Rose & Smereker, 2003; Vasey, 2002).
   c) No proven pharmacologic intervention currently is available for neurotoxicity prevention. Clinical trials using amifostine and glutamine have been equivocal (Moore et al., 2003; Vahdat et al., 2001).
   d) Manage concomitant medical conditions known to cause and increase chemother-

apy-related neurotoxicity (e.g., diabetes, vitamin B_{12} cachexia, Charcot-Marie-Tooth disease) (Armstrong & Gilbert, 2002).
   e) Use of vitamins and minerals to treat neurotoxic side effects
      (1) Vitamin E is an antioxidant believed to protect against cellular oxidative damage and side effects such as numbness, tingling, burning, and pain in peripheral extremities produced by cisplatin and other cytotoxic drugs (Visovsky, Collins, Abbott, Aschenbrenner, & Hart, 2007).
      (2) Calcium and magnesium infusions were used in patients receiving oxaliplatin. Oxalate, an oxaliplatin metabolite, seeks and binds to calcium and magnesium (Gamelin et al., 2004). This is responsible for the neurotoxic effects of oxaliplatin therapy. Following infusion of calcium and magnesium, patients experienced

improvements in pseudolaryngospasm and other clinical manifestations of acute neurotoxicity (Gamelin et al.). As noted in Table 5, however, oxaliplatin should be prepared with D5W solution rather than chloride-containing solutions.

(3) Both of these studies were done with a small sample and will need to be tested further in larger RCCTs.

f) Administer analgesic medications. The three most commonly used are NSAIDs, opioids, and adjuvant agents such as tricyclic antidepressants and corticosteroids (de Leon-Casasola & Lema, 2003).

g) Administer tricyclic antidepressants (e.g., amitriptyline, imipramine, nortriptyline) or anticonvulsants (e.g., gabapentin, phenytoin, carbamazepine) to treat pain related to peripheral neuropathy (Smith, Whedon, & Bookbinder, 2002; Voss & Wilkes, 1999).

h) Consider consultation with neurologist; occupational, physical, or speech therapist; or audiologist.

i) Consider nonpharmacologic management (e.g., exercise, relaxation techniques—yoga, meditation, acupuncture, deep breathing, guided imagery) (Richardson, Sandman, & Vela, 2001; Voss & Wilkes, 1999). Neuropathic pain usually does not respond to analgesics alone. In these patients, mind-body techniques may be especially worthwhile, as they may alter the perception of pain (Deng & Cassileth, 2005). Physical activity and exercise interventions have not been studied in the prevention or treatment of peripheral neuropathy in patients with cancer. Studies with small sample sizes have examined progressive resistance exercise, aerobic exercise, and stretching exercises in the treatment of diabetic neuropathy and myotonic dystrophy. All three found significant improvements in outcomes such as stance and functional reach (Balducci et al., 2006). Further RCCTs are needed with patients with cancer.

6. Patient and family education

a) Instruct patients and significant others that neurotoxicity is a possible side effect of selected cytotoxic agents. Teach strategies to manage symptoms of autonomic dysfunction (postural hypotension, constipation, and urinary retention), such as dangling legs prior to standing, increasing oral intake, and adding fiber (Vivosky et al., 2007).

b) Emphasize patient safety issues and provide educational materials (Almadrones & Arcot, 1999). Teach clients strategies for managing personal safety, such as using visual input to compensate for loss of lower extremity sensation in navigating changing terrains (Visovsky et al., 2007). Currently, the only interventions that can be recommended for nursing practice are education and support to preserve safety (Armstrong et al., 2005; Marrs & Newton, 2003; Paice, 2007).

c) Provide information regarding signs and symptoms of neurotoxicity, and instruct patients to report these symptoms to the physician and/or nurse if they occur.

d) Instruct patients about the risk for ischemic and thermal injuries resulting from loss of sensation in the extremities. Patients should protect body parts from cold and hot temperature extremes (Visovsky et al., 2007).

e) Provide information about the potential side effects of medications that can cause or change neurologic symptoms.

f) Educate patients and significant others regarding any needed referrals, support organizations, adaptations, and rehabilitative strategies.

g) Provide education regarding avoidance of behaviors (e.g., alcohol consumption) or medication that may alter neurologic status (Sandstrom, 1996).

h) For pediatric patients, provide information to parents regarding school reentry and intervention.

References

Ahles, T.A., & Saykin, A.J. (2001). Cognitive effects of standard dose chemotherapy in patients with cancer. *Cancer Investigation, 19*(8), 812–820.

Allen, J., Adlakha, A., & Bergethon, P. (2006). Reversible posterior leukoencephalopathy syndrome after bevacizumab/FOLFIRI regimen for metastatic colon cancer. *Archives of Neurology, 63*(10), 1475–1478.

Almadrones, L., & Arcot, R. (1999). Patient guide to peripheral neuropathy. *Oncology Nursing Forum, 26*(8), 1359–1360.

Almadrones, L., McGuire, D., Walczak, J.R., Florio, C., & Tian, C. (2004). Psychometric evaluation of two scales assessing functional status and peripheral neuropathy associated with chemotherapy for ovarian cancer: A Gynecologic Oncology Group study. *Oncology Nursing Forum, 31*(3), 615–623.

Ardavanis, A.S., Ioannidis, G.N., & Rigatos, G.A. (2005). Acute myopathy in a patient with lung adenocarcinoma treated with gemcitabine and docetaxel. *Anticancer Research, 25*(1B), 523–525.

Armstrong, T., Almadrones, L., & Gilbert, M.R. (2005). Chemotherapy-induced peripheral neuropathy. *Oncology Nursing Forum, 32*(2), 305–311.

Armstrong, T., & Gilbert, M. (2002). Chemotherapy-induced peripheral neuropathy. In W.T. Fetner (Ed.), *The female patient* (pp. 27–30). Chatham, NJ: Quadrant HealthCom.

Armstrong, T., Rust, D., & Kohtz, J.R. (1997). Neurologic, pulmonary, and cutaneous toxicities of high-dose chemotherapy. *Oncology Nursing Forum, 24*(Suppl. 1), 23–33.

Balducci, S., Iacobellis, G., Parisi, L., Di Biase, N., Calandriello, E., Leonetti, F., et al. (2006). Exercise training can modify the natural history of diabetic peripheral neuropathy. *Journal of Diabetes and Its Complications, 20*(4), 216–223.

Barker, E. (2008). *Neuroscience nursing: A spectrum of care* (3rd ed.). St. Louis, MO: Elsevier Mosby.

Battiato, L.A., & Wheeler, V. (2005). Biotherapy. In C.H. Yarbro, M.H. Frogge, & M. Goodman (Eds.), *Cancer nursing: Principles and practice* (6th ed., pp. 543–558). Sudbury, MA: Jones and Bartlett.

Bedford Laboratories. (2000). Methotrexate [Package insert]. Bedford, OH: Author.

Belka, C., Budach, W., Kortmann, R., & Bamberg, M. (2001). Radiation induced CNS toxicity—Molecular and cellular mechanisms. *British Journal of Cancer, 85*(9), 1233–1239.

Ben Venue Labs, Inc. (2007). Busulfex [Package insert]. Retrieved November 20, 2008, from http://www.fda.gov/cder/foi/label/2007/020954s008lbl.pdf

Brant, J.M. (1998). Cancer-related neuropathic pain. *Nurse Practitioner Forum, 9*(3), 154–162.

Buzaid, A., & Atkins, M. (2001). Practical guidelines for management of biochemotherapy-related toxicity in melanoma. *Clinical Cancer Research, 7*(9), 2611–2619.

Cassidy, J., & Misset, J.L. (2002). Oxaliplatin-related side effects: Characteristics and management. *Seminars in Oncology, 29*(Suppl. 15), 11–20.

Cata, J.P., Weng, H., Burton, A., Villareal, H., Girait, S., & Dougherty, P. (2007). Quantitative sensory findings in patients with bortezomib-induced pain. *Journal of Pain, 8*(4), 296–306.

Cavaletti, G., Beronio, A., Reni, L., Ghiglione, E., Schenone, A., Briani, C., et al. (2004). Thalidomide sensory neurotoxicity: A clinical and neurophysiologic study. *Neurology, 62*(12), 2291–2293.

Cavaletti, G., & Zanna, C. (2002). Current status and future prospects for the treatment of chemotherapy-induced peripheral neurotoxicity. *European Journal of Cancer, 38*(14), 1832–1837.

Celgene Corporation. (1998). Thalomid [Package insert]. Summit, NJ: Author.

Cella, D., Peterman, A., Hudgens, S., Webster, K., & Socinski, M. (2003). Measuring the side effects of taxane therapy in oncology. *Cancer, 98*(4), 822–831.

David, K.A., & Picus, J. (2005). Evaluating risk factors for the development of ifosfamide encephalopathy. *American Journal of Clinical Oncology, 28*(3), 277–280.

de Leon-Casasola, O.A. (2008). Implementing therapy with opioids in patients with cancer. *Oncology Nursing Forum, 35*(Suppl. 6), 7–12.

de Leon-Casasola, O.A., & Lema, M.J. (2003). Cancer pain. In T.J. Healy & P.R. Knight (Eds.), *Wylie and Churchill-Davidson's a practice of anesthesia* (7th ed., pp. 1255–1265). London: Arnold.

Deng, G., & Cassileth, B.R,. (2005). Integrative oncology: Complementary therapies for pain, anxiety and mood disturbance. *CA: A Cancer Journal for Clinicians, 55*(2), 108–116.

Denicoff, K.D., Rubinow, D.R., Papa, M.Z., Simpson, C., Seipp, C.A., Lotze, M.T., et al. (1987). The neuropsychiatric effects of treatment with interleukin-2 and lymphokine-activated killer cells. *Annals of Internal Medicine, 107*(3), 293–300.

Donelli, M., Zachetti, M., Munzone, E., D'Incalci, M., & Crosignani, A. (1998). Pharmacokinetics of anticancer agents in patients with impaired liver function. *European Journal of Cancer, 34*(1), 33–46.

Dormann, A., Grunewald, T., Wigginhaus, B., & Huchzermeyer, H. (1998). Gemcitabine-associated autonomic neuropathy. *Lancet, 351*(9103), 644.

du Bois, A., Schlaich, M., Luck, H.J., Mollenkopf, A., Wechsel, U., Rauchholz, M., et al. (1999). Evaluation of neurotoxicity induced by paclitaxel second-line chemotherapy. *Supportive Care in Cancer, 7*(5), 354–361.

Forsyth, P.A., & Cascino, T.L. (1995). Neurological complications of chemotherapy. In R.G. Wiley (Ed.), *Neurologic complications of cancer* (pp. 241–266). New York: Marcel Dekker.

Friedlander, P.A., Bansal, R., Schwartz, L., Wagman, R., Posner, J., & Kemeny, N. (2004). Gemcitabine-related radiation recall preferentially involves internal tissue and organs. *Cancer, 100*(9), 1793–1799.

Friedman, J.H., & Shetty, N. (2001). Permanent cerebellar toxicity of Ara-C in a young woman. *Movement Disorders, 16*(3), 575–577.

Gamelin, E., Gamelin, L., Bossi, L., & Quasthoff, S. (2002). Clinical aspects and molecular basis of oxaliplatin neurological management and development of preventative measures. *Oncology, 29*(Suppl. 15), 21–33.

Gamelin, L., Boistron-Celle, M., Delva, R., Guerin-Mayer, V., Ifrah, N., Morel, A., et al. (2004). Prevention of oxaliplatin-related neurotoxicity by calcium and magnesium infusions: A retrospective study of 161 patients receiving oxaliplatin combined with 5-fluorouracil and leucovorin for advanced colorectal cancer. *Clinical Cancer Research, 10*(12, Pt. 1), 4055–4061.

Gidal, B.E. (2006). New and emerging treatment options for neuropathic pain. *American Journal of Managed Care, 12*(Suppl. 9), S269–S278.

Gilbert, M.R. (2000). Neurologic complications. In M.D. Abeloff, J.O. Armitage, A.S. Lichter, & J.E. Neiderhuber (Eds.), *Clinical oncology* (2nd ed., pp. 89–105). New York: Churchill Livingstone.

Greimel, E., Bottomley, A., Cull, A., Waldenstrom, A., Arraras, L., Chauvenet, L., et al. (2003). An international field study of the reliability and validity of a disease-specific questionnaire module (the QLQ-OV28) in assessing the quality of life of patients with ovarian cancer. *European Journal of Cancer, 39*(10), 1402–1408.

Grigsby, J., Kaye, K., Kowalsky, J., & Kramer, A.M. (2002). Association of behavioral self-regulation with concurrent functional capacity among stroke rehabilitation patients. *Journal of Clinical Geropsychology, 8*(1), 25–33.

Hensley, M., Peterson, B., Silver, R., Larson, R.A., Schiffer, C.A., & Szatrowski, T.P. (2000). Risk factors for severe neuropsychiatric toxicity in patients receiving interferon alfa-2b and low dose cytarabine for chronic myelogenous leukemia: Analysis of Cancer and Leukemia Group B 9013. *Journal of Clinical Oncology, 18*(6), 1301–1308.

Hickey, J.V. (2003). *The clinical practice of neurological and neurosurgical nursing* (5th ed.). Philadelphia: Lippincott Williams & Wilkins.

Hilkens, P.H., Van der Burg, M.E., Moll, J.W., Planting, A.S., van Putten, W.L., Vecht, C.J., et al. (1995). Neurotoxicity is not enhanced by increased dose interval administration. *European Journal of Cancer, 31A*(5), 677–678.

Hughes, R.C. (2002). Regular review: Peripheral neuropathy. *BMJ, 324*(7335), 466–469.

Jagganath, S., Barlogie, B., Berenson, J., Siegel, D., Irwin, D., Richardson, P.G., et al. (2004). A phase II study of two doses of bortezomib in relapsed or refractory multiple myeloma. *British Journal of Haematology, 127*(2), 165–172.

Keime-Guibert, F., Napolitano, M., & Delattre, J.Y. (1998). Neurological complications of radiotherapy and chemotherapy. *Journal of Neurology, 245*(11), 695–708.

Kronfol, Z., & Remick, D.G. (2000). Cytokines and the brain: Implications for clinical psychiatry. *American Journal of Psychiatry, 157*(5), 683–694.

La Pier, T.K. (1997). Glucocorticoid-induced muscle atrophy. The role of exercise in treatment and prevention. *Journal of Cardiopulmonary Rehabilitation, 17*(2), 76–84.

Lee, J., & Swain, S.M. (2006). Peripheral neuropathy induced by microtubule stabilizing agents. *Journal of Clinical Oncology, 24*(10), 1633–1642.

Legha, S.S. (1986). Vincristine neurotoxicity: Pathophysiology and management. *Medical Toxicology, 1*(6), 421–427.

Lehky, T.J., Leonard, G.D., Wilson, R.H., Grem, J.L., & Floeter, M.K. (2004). Oxaliplatin-induced neurotoxicity: Acute hyperexcitability neuropathy. *Muscle and Nerve, 29*(3), 387–392.

Li, Y., Womer, R.B., & Silber, J.H. (2004). Predicting cisplatin toxicity in children: The influence of age. *Cancer, 40*(16), 2445–2451.

Low, W.K., Toh, S.T., Wee, J., Fook-Chong, S.M., & Wang, D.Y. (2006). Sensorineural hearing loss after radiotherapy and chemoradiotherapy randomized study. *Journal of Clinical Oncology, 24*(12), 1904–1909.

Maier, S.F., & Watkins, L.R. (2003). Immune-to-central nervous system communication and its role in modulating pain and cognition. Implications for cancer and cancer treatments. *Brain, Behavior and Immunity, 17*(Suppl. 1), S125–S131.

Marrs, J., & Newton, S. (2003). Updating your peripheral neuropathy "know how." *Clinical Journal of Oncology Nursing, 7*(3), 299–303.

Meyers, C.A., Obbens, E.A., Schiebel, R.S., & Moser, R.P. (1991). Neurotoxicity of intraventricularly administered interferon for leptomeningeal disease. *Cancer, 68*(1), 88–92.

Mileshkin, L., Stark, R., Day, B., Seymour, J.F., Zeldis, J.B., & Prince, H.M. (2006). Development of neuropathy in patients with multiple myeloma treated with thalidomide: Patterns of occurrence and the role of electrophysiologic monitoring. *Journal of Clinical Oncology, 24*(27), 4507–4514.

Moore, D.H., Donnelly, J., McGuire, W.P., Almadrones, L., Cella, D., Herzog, T.J., et al. (2003). Limited access trial using amifostine for protection against cisplatin- and three-hour paclitaxel-induced neurotoxicity: A phase II study of the Gynecologic Oncology Group. *Journal of Clinical Oncology, 21*(22), 4207–4213.

Myers, J.S., Pierce, J., & Pazdernick, T. (2008). Neurotoxicology of chemotherapy in relation to cytokine release, the blood-brain barrier, and cognitive impairment. *Oncology Nursing Forum, 35*(6), 916–920.

National Cancer Institute Cancer Therapy Evaluation Program. (2006). *Common terminology criteria for adverse events* (version 3.0). Bethesda, MD: National Cancer Institute.

National Comprehensive Cancer Network. (2007). *NCCN Clinical Practice Guidelines in Oncology™: Adult cancer pain* [v.1.2007]. Retrieved August 1, 2007, from http://www.nccn.org/professionals/physician/gls/PDF/pain.pdf

Oldenburg, J., Kraaggerud, S.M., Cvancarova, M., Lothe, R.A., & Fossa, S.D. (2007). Cisplatin-induced long-term hearing impairment is associated with specific glutathione s-transferrase genotypes in testicular cancer survivors. *Journal of Clinical Oncology, 25*(6), 708–714.

Ozcan, C., Wong, S., & Hari, P. (2006). Reversible posterior leukoencephalopathy syndrome and bevacizumab. *New England Journal of Medicine, 354*(9), 980–982.

Paice, J.A. (2007). Peripheral neuropathy: Experimental findings, clinical approaches. *Supportive Oncology, 5*(2), 61–63.

Parnet, P., Kelley, K.W., Bluthe, R.M., & Dantzer, R. (2002). Expression and regulation of interleukin-1 receptors in the brain. Role in cytokines-induced sickness behavior. *Journal of Neuroimmunology, 125*(1–2), 5–14.

Payne, R. (1987). Anatomy, physiology, and neuropharmacology of cancer pain. *Medical Clinics of North America, 71*(2), 153–167.

Pirzada, N.A., Ali, L., & Dafer, R.M. (2000). Fluorouracil-induced neurotoxicity. *Annals of Pharmacology, 34*(1), 35–38.

Pollmacher, T., Haack, M., Schuld, A., Reichenberg, A., & Yirmiya, R. (2002). Low levels of circulating inflammatory cytokines: Do they affect human brain functions? *Brain, Behavior, and Immunity, 16*(5), 525–532.

Posner, J.B. (2001). Neurotoxicity caused by chemotherapeutic agents. In D. Dale & D. Federman (Eds.), *Scientific American Medicine* (pp. 1–14). New York: WebMD.

Postma, T.J., & Heimans, J.J. (2000). Grading of chemotherapy-induced peripheral neuropathy. *Annals of Oncology, 11*(5), 509–513.

Quasthoff, S., & Hartung, H.P. (2002). Chemotherapy-induced peripheral neuropathy. *Journal of Neurology, 249*(1), 9–17.

Renouf, D., & Gill, S. (2006). Capecitabine-induced cerebellar toxicity. *Clinical Colorectal Cancer, 6*(1), 70–71.

Richardson, J.K., Sandman, D., & Vela, S. (2001). A focused exercise regimen improves clinical measures of balance in patients with peripheral neuropathy. *Archives of Physical Medicine and Rehabilitation, 82*(2), 205–209.

Richardson, P.G., Barlogie, B., Berenson, J., Singhal, S., Jagannath, S., Irwin, D., et al. (2003). A phase 2 study of bortezomib in relapsed, refractory myeloma. *New England Journal of Medicine, 348*(26), 2609–2617.

Rose, P.G., & Smereker, M. (2003). Improvement of paclitaxel-induced neuropathy by substitution of docetaxel for paclitaxel. *Gynecologic Oncology, 91*(2), 423–425.

Rutkove, S.B. (1997). An unusual axonal polyneuropathy induced by low-dose interferon alfa-2a. *Archives of Neurology, 54*(7), 907–908.

Sandstrom, S.K. (1996). Nursing management of patients receiving biological therapy. *Seminars in Oncology Nursing, 12*(2), 152–162.

Saykin, A.J., Ahles, T.A., & McDonald, B.C. (2003). Mechanisms of chemotherapy-induced cognitive disorders. Neuropsychological, pathophysiological and neuroimaging perspectives. *Seminars in Clinical Neuropsychiatry, 8*(4), 201–216.

Seidel, H.M., Ball, J.W., Dains, J.E., & Benedict, G.W. (1999). *Mosby's guide to physical examination* (4th ed., pp. 755–804). St. Louis, MO: Mosby.

Shapiro, P.J., Jacobs, A.R., Palmer, S.C., Coyne, J.C., Meadows, A.T., & Vaughn, D.J. (2005). Neurocognitive function in long-term survivors of testicular cancer. Report of a workshop. *Journal of Clinical Oncology, 23*(11), 2233–2239.

Smith, E.L., Whedon, M.B., & Bookbinder, M. (2002). Quality improvement of painful peripheral neuropathy. *Seminars in Oncology Nursing, 18*(1), 36–43.

Smith, G.A., Damon, L.E., Rugo, H.S., Ries, C.A., & Linker, C.A. (1997). High-dose cytarabine dose modification reduces the incidence of neurotoxicity in patients with renal insufficiency. *Journal of Clinical Oncology, 15*(2), 833–839.

Tannock, I.F., Ahles, T.A., Ganz, P.A., & Van Dam, F.S. (2004). Cognitive impairment associated with chemotherapy for cancer. Report of a workshop. *Journal of Clinical Oncology, 23*(11), 2233–2239.

Tosi, P., Zamagni, E., Cellini, C., Plasmati, R., Cangini, D., Tacchetti, P., et al. (2005). Neurological toxicity of long term (> 1 yr) thalidomide therapy in patients with multiple myeloma. *European Journal of Haematology, 74*(3), 212–216.

Tuxen, M.K., & Hansen, S.W. (1994). Neurotoxicity secondary to antineoplastic drugs. *Cancer Treatment Reviews, 20*(2), 191–214.

Vahdat, L., Papadopoulos, K., Lange, D., Lewin, S., Kaufman, E., Donovan, D., et al. (2001). Reduction of paclitaxel-induced peripheral neuropathy with glutamine. *Clinical Cancer Research, 7*(5), 1192–1197.

Van der Hoop, R.G., Van der Burg, M.E., ten Bokkel Huinink, W.W., van Houwelingen, C., & Neijt, J.P. (1990). Incidence of neuropathy in 395 patients with cancer treated with or without cisplatin. *Cancer, 66*(8), 1697–1702.

Vasey, P.A. (2002). Survival and longer-term toxicity results of the SCOTROC study: Docetaxel-carboplatin (DC) vs. paclitaxel-carboplatin (PC) in epithelial ovarian cancer (EOC). *Proceedings of the American Society of Clinical Oncology, 21,* Abstract 804.

Verstappen, C.C., Heimans, J.J., Hockman, K., & Postma, T.J. (2003). Neurotoxic complications of chemotherapy in patients with cancer: Clinical signs and symptoms and optimal management. *Drugs, 63*(15), 1549–1563.

Verstappen, C.C., Koeppen, S., Heiman, J.J., Huijgens, P.C., Scheulen, M.E., Strumberg, D., et al. (2005). Dose-related vincristine-induced peripheral neuropathy with unexpected off-therapy worsening. *Neurology, 64*(6), 1076–1077.

Videnovic, A., Semonov, I., Chua-Adajar, R., Baddi, L., Blumenthal, D.T., Beck, A.C., et al. (2005). Capecitabine-induced multifocal encephalopathy: A report of five cases. *Neurology, 65*(11), 1792–1794.

Visovsky, C., Collins, M., Abbott, L., Aschenbrenner, J., & Hart, C. (2007). Putting evidence into practice: Evidence-based interventions for chemotherapeutic-induced peripheral neuropathy. *Clinical Journal of Oncology Nursing, 11*(6), 901–909.

Voss, M.A.B., & Wilkes, G.M. (1999). Neurotoxicities. *American Journal of Nursing, 99*(Suppl. 4), 20–23.

Wilkes, G.M., & Barton-Burke, M. (2007). *2007 oncology nursing drug handbook.* Sudbury, MA: Jones and Bartlett.

Wilson, C.T., Finch, C.E., & Cohen, H.J. (2002). Cytokines and cognition: The case for a head-to-toe inflammatory paradigm. *Journal of the American Geriatrics Society, 50*(12), 2041–2056.

Wong, E.T., & Berkenblit, A. (2004). The role of topotecan in the treatment of brain metastases. *Oncologist, 9*(1), 68–79.

Zochodone, D. (1998). Myopathies in the ICU. *Cancer Journal of Neurological Sciences, 25*(1), 540–542.

    K. Cancer treatment–related cognitive changes: Cognitive function is an outcome of healthy brain performance, encompassing multiple domains that are so inextricably linked that impairment in one invariably affects another. Cognitive domains include attention and concentration, executive function, information processing speed, language, motor function, visuospatial skill, learning, and memory (Jansen, Miaskowski, Dodd, Dowling, & Kramer, 2005a). Several meta-analyses have concluded that evidence for cancer treatment–related cognitive changes exists, but they have also highlighted methodologic issues in the studies included in their analyses (Anderson-Hanley, Sherman, Riggs, Agocha, & Compass, 2003; Falleti, Sanfilippo, Maruff, Weih, & Phillips, 2005; Jansen, Miaskowski, Dodd, Dowling, & Kramer, 2005b; Stewart, Bielajew, Collins, Parkinson, & Tomiak, 2006). Identifying cognitive changes associated with cancer treatments is challenging, as cognitive function is influenced by various factors that are independent of treatment. The science defining the phenomena, potential mechanisms, and sensitive neuropsychological measures is ongoing.

1. Pathophysiology: The precise mechanisms of cancer treatment–related cognitive changes are not fully understood, but they are most likely multifactorial, and experts have suggested several etiologies.

 a) DNA damage (Ahles & Saykin, 2007).

 b) Direct neurotoxic effects (Dietrich, Han, Yang, Mayer-Proschel, & Nobel, 2006; Reiriz et al., 2006; Winocur, Vardy, Binns, Kerr, & Tannock, 2006)

 c) Leukoencephalopathy: Structural alterations in cerebral white matter can occur with cranial irradiation (Filley, 1999) and have been reported with various chemotherapy agents (Inagaki et al., 2006; Jansen et al., 2005a; Saykin, Ahles, & McDonald, 2003). Cognitive deficits caused by leukoencephalopathy are dependent upon the degree of myelin and axon damage (Filley & Kleinschmidt-DeMasters, 2001).

 d) Cytokines are proteins that have a role in neural function and repair, as well as the metabolism of neurotransmitters, and therefore have the potential to cause cognitive changes (Wilson, Finch, & Cohen, 2002). Although evidence for treatment-related increases in cytokine levels exists for standard-dose chemotherapy (Jansen et al., 2005a) and biologics, such as IFN alfa and IL-2 (Capuron, Ravaud, & Dantzer, 2001; Scheibel, Valentine, O'Brien, & Meyers, 2004), increased levels also have been found prior to treatment (Meyers, Albitar, & Estey, 2005).

e) Anemia related to chemotherapy has been associated with cognitive changes (Jacobsen et al., 2004).

f) Changes in hormonal levels and/or menopausal status: Reproductive hormones are known to influence cognition. Women who become menopausal as a result of chemotherapy experience a more rapid drop in estrogen than they would during natural menopause. But, whether the accelerated decrease causes cognitive changes is still not clear (Shilling, Jenkins, Fallowfield, & Howell, 2001).

2. The incidence of treatment-related cognitive changes is difficult to determine because of many factors that can influence cognition, including predisposing factors, presence of impairment prior to treatment, use of combination therapies, differences in sample characteristics, and study designs of current research (see Table 32).

a) For example, although chemotherapy-related cognitive changes have been most extensively studied in breast cancer, evidence to support whether chemotherapy-induced cognitive changes exist or are due solely to chemotherapy are inconsistent.

b) To further complicate the picture, evidence of cognitive impairment has been found prior to treatment in 11%–35% of patients with breast cancer (Ahles et al., 2007; Hermelink et al., 2007; Hurria et al., 2006; Jansen, Dodd, Miaskowski, Dowling, & Kramer, 2008; Wefel, Lenzi, Theriault, Buzdar, et al., 2004), 70%–80% of patients with lung cancer (Meyers, Byrne, & Komaki, 1995), and 40% of patients with acute myeloid leukemia (Meyers et al., 2005).

3. Risk factors

a) Predisposing factors that influence cognitive function

(1) Gender: Women excel in language, information processing speed, and motor function, whereas men perform better in visuospatial skills and mathematics (Bender, Paraska, Sereika, Ryan, & Berga, 2001; Lezak, Howieson, & Loring, 2004).

(2) Age: Cognitive decline occurs with aging. However, normative data for neuropsychological tests are based on age.

(3) Intelligence and educational levels: These have strong, positive relationships with neuropsychological test performances and have been found to be protective against cognitive impair-

ments associated with brain trauma (Lezak et al., 2004). Cognitive changes in highly functioning individuals may bring them into normal test ranges (Tannock, Ahles, Ganz, & van Dam, 2004).

(4) Genetics: The presence of the apolipoprotein E (APOE) ε4 gene has been associated with decreased cognitive function. One study of cancer survivors found a greater risk for deficits in visual memory and visuospatial skills in those patients who had at least one ε4 allele of APOE (Ahles et al., 2003). Several other candidate genes are being studied for their potential role in chemotherapy-induced cognitive changes (Ahles & Saykin, 2007).

(5) Psychological factors such as stress, anxiety, and depression can affect performance on neuropsychological testing (Lezak et al., 2004).

(6) Fatigue can negatively affect cognitive function and was found in one study to cause impairments in information processing speed (Servaes, Verhagen, & Bleijenberg, 2002).

b) Factors related to cancer treatments

(1) Regimens: Because most patients receive multimodal therapy, it is difficult to determine if specific drugs or regimens promote higher incidences of cognitive changes.

(2) Dose intensity: Cognitive changes in patients who receive cranial radiation are related to the total dose received (Meyers, Geara, Wong, & Morrison, 2000). Although two studies provided evidence that high-dose chemotherapy regimens cause greater decreases in cognitive function than standard-dose regimens (Schagen, Muller, Boogerd, Mellenberg, & van Dam, 2006; van

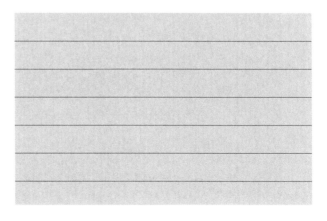

Table 32. Evidence of Cancer Treatment–Related Cognitive Changes

Type of Cancer	Author and Year Published	Treatment Specifics	Sample Characteristics and Study Designs	Cognitive Domains Assessed	Results and Conclusions
Breast	Bender et al., 2006	Chemotherapy and hormonal therapy: Multiple chemotherapy regimens included CMF, AC, and ACT. One group also received tamoxifen.	N = 58 Mean age (standard deviation): 42.6 (5.4) Cognitive testing prior to chemotherapy, as well as 1 week and a year after completion of chemotherapy	AC, EF, MF, VerM, VisM, VS	Significant declines compared to controls were found in VerM for women who received chemotherapy alone. Women who received tamoxifen in addition to chemotherapy had significant declines in both VerM and VisM. In general, cognitive changes were not related to anxiety, depression, or fatigue.
	Bender et al., 2007	Hormonal therapy: 48% anastrozole, 52% tamoxifen	N = 31 Mean age (standard deviation): 52.7 (6.7) Cognitive testing after patients had received at least 3 months of hormonal therapy	AC, EF, IPS, MF, VerM, VisM, VS	Women who received anastrozole had significantly poorer VerM and VisM than women who received tamoxifen. Differences in cognitive function were not related to anxiety, depression, or fatigue. However, this was difficult to interpret, as many of these women received chemotherapy prior to their hormonal therapy.
	Brezden et al., 2000	Chemotherapy and hormonal therapy: Chemotherapy regimens included CMF, CEF, and others; 45% of the survivor group was treated with tamoxifen.	N = 107; 31 current chemotherapy, 40 survivors, 36 controls Median age: 49 current chemotherapy, 46 survivors, 41.5 controls At time of cognitive testing, median time since treatment for survivors was 25 months.	AC, EF, L, MF, VerM, VS	No differences were seen among groups for AC, EF, or VS. Significantly lower cognitive scores were found for L in current chemotherapy and survivor groups compared to controls (p = 0.03 for current chemotherapy; p = 0.05 for survivors) and MF for survivors compared to controls (p = 0.02), and VerM in the current chemotherapy group compared to the control group (p = 0.02). Differences in cognitive function were not related to anxiety or depression. Differences in group ages as well as menopausal status may have influenced results. Results are difficult to interpret because of lack of baseline data.
	Castellon et al., 2004	Chemotherapy and hormonal therapy: Chemotherapy regimens included CMF, AC, CMF + AC, and ACT	N = 72; 36 survivors (50% received only chemotherapy, 50% also received tamoxifen), 17 breast cancer controls, and 19 healthy controls Mean age (standard deviation): 46.8 (6.3) survivors (± tamoxifen), 48.3 (4.0) survivors without treatment, 49.2 (6.0) healthy controls Cognitive testing 2–5 years after diagnosis	AC, EF, IPS, L, VerM, VisM, VS	No significant differences among groups were found for AC, EF, IPS, or VerM. Significant decrease was found in L (p = 0.03), VS (p = 0.02), and VisM (p = 0.03) in survivors who received treatment compared to the controls. Differences in cognitive function were not related to anxiety, depression, or fatigue. Results are difficult to interpret because of lack of baseline testing, multiple regimens of chemotherapy, and variable time periods since treatment.

(Continued on next page)

Table 32. Evidence of Cancer Treatment–Related Cognitive Changes *(Continued)*

Type of Cancer	Author and Year Published	Treatment Specifics	Sample Characteristics and Study Designs	Cognitive Domains Assessed	Results and Conclusions
Breast *(cont.)*	Donovan et al., 2005	Chemotherapy: Chemotherapy regimens included AC, ACT, AD, AC-D, CMF.	N = 143, 60 chemotherapy, 83 radiation therapy only. Mean age (standard deviation): 52.3 (8.1) chemotherapy, 57.7 (9.1) radiation only. Cognitive testing was done 6 months after therapy.	AC, EF, IPS, L, MF, VerM, VisM	No differences between groups were found in any cognitive domain. Difficult to interpret the results because of lack of baseline testing and multiple regimens of chemotherapy.
	Freeman & Broshek, 2002	Chemotherapy: Specific regimens were not reported (however, included doxorubicin ± a taxane).	N = 17; 8 current chemotherapy, 9 survivors. Mean age (standard deviation): 52.6 (7.0) current chemotherapy, 51.1 (7.0) survivors. Current treatment patients had received at least 4 cycles of therapy. Survivors were tested within 6–12 months of treatment.	AC, EF, IPS, L, MF, VerM, VisM, VS	No differences were found in AC, IPS, L, MF, VerM, and VisM. Survivor group scored significantly lower than the current chemotherapy group (p = 0.03) for one measure of EF. Significantly lower scores were found in the current chemotherapy group for VS compared to survivors (p = 0.002). Differences in cognitive function were not related to depression. Difficult to interpret this type of comparison.
	Hermelink et al., 2007	Chemotherapy: SD or DD ECT or CMF	N = 109. Mean age (standard deviation): 48.6 (9.7). Cognitive testing prior to chemotherapy and between the last two chemotherapy cycles	AC, EF, IPS, L, VerM	31% of patients had cognitive impairment prior to initiation of chemotherapy in AC, EF, and/or L. Significant improvement was found in AC, IPS, and VerM after chemotherapy. Cognitive changes were not related to anxiety or depression. Difficult to compare results with other studies because of lack of rigid inclusion criteria.
	Hurria et al., 2006	Chemotherapy and hormonal therapy: Chemotherapy regimens included CMF, AC (SD or DD), ACT, ACT-H. 89% received adjuvant hormonal therapy after completion of chemotherapy.	N = 28. Mean age (standard deviation): 71.0 (5.0). Cognitive testing done prior to chemotherapy and 6 months after completion	AC, EF, L, MF, VerM, VisM, VS	No differences were found for AC, EF, L, MF, and VerM after chemotherapy. However, a significant improvement was found in VisM as well as a significant decline in IPS. Cognitive decline was not related to depression.

(Continued on next page)

Table 32. Evidence of Cancer Treatment–Related Cognitive Changes *(Continued)*

Type of Cancer	Author and Year Published	Treatment Specifics	Sample Characteristics and Study Designs	Cognitive Domains Assessed	Results and Conclusions
Breast *(cont.)*	Jansen et al., 2008	Chemotherapy: AC	N = 30 Mean age (standard deviation): 49.6 (9.0) Cognitive testing done prior to chemotherapy and approximately 1 week after 4 cycles of AC	AC, EF, L, M, MF, VS	13% of patients had cognitive impairment prior to initiation of chemotherapy in VS, L, and/or M. No cognitive changes were found for AC, L, MF, and M after chemotherapy. However, significant declines were found for VS and the total cognitive score. Although a significant improvement was found in EF, it is most likely the result of practice effects. Cognitive changes were not related to anemia, anxiety, depression, fatigue, or patient perception of cognitive functioning.
	Jenkins et al., 2006	Chemotherapy and hormonal therapy: Chemotherapy regimens included FEC, CMF, FEC-D, AC, EC, ECT, and E followed by either CMF or FEC. 93% of the breast cancer control group was on hormonal therapy (i.e., tamoxifen, anastrozole) as well as 71% of the chemotherapy group by the last testing.	N = 85 Mean age (standard deviation): 51.5 (9.6) chemotherapy group, 58.9 (7.3) breast cancer controls, 51.9 (6.9) healthy controls Cognitive testing done prior to chemotherapy, as well as 4 weeks and 6 months after completion	EF, IPS, VerM, VisM	No group differences were found for EF, IPS, VerM, or VisM. Despite the lack of cognitive changes, this study is difficult to interpret because of multiple chemotherapy regimens with or without hormonal therapy as well as significant differences in age and education between groups.
	Schagen et al., 1999	Chemotherapy and hormonal therapy: Chemotherapy regimen: CMF Approximately 50% were treated with tamoxifen for 3 years.	N = 73; survivors = 39, controls = 34 Mean age (standard deviation): 47.1 (6.9) survivors, 46.1 (5.2) controls Testing done approximately 2 years after completion of chemotherapy	AC, EF, IPS, L, MF, VerM, VisM, VS	No differences were found for VS. Survivors scored significantly lower than controls in tests of AC, EF, IPS, L, MF, VerM, and VisM. Differences in cognitive function were not related to anxiety, depression, or fatigue. Difficult to interpret because of lack of baseline data as well as differences in education and menopausal status between groups.
	Schagen et al., 2002	Chemotherapy and hormonal therapy: Chemotherapy regimens: SD CMF or FEC, HD FEC followed by CTC Hormonal therapy: tamoxifen	N = 103; SD survivors = 54, HD survivors = 22, controls = 27 Mean age (standard deviation): 50.4 (5.3) SD survivors, 47.0 (4.8) HD survivors, 48.4 (5.0) controls Testing done about 3 years after completion of chemotherapy	AC, EF, IPS, L, MF, VerM, VisM, VS	This study tested participants from Schagen et al., 1999, and van Dam et al., 1998, studies and found improvement in cognitive function. However, there was significant attrition, especially of patients who were impaired at the time of the previous testing, since original studies.

(Continued on next page)

Table 32. Evidence of Cancer Treatment–Related Cognitive Changes (Continued)

Type of Cancer	Author and Year Published	Treatment Specifics	Sample Characteristics and Study Designs	Cognitive Domains Assessed	Results and Conclusions
Breast (cont.)	Schagen et al., 2006	Chemotherapy and hormonal therapy: Chemotherapy regimens: FEC (SD) or CTC (HD) All chemotherapy patients received tamoxifen.	N = 164; 39 SD, 28 HD, 57 breast cancer controls; 60 healthy controls Mean age (standard deviation): 45.5 (6.6) SD, 45.2 (5.8) HD, 50.5 (7.7) breast cancer controls, 48.8 (6.0) healthy controls Cognitive testing was done prior to the start of chemotherapy and 6 months after completion.	AC, EF, IPS, MF, VerM, VisM	No differences were found between SD chemotherapy patients and the control groups. However, the percentage of HD chemotherapy patients with cognitive decline was significantly higher than control groups. Information was not given regarding which cognitive domains were most affected. There were significant differences between groups for age, postmenopausal status, and number in each group on tamoxifen treatment. However, cognitive changes were not related to anxiety, depression, fatigue, or menopausal status.
	Scherwath et al., 2006	Chemotherapy and hormonal therapy: Chemotherapy regimens included EC followed by CMF or CTM Hormonal therapy: 44% of SD, 50% of HD, and 21% of controls used tamoxifen	N = 76, SD = 23, HD = 24, control = 29 Mean age (standard deviation): 51.8 (8.6) SD, 53.3 (7.1) HD, 54.6 (8.0) controls Cognitive testing was done approximately 5 years after chemotherapy	AC, EF, IPS, L, VerM, VisM	No differences were found between groups. However, it is difficult to interpret data because of the lack of baseline data and the small sample size for multiple chemotherapy regimens.
	Shilling et al., 2001	Hormonal therapy: anastrozole, tamoxifen	N = 129; hormonal therapy patients = 94, healthy controls = 35 Mean age (standard deviation): 63.1 (7.2) patients, 60.9 (9.3) controls Patients had been on hormonal therapy 12 and 60 months at the time of cognitive testing.	AC, IPS, VerM, VisM	No differences were found between groups for AC or VisM. Significant differences for IPS (p = 0.032) and VerM (p = 0.026) were found after controlling for previous hormonal replacement therapy. Depression was not related to differences in cognitive function. Difficult to interpret data because of the lack of baseline data and wide range in time on hormonal therapy.
	Stewart et al., 2008	Chemotherapy and hormonal therapy Chemotherapy regimens: FEC, AC, CEF, FAC, ACT, ECT, AP Hormonal therapies: tamoxifen, anastroxole, letrozole	N = 112; chemotherapy = 61 (80% also received hormonal therapy), hormonal therapy = 51 Mean age (standard deviation): 57.5 (3.7) chemotherapy group, 57.9 (4.4) hormonal group Cognitive testing was done prior to the start of and after the last cycle of chemotherapy and at comparable intervals for hormonal therapy group.	EF, IPS, L, MF, VerM, VS	No differences were found between groups for any cognitive domain. Although the authors stated that the analysis of individual cognitive changes revealed that chemotherapy patients were 3.3 times more likely to have cognitive decline, it is difficult to interpret the data because 80% of the chemotherapy group also received hormonal therapy.

(Continued on next page)

Table 32. Evidence of Cancer Treatment–Related Cognitive Changes (Continued)

Type of Cancer	Author and Year Published	Treatment Specifics	Sample Characteristics and Study Designs	Cognitive Domains Assessed	Results and Conclusions
Breast (cont.)	Tchen et al., 2003	Chemotherapy: Chemotherapy regimens included CEF, AC, CMF, and other (5% of patients were also taking tamoxifen).	N = 200; current chemotherapy = 100, controls = 100 Median age: 48 current chemotherapy, 47 controls Cognitive testing was done after 3–7 cycles of chemotherapy.	AC, EF, L, MF, VerM, VS	No differences were found for AC, EF, MF, VS, or VerM. However, the chemotherapy group had significant decreases in L compared to the control group (p = 0.005). Difficult to interpret because of lack of baseline data, variable number of treatment cycles, and small percentage of patients who were also taking hormonal therapy.
	van Dam et al., 1998	Chemotherapy and hormonal therapy: Chemotherapy regimens: SD FEC, HD FEC followed by CTC Survivors received tamoxifen for two years.	N = 104; SD survivors = 36, HD survivors = 34, controls = 34 Mean age (standard deviation): 48.1 (6.8) SD, 46.5 (6.8) HD, 46.1 (5.2) controls Testing occurred about 1.9 (SD) and 1.6 (HD) years after completion of chemotherapy.	AC, EF, IPS, L, MF, VerM, VisM, VS	No differences were found for EF, L, VS, or VerM. HD survivors scored significantly lower than controls in tests of AC, IPS, MF, and VisM. Differences in cognitive function were not related to anxiety, depression, or fatigue. Difficult to interpret the data because of lack of baseline testing.
	Wefel, Lenzi, Theriault, Davis, et al., 2004	Chemotherapy: Chemotherapy regimen: CAF	N = 18 Mean age (standard deviation): 45.4 (6.7) Testing occurred prior to the start of chemotherapy as well as 3 weeks and 1 year after completion.	AC, EF, IPS, MF, VerM, VisM, VS	No differences were found for AC or MF. Women had significantly decreased EF, IPS, VS, VerM, and VisM three weeks post-chemotherapy compared to baseline, but these cognitive changes were not found one year after chemotherapy completion. Cognitive changes were not related to anxiety or depression.
	Wieneke & Dienst, 1995	Chemotherapy: Chemotherapy regimens: CMF, CAF, CMF + CAF 39% of patients were on tamoxifen.	N = 28 Mean age (standard deviation): 42 (6.7) Testing was done approximately 6.6 months after completion of chemotherapy.	AC, EF, IPS, L, MF, VerM, VisM, VS	No differences were found for EF. Survivors had significantly lower scores compared to test norms in AC, IPS, L, MF, VS, VerM, and VisM. Deficits in cognitive function compared to normative data were not related to depression or type of chemotherapy; however, they were related to length of treatment. Difficult to interpret this data because of lack of baseline testing or a control group for comparison.
Colorectal	Vardy et al., 2007	Chemotherapy: Specific regimens not reported	N = 182; 127 chemotherapy patients, 52 colorectal patient controls Median age: 57 Cognitive testing was done prior to chemotherapy as well as 6 and 12 months after completion of therapy.	Not reported	At baseline, 30% of the sample had cognitive impairment. No differences were found in cognitive function over time. Unable to interpret data as information regarding specific regimens not available.

(Continued on next page)

Table 32. Evidence of Cancer Treatment–Related Cognitive Changes (Continued)

Type of Cancer	Author and Year Published	Treatment Specifics	Sample Characteristics and Study Designs	Cognitive Domains Assessed	Results and Conclusions
Colorectal (cont.)	Walker et al., 1996	Chemotherapy and biotherapy: Chemotherapy: 5-FU and leucovorin Biotherapy: IL-2	N = 17; 9 chemotherapy + biotherapy, 8 IL-2 only Mean age (standard deviation): 56 (10) chemotherapy + IL-2, 59 (12) IL-2 only Cognitive testing done daily for 8 days every 4 weeks as well as weekly in between	AC, IPS, VerM, VisM	No differences were found in AC or VerM over time. However, patients who received a combination of chemotherapy and biotherapy had cognitive declines in IPS and VisM, which returned to baseline approximately 10 days after IL-2. Cognitive scores were not related to anxiety or depression. Difficult to interpret results because of small sample size.
	Walker et al., 1997	Chemotherapy and biotherapy: Chemotherapy: 5-FU and leucovorin Biotherapy: IL-2	N = 17; 9 chemotherapy + biotherapy, 8 IL-2 only Mean age (standard deviation): 56 (10) chemotherapy + IL-2, 59 (12) IL-2 only Cognitive testing done prior to the start of therapy then weekly for 4 weeks	EF, IPS, VisM	No differences were found in VisM. However, patients who received chemotherapy and IL-2 had significant declines in EF and IPS. Difficult to interpret results because of small sample size and significant differences between groups for depression, with patients receiving IL-2 having higher depression scores.
Leukemia	Scheibel et al., 2004	Chemotherapy and biotherapy: Chemotherapy regimens: low-dose cytarabine or hydroxyurea Biotherapy: IFN alfa	N = 30 patients with chronic myeloid leukemia Mean age (standard deviation): 45.5 (16.6) IFN alfa alone, 46.5 (9.6) chemotherapy with IFN alfa Cognitive testing was done prior to the start of treatment and at a median of 13.4 weeks for patients treated with IFN alfa alone and 24.4 weeks for those on combination therapy.	EF, IPS, L, VerM	Significant declines were found over time in EF and IPS for patients who received IFN alfa alone and in L and VerM for patients who received combination therapy. Results are difficult to interpret because of significant differences in educational level, weeks on treatment, and cumulative dose between groups as well as the lack of a non-treated control group.
Lung	Kaasa et al., 1988	Chemotherapy: EP	N = 95; 44 chemotherapy, 51 controls (local radiation therapy only) Median age: 61 chemotherapy, 62 controls Cognitive testing was done before treatment and about 14 weeks after the initiation of treatment (i.e., 11 weeks after radiation therapy and 5 weeks after chemotherapy completion).	EF, IPS, VerM, VisM	No differences were found between patients who received chemotherapy versus radiation therapy. Approximately 20% of patients died prior to the second testing. Results suggest that cognitive changes do not occur with EP chemotherapy.
	Meyers et al., 1995	Chemotherapy: VIP	N = 46; 25 chemotherapy, 21 untreated patients Median age: 54.7 chemotherapy, 54.9 untreated patients Cognitive testing was done prior to chemoradiation in untreated patients and after attaining a complete response, but prior to cranial irradiation in chemotherapy patients.	AC, EF, IPS, L, MF, VerM, VisM, VS	No difference was found between groups in any cognitive domain. However, cognitive impairment, compared to normative data, was found in both groups in EF, MF, and VerM. Results are difficult to interpret because of lack of baseline data.

(Continued on next page)

Table 32. Evidence of Cancer Treatment–Related Cognitive Changes *(Continued)*

Type of Cancer	Author and Year Published	Treatment Specifics	Sample Characteristics and Study Designs	Cognitive Domains Assessed	Results and Conclusions
Lung *(cont.)*	van Oosterhout et al., 1996	Chemotherapy and/or cranial irradiation: Chemotherapy regimens: 9 different regimens, including CAE, CAV	N = 78; 19 chemotherapy alone, 19 prophylactic cranial irradiation after chemotherapy, 11 prophylactic cranial irradiation concurrent with chemotherapy, 29 healthy controls Cognitive testing was performed 2 or more years after diagnosis.	AC, EF, IPS, VerM	No differences were found between treatment groups in any cognitive domain. Patients who were treated with either chemotherapy alone or in combination with radiation therapy scored significantly worse than healthy controls in AC, EF, IPS, and VerM. Results are difficult to interpret because of lack of baseline data and length of time since treatment completion.
Lymphoma	Cull et al., 1996	Chemotherapy: Information regarding specific regimens not provided	N = 91; 27 did not receive chemotherapy, 11 received a single agent, and 51 recieved combination chemotherapy Mean age (standard deviation): 55 (15.9) Testing done at a median of 43 months after treatment completion.	IPS, VerM	Patients scored significantly lower than test norms for IPS. Data are difficult to interpret because of the lack of baseline data, multiple treatment regimens, and wide range of time (6–243 months) since last treatment.
Melanoma	Bender et al., 2000	IFN (low-dose versus HD)	N = 18 Age not reported Cognitive testing was done prior to start of treatment and repeated every 3 months for a total of 6 times.	AC, EF, IPS, MF	Significant attrition over time due to disease extension or IFN toxicity caused researchers to only report results of baseline versus 3 months testing. No differences were found over time; however, the study had a very small sample size, especially for 3 different dosing schedules.
Ovarian	Hensley et al., 2006	Chemotherapy: paclitaxel, gemcitabine, and carboplatin	N = 26 Median age: 54 Cognitive testing was done prior to chemotherapy, after cycles 3 and 6, as well as 6 months after chemotherapy completion.	AC, EF, IPS	No differences were found in AC, EF, or IPS over time. Cognitive scores were not related to depression. Use of a control group may have helped to determine if lack of cognitive decline was caused by practice effects with multiple testing.
Ovarian	Mayerhofer et al., 2000	Chemotherapy: paclitaxel and carboplatin	N = 28 Median age: 63 Cognitive testing was done prior to the start of chemotherapy, after 3 cycles, and at the completion of therapy.	AC	Patients scored below normal at baseline but had significant improvement by the last testing. Although paclitaxel and carboplatin do not appear to cause cognitive changes, a larger sample size, control group, and measurement of other cognitive domains would be worthwhile to confirm these findings.
Prostate	Jenkins et al., 2005	Hormonal therapy: LHRH	N = 50; 32 patients, 18 healthy controls Mean age (standard deviation): 67.5 (4.7) patients, 65.4 (5.3) controls Cognitive testing was done prior to the start of drug treatment, 3 months after completion of drug treatment, and 9 months later.	AC, IPS, L, VS, VerM	No differences were found between groups for any cognitive domain. However, a significant decline was found in VS for patients who received hormonal therapy. This study is limited by its small sample size.

(Continued on next page)

ant рос

Table 32. Evidence of Cancer Treatment–Related Cognitive Changes (Continued)

Type of Cancer	Author and Year Published	Treatment Specifics	Sample Characteristics and Study Designs	Cognitive Domains Assessed	Results and Conclusions
Prostate (cont.)	Joly et al., 2006	Hormonal therapy: LHRH ± an antiandrogen	N = 108; 57 patients, 51 healthy controls. Median age: 73 patients, 72 controls. Cognitive testing was done in patients after they had been on therapy for at least 3 months (median 1.8 years).	AC, EF, L, VerM, VS	Despite significantly greater anemia in patients, no differences were found in any cognitive domain between patients and controls. This study is limited by the lack of baseline data and wide range in time on treatment (3 months to over 7 years) for patients.
	Salminen et al., 2003	Hormonal therapy: flutamide and LHRH	N = 77; 25 patients, 52 healthy controls. Mean age (standard deviation): 64.4 (6.5) patients, 65.3 (6.6) controls. Cognitive testing was done prior to the initiation of treatment and at 6 and 12 months.	AC, EF, IPS, L, VerM, VisM, VS	Patients with prostate cancer had significantly lower scores than controls in AC, IPS, and L prior to the start of therapy. After starting therapy, patients had significant improvements in EF and VerM compared to their own baseline scores. It is difficult to determine how much of this improvement was caused by practice effects since controls were only tested at baseline.
	Salminen et al., 2005	Hormonal therapy: flutamide and LHRH	N = 23 patients. Median age: 65. Cognitive testing was done prior to the initiation of treatment as well as at 6 and 12 months.	AC, EF, IPS, L, VerM, VisM, VS	No differences were found in any cognitive domain over time. However, there were significant associations between estradiol levels and improvement in L as well as declines in IPS and VisM over time. These results are difficult to interpret because of the small sample size and lack of a control group.
Testicular	Schagen et al., 2008	Chemotherapy: BEP	N = 182; 70 chemotherapy, 57 radiation therapy, 55 surgery-only patients. Mean age (standard deviation): 32.1 (7.6) chemotherapy, 38.9 (8.4) radiation therapy, 34.4 (9.5) surgery-only patients. Cognitive testing was performed about 3 years after completion of therapy.	AC, EF, IPS, MF, VerM, VisM	No differences among groups were found in any cognitive domain. Cognitive function was not related to time since treatment, anxiety, depression, or fatigue. Despite the use of a control group, these results are difficult to interpret because of the lack of baseline data. In addition, radiation therapy patients were significantly older than patients in the chemotherapy or surgery-only groups.

Mixed cancer populations

Type of Cancer	Author and Year Published	Treatment Specifics	Sample Characteristics and Study Designs	Cognitive Domains Assessed	Results and Conclusions
Breast and hematologic	Ahles et al., 1996	Chemotherapy: Multiple (8) BMT regimens	N = 54. Median age: 39.2. Cognitive testing done prior to BMT, 1–3 days after bone marrow infusion and within 1–2 days before discharge	EF, L, VisM, VS	No differences were found in VisM over time. However, cognitive declines were found in EF, L, and VS over time. Study results must be interpreted with caution because of significant attrition over time (38%), small sample size for multiple diagnoses with varying treatment regimens, and some patients with history of receiving cranial irradiation and/or intrathecal chemotherapy.

(Continued on next page)

Table 32. Evidence of Cancer Treatment–Related Cognitive Changes *(Continued)*

Type of Cancer	Author and Year Published	Treatment Specifics	Sample Characteristics and Study Designs	Cognitive Domains Assessed	Results and Conclusions
Breast and hematologic *(cont.)*	Jacobs et al., 2007	Chemotherapy: Specific chemotherapy regimens not reported	N = 288 Mean age (standard deviation): 50.07 (12.43) Cognitive testing was done prior to transplant as well as 6 and 12 months after transplantation.	AC, EF, MF, VerM, VisM	No differences were found in any cognitive domain, and performance actually improved by 12 months after BMT. This study is limited by numerous diagnoses but even more so by significant attrition (almost 70%). Need to consider that patients lost to attrition may have been those who had greater cognitive declines.
Breast and lymphoma	Ahles et al., 2002	Chemotherapy: Breast: CMF, CAF, AC, other 37% of survivors and 14% of controls had taken tamoxifen. Lymphoma: 15 different regimens including ABVD, CHOP, MOPP	N = 128, 70 breast (35 survivors who had received chemotherapy, 35 controls), 58 lymphoma (36 survivors and 22 controls) Mean age (standard deviation): breast survivors 59.1 (10.7), controls 60.6 (12.1); lymphoma survivors 55.9 (12.1), controls 48.7 (11.7) Cognitive testing was done approximately 9.5 years after treatment.	AC, IPS, L, MF, VerM, VisM, VS	No differences were found in AC, EF, L, VS, MF, and VisM between groups of chemotherapy patients versus controls. Survivors had significantly poorer overall IPS (p = 0.05) for breast cancer and VerM (p = 0.05) for lymphoma patients compared to controls. Differences in cognitive function were not related to anxiety, depression, or fatigue. Results were difficult to interpret because of lack of baseline data and small sample size for multiple regimens as well as variability in time since last treatment.
	Ahles et al., 2003	Chemotherapy: Multiple chemotherapy regimens (see Ahles et al., 2002)	N = 80 Mean age (standard deviation): APOE ε4 allele carriers 58.0 (10.4); non-carriers 55.3 (9.7)	AC, L, MF, VerM, VisM, VS	No differences were found in AC, L, MF, or VerM. However, APOE ε4 allele carriers had significantly poorer scores in VS (p = 0.03) and VisM (p < 0.05). Differences in cognitive function were not related to anxiety, depression, or fatigue. These results are preliminary and will require baseline data and larger samples to validate these findings.
Hematologic	Andrykowski et al., 1992	Chemotherapy ± cranial irradiation Actual regimens not reported	N = 55 Mean age (standard deviation): 35.9 (9.5) Cognitive testing done prior to BMT, but after a minimum of 1 course of chemotherapy	AC, EF, IPS, MF, VerM, VisM	Cognitive deficits were found in EF, MF, VerM, and VisM. However, these results are difficult to interpret because of the small sample size, especially with multiple cancer diagnoses, a wide variety of previous chemotherapy regimens including HD or intrathecal drugs, variable number of previous cycles of chemotherapy, some patients had cranial irradiation, and the lack of baseline data or a control group to compare results.

(Continued on next page)

Table 32. Evidence of Cancer Treatment–Related Cognitive Changes (Continued)

Type of Cancer	Author and Year Published	Treatment Specifics	Sample Characteristics and Study Designs	Cognitive Domains Assessed	Results and Conclusions
Hematologic (cont.)	Harder et al., 2002	Chemotherapy: Chemotherapy regimens: HD cyclophosphamide ± either cytarabine or etoposide. Some patients received TBI.	N = 40 Mean age (standard deviation): 40.8 (10.3) Cognitive testing was done 22–82 months after completion of BMT.	AC, EF, IPS, L, VS, MF, VerM, VisM	Deficits were not found in L, VS, or MF as compared to normative data. However, cognitive impairments were found in AC, EF, IPS, VerM, and VisM. Difficult to interpret results because of lack of baseline testing, small sample size for multiple diagnoses, as well as chemotherapy regimens (prior to and including transplant) and wide range for time of testing.
	Harder et al., 2006	Chemotherapy: HD cyclophosphamide followed by TBI was most common conditioning regimen. Previous regimens were not reported.	N = 25 Median age: 47 Cognitive testing was done prior to BMT and 1 year later.	AC, EF, IPS, L, VS, MF, VerM, VisM	Cognitive deficits were found in AC, EF, IPS, and MF at baseline. Cognitive declines were not found in any domain a year after BMT. However, these results are limited because of the small sample size with significant attrition (64%) and the lack of a control group for comparison.
	Harder et al., 2007	Chemotherapy: Specific chemotherapy regimens not reported; HD cyclophosphamide followed by TBI was most common conditioning regimen.	N = 183: 101 BMT group, 82 patient controls Mean age (standard deviation): 42.0 (12.1) BMT group, 39.2 (13.1) controls Cognitive testing was done prior to BMT and at 8 and 20 months after baseline.	AC, EF, IPS, VS, MF, VerM, VisM	No differences were found between groups in any domain of cognitive function at baseline. However, significant cognitive decline was found in AC, EF, IPS, and MF over time. Increased age, female gender, and lower educational levels were associated with cognitive declines in AC and EF. In addition, TBI was associated with declines in IPS and MF. Despite significant attrition over time (50% in BMT group and 30% in patient controls), it appears that cognitive declines occur with BMT in multiple domains.
	Meyers et al., 1994	Chemotherapy: BMT and previous treatment regimens not reported	N = 61 Median age: 37.5 Cognitive testing was done prior to BMT, after 2 weeks, at discharge, and at 8 months after BMT.	AC, EF, VS, VerM	Patients scored within normal ranges at all time periods. However, significant declines in EF and VerM were found over time. Pretreatment anxiety was correlated to decreases in cognitive function after transplant. In contrast, depression was not related to cognitive function. Difficult to interpret results because of significant attrition (about 66%), lack of baseline data prior to any therapy, as well as multiple diagnoses and treatment regimens.

(Continued on next page)

Table 32. Evidence of Cancer Treatment–Related Cognitive Changes *(Continued)*

Type of Cancer	Author and Year Published	Treatment Specifics	Sample Characteristics and Study Designs	Cognitive Domains Assessed	Results and Conclusions
Leukemia and myelo-dysplastic syndrome	Meyers et al., 2005	Chemotherapy: lipodaunocin + cyclophosphamide topotecan ± thalidomide	N = 54 Median age: 60.2 Cognitive testing was done prior to the start of chemotherapy and 1 month after treatment.	AC, EF, IPS, L, MF, VerM	Cognitive impairments were found in EF, IPS, L, MF, and M prior to the initiation of chemotherapy. However, significant declines were found in MF only after treatment. Of note, higher IL-6 levels were associated with poorer EF, and higher IL-8 levels were associated with better performance in M tests. Cognitive function was not associated with depression. Significant attrition of more than half of the sample makes it difficult to interpret data.
Renal cell and mela-noma	Caputon et al., 2001	Biotherapy: IL-2, IFN alfa	N = 47; 17 IL-2 only, 7 IL-2 and IFN alfa, 7 low-dose IFN alfa, 16 HD IFN alfa Mean age (standard deviation): 56 (11) IL-2 only group, 51 (10) IL-2 + IFN alfa group, 57 (10) low-dose IFN alfa group, 41 (15) HD IFN alfa group Cognitive testing was done before start of treatment, on the fifth day of treatment, and at the end of the last week of treatment (i.e., 3–4 weeks).	EF, IPS, VisM	Patients receiving IL-2 had significant declines in EF and VisM at the second testing. Patients receiving either low-dose or HD IFN alfa experienced persistent declines in IPS at both the second and final testing. Cognitive changes were not related to depression or fatigue. It was difficult to interpret results because of small sample size for multiple regimens and lack of a control group.

Therapy: ABVD—doxorubicin, bleomycin, vinblastine, and dacarbazine; AC—doxorubicin and cyclophosphamide; AC-D—doxorubicin and cyclophosphamide followed by docetaxel; ACT—doxorubicin and cyclophosphamide followed by paclitaxel; ACT-H—doxorubicin and cyclophosphamide followed by paclitaxel and trastuzumab; AD—doxorubicin and docetaxel; AP—doxorubicin and cisplatin; APOE—apolipoprotein E; BEP—bleomycin, etoposide, and cisplatin; BMT—bone marrow transplant; CAE—cyclophosphamide, doxorubicin, and etoposide; CAF—cyclophosphamide, doxorubicin, and 5-fluorouracil; CAV—cyclophosphamide, doxorubicin, and vincristine; CEF—cyclophosphamide, epirubicin, and 5-fluorouracil; CHOP—cyclophosphamide, doxorubicin, vincristine, and prednisone; CMF—cyclophosphamide, methotrexate, and 5-fluorouracil; CTC—cyclophosphamide, thiotepa, and carboplatin; CTM—cyclophosphamide, thiotepa, and mitoxantrone; DD—dose-dense; E—epirubicin; EC—epirubicin and cyclophosphamide; ECT—epirubicin and cyclophosphamide followed by paclitaxel; EP—etoposide and cisplatin; FAC—fluorouracil, doxorubicin, and cyclophosphamide; FEC—5-fluorouracil, epidoxorubicin, and cyclophosphamide; FEC-D—5-fluorouracil, epidoxorubicin, and cyclophosphamide followed by docetaxel; 5-FU—5-fluorouracil; HD—high-dose; IFN—interferon; IL—interleukin; LHRH—luteinizing hormone–releasing hormone agonist; MOPP—mechlorethamine, vincristine, procarbazine, and prednisone; SD—standard dose; TBI—total body irradiation; VIP—etoposide, ifosfamide, and cisplatin

Cognitive domains: AC—attention/concentration; EF—executive function; IPS—information processing speed; L—language; M—memory; MF—motor function; VerM—verbal memory; VisM—visual memory; VS—visuospatial skill

Dam et al., 1998), one other did not (Scherwath et al., 2006).

(3) Cumulative effects: Although the cumulative effects of chemotherapy on cognitive function have not been studied, a single study found an association with cognitive impairment and the number of chemotherapy cycles received (Ahles & Saykin, 2002).

c) Concomitant medications (e.g., steroids)

4. Assessment: An array of neuropsychological tests are available to measure cognitive function.

a) Test selection should be based on the following factors (Lezak et al., 2004).

(1) Specific cognitive domain to be measured

(2) Appropriateness of test for the domain being studied

(3) Reliability and validity of the test and availability of normative data

(4) Sensitivity and specificity to measure cancer treatment–related cognitive changes (Jansen, Miaskowski, Dodd, & Dowling, 2007)

(5) Availability of parallel forms or resistance to practice effects for use with repeated measures

(6) Feasibility of instrument for clinical use

b) Baseline neuropsychological assessment prior to the initiation of treatment is necessary to determine if changes occur after treatment. Changes may be difficult to assess because they may be subtle (e.g., patients test within normal limits, but lower than non-chemotherapy-treated patients), or preexisting risk factors may influence results.

c) Assess coexisting medical conditions and current medications as well as any potential influencing factors, such as anxiety, depression, fatigue, or menopausal status.

5. Collaborative management: No proven pharmacologic interventions are available to prevent or treat cognitive changes. Although the mechanisms of cancer treatment–related cognitive changes are still unclear, several interventions have been evaluated.

a) Erythropoietin was found, in one study, to improve some measures of cognitive function after four cycles but not at six months after chemotherapy completion (O'Shaughnessy et al., 2005).

b) Methylphenidate, 10 mg twice daily, was found to improve cognitive function in patients with brain tumors (Meyers, Weitzner,

Valentine, & Levin, 1998), but not in patients receiving chemotherapy (Lower et al., 2005; Mar Fan, Chemerynsky, Xu, Clemons, & Tannock, 2008).

c) Donepezil was found to improve cognitive function in patients with brain tumors after cranial irradiation (Shaw et al., 2006), but no differences were found between donepezil with vitamin E versus placebo in a small underpowered study of patients with lung cancer who had completed chemotherapy and/or cranial irradiation (Jatoi et al., 2005).

6. Patient and family education: Patients should be informed that cognitive changes are a possible side effect of treatment of which little is known. Studies elucidating this phenomenon, its mechanisms, and subsequent interventions are ongoing.

a) Acknowledge, validate, and record patient reports of cognitive changes.

b) Encourage practical solutions, such as the following.

(1) Ensure adequate sleep and rest.

(2) Engage in physical exercise.

(3) Exercise the brain (e.g., learn new skills, solve puzzles, work out math problems).

(4) Use a daily planner, write reminders, and use voice recorders to overcome cognitive changes.

References

Ahles, T.A., & Saykin, A.J. (2002). Breast cancer chemotherapy-related cognitive dysfunction. *Clinical Breast Cancer, 3*(Suppl. 3), S84–S90.

Ahles, T.A., & Saykin, A.J. (2007). Candidate mechanisms for chemotherapy-induced cognitive changes. *Nature, 7*(3), 192–201.

Ahles, T.A., Saykin, A.J., Furstenberg, C.T., Cole, B., Mott, L.A., Skalla, K., et al. (2002). Neuropsychologic impact of standard-dose systemic chemotherapy in long-term survivors of breast cancer and lymphoma. *Journal of Clinical Oncology, 20*(2), 485–493.

Ahles, T.A., Saykin, A.J., McDonald, B.C., Furstenberg, C.T., Cole, B.F., Hanscom, B.S., et al. (2007). Cognitive function in breast cancer patients prior to adjuvant treatment. *Breast Cancer Research and Treatment, 110*(1), 143–152.

Ahles, T.A., Saykin, A.J., Noll, W.W., Furstenberg, C.T., Guerin, S., Cole, B., et al. (2003). The relationship of APOE genotype of neuropsychological performance in long-term cancer survivors treated with standard dose chemotherapy. *Psycho-Oncology, 12*(6), 612–619.

Ahles, T.A., Tope, D.M., Furstenberg, C., Hann, D., & Mills, L. (1996). Psychological and neuropsychologic impact of autologous bone marrow transplantation. *Journal of Clinical Oncology, 14*(5), 1457–1462.

Anderson-Hanley, C., Sherman, M.L., Riggs, R., Agocha, V.B., & Compass, B.E. (2003). Neuropsychological effects of treatments for adults with cancer: A meta-analysis and review of the literature. *Journal of the International Neuropsychological Society, 9*(7), 967–982.

Andrykowski, M.A., Schmitt, F.A., Gregg, M.E., Brady, M.J., Lamb, D.G., & Henslee-Downey, P.J. (1992). Neuropsychologic impairment in adult bone marrow transplant candidates. *Cancer, 70*(9), 2288–2297.

Bender, C.M., Paraska, K.K., Sereika, S.M., Ryan, C.M., & Berga, S.L. (2001). Cognitive function and reproductive hormones in adjuvant therapy for breast cancer: A critical review. *Journal of Pain and Symptom Management, 21*(5), 407–424.

Bender, C.M., Sereika, S.M., Berga, S.L., Vogel, V.G., Brufsky, A.M., Paraska, K.K., et al. (2006). Cognitive impairment associated with adjuvant therapy in breast cancer. *Psycho-Oncology, 15*(5), 422–430.

Bender, C.M., Sereika, S.M., Brufsky, A.M., Ryan, C.M., Vogel, V.G., Rastogi, P., et al. (2007). Memory impairments with adjuvant anastrozole versus tamoxifen in women with early-stage breast cancer. *Menopause, 14*(6), 995–998.

Bender, C.M., Yasko, J.M., Kirkwood, J.M., Ryan, C., Dunbar-Jacob, J., & Zullo, T. (2000). Cognitive function and quality of life in interferon therapy for melanoma. *Clinical Nursing Research, 9*(3), 352–363.

Brezden, C.B., Phillips, K.A., Abdolell, M., Bunston, T., & Tannock, I.F. (2000). Cognitive function in breast cancer patients receiving adjuvant chemotherapy. *Journal of Clinical Oncology, 18*(14), 2695–2701.

Capuron, L., Ravaud, A., & Dantzer, R. (2001). Timing and specificity of the cognitive changes induced by interleukin-2 and interferon-alpha treatments in cancer patients. *Psychosomatic Medicine, 63*(3), 376–386.

Castellon, S.A., Ganz, P.A., Bower, J.E., Petersen, L., Abraham, L., & Greendale, G. (2004). Neurocognitive performance in breast cancer survivors exposed to adjuvant chemotherapy and tamoxifen. *Journal of Clinical and Experimental Neuropsychology, 26*(7), 955–969.

Cull, A., Hay, C., Love, S.B., Mackie, M., Smets, E., & Stewart, M. (1996). What do patients mean when they complain of concentration and memory problems? *British Journal of Cancer, 74*(10), 1674–1679.

Dietrich, J., Han, R., Yang, Y., Mayer-Proschel, M., & Noble, M. (2006). CNS progenitor cells and oligodendrocytes are targets of chemotherapeutic agents in vitro and in vivo. *Journal of Biology, 5*(7), 22.

Donovan, K.A., Small, B.J., Andrykowski, M.A., Schmitt, F.A., Munster, P., & Jacobsen, P.B. (2005). Cognitive functioning after adjuvant chemotherapy and/or radiotherapy for early-stage breast carcinoma. *Cancer, 104*(11), 2499–2507.

Falleti, M.G., Sanfilippo, A., Maruff, P., Weih, L., & Phillips, K.A. (2005). The nature and severity of cognitive impairment associated with adjuvant chemotherapy in women with breast cancer: A meta-analysis of the current literature. *Brain and Cognition, 59*(1), 60–70.

Filley, C.M. (1999). Toxic leukoencephalopathy. *Clinical Neuropharmacology, 22*(5), 249–260.

Filley, C.M., & Kleinschmidt-DeMasters, B.K. (2001). Toxic leukoencephalopathy. *New England Journal of Medicine, 345*(6), 425–432.

Freeman, J.R., & Broshek, D.K. (2002). Assessing cognitive dysfunction in breast cancer: What are the tools? *Clinical Breast Cancer, 3*(Suppl. 3), S91–S99.

Harder, H., Cornelissen, J.J., Van Gool, A.R., Duivenvoorden, H.J., Eijkenboom, W.M.H., & van den Bent, M.J. (2002). Cognitive functioning and quality of life in long-term adult survivors of bone marrow transplantation. *Cancer, 95*(1), 183–192.

Harder, H., Duivenvoorden, H.J., Van Gool, A.R., Cornelissen, J.J., & van den Bent, M.J. (2006). Neurocognitive functions and quality of life in haematological patients receiving haematopoietic stem cell grafts: A one-year follow-up pilot study. *Journal of Clinical and Experimental Neuropsychology, 28*(3), 283–293.

Harder, H., Van Gool, A.R., Duivenvoorden, H.J., Cornelissen, J.J., Eijkenboom, W.M.H., Barge, M.Y., et al. (2007). Case-referent comparison of cognitive functions in patients receiving haematopoietic stem-cell transplantation for haematological malignancies: Two-year follow-up results. *European Journal of Cancer, 43*(14), 2052–2059.

Hensley, M.L., Correa, D.D., Thaler, H., Wilton, A., Venkatraman, E., Sabbatini, P., et al. (2006). Phase I/II study of weekly paclitaxel plus carboplatin and gemcitabine as first-line treatment of advanced-stage ovarian cancer: Pathologic complete response and longitudinal assessment of impact on cognitive functioning. *Gynecologic Oncology, 102*(2), 270–277.

Hermelink, K., Untch, M., Lux, M.P., Kreienberg, R., Beck, T., Bauerfeind, I., et al. (2007). Cognitive function during neoadjuvant chemotherapy for breast cancer: Results of a prospective multicenter longitudinal study. *Cancer, 109*(9), 1905–1913.

Hurria, A., Rosen, C., Hudis, C., Zuckerman, E., Panageas, K.S., Lachs, M.S., et al. (2006). Cognitive function of older patients receiving adjuvant chemotherapy for breast cancer: A pilot prospective longitudinal study. *Journal of the American Geriatrics Society, 54*(6), 926–931.

Inagaki, M., Yoshikawa, E., Matsuoka, Y., Sugawara, Y., Nakano, T., Akechi, T., et al. (2006). Smaller regional volumes of brain gray and white matter demonstrated in breast cancer survivors exposed to adjuvant chemotherapy. *Cancer, 109*(1), 146–156.

Jacobs, S.R., Small, B.J., Booth-Jones, M., Jacobsen, P.B., & Fields, K.K. (2007). Changes in cognitive functioning in the year after hematopoietic stem cell transplantation. *Cancer, 110*(7), 1546–1567.

Jacobsen, P.B., Garland, L.L., Booth-Jones, M., Donovan, K.A., Thors, C.L., Winters, E., et al. (2004). Relationship of hemoglobin levels to fatigue and cognitive functioning among cancer patients receiving chemotherapy. *Journal of Pain and Symptom Management, 28*(1), 7–18.

Jansen, C., Miaskowski, C., Dodd, M., Dowling, G., & Kramer, J. (2005a). Potential mechanisms for chemotherapy-induced impairments in cognitive function. *Oncology Nursing Forum, 32*(6), 1151–1163.

Jansen, C.E., Dodd, M.J., Miaskowski, C.A., Dowling, G.A., & Kramer, J. (2008, May 27). Preliminary results of a longitudinal study of changes in cognitive function in breast cancer patients undergoing chemotherapy with doxorubicin and cyclophosphamide. *Psycho-Oncology.* Retrieved October 19, 2008, from http://www3.interscience.wiley.com/journal/119230035/abstract?CRETRY=1&SRETRY=0

Jansen, C.E., Miaskowski, C., Dodd, M., Dowling, G., & Kramer, J. (2005b). A meta-analysis of studies of the effects of cancer chemotherapy on various domains of cognitive function. *Cancer, 104*(10), 2222–2233.

Jansen, C.E., Miaskowski, C.A., Dodd, M.J., & Dowling, G.A. (2007). A meta-analysis of the sensitivity of various neuropsychological tests used to detect chemotherapy-induced cognitive impairment in patients with breast cancer. *Oncology Nursing Forum, 34*(5), 997–1005.

Jatoi, A., Kahanic, S.P., Frytak, S., Schaefer, P., Foote, R.L., Sloan, J., et al. (2005). Donepezil and vitamin E for preventing cognitive dysfunction in small cell lung cancer patients: Preliminary results and suggestions for future study designs. *Supportive Care in Cancer, 13*(1), 66–69.

Jenkins, V., Shilling, V., Deutsch, G., Bloomfield, D., Morris, R., Allan, S., et al. (2006). A 3-year prospective study of the effects of adjuvant treatments on cognition in women with early stage breast cancer. *British Journal of Cancer, 94*(6), 828–834.

Jenkins, V.A., Bloomfield, D.J., Shilling V.M., & Edginton, T.L. (2005). Does neoadjuvant hormone therapy for early prostate cancer affect cognition? Results from a pilot study. *British Journal of Urology, 96*(1), 48–53.

Joly, F., Alibhai, S.M., Galica, J., Park, A., Yi, Q.L., Wagner, L., et al. (2006). Impact of androgen deprivation therapy on physical and cognitive function, as well as quality of life of patients with nonmetastatic prostate cancer. *Journal of Urology, 176*(6, Pt. 1), 2443–2447.

Kaasa, S., Olsnes, B.T., & Mastekaasa, A. (1988). Neuropsychological evaluation of patients with inoperable non-small cell lung cancer treated with combination chemotherapy or radiotherapy. *Acta Oncologica, 27*(3), 241–246.

Lezak, M.D., Howieson, D.B., & Loring, D.W. (2004). *Neuropsychological assessment* (4th ed.). New York: Oxford University Press.

Lower, E., Fleishman, S., Cooper, A., Zeldis, J., Faleck, H., & Mannaing, D. (2005). A phase III, randomized placebo-controlled trial of the safety and efficacy of d-MPH as new treatment of fatigue and "chemobrain" in adult cancer patients. *Journal of Clinical Oncology, 23*(16S), 8000.

Mar Fan, H.G., Chemerynsky, I., Xu, W., Clemons, M., & Tannock, I.F. (2008). A randomized, placebo-controlled, double-blind trial of the effects of d-methylphenidate on fatigue and cognitive dysfunction in women undergoing adjuvant chemotherapy for breast cancer. *Supportive Care in Cancer, 16*(6), 577–583.

Mayerhofer, K., Bodner-Adler, B., Bodner, K., Saletu, B., Schindl, M., Kaiser, A., et al. (2000). A paclitaxel-containing chemotherapy does not cause central nervous adverse effects: A prospective study in patients with ovarian cancer. *Anticancer Research, 20*(5C), 4051–4055.

Meyers, C.A., Albitar, M., & Estey, E. (2005). Cognitive impairment, fatigue, and cytokine levels in patients with acute myelogenous leukemia or myelodysplastic syndrome. *Cancer, 104*(4), 788–793.

Meyers, C.A., Byrne, K.S., & Komaki, R. (1995). Cognitive deficits in patients with small cell lung cancer before and after chemotherapy. *Lung Cancer, 12*(3), 231–235.

Meyers, C.A., Geara, F., Wong, P.F., & Morrison, W.H. (2000). Neurocognitive effects of therapeutic irradiation for base of skull tumors. *International Journal of Radiation Oncology, Biology, Physics, 46*(1), 51–55.

Meyers, C.A., Weitzner, M., Byrne, K., Valentine, A., Champlin, R.E., & Przepiorka, D. (1994). Evaluation of the neurobehavioral functioning of patients before, during, and after bone marrow transplantation. *Journal of Clinical Oncology, 12*(4), 820–826.

Meyers, C.A., Weitzner, M.A., Valentine, A.D., & Levin, V.A. (1998). Methylphenidate therapy improves cognition, mood, and function of brain tumor patients. *Journal of Clinical Oncology, 16*(7), 2522–2527.

O'Shaughnessy, J.A., Vukelja, S.J., Holmes, F.A., Savin, M., Jones, M., Royall, D., et al. (2005). Feasibility of quantifying the effects of epoetin alfa therapy on cognitive function in women with breast cancer undergoing adjuvant or neoadjuvant chemotherapy. *Clinical Breast Cancer, 5*(6), 439–446.

Reiriz, A.B., Reolon, G.K., Preissler, T., Rosado, J.O., Henriques, J.A., Roesler, R., et al. (2006). Cancer chemotherapy and cognitive function in rodent models: Memory impairment induced by cyclophosphamide in mice. *Clinical Cancer Research, 12*(16), 5000.

Salminen, E., Portin, R., Korpela, J., Backman, H., Parvinen, L.M., Helenius, H., et al. (2003). Androgen deprivation and cognition in prostate cancer. *British Journal of Cancer, 89*(6), 971–976.

Salminen, E., Portin, R., Koskinen, A.I., Helenius, H., & Nurmi, M.J. (2005). Estradiol and cognition during androgen deprivation in men with prostate carcinoma. *Cancer, 103*(7), 1381–1387.

Saykin, A.J., Ahles, T.A., & McDonald, B.C. (2003). Mechanisms of chemotherapy-induced cognitive disorders: Neuropsychological, pathophysiological, and neuroimaging perspectives. *Seminars in Clinical Neuropsychiatry, 8*(4), 201–216.

Schagen, S.B., Boogerd, W., Muller, M.J., Huinink, W.T., Moonen, L., Meinhardt, W., et al. (2008). Cognitive complaints and cognitive impairment following BEP chemotherapy in patients with testicular cancer. *Acta Oncologica, 47*(1), 63–70.

Schagen, S.B., Muller, M.J., Boogerd, W., Mellenberg, G.J., & van Dam, F.S.A.M. (2006). Change in cognitive function after chemotherapy: A prospective longitudinal study in breast cancer patients. *Journal of the National Cancer Institute, 98*(23), 1742–1745.

Schagen, S.B., Muller, M.J., Boogerd, W., Rosenbrand, R.M., van Rhijn, D., Rodenhuis, S., et al. (2002). Late effects of adjuvant chemotherapy on cognitive function: A follow-up study in breast cancer patients. *Annals of Oncology, 13*(9), 1387–1397.

Schagen, S.B., van Dam, F.S., Muller, M.J., Boogerd, W., Lindeboom, J., & Bruning, P.F. (1999). Cognitive deficits after postoperative adjuvant chemotherapy for breast carcinoma. *Cancer, 85*(3), 640–650.

Scheibel, R.S., Valentine, A.D., O'Brien, S., & Meyers, C.A. (2004). Cognitive dysfunction and depression during treatment with interferon-alpha and chemotherapy. *Journal of Neuropsychiatry and Clinical Neuroscience, 16*(2), 185–191.

Scherwath, A., Mehnert, A., Schleimer, B., Schirmer, L., Fehlauer, F., Kreienberg, R., et al. (2006). Neuropsychological function in high-risk breast cancer survivors after stem-cell supported high-dose therapy versus standard-dose chemotherapy: Evaluation of long-term treatment effects. *Annals of Oncology, 17*(3), 415–423.

Servaes, P., Verhagen, C.A., & Bleijenberg, G. (2002). Relations between fatigue, neuropsychological functioning, and physical activity after treatment for breast carcinoma: Daily self-report and objective behavior. *Cancer, 95*(9), 2017–2026.

Shaw, E.G., Rosdhal, R., D'Agostino, R.B., Lovato, J., Naughton, M.J., Robbins, M.E., et al. (2006). Phase II study of donepezil in irradiated brain tumor patients: Effect on cognitive function, mood, and quality of life. *Journal of Clinical Oncology, 24*(9), 1415–1420.

Shilling, V., Jenkins, V., Fallowfield, L., & Howell, A. (2001). The effects of oestrogens and anti-oestrogens on cognition. *Breast, 10*(6), 484–491.

Stewart, A., Bielajew, C., Collins, B., Parkinson, M., & Tomiak, E. (2006). A meta-analysis of the neuropsychological effects of adjuvant chemotherapy treatment in women treated for breast cancer. *Clinical Neuropsychologist, 20*(1), 76–89.

Stewart, A., Collins, B., MacKenzie, J., Tomiak, E., Verma, S., & Bielajew, C. (2008). The cognitive effects of adjuvant chemotherapy in early stage breast cancer: A prospective study. *Psycho-Oncology, 17*(2), 122–130.

Tannock, I.F., Ahles, T.A., Ganz, P.A., & van Dam, F.S. (2004). Cognitive impairment associated with chemotherapy for cancer: Report of a workshop. *Journal of Clinical Oncology, 22*(11), 2233–2239.

Tchen, N., Juffs, H.G., Downie, F.P., Yi, Q.L., Hu, H., Chemerynsky, I., et al. (2003). Cognitive function, fatigue, and menopausal symptoms in women receiving adjuvant chemotherapy for breast cancer. *Journal of Clinical Oncology, 21*(22), 4175–5183.

van Dam, F.S.A.M., Schagen, S.B., Muller, M.J., Boogerd, W., Wall, E.V.D., Fortuyn, M.E.D., et al. (1998). Impairment of cognitive function in women receiving adjuvant treatment for high-risk breast cancer: High-dose versus standard-dose chemotherapy. *Journal of the National Cancer Institute, 90*(3), 210–218.

van Oosterhout, A.G.M., Ganzevles, P.G.J., Wilmink, J.T., De Geus, B.W.J., van Vonderen, R.G.M.W., & Twijnstra, A. (1996). Sequelae in long-term survivors of small cell lung cancer. *International Journal of Radiation Oncology, Biology, Physics, 34*(5), 1037–1044.

Vardy, J.S., Rourke, S., Pond, G.R., Galica, J., Park, A., Dhillon, H.P., et al. (2007). Cognitive function and fatigue in cancer patients after chemotherapy: A longitudinal cohort study in patients with colorectal cancer. *Journal of Clinical Oncology, 25*(18S), Abstract 9099.

Walker, L.G., Walker, M.B., Heys, S.D., Lolley, J., Wesnes, K., & Eremin, O. (1997). The psychological and psychiatric effects of IL-2 therapy: A controlled clinical trial. *Psycho-Oncology, 6*(4), 290–301.

Walker, L.G., Wesnes, K.P., Heys, S.D., Walker, M.D., Lolley, J., & Eremin, O. (1996). The cognitive effects of recombinant interleukin-2 (rIL-2) therapy: A controlled clinical trial using computerized assessments. *European Journal of Cancer, 32A*(13), 2275–2283.

Wefel, J.S., Lenzi, R., Theriault, R.L., Buzdar, A.U., Cruickshank, S., & Meyers, C.A. (2004). Chemobrain in breast carcinoma? A prologue. *Cancer, 101*(3), 466–475.

Wefel, J.S., Lenzi, R., Theriault, R.L., Davis, R.N., & Meyers, C.A. (2004). The cognitive sequelae of standard-dose adjuvant chemotherapy in women with breast carcinoma. *Cancer, 100*(11), 2292–2299.

Wieneke, M.M., & Dienst, E.R. (1995). Neuropsychological assessment of cognitive functioning following chemotherapy for breast cancer. *Psycho-Oncology, 4*(1), 61–66.

Wilson, C.J., Finch, C.E., & Cohen, H.J. (2002). Cytokines and cognition: The case for a head-to-toe inflammatory paradigm. *Journal of the American Geriatrics Society, 50*(12), 2041–2056.

Winocur, G., Vardy, J., Binns, M.A., Kerr, L., & Tannock, I. (2006). The effects of the anti-cancer drugs, methotrexate and 5-fluorouracil on cognitive function in mice. *Pharmacological and Biochemical Behavior, 85*(1), 66–75.

L. Ocular toxicity
  1. Pathophysiology
    a) The causes of ocular toxicity are not fully understood. They may include the following.
      (1) Damage to the eye or eye structures related directly to treatment (e.g., distribution of cytotoxic drugs in tears, direct vascular injury during intracarotid administration, direct nerve injury from chemotherapy or radiation therapy) (DeAngelis, 2006; Fraunfelder & Fraunfelder, 2001)
      (2) EGFRIs: EGFR is a normal part of epidermal cells. Inhibiting EGFR can lead to damage to the epidermal cells found in the ocular region (eye and surrounding skin) (Garibaldi & Adler, 2007). Examples of EGFRI are tear film dysfunction and unusual hyper- or hypopigmentation (Zhang, Basti, & Jampol, 2007). EGFR also has a crucial role in the regulation of the hair growth cycle. An EGFRI can hinder this cycle, leading to loss of eyelashes and/or eyebrows (Robert et al., 2005; Zhang et al., 2007) or an accelerated growth and curling of the eyelashes, leading to tortuous eyelashes or eyelash trichomegaly (Robert et al.). For symptom management related to EGFRI medications for ocular toxicity, see Table 33.
      (3) A secondary process related to treatment (e.g., eye irritation caused by loss of eyelashes in the presence of neutropenia)
      (4) A secondary process related to concurrent disease (e.g., diabetes or Graves disease leading to diplopia or ptosis) (DeAngelis, 2006)
      (5) Metastases to the eyes or CNS resulting in increased intracranial pressure
      (6) Factors unrelated to cytotoxic therapy (e.g., head trauma or drug toxicity from narcotics or anticonvulsants leading to diplopia) (DeAngelis, 2006)
    b) A broad spectrum of disorders has been documented, including inflammatory conditions (e.g., uveitis, conjunctivitis, keratitis, blepharitis, iritis), development of retinal opacities, cataract formation, lid and lacrimation disorders, optic neuritis, and other neurologic injuries (Fraunfelder & Fraunfelder, 2001). For site-specific disorders, see Table 34.
    c) Ocular effects are becoming more common because of the use of more aggressive regimens as well as new agents and new drug combinations (al-Tweigeri, Nabholtz, & Mackey, 1996).
    d) With frequent use of combination therapy, determining which specific drug is causing complications may be difficult (Fraunfelder & Fraunfelder, 2001).
    e) Patients may experience toxicity-related visual impairment during chemotherapy

Table 33. Ocular Toxicity Symptom Management Related to Epidermal Growth Factor Receptor (EGFR) Inhibitors

Adverse Event	Symptoms	Management Strategy
Corneal epithelial defect	Significant eye pain, sensitivity to light	Refer to an ophthalmologist.
Eyelid skin changes (i.e., squamous blepharitis)	Hyperemia, papulopustular rash, crusting	Acute reactions: Apply fluorometholone (0.1%) ointment to eyelid (both skin and lid margin) for 1 week. DO NOT use for more than 2 weeks. An ophthalmologist must examine patient within 4 weeks. Chronic reactions: Apply tacrolimus (0.03%) ointment or pimecrolimus cream BID to skin of eyelid only. If treatment is minimally effective or not effective at all, try tacrolimus (0.1%). This treatment should not be used for more than 6 months.
Iridocyclitis	Sensitivity to light, sustained eye pain, decrease in vision	Refer to an ophthalmologist. Treatment involves use of anti-inflammatory medications.
Meibomitis (meibomian gland dysfunction)	Fluctuations in vision (varying degrees), burning sensation in the eye, some mucus discharge, and eye redness (may occur only on awakening)	Perform lid scrubs and apply warm compresses to the eyelid for at least 5 minutes BID. If lid scrubs and warm compresses are ineffective, give PO doxycycline 50 mg BID for 2 weeks, followed by 50 mg Q day for 4 weeks.
Tear film changes (dysfunctional tear syndrome)	Fluctuating or mild decrease in vision, transient eye pain, burning or foreign body sensation in the eye, eye fatigue	Mild symptoms: Apply supplemental tears 4–6 times a day. Severe or no relief: Refer to an ophthalmologist (treatment may consist of punctal plugs and/or anti-inflammatory medications).
Trichomegaly	Lengthening of the eyelashes or eyebrows, "patchy" lashes, misdirected lashes	Elongated or "patchy": No specific treatment. Will return to normal after EGFR inhibitor is completed. While many researchers (Braiteh et al., 2008; Eaby et al., 2008; Esper et al., 2007) agree that for patients experiencing trichomegaly, an ophthalmologist should be seen if eye irritations occur, and eyelashes may be carefully and safely trimmed, only Basti (2007) advises patients to not cut their lashes or have them cut. Waxing or electrolysis may be recommended (Braiteh et al., 2008; Segaert & Van Cutsem, 2005). Misdirected lashes: This is infrequent. Refer to an ophthalmologist. Do NOT remove misdirected lashes.

Note. From "Ocular Toxicities of Epidermal Growth Factor Receptor Inhibitors and Their Management," by S. Basti, 2007, *Cancer Nursing, 30*(Suppl. 4), p. S14. Copyright 2007 by Lippincott Williams & Wilkins. Adapted with permission.

and up to two weeks after chemotherapy (Kende, Sirkin, Thomas, & Freeman, 1979). Neurologic damage to the eye has occurred up to 43 days following chemotherapy (Warrell & Berman, 1986).

f) Ocular changes may go unnoticed until damage is irreversible.

g) Ocular signs and symptoms may precede the development of peripheral neuropathies and, thus, may be an important marker of neurologic status (Burns, 2001).

h) The presence of ocular signs or symptoms may predict development of GVHD in patients who have received allogeneic BMT (Kim et al., 2002).

i) Ocular changes may be incorrectly attributed to the aging process.

2. Incidence: Incidence varies according to drug classification, dose, and route of administration (see Table 35).

3. Risk factors: Causal relationships between agents and ocular toxicities are difficult to establish. Risk factors are equally difficult to establish.

4. Clinical manifestations: See Table 35.

5. Assessment: Ask patient about a history of any eye disturbance. In addition, assess the following (Bickley, 2007).

a) Visual acuity: Use a Snellen eye chart if possible. Position the patient 20 feet from the chart. Have the patient wear glasses or contacts for the examination if the corrective lenses are normally used other than for reading. Ask the patient to cover one eye with a card and to read the smallest line possible. Have the patient repeat with the other eye. You

Table 34. Specific Ocular Toxicities by Anatomic Site

Site	Ocular Toxicity
Orbit	Arteriovenous shunts, cavernous sinus syndrome, edema, exophthalmos, pallor, pain
Lids	Cicatricial ectropion, ankyloblepharon, increased lid necrosis after cryotherapy, hyperpigmentation
Lacrimal drainage	Tear duct fibrosis and punctal occlusion
Lacrimal gland	Keratoconjunctivitis sicca
Conjunctiva	Conjunctivitis
Sclera	Discoloration
Cornea	Keratopathy, keratitis
Pupil	Pinpoint pupils, internal ophthalmoplegia
Uvea	Uveitis
Trabecular meshwork and/or ciliary body	Increased intraocular pressure
Lens	Cataract
Retina	Toxic retinopathy
Vitreous	Opacification
Optic nerve	Disc edema, optic neuritis, optic atrophy
Cranial nerves III, IV, V, VI	Ptosis, paresis with or without diplopia, corneal hypesthesia
Extraocular muscles	Fibrosis
Central nervous system	Cortical blindness, internuclear ophthalmoplegia, blepharospasm

Note. Based on information from Murtha, 2000.

can also assess acuity using a near-vision card held at arm's length; patients who wear glasses or contact lenses should remove them. Record any visual disturbances.

b) Visual fields: Sit or stand in front of the patient and have the patient look with both eyes into your eyes. While the patient gazes into your eyes, place your hands two feet apart, lateral to the patient's ears. Instruct the patient to point to your fingers as soon as they are seen. Slowly move your fingers along an imaginary bowl and toward the line of gaze until the patient identifies them. Repeat this pattern in upper and lower temporal quadrants.

c) Position of eyes, eyebrows, and eyelids: While standing or sitting in front of the patient, observe the eyes for position and alignment with each other. Also inspect the eyebrows, noting their quantity and distribution and any flaking of the underlying skin. You also should survey the eyelids, observing and palpating for signs of erythema and edema. Assess for signs of exudates, crusting, and presence of ptosis. Observe condition of lashes.

d) Lacrimation: Note dryness, foreign-body sensation, excessive tearing, and/or swelling of the lacrimal sac.

e) Conjunctiva and sclera: Ask the patient to look up as you depress both lower lids with your thumbs, exposing the sclera and conjunctiva. Inspect both for color, vascular pattern, any discharge, and any nodules or swelling.

f) Cornea, lens, iris, and pupils: Observe the cornea and lens for smooth appearance, clarity, and any opacities in the lens. Test corneal reflex by gently touching a cotton swab to corneal surface. Observe iris and pupils. Margins should be clearly identified. Also observe the pupils for size, shape, and symmetry. If the pupils are > 5 mm or < 3 mm, then measure the pupils with a pupil guide (a card or pen light with black circles of varying sizes). Also test the pupils for light reaction, observing for direct reaction (pupillary constriction in the same eye), and consensual reaction (pupillary constriction in the opposite eye). Note pain and photophobia.

g) Extraocular muscles (CNs): Observe for light reflex (shining a light in the patient's eyes and inspecting the reflections in the corneas) and extraocular movement by having the patient follow finger movements in six planes and convergence. Note any unilateral movement, lack of movement, nystagmus, lid lag, or other abnormal movements.

6. Collaborative management
   a) Refer to an ophthalmologist for further evaluation and treatment (Burns, 2001).
   b) Instruct patient to use pharmacologic management as appropriate (e.g., antibiotics, steroids, artificial tears).
   c) Prevent further damage: Discontinue causative agent and promote symptom management.
   d) Surgical interventions may be necessary (e.g., cataract surgery, dilatation for punctal stenosis, enucleation).

7. Patient and family education
   a) Teach patients self-examination techniques emphasizing the importance of close monitoring and prompt reporting of any

Table 35. Ocular Toxicities Associated With Chemotherapy and Biotherapy

Classification	Agent	Ocular Toxicity	Comments
Alkylating agent	Busulfan	Long-standing reports of cataract formation and blurred vision (Burns, 2001; Murtha, 2000); rare cases of keratoconjunctivitis sicca (Murtha; Sidi et al., 1977)	Toxic effects are believed to act on proliferating lens epithelial cells (Burns, 2001).
	Carboplatin	*IV:* Rare cases of blurred vision, eye pain (al-Tweigeri et al., 1996); reports of maculopathy and optic neuropathy with transient cortical blindness when given to patients with renal dysfunction (O'Brien et al., 1992) *Intracarotid:* Reports of severe ocular and orbital toxicity in ipsilateral eye following intracarotid injection (Watanabe et al., 2002)	—
	Chlorambucil	Keratitis, diplopia, bilateral papilledema, retinal hemorrhages (al-Tweigeri et al., 1996; Burns, 2001); oculomotor disturbance, disc edema, retinopathy (Murtha, 2000)	Ocular toxicity is rare (Burns, 2001).
	Cisplatin	*IV:* Blurred vision, altered color perception, papilledema, decreased visual acuity, retrobulbar neuritis, transient cortical blindness, disc edema, retinopathy, electroretinogram abnormalities, cavernous sinus syndrome, color blindness (Becher et al., 1980; Murtha, 2000; Prager et al., 1998) *Intracarotid:* Ipsilateral visual loss (15%–60%) from retinal and/or optic nerve ischemia; possibly prevented by infusion distal to ophthalmic artery (Prager et al., 1998); optic neuropathy, unilateral vision loss (DeAngelis, 2006); retinal pigment disturbances, altered color perception, cotton wool spots, and intraretinal hemorrhages (Kwan et al., 2006)	—
	Cyclophosphamide	Blurred vision (reversible), keratoconjunctivitis sicca, pinpoint pupils (Jack & Hicks, 1981; Kende et al., 1979; Murtha, 2000)	—
	Ifosfamide	Blurred vision (reversible), conjunctivitis (Choonara et al., 1987; Murtha, 2000)	—
	Mechlorethamine	*Intracarotid:* Rare reports of ipsilateral necrotizing uveitis and necrotizing vasculitis of choroids (Burns, 2001)	No reports of ocular toxicity with IV administration (Burns, 2001)
Antimetabolite	Capecitabine	Ocular irritation, decreased vision, corneal deposits (Walkhom et al., 2000)	Ocular effects are seen in 10%–15% of patients (Fraunfelder & Fraunfelder, 2001).
	Cytarabine	*IV:* Keratitis (40%–100%), blurred vision with evidence of bilateral conjunctival hyperemia, ocular pain, photophobia, and foreign body sensation at high doses (al-Tweigeri et al., 1996; Burns, 2001); case reports of corneal toxicity with low dose of cytarabine (Lochhead et al., 2003) *Intrathecal:* Optic neuropathy leading to severe visual loss (may be potentiated by cranial radiation therapy) (Hopen et al., 1981; Margileth et al., 1977)	Hydrocortisone or dexamethasone eye drops may prevent keratitis. It is recommended to start eye drops the evening before therapy begins (Cleri & Haywood, 2002; Higa et al., 1991).

(Continued on next page)

Table 35. Ocular Toxicities Associated With Chemotherapy and Biotherapy (Continued)

Classification	Agent	Ocular Toxicity	Comments
Antimetabolite (cont.)	5-fluorouracil	25%–35% of patients have ocular side effects (Fraunfelder & Fraunfelder, 2001), including conjunctivitis (Christophidis et al., 1979); excessive lacrimation (Hamersley et al., 1973); tear duct fibrosis (Haidak et al., 1978); and blepharitis (Fraunfelder & Fraunfelder, 2001). Other ocular toxicities include keratoconjunctivitis, cicatricial ectropion, ankyloblepharon, blepharospasm, punctal occlusion, oculomotor disturbances, blurred vision, photophobia, nystagmus, increased lid necrosis after cryotherapy, ocular pain, and circumorbital edemas (Jansman et al., 2001; Murtha, 2000).	Loprinzi et al. (1994) studied the use of ice packs to decrease ocular irritation; this was reinforced by North Central Cancer Treatment Group (ice applied for 30 minutes, 5 minutes before infusion). Also the use of dexamethasone eye drops decreased ocular toxicities (Jansman et al., 2001).
	Fludarabine	Decreased visual acuity (most common presenting sign before development of progressive encephalopathy); rare cases of diplopia, photophobia, and optic neuritis (al-Tweigeri et al., 1996; Chun et al., 1986; Murtha, 2000; Warrell & Berman, 1986)	Effects are dose-dependent (Burns, 2001).
	Methotrexate	*IV:* Blepharitis, conjunctival hyperemia, increased lacrimation, periorbital edema, photophobia, optic pain (Murtha, 2000) *IT:* With concurrent radiation, case report of bilateral ophthalmoplegia with exotropia; optic nerve atrophy *Intra-arterial:* Retinal changes in ipsilateral eye (Fraunfelder & Fraunfelder, 2001)	Up to 25% of patients may develop ocular toxicity (al-Tweigeri et al., 1996); toxicity is more common with higher doses (Burns, 2001). Drug is found in tears (Fraunfelder & Fraunfelder, 2001).
	Pentostatin	Keratitis, conjunctivitis (Burns, 2001)	Mild to moderate, transient in nature (Burns, 2001)
Antitumor antibiotic	Doxorubicin	Conjunctivitis, increased lacrimation (Curran & Luce, 1989; Murtha, 2000); increased lacrimation occurs in up to 25% of patients receiving doxorubicin (Blum, 1975).	Serious ocular side effects are rare (Burns, 2001).
	Mitomycin-C	*IV:* Blurred vision (al-Tweigeri et al., 1996; Murtha, 2000) *Topical:* Keratoconjunctivitis (Burns, 2001)	—
	Mitoxantrone	Conjunctivitis, discoloration of sclera (Fraunfelder & Fraunfelder, 2001)	Drug is secreted in tears (Fraunfelder & Fraunfelder, 2001).
Biotherapy agents	BCG live vaccine	Uveitis, conjunctivitis, iritis, keratitis, granulomatous chorioretinitis (Murtha, 2000; Sanofi Pasteur, 2006)	Ocular side effects rare, more common in patients who are positive for HLA-B27 (Sanofi Pasteur, 2006)
	G-CSF, GM-CSF	Case report of acute iritis in healthy stem cell donor taking G-CSF (Parkkali et al., 1996); marginal keratitis and mild uveitis in healthy stem cell donor following both G-CSF and GM-CSF (Esmaeli et al., 2002)	—
	IFN alfa, IFN beta, IFN gamma	Retinopathy, primarily retinal hemorrhages; cotton wool spots (Esmaeli, Koller, et al., 2001; Wilson, 2004); disc edema (Murtha, 2000) Visual loss from IFN alfa (DeAngelis, 2006)	Incidence is 50% or higher (Kawano et al., 1996). Risk is increased in patients with hypertension or diabetes and those receiving higher doses (Fraunfelder & Fraunfelder, 2001).
	IL-2	Neuro-ophthalmic effects including scotoma, diplopia, transient blindness, visual hallucinations (Fraunfelder & Fraunfelder, 2001)	—

(Continued on next page)

Table 35. Ocular Toxicities Associated With Chemotherapy and Biotherapy (Continued)

Classification	Agent	Ocular Toxicity	Comments
Biotherapy agents (cont.)	Retinoid	Blepharoconjunctivitis, corneal opacities, papilledema, pseudotumor cerebri, night blindness (al-Tweigeri et al., 1996)	Avoid concurrent use of tetracyclines and drugs causing intracranial hypertension (Fraunfelder & Fraunfelder, 2004).
Miscellaneous	Bisphosphonates	Conjunctivitis, uveitis, scleritis (Fraunfelder & Fraunfelder, 2004)	Bisphosphonates must be discontinued for symptoms to resolve (Fraunfelder & Fraunfelder, 2004).
	Corticosteroids	Posterior subcapsular cataracts, glaucoma, retinal hemorrhage (Loredo et al., 1972), opportunistic eye infections, visual field defects, blurred vision, diplopia, exophthalmos, scleral discoloration (Murtha, 2000)	—
	Cyclosporine A	Optic neuropathy (Mejico et al., 2000), blurred vision, retinopathy, case reports of cortical blindness (Burns, 2001)	Combination of cyclosporine A and TBI may increase susceptibility to develop radiation-induced optic neuropathy; patients' symptoms improved to some extent when cyclosporine was discontinued (Mejico et al., 2000).
	Deferoxamine mesylate/desferrioxamine	Night blindness, visual field constriction, cataracts, pigmentary retinopathy, optic neuropathy (Arora, 2004); blurring vision, decreased visual acuity, vision loss, visual defects, scotoma, impaired peripheral, color, and night vision, optic neuritis, corneal opacities (Novartis Pharmaceuticals Corp., 2007)	Ocular side effects related to prolonged use, high doses, or in patients with low ferritin levels; ocular disturbances were reversible upon cessation of treatment (Arora, 2004; Novartis Pharmaceuticals Corp., 2007).
	Ethambutol hydrochloride	Decrease in visual acuity, color blindness, visual defect, possible irreversible blindness, optic neuritis (Dura Pharmaceuticals, 2003)	Ocular toxicity can happen at any dose, but increased at > 50 mg/kg (Donald et al., 2006); change in visual acuity can be unilateral or bilateral. Testing for visual acuity should be performed before treatment begins and periodically during treatment, unless dose is > 15 mg/kg/day, then monthly testing is needed (Dura Pharmaceuticals, 2003).
	Mannitol	Blurred vision (Baxter, 2005), cataracts (Murtha, 2000)	Because of fluid and electrolyte shift, side effects can be prevented with close monitoring and test dose to evaluate degree of renal failure when indicated (Baxter, 2005).
	Mitotane	Visual blurring, diplopia, lens opacity, toxic retinopathy (Bristol-Myers Squibb, 2006; Murtha, 2000)	Ocular side effects are infrequent (Bristol-Myers Squibb, 2006).
	Procarbazine hydrochloride	Retinal hemorrhage, papilledema, photophobia, diplopia, inability to focus (Sigma-Tau Pharmaceuticals, 2004); retinopathy, nystagmus, disc edema (Murtha, 2000)	Ophthalmic side effects are rare (Cleri & Haywood, 2002).
	Radiation therapy	Xerophthalmia, keratoconjunctivitis (dry eye syndrome), pain, sensation of a foreign body in the eye, corneal ulceration (Brigden & McKenzie, 2000)	Xerophthalmia effect is caused by the radiation effect on the lacrimal and other adnexal glands that contribute to tear production. Lubricants and an ophthalmologic consultation are helpful (Brigden & McKenzie, 2000).
	Tacrolimus (FK506)	Optic neuropathy (Mejico et al., 2000); rare cortical blindness (Burns, 2001)	—

(Continued on next page)

Table 35. Ocular Toxicities Associated With Chemotherapy and Biotherapy *(Continued)*

Classification	Agent	Ocular Toxicity	Comments
Miscellaneous *(cont.)*	Tamoxifen	Cataracts and decreased color vision; increased risk with doses greater than 20 mg/day (DeAngelis, 2006; Gorin et al., 1998; Fraunfelder & Fraunfelder, 2001; retinal toxicity (small refractile or crystalline dot-like yellowish deposits in the area surrounding the macula, in the nerve, and in plexiform layers) (Gianni et al., 2006; Lazzaroni et al., 1998; Tsai et al., 2003); corneal opacities, retinopathy (Murtha, 2000)	A baseline ophthalmic examination is recommended within the first year (Gorin et al., 1998); visual acuity may improve with tamoxifen withdrawal along with macular edema, but retinal deposits often do not (Gianni et al., 2006).
Nitrosourea	Carmustine Lomustine	Optic neuritis and atrophy, hyperemia, orbital pain, retinopathy, corneal opacities and edema, orbital IV shunts, secondary glaucoma, internal ophthalmoplegia, blurred vision, vitreal opacification, extraocular muscle fibrosis, diplopia (Murtha, 2000) *IV:* Rare reports of delayed blurred vision and loss of depth perception (Burns, 2001) *Intracarotid:* Severe, ipsilateral occurrences including arterial narrowing, disc edema, and intraretinal hemorrhages (Greenberg et al., 1984; Shingleton et al., 1982)	—
Targeted therapy	Cetuximab	Relatively common: Loss of eyelashes (madarosis)/eyebrows and/or cicatricial ectropion, on, loss of color of the skin around the eye with weekly infusions (Garibaldi & Adler, 2007); trichomegaly (Basti, 2007; Robert et al., 2005) Very rare: Bilateral ocular discomfort with itchiness around both eyelids, foreign body sensation, tearing associated with exfoliated skin, oil secretions, and crusty scaling (Tonini et al., 2005)	Madarosis and cicatricial ectropion resolved after discontinuation of cetuximab (Garibaldi & Adler, 2007). Ocular discomfort cleared up with topical antibiotics and holding therapy (Tonini et al., 2005). While many researchers (Braiteh et al., 2008; Eaby et al., 2008; Esper et al., 2007) agree that for patients experiencing trichomegaly, an ophthalmologist should be seen if eye irritations occur, and eyelashes may be carefully and safely trimmed, only Basti (2007) advises patients to not cut their lashes or have them cut. Waxing or electrolysis may be recommended (Braiteh et al.; Segaert & Van Cutsem, 2005).
	Erlotinib	Periorbital rash, conjunctivitis, and eyelid ectropion (Methvin & Gausas, 2007); eyelash trichomegaly (Robert et al., 2005)	Side effects resolved within 6 weeks after treatment stopped (Methvin & Gausas, 2007). See cetuximab for comments regarding trichomegaly.
	Gefitinib	Trichomegaly (Basti, 2007; Eaby et al., 2008; Robert et al., 2005); eye pain, conjunctivitis (VHA Pharmacy Benefits Management Strategic Healthcare Group & Medical Advisory Panel, 2003); dry blepharitis (Tullo et al., 2005); visual disturbances, eye pain, eye itchiness, or redness (Dawson et al., 2004)	Resolves after EGFR treatment is stopped. While many researchers (Braiteh et al., 2008; Eaby et al., 2008; Esper et al., 2007) agree that for patients experiencing trichomegaly, an ophthalmologist should be seen if eye irritations occur, and eyelashes may be carefully and safely trimmed, only Basti (2007) advises patients to not cut their lashes or have them cut. Waxing or electrolysis may be recommended (Braiteh et al., 2008; Segaert & Van Cutsem, 2005). If therapy is interrupted because of symptoms, gefitinib may be restarted once symptoms have resolved (Dawson et al., 2004; VHA Pharmacy Benefits Management Strategic Healthcare Group & Medical Advisory Panel, 2003).

(Continued on next page)

Table 35. Ocular Toxicities Associated With Chemotherapy and Biotherapy (Continued)

Classification	Agent	Ocular Toxicity	Comments
Targeted therapy (cont.)	Imatinib	Periorbital edema (Robert et al., 2005)	Resolves after EGFR treatment is stopped
	Panitumumab	Conjunctivitis, ocular hyperemia, increased lacrimation, eye/eyelid irritation (Amgen Inc., 2007)	Onset of ocular symptoms is 14–15 days after first dose of panitumumab. Symptoms resolved after panitumumab was stopped. Median time of resolution is 84 days (Amgen Inc., 2007).
	Sunitinib	Periorbital edema (Robert et al., 2005)	Resolves after EGFR treatment is stopped
Taxanes	Docetaxel	Epiphora, canalicular stenosis (Esmaeli, Valero, et al., 2001); successful treatment with bicanalicular silicone intubation (Ahmadi & Esmaeli, 2001)	Drug is secreted in tears (Esmaeli et al., 2002).
	Paclitaxel	Scintillating scotomas or "shooting lights" occur in 20% of cases; resolved spontaneously (Capri et al., 1994).	Scotomas usually occur toward the end of 3-hour infusion (Fraunfelder & Fraunfelder, 2001).
Vinca alkaloids	Etoposide	*Intracarotid:* Optic neuritis, transient cortical blindness (Lauer et al., 1999)	Given in combination with carboplatin (Lauer et al., 1999)
	Vinblastine	Extraocular muscle palsies (Fraunfelder & Fraunfelder, 2001)	–
	Vincristine	Cranial nerve palsies, optic neuropathy, case reports of transient cortical blindness (Burns, 2001; Murtha, 2000); diplopia (DeAngelis, 2006)	80% of toxicities are reversible (Fraunfelder & Fraunfelder, 2001); usually reversible after discontinuation of the vincristine (DeAngelis, 2006)

BCG—bacillus Calmette-Guérin; EGFR—epidermal growth factor receptor; G-CSF—granulocyte–colony-stimulating factor; GM-CSF—granulocyte macrophage–colony-stimulating factor; HLA—human leukocyte antigen; IFN—interferon; IL—interleukin; IT—intrathecal; IV—intravenous; TBI—total body irradiation

Wilson, R.A. (2004). Visual side effects of pegylated interferon during therapy for chronic hepatitis C infection. *Journal of Clinical Gastroenterology, 38*(8), 717–722.

Zhang, G., Basti, S., & Jampol, L.M. (2007). Acquired trichomegaly and symptomatic external ocular changes in patients receiving epidermal growth factor receptor inhibitors: Case reports and a review of literature. *Cornea, 26*(7), 858–860.

M. Pancreatitis: Inflammation of the pancreas
1. Pathophysiology (Hruban & Wilentz, 2005)
   a) Pancreatitis is a group of disorders ranging from mild, transient changes to life-threatening inflammatory process and irreversible loss of function.
   b) Causes are secondary to ductal obstruction (e.g., cholelithiasis), acinar cell injury (e.g., drugs, viruses), or defective intracellular transport (e.g., alcohol).
2. Risk factors (Ellsworth-Wolk, 1998; Hruban & Wilentz, 2005)
   a) Chemotherapy drugs, including asparaginase, mercaptopurine, all-trans-retinoic acid, tamoxifen, and cytosine arabinoside
   b) Hypertriglyceridemia, hypercalcemia
   c) TLS
   d) Post–endoscopic retrograde cholangiopancreatography, abdominal surgery
   e) Alcohol abuse
   f) Illicit drug use
   g) Cholelithiasis
   h) Pediatrics: Post-BMT
   i) Infection
3. Clinical manifestations (Swaroop, Chari, & Clain, 2004)
   a) Epigastric, periumbilical, or left/right upper abdominal pain
   b) Pain radiating to the back
   c) Fever, tachycardia
   d) Severe nausea and vomiting
   e) Jaundice
   f) Signs and symptoms of shock with severe or acute pancreatitis
   g) Hypoactive bowel sounds, ileus
   h) Increased serum levels of pancreatic enzymes (amylase, lipase)
   i) Elevated LFTs
   j) Frequently elevated WBC count
4. Assessment: Physical examination must be performed to find and document the preceding clinical manifestations.
5. Collaborative management (Bryant, 2006; Forsmark & Baillie, 2007): Treatment is aimed at correcting underlying predisposing conditions and decreasing pancreatic inflammation.
   a) Hold or discontinue any agent that may be the cause of the condition.
   b) Insert a nasogastric tube if patient has nausea and vomiting or ileus to rest the gut during the acute phase of pancreatitis.
   c) If NPO (nothing by mouth) more than three to five days, consider total parenteral nutrition to prevent malnutrition.
   d) Administer vigorous hydration with electrolyte monitoring and replacement (e.g., calcium, potassium, magnesium) as indicated.
   e) Monitor serum lipase, amylase, and electrolyte levels and LFTs.
   f) Provide effective pain control.
   g) Anticipate orders for diagnostic imaging of the abdomen (e.g., abdominal flat plate and upright to detect ileus; ultrasound to visualize gallbladder and biliary tree for stones, edema, dilation; CT scan to image pancreas).
   h) Administer antibiotic therapy.
   i) Ensure bed rest.
   j) Monitor vital signs, including oxygen saturation, level of consciousness, and condition carefully for signs of hypovolemic shock (hypotension occurs because of sequestration of protein-rich fluids into the pancreas, retroperitoneal space, and abdominal cavity in severe acute pancreatitis).
   k) When food is reintroduced, provide a lipid-restricted diet (Bryant, 2006).
6. Patient and family education
   a) Instruct patients to use analgesics for pain control.
   b) Implement effective oral and nasal care while NPO with a nasogastric tube.
   c) Ensure that patients know the importance of adherence to dietary, pharmacologic, and lifestyle recommendations.
   d) Ensure that patients and significant others can recognize the early symptoms of pancreatitis, and instruct them to seek medical intervention when these appear.

References

Bryant, G. (2006). Pancreatitis. In D. Camp-Sorrell & R.A. Hawkins (Eds.), *Clinical manual for the oncology advanced practice nurse* (2nd ed., pp. 567–571). Pittsburgh, PA: Oncology Nursing Society.

Ellsworth-Wolk, J. (1998). Acute pancreatitis. In C.C. Chernecky & B.J. Berger (Eds.), *Advanced and critical care oncology nursing: Managing primary complications* (pp. 26–38). Philadelphia: Saunders.

Forsmark, C.E., & Baillie, J. (2007). AGA Institute technical review on acute pancreatitis. *Gastroenterology, 132*(5), 2022–2044.

Hruban, R.H., & Wilentz, R.E. (2005). The pancreas. In V. Kumar, A.K. Abbas, & N. Fausto (Eds.), *Robbins & Cotran pathologic basis of disease* (7th ed., pp. 939–953). Philadelphia: Elsevier.

Swaroop, V.S., Chari, S.T., & Clain, J.E. (2004). Severe acute pancreatitis. *JAMA, 291*(23), 2865–2868.

N. Fatigue: "Cancer-related fatigue is a distressing, persistent, subjective sense of physical, emotional, or cognitive tiredness or exhaustion related to cancer or cancer treatment that is not proportional to recent activity and interferes with usual functioning" (NCCN, 2008, p. FT-1). It is a complex concept that is multidimensional and multicausal (Sura, Murphy, & Gonzales, 2006). Fatigue is underreported, underdiagnosed, and undertreated. Cancer-related fatigue is the most common and distressing side effect of cancer treatment and has a profound effect on ADLs and QOL (Stricker, Drake, Hoyer, & Mock, 2004). NCCN guidelines recommend that all patients be screened for fatigue at their initial visit and at regular intervals during the cancer treatment continuum and that fatigue should be treated promptly in both children and adults.

1. Pathophysiology: Exact mechanisms are unknown. Numerous hypotheses regarding the etiologies have been studied, largely based on evidence from chronic fatigue syndrome and exercise fatigue (Ryan et al., 2007) (see Figure 34).

    a) Underlying causes of cancer-related fatigue are believed to involve several physiologic and biochemical systems. These include (Ryan et al., 2007)
        (1) 5HT neurotransmitter dysregulation
        (2) Vagal afferent activation
        (3) Alterations in muscle and ATP metabolism
        (4) Hypothalamic-pituitary-adrenal axis dysfunction
        (5) Circadian rhythm disruption
        (6) Cytokine dysregulation.

    b) Accumulation of muscle metabolites (NCCN, 2008)

    c) Proinflammatory cytokines: IL-1, IL-6, and TNF may act on the CNS causing fatigue, sleep disturbances, depressed mood, and decreased activity (Schwartz, 2007).

    d) Treatment-related causes: Chemotherapy, hormone therapy, radiation therapy, and combined modality therapies have all been implicated with exacerbating fatigue (Lipman & Lawrence, 2004). Travel to and from a clinic for treatment adds to a patient's fatigue, as well as the therapy itself.

    e) Disease process and comorbid conditions including metabolic disorders
        (1) Hypothyroidism
        (2) Electrolyte imbalances
        (3) Infection

    f) Uncontrolled pain, nausea, and vomiting

    g) Anxiety

    h) Sleep disturbances, such as (NCCN, 2008)
        (1) Obstructive sleep apnea
        (2) Restless leg syndrome
        (3) Narcolepsy
        (4) Insomnia

    i) Mood disturbances

    j) Anemia: A relationship clearly exists between Hgb and fatigue. Fatigue is more frequent in patients with lower Hgb. Even small increases in Hgb levels can alleviate fatigue and anemia-related symptoms (Cella, 2006).

    k) Nutritional deficiencies (e.g., vitamin B_{12}, folic acid, iron, protein) (Madden & Newton, 2006)

    l) Physical deconditioning and activity level: Reduced functional capacity and physical strength contributes to sedentary behavior. Inactivity can lead to debilitation. Routine tasks become fatiguing (Schwartz, 2007).

    m) Stress

    n) Depression

2. Incidence: The prevalence of fatigue is reported as high as 61%–100% in studies of patients with cancer. Often, patients report fatigue being more disturbing and disruptive than pain. More than 75% of patients with metastatic disease report fatigue, and even cancer survivors report fatigue as a continuing distressing symptom months to years after completion of treatment (Stricker et al., 2004).

3. Assessment

    a) Utilization of a fatigue scale; this is particularly beneficial to evaluate the effectiveness of interventions. The 0–10 scale, a visual analog scale, or Likert scales all have been used with success (Lipman & Lawrence, 2004).
        (1) On a 0–10 scale (zero = no fatigue and 10 = worst fatigue imaginable), mild fatigue is given a score of 1–3, moderate fatigue 4–6, and severe fatigue 7–10.

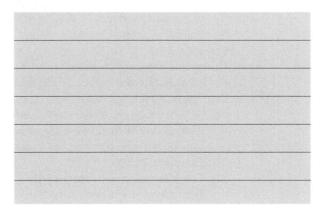

Figure 34. Treatable Contributing Factors for Cancer-Related Fatigue Based on National Comprehensive Cancer Network Guidelines

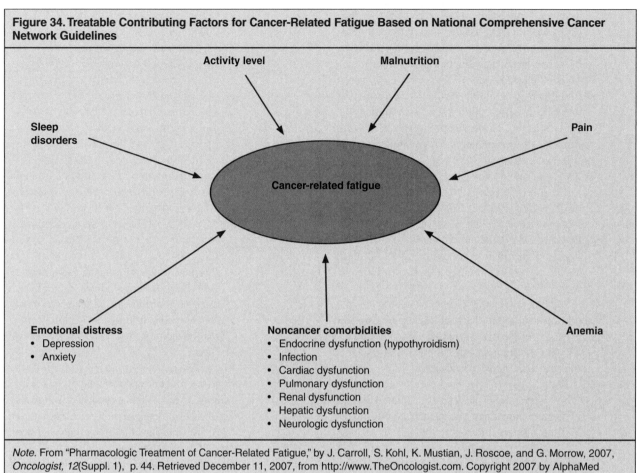

Activity level

Malnutrition

Sleep disorders

Pain

Cancer-related fatigue

Emotional distress
- Depression
- Anxiety

Noncancer comorbidities
- Endocrine dysfunction (hypothyroidism)
- Infection
- Cardiac dysfunction
- Pulmonary dysfunction
- Renal dysfunction
- Hepatic dysfunction
- Neurologic dysfunction

Anemia

Note. From "Pharmacologic Treatment of Cancer-Related Fatigue," by J. Carroll, S. Kohl, K. Mustian, J. Roscoe, and G. Morrow, 2007, *Oncologist, 12*(Suppl. 1), p. 44. Retrieved December 11, 2007, from http://www.TheOncologist.com. Copyright 2007 by AlphaMed Press. Reprinted with permission.

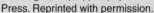

(2) Fatigue measurement in children is simplified. Young children (age < 6) may just be asked if they are "tired" or "not tired." Valid and reliable instruments are available to measure fatigue in children and adolescents (NCCN, 2008).

(3) If mild levels (1–3) are determined, patients and family members should receive education about fatigue and common strategies for management.

(4) When fatigue is rated as moderate to severe (4–10), a more focused history and physical examination should be conducted as part of the primary evaluation phase.

b) Disease status

c) Disease recurrence or progression

d) Current medications or medication changes that may contribute to fatigue

(1) Polypharmacy is common in patients with cancer. Many drugs alone or in combination can contribute to fatigue (Schwartz, 2007).

(2) Tricyclic antidepressants, opioids, antinausea medications, and sleep aids all can cause sedation. Combined use can cause prolonged sedation, leading to limited activity and overall fatigue.

e) Complete review of systems

f) Onset, pattern, and duration of fatigue

g) Nutritional and metabolic evaluation; often, fatigue symptoms can be improved by improving dietary intake, with appropriate caloric intake.

(1) A dietitian can design a patient-specific plan to improve nutritional status. Fluids and electrolytes should be assessed. Specifically, imbalances in sodium, potassium, calcium, and magnesium can be reversed with appropriate supplementation, which may improve fatigue (NCCN, 2008).

(2) Nausea and vomiting, taste changes, and bowel changes (e.g., obstruction, constipation, diarrhea) will interfere with nutritional intake and affect fatigue level.

h) Activity level

i) Associated or alleviating factors (e.g., rest, energy conservation, balancing activities with rest periods)

4. Collaborative management

   a) General

     (1) Energy conservation: Defined by NCCN (2008) as "the deliberately planned management of one's personal energy resources to prevent their depletion" (p. MS-13). Patients need to balance energy demands with planned activities. This is a learned process for each patient and is dictated by each patient's disease experience.

     (2) Instruct patients to delegate activities, pace themselves, take extra rest periods, plan high-energy activities at times of peak energy, and conserve energy for valued activities (NCCN, 2008).

     (3) Recommend energy-saving devices (e.g., raised toilet seats, grabber tools, seated walkers, wheelchairs).

   b) Pharmacologic: Because the exact pathophysiology of cancer-related fatigue is obscure, pharmacotherapy is empiric or geared toward reversing possible contributing factors (Lipman & Lawrence, 2004).

     (1) Erythropoiesis-stimulating agents (Epogen®, Procrit®, and Aranesp®) have been under intense scrutiny. These agents, when used appropriately, will reduce transfusion requirements and improve anemia. However, correcting anemia does not always improve fatigue, and many patients with cancer experiencing fatigue are not anemic (Schwartz, 2007).

     (2) Antidepressants have been recommended as treatment for fatigue because depression was suggested as a causal factor. In particular, paroxetine (Paxil®) and bupropion (Wellbutrin®) are used.

       (a) While these drugs are helpful in alleviating depression, they can cause sedation and have a delayed onset of action. Several randomized placebo-controlled trials have not shown improvement in fatigue with the addition of these drugs (Mitchell, Beck, Hood, Moore, & Tanner, 2007).

       (b) Antidepressants might have a greater effect on cancer survivors, in whom fatigue and depression are prevalent and often coexist (Lipman & Lawrence, 2004).

(3) Psychostimulants

   (a) Methylphenidate (Ritalin®): Several small, open-label, single-arm studies have examined use of methylphenidate in reducing fatigue. All reported improvement in fatigue, but side effects of insomnia, agitation, anorexia, nausea and vomiting, and dry mouth have been reported.

   (b) Dextromethylphenidate was used in early trials. Preliminary results demonstrated safety and efficacy as well as improved fatigue and memory. Trials with larger sample sizes are needed to determine generalizable efficacy of these drugs on fatigue (Schwartz, 2007).

   (c) Modafinil (Provigil®) is a wakefulness-promoting agent. It is indicated for narcolepsy. It has been used in a small open-label study with a group of breast cancer survivors. 83% reported a reduction in fatigue. A similar trial involving adults with brain tumors showed that modafinil is safe and effective when used to treat fatigue in patients with cancer (NCCN, 2008). RCCTs of modafinil for cancer-related fatigue are ongoing.

(4) Glucocorticoids

   (a) Preliminary studies with methylprednisolone and prednisone reported improvements in symptoms, especially pain, and showed improved QOL and reduced fatigue in patients with metastatic disease. Decreased fatigue and increased energy levels, appetite, and feelings of well-being were demonstrated. Studies were of

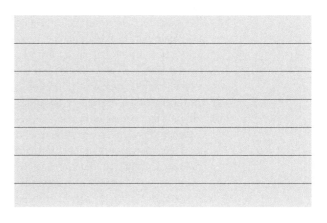

short duration (10–14 days), but considering the outcomes, more clinical trials of longer duration are needed (Carroll, Kohli, Mustian, Roscoe, & Morrow, 2007).

(b) Megestrol acetate (Megace®), widely used for appetite improvement, has demonstrated a dose-dependent improvement in fatigue and well-being (Carroll et al., 2007). The NCCN guidelines (2008) recommend use of megestrol acetate over dexamethasone if long-term use is anticipated because it has a more favorable side effect profile. Safety and efficacy of megestrol acetate have been confirmed for patients with cancer (NCCN).

(5) The supplement L-carnitine has been studied in several open-label studies. Carnitine is a micronutrient important in the processing of long-chain fatty acids and energy production in mammalian cells. Treatment with L-carnitine (500–600 mg/day) for one to four weeks in nonanemic patients with cancer increased plasma-free carnitine and significantly improved fatigue and QOL measures (Carroll et al., 2007). Micronutrient deficiency may be responsible for fatigue in patients with advanced cancer. Although the work with this is still preliminary, carnitine supplement may prove beneficial for fatigue management (NCCN, 2008).

(6) Complementary/alternative therapies

(a) Limited studies of herbal supplements have been conducted with regard to fatigue in patients with cancer. Current data are insufficient to warrant recommendation of these agents; therefore,

additional controlled studies are being conducted to further understand the effects of these products (Schwartz, 2007).

(b) Ginkgo biloba and mistletoe extract have demonstrated some positive effect on cancer-related fatigue.

(7) Nonpharmacologic interventions

(a) Exercise: Cumulative evidence is strong in support of exercise as an intervention to manage cancer-related fatigue. All patients with cancer should be encouraged to maintain an optimum level of physical activity during and following cancer treatment. Many studies have been conducted focusing on the effect of exercise on cancer-related fatigue. The majority involved patients with nonmetastatic breast cancer; however, numerous ongoing trials involving patients with multiple myeloma, prostate cancer, and melanoma show promising evidence that exercise may be beneficial in other cancer populations (Hanna, Avila, Meteer, Nicholas, & Kaminsky, 2008).

i) Exercise interventions should be individualized and based on the patient's specific disease and treatment (Stricker et al., 2004). Patients with comorbidities or substantial deconditioning should be referred to physical therapy or physical medicine and rehabilitation for assessment and exercise prescription.

ii) Exercise programs must be undertaken with caution for patients with bone metastasis, immunosuppression or neutropenia, fever, thrombocytopenia, anemia, or other treatment complications.

iii) Programs should be initiated slowly to assess the patient's tolerance and can be modified as time progresses (NCCN, 2008). Generally, exercise activities such as walking, cycling, swimming, resistive exercise, and low-to-moderate-intensity aerobic exercise occurring several times per week can be effective in reducing fatigue in patients (Mitchell et al., 2007).

(b) Complementary therapies: Yoga, acupuncture, expressive writing, aromatherapies, lavender foot soak, and reflexology have been evaluated in small pilot studies. Although the sample sizes were small, the study results suggest that such complementary therapies have potential in treating fatigue in patients with cancer (Mitchell et al., 2007).

5. Patient and family education

a) Management of fatigue originates with the primary oncology team who assess fatigue as a symptom related to treatment and disease status. This begins with the initial screening and then expands to a more focused evaluation for moderate to higher levels of fatigue (NCCN, 2008).

b) Patients and family members need to be made aware that fatigue is a major symptom related to the disease and treatment process and that patterns of fatigue are variable. For some adults, fatigue may be characterized as constant and unrelenting; for others, it is unpredictable and may come on suddenly (NCCN, 2008). Knowledge is a powerful tool. Knowing that fatigue is a common side effect of cancer and awareness of its treatment can help patients to feel less worried about it (Schwartz, 2007).

c) Psychosocial interventions, including education, individual counseling, and support groups, should be utilized. These methods teach coping and stress management techniques and ultimately reassure patients and caregivers that they are not alone. Additionally, they provide interventions that help to improve energy and reduce fatigue (Schwartz, 2007).

d) Nutritional consults with a registered dietitian will inform patients and caregivers of the best strategies to improve dietary intake. This knowledge empowers patients to take charge of this aspect of treatment for cancer-related fatigue.

References

Carroll, J., Kohli, S., Mustian, K., Roscoe, J., & Morrow, G. (2007). Pharmacologic treatment of cancer-related fatigue. *Oncologist, 12*(Suppl. 1), 43–51. Retrieved December 11, 2007, from http:// www.TheOncologist.com

Cella, D. (2006). Quality of life and clinical decisions in chemotherapy-induced anemia. *Oncology, 20*(8, Suppl. 6), 25–28.

Hanna, L., Avila, P., Meteer, J., Nicholas, D., & Kaminsky, L. (2008). The effects of a comprehensive exercise program on physical function, fatigue, and mood in patients with various types of cancer. *Oncology Nursing Forum, 35*(5), 461–469.

Lipman, A., & Lawrence, D. (2004). The management of fatigue in cancer patients. *Oncology, 18*(12), 1527–1535.

Madden, J., & Newton, S. (2006). "Why am I so tired all the time?" Understanding cancer-related fatigue. *Clinical Journal of Oncology Nursing, 10*(5), 659–661.

Mitchell, S., Beck, S., Hood, L., Moore, K., & Tanner, E. (2007). Putting Evidence Into Practice: Evidence-based interventions for fatigue during and following cancer and its treatment. *Clinical Journal of Oncology Nursing, 11*(1), 99–113.

National Comprehensive Cancer Network. (2008). *Clinical Practice Guidelines in Oncology™: Cancer-related fatigue* [v.1.2008]. Retrieved July 5, 2008, from http://www.nccn.org/professionals/ physician_gls/PDF/fatigue.pdf

Ryan, J., Carroll, J., Ryan, E., Mustian, K., Fiscella, K., & Morrow, G. (2007). Mechanisms of cancer-related fatigue. *Oncologist, 12*(Suppl. 1), 22–34. Retrieved December 11, 2007, from http:// www.TheOncologist.com

Schwartz, A. (2007). Understanding and treating cancer-related fatigue. (2007). *Oncology, 21*(Suppl. 11, Nurse Ed.), 30–34.

Stricker, C., Drake, D., Hoyer, K., & Mock, V. (2004). Evidence-based practice for fatigue management in adults with cancer: Exercise as an intervention. *Oncology Nursing Forum, 31*(5), 963–974.

Sura, W., Murphy, S., & Gonzales, I. (2006). Level of fatigue in women receiving dose-dense versus chemotherapy for breast cancer: A pilot study. *Oncology Nursing Forum, 33*(5), 1015–1021.

O. Alterations in sexuality

1. Pathophysiology

a) Female: Ovarian function is affected by chemotherapy.

(1) Altered production of female sex hormones (estrogen, progesterone, and testosterone) (Speer et al., 2005)

(2) Varying effects on sexuality (Davison, Bell, Donath, Montalto, & Davis, 2005)

(3) No association found between specific androgen levels and low sexual function (Davis, Davison, Donath, & Bell, 2005)

b) Male

(1) Testosterone is involved in

(a) Development of secondary sex characteristics

(b) Development of sperm

(c) Secretion of fluid from the prostate gland, seminal vesicles, and Cowper's glands.

(2) Prolactin is secreted by the pituitary gland.

(a) Maintains the production of testosterone

(b) At high levels, suppresses production in a negative feedback loop (Robinson & Huether, 2002)

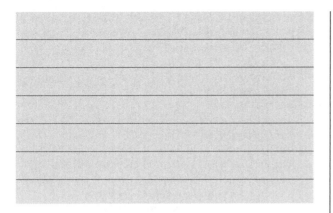

2. Incidence: Almost half of cancer survivors report ongoing problems with sexual functioning (Baker, Denniston, Smith, & West, 2005). These issues are global and reflect changes in body image, sexual self-image, and reentering life as a cancer survivor (Holland & Reznik, 2005).
   a) Females
      (1) Desire (Barni & Mondin, 1997)
         (a) 64% report no sexual desire at all.
         (b) 48% report low desire.
      (2) Dyspareunia
         (a) Painful intercourse is a common complaint caused by vaginal dryness as a result of reduced estrogen levels (Knobf, 2001).
         (b) 80% of women in one large study (n = 863) reported some change in sexual functioning up to five years after treatment (Meyerowitz, Desmond, Rowland, Wyatt, & Ganz, 1999).
      (3) Arousal and orgasm
         (a) Dysfunction is worse for women younger than 50 years old.
         (b) Women report satisfaction in their relationship in spite of ongoing sexual challenges (Ganz, Rowland, Desmond, Meyerowitz, & Wyatt, 1998).
         (c) Long-term sexual difficulties are strongly associated with vaginal dryness (Broeckel, Thors, Jacobsen, Small, & Cox, 2002).
   b) Males
      (1) Desire: 54% of men on androgen-deprivation therapy reported no desire after one year of treatment (Potosky et al., 2002).
      (2) 80%–90% of men developed erectile difficulties one or more years after starting androgen-deprivation therapy (Helgason et al., 1997).

3. Chemotherapy agents that affect sexual function: There is very little information in the literature directly related to the effects of chemotherapy on sexual functioning beyond agents that are known to target the gonads. Much of what is known comes from anecdotal evidence from qualitative studies where participants may mention alterations in sexual functioning while on chemotherapy. All of the following agents are used in various combinations; thus, the side effects may be cumulative (Lubejko & Ashley, 1998).
   a) Alkylating agents (e.g., busulfan, cyclophosphamide, ifosfamide, nitrogen mustard) cause nausea and vomiting, which significantly decreases desire.
   b) Antimetabolites (e.g., cladribine, cytarabine, hydroxyurea, methotrexate) cause general malaise, mucositis, nausea, and vomiting.
   c) Antitumor antibiotics (e.g., daunorubicin, doxorubicin, mitoxantrone) cause nausea, vomiting, and mucositis.
   d) Plant alkaloids (e.g., vincristine) cause peripheral neuropathy, which may affect sensation in the hands and fingers (Schwartz & Plawecki, 2002).
   e) Hair loss is a common side effect of chemotherapy. The loss of hair makes both men and women feel less attractive.
4. Contributing factors
   a) Endocrine manipulation: Tamoxifen
      (1) Side effects appear to be most severe in premenopausal women.
      (2) Postmenopausal women experience negative side effects of this drug to a lesser degree (Ganz et al., 1998).
      (3) Decrease in libido has been reported.
      (4) Tamoxifen produces mildly estrogenic effects on the vagina. Some women find relief from the vaginal dryness experienced as a result of chemotherapy-induced atrophy (Rogers & Kristjanson, 2002), whereas others think that the dryness has resulted from tamoxifen use (Hunter et al., 2004).
   b) Endocrine manipulation: Aromatase inhibitors cause vaginal dryness (Bentrem & Jordan, 2002).
   c) Body image changes related to ability to engage in sexually pleasurable activities: A woman's comfort with her body after treatment; the reaction of her sexual partner to her body (Wilmoth & Ross, 1997); weight gain (McInnes & Knobf, 2001)
5. Clinical manifestations

a) Females: Alterations in sexual functioning can occur at all stages of the sexual response cycle for women treated for cancer. Fatigue, weight gain, and altered sexuality occur as a cluster of symptoms, which magnifies the impact of each more than if they were viewed individually (Wilmoth, Coleman, Smith, & Davis, 2004).

(1) Dyspareunia leading to vaginismus (Barni & Mondin, 1997)

(2) Urinary tract infections after attempts at sexual intercourse (Ponzone et al., 2005); this can set up a negative feedback loop with decreased interest in sex if the result is a painful infection.

(3) Mucositis manifested as vaginal irritation or vaginitis, vulvar irritation, itching, discharge, soreness, bleeding, and odor; this usually occurs 3–5 days after chemotherapy administration and lasts for up to 10 days.

(4) Other factors contributing to decreased sexual desire

(a) Mood, fatigue, and nausea (Taylor, Basen-Engquist, Shinn, & Bodurka, 2004)

(b) Loss of hair, particularly pubic hair (Fitch, 2003)

(c) Distress at role inadequacy (Lammers, Schaefer, Ladd, & Echenberg, 2000)

(d) Fear that lack of sexual activity may cause problems in the relationship (Sun et al., 2005)

b) Males

(1) Androgen-deprivation therapy causes

(a) Absence of sexual dreams; cessation of fantasies

(b) Lack of interest in anything sexual

(c) Cessation of any sexual pleasure (Navon & Morag, 2003)

(d) Changes in body image and perception of masculinity

(e) Alterations in spousal relationships (Clark et al., 1997)

(f) Erectile dysfunction

(g) Feminization

(h) Gynecomastia (increase in volume of breast tissue) (Anderson, 2001).

(2) Treatment for testicular cancer: Up to one-third of men experience loss of libido, orgasmic and ejaculatory problems, and a subsequent decrease in sexual activity (Jonker-Pool et al., 2001). These problems appear to persist for at least the first six months after completion of treatment (Heidenreich & Hofmann, 1999). Inability to perform sexually can impact the man's confidence in himself as a sexual partner and may have psychological consequences that last for a significant period of time.

6. Collaborative management

a) Female

(1) Provision of anticipatory guidance at all stages of the disease trajectory (Rustoen & Begnum, 2000)

(a) Individual women will have unique needs for information at different points in time.

(b) A great deal of information is given at the time of diagnosis, when the woman cannot assimilate and integrate the new information (Koinberg, Holmberg, & Fridlund, 2001).

(c) Only a small proportion of women with breast cancer discussed sexual issues with their physician (Barni & Mondin, 1997).

(d) Most women have never been asked if sexual problems occurred as a result of treatment (Young-McCaughan, 1996).

(e) Some women may be reluctant to talk about intimate sexual matters with healthcare providers (Knobf, 2001).

(f) Women have reported that their physicians were not understanding or helpful when sexual dysfunction was identified as a problem (Wilmoth & Ross, 1997).

(g) Older women may be more reluctant to state their needs for information than younger women (Gray, Goel, Fitch, Franssen, & Labrecque, 2002).

(2) A modified form of sensate focus exercises can help the woman and her partner to learn a new way of dealing with the changes from treatment. Refer patients to a sexuality counselor or sex therapist for assistance.

(3) Instruct patient to prevent or manage vaginitis or vulvar irritation.

    (a) Focus on prevention, with avoidance of tight-fitting pants and pantyhose.

    (b) Wear cotton underwear.

    (c) Employ fastidious personal hygiene; use a mild soap with water for cleansing.

    (d) Avoid bubble baths, douching, and chemical irritants such as genital deodorant sprays.

    (e) Utilize cool sitz baths and warm compresses to provide local relief.

    (f) Treat concomitant bacterial infections such as *Candida albicans* or *Trichomonas vaginitis*, if present.

(4) A number of lubricants are available to help women feel more comfortable with sexual activity.

    (a) Water- and glycerin- or silicone-based lubricants are the safest to use.

    (b) Numerous lubricants are dye- and perfume-free and will be less irritating.

    (c) Instruct patients to avoid the use of oil-based products or anything that is colored, scented, or not designed specifically for sexual activity, such as hand lotion.

b) Male: A thorough assessment of prediagnostic and pretreatment sexual functioning is important to establish the man's current level of functioning.

(1) It is common for men 75 years and older who have prostate cancer to have diminished levels of sexual interest and functioning before treatment begins.

(2) Other men may have erectile difficulties before the diagnosis of cancer (Iversen, Melezinek, & Schmidt, 2001) as a result of cardiac disease, diabetes, and medications (Helgason et al., 1997).

(3) Obtaining an accurate description of pretreatment erectile functioning and sexual activity is crucial so that the patient has realistic expectations of what treatment can do.

(4) Treatment of erectile dysfunction includes oral therapies (phosphodiesterase-5 [PDE5] inhibitors), vacuum devices, intraurethral pellets (MUSE®), intracorporeal injections (Caverject®), and penile implants. Each has benefits and disadvantages. All require a prescription, extensive patient education, and varied degrees of motivation on the part of both the man and his partner. Men who used erectile aids after surgery (penile implants, PDE5 inhibitors such as sildenafil, tadalafil, or vardenafil, or vacuum devices) reported greater satisfaction with their sex lives than those who did not use any aids (Perez et al., 1997).

7. Patient/couple education: A number of models are helpful in communicating with patients about sexuality. The most frequently used model is the PLISSIT model (Annon, 1974). A more recent model specifically designed for the oncology population is the BETTER model (Mick, Hughes, & Cohen, 2003).

a) PLISSIT

(1) The first level in this model involves giving the patient or client *permission* to talk about sexual issues.

(2) The second level, *limited information*, refers to factual information given to the patient in response to a question or observation.

(3) The third level involves making a *specific suggestion* to the client or patient.

(4) The fourth level refers to *intensive therapy* needed for severe or more long-standing sexual problems.

b) BETTER

(1) The first level of intervention involves *bringing up* the topic.

(2) The second level involves *explaining* that sexuality is part of QOL, and patients should be aware that they can talk about this with the nurse.

(3) Care providers should then *tell* the patient that appropriate resources will be found to address their concerns.

(4) While the *timing* may not be appropriate now, they can ask for information at any time.

(5) Patients should be *educated* about the sexual side effects of their treatment.

(6) Finally, a *record* should be made in the patient's medical record to report that this topic has been discussed.

c) Sexual intercourse is not always the end goal of sexual touch. Patients and their partners should be encouraged to find other ways of sexual pleasuring that are not fatigue- or nausea-provoking for patients and that satisfy both individuals' needs and desires for intimate touch.

d) Encourage patients to avoid intercourse when neutrophil and platelet counts are low (Camp-Sorrell, 2005). Recommend use of condoms to prevent transmission of infection and exposure of the partner to chemotherapeutic agents in the body fluids of the patient. Caution should be used in the type of condom chosen, as those that are lubricated usually contain nonoxynol-9, which can be irritating to vaginal tissue.

References

Anderson, J. (2001). Quality of life aspects of treatment options for localized and locally advanced prostate cancer. *European Urology, 40*(Suppl. 2), 24–30.

Annon, J. (1974). *The behavioral treatment of sexual problems.* Honolulu, HI: Enabling Systems.

Baker, F., Denniston, M., Smith, T., & West, M.M. (2005). Adult cancer survivors: How are they faring? *Cancer, 104*(Suppl. 11), 2565–2576.

Barni, S., & Mondin, R. (1997). Sexual dysfunction in treated breast cancer patients. *Annals of Oncology, 8*(2), 149–153.

Bentrem, D., & Jordan, C. (2002). Role of antiestrogens and aromatase inhibitors in breast cancer treatment. *Current Opinion in Obstetrics and Gynecology, 14*(1), 5–12.

Broeckel, J.A., Thors, C.L., Jacobsen, P.B., Small, M., & Cox, C.E. (2002). Sexual functioning in long-term breast cancer survivors treated with adjuvant chemotherapy. *Breast Cancer Research and Treatment, 75*(3), 241–248.

Camp-Sorrell, D. (2005). Chemotherapy: Toxicity management. In C.H. Yarbro, M.H. Frogge, & M. Goodman (Eds.), *Cancer nursing: Principles and practice* (6th ed., pp. 412–457). Sudbury, MA: Jones and Bartlett.

Clark, J., Wray, N., Brody, B., Ashton, C., Giesler, B., & Watkins, H. (1997). Dimensions of quality of life expressed by men treated for metastatic prostate cancer. *Social Science and Medicine, 45*(8), 1299–1309.

Davis, S., Davison, S., Donath, S., & Bell, R. (2005). Circulating androgen levels and self-reported sexual function in women. *JAMA, 294*(1), 91–96.

Davison, S., Bell, R., Donath, S., Montalto, J., & Davis, S. (2005). Androgen levels in adult females: Changes with age, menopause, and oophorectomy. *Journal of Clinical Endocrinology and Metabolism, 90*(7), 3847–3853.

Fitch, M.I. (2003). Psychosocial management of patients with recurrent ovarian cancer: Treating the whole patient to improve quality of life. *Seminars in Oncology Nursing, 19*(3, Suppl. 1), 40–53.

Ganz, P.A., Rowland, J.H., Desmond, K., Meyerowitz, B.E., & Wyatt, G.E. (1998). Life after breast cancer: Understanding women's health-related quality of life and sexual functioning. *Journal of Clinical Oncology, 16*(2), 501–514.

Gray, R., Goel, V., Fitch, M., Franssen, E., & Labrecque, M. (2002). Supportive care provided by physicians and nurses to women with breast cancer. *Supportive Care in Cancer, 10*(8), 647–652.

Heidenreich, A., & Hofmann, R. (1999). Quality-of-life issues in the treatment of testicular cancer. *World Journal of Urology, 17*(4), 230–238.

Helgason, A.R., Adolfsson, J., Dickman, P., Arver, S., Fredrikson, M., & Steineck, G. (1997). Factors associated with waning sexual function among elderly men and prostate cancer patients. *Journal of Urology, 158*(1), 155–159.

Holland, J., & Reznik, I. (2005). Pathways for psychosocial care of cancer survivors. *Cancer, 104*(Suppl. 11), 2624–2637.

Hunter, M., Grunfeld, E., Mittal, S., Sikka, P., Ramirez, A., Fentiman, I., et al. (2004). Menopausal symptoms in women with breast cancer: Prevalence and treatment preferences. *Psycho-Oncology, 13*(11), 769–778.

Iversen, P., Melezinek, I., & Schmidt, A. (2001). Nonsteroidal antiandrogens: A therapeutic option for patients with advanced prostate cancer who wish to retain sexual interest and function. *BJU International, 87*(1), 47–56.

Jonker-Pool, G., van de Wiel, H.B., Hoekstra, H.J., Sleijfer, D.T., Van Driel, M.F., Van Basten, J.P., et al. (2001). Sexual functioning after treatment for testicular cancer—Review and meta-analysis of 36 empirical studies between 1975–2000. *Archives of Sexual Behavior, 30*(1), 55–74.

Knobf, M.T. (2001). The menopausal symptom experience in young mid-life women with breast cancer. *Cancer Nursing, 24*(3), 201–210.

Koinberg, I., Holmberg, L., & Fridlund, B. (2001). Satisfaction with routine follow-up visits to the physician. *Acta Oncologica, 40*(4), 454–459.

Lammers, S.E., Schaefer, K.M., Ladd, E.C., & Echenberg, R. (2000). Caring for women living with ovarian cancer: Recommendations for advanced practice nurses. *Journal of Obstetric, Gynecologic, and Neonatal Nursing, 29*(6), 567–573.

Lubejko, B., & Ashley, B. (1998). Chemotherapy. In C. Ziegfeld, B. Lubejko, & B. Shelton (Eds.), *Manual of cancer care* (pp. 30–47). Philadelphia: Lippincott.

McInnes, J.A., & Knobf, M.T. (2001). Weight gain and quality of life in women treated with adjuvant chemotherapy for early-stage breast cancer. *Oncology Nursing Forum, 28*(4), 675–684.

Meyerowitz, B.E., Desmond, K.A., Rowland, J.H., Wyatt, G.E., & Ganz, P.A. (1999). Sexuality following breast cancer. *Journal of Sex and Marital Therapy, 25*(3), 237–250.

Mick, J., Hughes, M., & Cohen, M. (2003). Sexuality and cancer: How oncology nurses can address it BETTER. *Oncology Nursing Forum, 30*(Suppl. 2), 152–153.

Navon, L., & Morag, A. (2003). Advanced prostate cancer patients' relationships with their spouses following hormonal therapy. *European Journal of Oncology Nursing, 7*(2), 73–80.

Perez, M.A., Meyerowitz, B.E., Lieskovsky, G., Skinner, D.G., Reynolds, B., & Skinner, E.C. (1997). Quality of life and sexuality following radical prostatectomy in patients with prostate cancer who use or do not use erectile aids. *Urology, 50*(5), 740–746.

Ponzone, R., Biglia, N., Jacomuzzi, M.E., Maggiorotto, F., Mariani, L., & Sismondi, P. (2005). Vaginal oestrogen therapy after breast cancer: Is it safe? *European Journal of Cancer, 41*(17), 2673–2681.

Potosky, A.L., Reeve, B.B., Clegg, L.X., Hoffman, R.M., Stephenson, R.A., Albertsen, P.C., et al. (2002). Quality of life following localized prostate cancer treated initially with androgen deprivation therapy or no therapy. *Journal of the National Cancer Institute, 94*(6), 430–437.

Robinson, K., & Huether, S. (2002). Structure and function of the reproductive systems. In K. McCance & S. Huether (Eds.), *Pathophysiology: The biologic basis for disease in adults and children* (4th ed., pp. 670–704). Philadelphia: Mosby.

Rogers, M., & Kristjanson, L.J. (2002). The impact on sexual functioning of chemotherapy-induced menopause in women with breast cancer. *Cancer Nursing, 25*(1), 57–65.

Rustoen, T., & Begnum, S. (2000). Quality of life in women with breast cancer. *Cancer Nursing, 23*(6), 416–421.

Schwartz, S., & Plawecki, H.M. (2002). Consequences of chemotherapy on the sexuality of patients with lung cancer. *Clinical Journal of Oncology Nursing, 6*(4), 212–216.

Speer, J.J., Hillenberg, B., Sugrue, D.P., Blacker, C., Kresge, C.L., Decker, V.B., et al. (2005). Study of sexual functioning determinants in breast cancer survivors. *Breast Journal, 11*(6), 440–447.

Sun, C.C., Bodurka, D.C., Weaver, C.B., Rasu, R., Wolf, J.K., Bevers, M.W., et al. (2005). Rankings and symptom assessments of side effects from chemotherapy: Insights from experienced patients with ovarian cancer. *Supportive Care in Cancer, 13*(4), 219–227.

Taylor, C.L., Basen-Engquist, K., Shinn, E.H., & Bodurka, D.C. (2004). Predictors of sexual functioning in ovarian cancer patients. *Journal of Clinical Oncology, 22*(5), 881–889.

Wilmoth, M.C., Coleman, E.A., Smith, S.C., & Davis, C. (2004). Fatigue, weight gain, and altered sexuality in patients with breast cancer: Exploration of a symptom cluster. *Oncology Nursing Forum, 31*(6), 1069–1075.

Wilmoth, M.C., & Ross, J.A. (1997). Women's perception. Breast cancer treatment and sexuality. *Cancer Practice, 5*(6), 353–359.

Young-McCaughan, S. (1996). Sexual functioning in women with breast cancer after treatment with adjuvant therapy. *Cancer Nursing, 19*(4), 308–319.

P. Reproductive alterations
   1. Pathophysiology
      a) Female
         (1) Chemotherapy results in
             (a) Damage to ovarian follicles
             (b) Decreased ovarian volume
             (c) Ovarian fibrosis.
         (2) Manifested as
             (a) Amenorrhea (permanent or reversible)
             (b) Menopausal symptoms
             (c) Eventual bone loss
         (3) Related to
             (a) Age
             (b) Dosage and duration of treatment (Knobf, 2006)
      b) Male: Chemotherapy results in
         (1) Primary or secondary hormonal changes from damage to the hypothalamic-pituitary axis
         (2) Damage to germinal stem cells in the testes (Maltaris et al., 2006).
   2. Incidence
      a) Female
         (1) Women older than age 30: Risk of permanent amenorrhea increases.
         (2) Breast cancer: 15% of premenopausal women treated with an alkylating agent developed long-term amenorrhea (Fornier, Modi, Panageas, Norton, & Hudis, 2005).
         (3) Childhood cancer survivors: < 20% will develop premature ovarian failure (Larsen, Muller, Schmiegelow, Rechnitzer, & Andersen, 2006).
      b) Male: Testicular cancer
         (1) 75% have decreased sperm production at the time of diagnosis (Spermon et al., 2003).
         (2) 70% who have retroperitoneal lymph node dissection will be unable to ejaculate and will notice a decrease in semen volume or experience a "dry ejaculate" (Arai, Kawakita, Okada, & Yoshida, 1997).
   3. Agents
      a) Alkylating agents (e.g., cyclophosphamide, cisplatin, chlorambucil, melphalan, busulfan, nitrogen mustard, dacarbazine, ifosfamide, procarbazine) (Marhhom & Cohen, 2006) have the greatest effect on both female and male fertility (Maltaris et al., 2006).
      b) Nitrosoureas (e.g., carmustine, lomustine) affect the ovaries (Blatt, 1999).
      c) Anthracycline antibiotics affect fertility.
      d) Vinca alkaloids affect fertility (Maltaris et al., 2007).
      e) Taxanes increase the risk of chemotherapy-induced amenorrhea (Tham et al., 2007).
   4. Contributing factors
      a) Age
         (1) Older women are more likely to experience complete ovarian failure and permanent infertility (Maltaris et al., 2007).

(2) The adult testis is more susceptible than the testis of the prepubescent boy (Tomao, Miele, Spinelli, & Tomao, 2006).

b) Combination therapy: The addition of radiation to the treatment regimen significantly increases the risk of permanent infertility (Davis, 2006b).

c) Preexisting disease
(1) Men with cancer commonly have reduced fertility before diagnosis and treatment.
(2) This reduced fertility is thought to be a result of anatomic or endocrine changes (Maltaris et al., 2006).

d) Treatment effect: Lymph node or tumor resection results in retrograde ejaculation, which affects fertility (Spermon et al., 2003).

5. Clinical manifestations
a) Female
(1) Amenorrhea (permanent or temporary)
(2) Signs of premature menopause in younger women: These may be more severe than in naturally menopausal women.
(a) Hot flashes
(b) Urogenital atrophy
(c) Osteoporosis (late-stage symptom)
(3) Psychosocial distress: 57% of young women in one study identified significant concerns about infertility (Partridge et al., 2004).

b) Male: Alterations in spermatogenesis
(1) Low sperm counts
(2) Poor sperm motility
(3) Altered morphology (Maltaris et al., 2006)

6. Collaborative management
a) Female
(1) Cryopreservation of embryos
(a) Most effective intervention in terms of successful pregnancies
(b) May result in a delay of two to six weeks in starting chemotherapy (Oktay, 2005)
(c) Requires ovarian stimulation; may be contraindicated with estrogen-sensitive cancers (Marhhom et al., 2006)
(d) Tamoxifen and letrozole may be used to stimulate ovaries with estrogen-sensitive tumors (Marhhom et al., 2006). Tamoxifen cannot be used for women with endometrial cancer (Marhhom et al.).

(2) Oocyte cryopreservation (surgical)
(a) Regarded as experimental
(b) May be offered to single women with no male partner
(c) Pregnancy rates are low (Marhhom et al., 2006).

(3) Cryopreservation of ovarian tissue (surgical)
(a) New experimental technique that may offer some hope to women who do not have the time for ovarian stimulation
(b) Concerns about introducing malignant cells when the preserved ovarian tissue is transplanted back into the woman

(4) Nonsurgical: Monthly injections of gonadotropin analogs (e.g., leuprolide) to reduce the rate of ovarian follicle atresia (Davis, 2006a)

(5) The return of menstrual periods does not necessarily indicate good ovarian function, and in turn, lack of menstruation does not mean that ovarian function has ceased (Del Mastro, Catzeddu, & Venturini, 2006).

b) Male
(1) Cryopreservation: Sperm cryopreservation before treatment is highly effective, as sperm remain viable after freezing and can be used to fertilize ovum (Spermon et al., 2003).
(2) New reproductive technologies may be useful in causing pregnancy.
(a) Testicular sperm extraction
(b) In vitro fertilization
(c) Intracytoplasmic sperm injection (Krumm & Lamberti, 1993)

7. Chemotherapy-induced menopause
a) Symptoms of chemically induced menopause are dramatic.

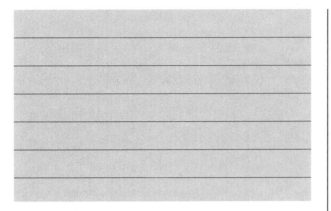

(1) Menstrual cycle changes, with eventual cessation
(2) Hot flashes, insomnia
(3) Vaginal dryness
(4) Dyspareunia
(5) Weight gain (Deniz, Liebens, Carly, Pastijn, & Rozenberg, 2007)

b) Severity
(1) Symptoms may be worse for women who are premenopausal when diagnosed (Rogers & Kristjanson, 2002).
(2) Postmenopausal women also suffer severe symptoms (Crandall, Petersen, Ganz, & Greendale, 2004).

c) Treatment: Women experiencing chemotherapy-induced menopause benefit from a coordinated, multidisciplinary approach to managing symptoms.
(1) Hormonal: There is no consensus on the safety of hormone therapy for women with breast cancer, especially if it is estrogen receptor–positive (Hickey, Saunders, & Stuckey, 2005, 2007; Ponzone et al., 2005). Those with hormone-dependent cancer should make a decision based on a consultation with an oncologist (North American Menopause Society, 2007).
(a) Local estrogen therapy for vaginal atrophy
    i) Vaginal dryness can be significantly reduced with the use of vaginal estrogen creams, pessaries, or rings.
    ii) Systemic absorption is minimal (Ponzone et al., 2005).
(b) Systemic therapy: Three to five years of hormone replacement therapy may be considered if menopausal symptoms are refractory to other treatments (Xydakis, Sakkas, & Mastorakos, 2006).

(2) Nonhormonal
(a) Clonidine (an antihypertensive) and gabapentin (an anticonvulsant) may reduce the severity and frequency of hot flashes (Molina, Barton, & Loprinzi, 2005).
(b) Selective serotonin reuptake inhibitors (SSRIs)
    i) These agents have been effective in reducing the frequency and severity of hot flashes (Hickey et al., 2007).
    ii) Venlafaxine and paroxetine have been suggested as the most effective nonhormonal treatments for women with breast cancer (Bordeleau, Pritchard, Goodwin, & Loprinzi, 2007).
    iii) Safety of SSRIs in women with cancer is not yet established (Antoine, Liebens, Carly, Pastijn, & Rozenberg, 2007). Recent evidence suggests that these drugs may decrease the effectiveness of tamoxifen.
(c) Vitamin E may be effective in reducing hot flashes (Hickey et al., 2007).
(d) Vaginal moisturizers such as Replens® may help women experiencing vaginal dryness (Davis, Zinkand, & Fitch, 2000).

(3) Complementary therapies
(a) Phytoestrogens: Long-term effectiveness has not been established (Hickey et al., 2007).
(b) Acupuncture may reduce the severity but not the frequency of hot flashes (Nir, Huang, Schnyer, Chen, & Manber, 2007).
(c) Relaxation exercises are also effective in reducing hot flashes (Zaborowska et al., 2007).

8. Patient/family education: Decisions about treatments that affect fertility have to be made when the patient is trying to cope with the diagnosis of cancer; priorities may change over time. It is important to educate patients honestly and directly, as they may assume that modern reproductive technologies will result in a future pregnancy.
a) Parents of a child with cancer may have to make decisions about treatment for their child and may not be capable of discussing sperm banking or ovary preservation with their child or healthcare providers, as their priority is to save the life of their child.

b) Because of the average young age of those affected with testicular cancer, many will not be in a relationship at the time of diagnosis, and thoughts of parenthood may be remote and not a priority.

(1) Men who are young, unmarried, and childless experience more infertility-related distress than those who have fathered children and are in a supportive relationship. This needs to be taken into consideration when informing patients of the consequences of treatment.

(2) Sperm samples can be collected with 24–48 hours between collections (Brown, 2003), which allows for minimal delay of chemotherapy treatment.

(3) However, men should be counseled honestly and directly that cryopreservation does not guarantee success despite advances in technique (Schmidt et al., 2004).

c) Women rate a discussion about fertility as more important than a discussion about menopausal information (Thewes et al., 2005).

(1) Many do not recall being told about alterations to reproductive health (Duffy, Allen, & Clark, 2005).

(2) Little is known about the efficacy and safety of in vitro fertilization (IVF) in women who have been treated for cancer (Maltaris et al., 2006); however, many women assume that IVF will be successful at a later date.

References

Antoine, C., Liebens, F., Carly, B., Pastijn, A., & Rozenberg, S. (2007). Safety of alternative treatments for menopausal symptoms after breast cancer: A qualitative systematic review. *Climacteric, 10*(1), 23–26.

Arai, Y., Kawakita, M., Okada, Y., & Yoshida, O. (1997). Sexuality and fertility in long-term survivors of testicular cancer. *Journal of Clinical Oncology, 15*(4), 1444–1448.

Blatt, J. (1999). Pregnancy outcome in long-term survivors of childhood cancer. *Medical and Pediatric Oncology, 33*(1), 29–33.

Bordeleau, L., Pritchard, K., Goodwin, P., & Loprinzi, C. (2007). Therapeutic option for the management of hot flashes in breast cancer survivors: An evidence-based review. *Clinical Therapy, 29*(2), 230–241.

Brown, C.G. (2003). Testicular cancer: An overview. *Medsurg Nursing, 12*(1), 37–43.

Crandall, C., Petersen, L., Ganz, P.A., & Greendale, G.A. (2004). Association of breast cancer and its therapy with menopause-related symptoms. *Menopause, 11*(5), 519–530.

Davis, C., Zinkand, J., & Fitch, M. (2000). Cancer treatment-induced menopause: Meaning for breast and gynecological cancer survivors. *Canadian Oncology Nursing Journal, 10*(1), 14–21.

Davis, M. (2006a). Fertility considerations for female adolescent and young adult patients following cancer therapy: A guide for counseling patients and their families. *Clinical Journal of Oncology Nursing, 10*(2), 213–219.

Davis, V. (2006b). Female gamete preservation. *Cancer, 107*(Suppl. 7), 1690–1694.

Del Mastro, L., Catzeddu, T., & Venturini, M. (2006). Infertility and pregnancy after breast cancer: Current knowledge and future perspectives. *Cancer Treatment Reviews, 32*(6), 417–422.

Deniz, G., Liebens, A., Carly, B., Pastijn, A., & Rozenberg, S. (2007). Treatment of premature menopause in breast cancer patients. *Acta Chirurgica Hungarica, 107*(3), 263–266.

Duffy, C., Allen, S., & Clark, M. (2005). Discussions regarding reproductive health for young women with breast cancer undergoing chemotherapy. *Journal of Clinical Oncology, 23*(4), 766–773.

Fornier, M., Modi, S., Panageas, K., Norton, L., & Hudis, C.A. (2005). Incidence of chemotherapy-induced, long-term amenorrhea in patients with breast carcinoma age 40 years and younger after adjuvant anthracycline and taxane. *Cancer, 104*(8), 1575–1579.

Hickey, M., Saunders, C.M., & Stuckey, B.G. (2005). Management of menopausal symptoms in patients with breast cancer: An evidence-based approach. *Lancet Oncology, 6*(9), 687–695.

Hickey, M., Saunders, C.M., & Stuckey, B.G. (2007). Non-hormonal treatments for menopausal symptoms. *Maturitas, 57*(1), 85–89.

Knobf, M.T. (2006). Reproductive and hormonal sequelae of chemotherapy in women. *American Journal of Nursing, 106*(Suppl. 3), 60–65.

Krumm, S., & Lamberti, J. (1993). Changes in sexual behavior following radiation therapy for cervical cancer. *Journal of Psychosomatic Obstetrics and Gynaecology, 14*(1), 51–63.

Larsen, E., Muller, J., Schmiegelow, K., Rechnitzer, C., & Andersen, A. (2006). Reduced ovarian function in long-term survivors of radiation- and chemotherapy-treated childhood cancer. *Journal of Clinical Endocrinology and Metabolism, 88*(11), 5307–5314.

Maltaris, T., Koelbl, H., Seufert, R., Kiesewetter, F., Beckmann, M., Mueller, A., et al. (2006). Gonadal damage and options for fertility preservation in female and male cancer survivors. *Asian Journal of Andrology, 8*(5), 515–533.

Maltaris, T., Seufert, R., Fischl, F., Schaffrath, M., Pollow, K., Koelbl, H., et al. (2007). The effect of cancer treatment on female fertility and strategies for preserving fertility. *European Journal of Obstetrics, Gynecology, and Reproductive Biology, 130*(2), 148–155.

Marhhom, E., & Cohen, I. (2006). Fertility preservation options for women with malignancies. *Obstetrical and Gynecological Survey, 62*(1), 58–72.

Molina, J.R., Barton, D.L., & Loprinzi, C.L. (2005). Chemotherapy-induced ovarian failure: Manifestations and management. *Drug Safety, 28*(5), 401–416.

Nir, Y., Huang, M., Schnyer, R., Chen, B., & Manber, R. (2007). Acupuncture for postmenopausal hot flushes. *Maturitas, 56*(4), 383–395.

North American Menopause Society. (2007). The role of local vaginal estrogen for treatment of vaginal atrophy in post-menopausal women: 2007 position statement of The North American Menopause Society. *Menopause, 14*(3), 357–369.

Oktay, K. (2005). Fertility preservation: An emerging discipline in the care of young patients with cancer. *Lancet Oncology, 6*(4), 192–193.

Partridge, A., Gelber, S., Peppercorn, J., Sampson, E., Knudsen, K., Laufer, M., et al. (2004). Web-based survey of fertility issues in young women with breast cancer. *Journal of Clinical Oncology, 22*(20), 4174–4183.

Ponzone, R., Biglia, N., Jacomuzzi, M.E., Maggiorotto, F., Mariani, L., & Sismondi, P. (2005). Vaginal oestrogen therapy after breast cancer: Is it safe? *European Journal of Cancer, 41*(17), 2673–2681.

Rogers, M., & Kristjanson, L.J. (2002). The impact on sexual functioning of chemotherapy-induced menopause in women with breast cancer. *Cancer Nursing, 25*(1), 57–65.

Schmidt, K., Larsen, E., Bangsboll, S., Meinertz, H., Carlsen, E., & Andersen, A. (2004). Assisted reproduction in male cancer survivors: Fertility treatment and outcome in 67 couples. *Human Reproduction, 19*(12), 2806–2810.

Spermon, J.R., Kiemeney, L.A., Meuleman, E.J., Ramos, L., Wetzels, A.M., & Witjes, J.A. (2003). Fertility in men with testicular germ cell tumors. *Fertility and Sterility, 79*(Suppl. 3), 1543–1549.

Tham, Y., Sexton, K., Weiss, H., Elledge, R., Friedman, L., & Kramer, R. (2007). The rates of chemotherapy-induced amenorrhea in pa-tients treated with adjuvant doxorubicin and cyclophosphamide followed by a taxane. *American Journal of Clinical Oncology, 30*(2), 126–132.

Thewes, B., Meiser, B., Taylor, A., Phillips, K.A., Pendlebury, S., Capp, A., et al. (2005). Fertility- and menopause-related information needs of younger women with a diagnosis of early breast cancer. *Journal of Clinical Oncology, 23*(22), 5155–5165.

Tomao, F., Miele, E., Spinelli, G., & Tomao, S. (2006). Anticancer treatment and fertility effects. Literature review. *Journal of Experimental and Clinical Cancer Research, 25*(4), 475–481.

Xydakis, A., Sakkas, E., & Mastorakos, G. (2006, December). Hormone replacement therapy in breast cancer survivors. *Annals of the New York Academy of Sciences, 1092,* 349–360.

Zaborowska, E., Brynhildsen, J., Damberg, S., Fredriksson, M., Lindh-Astrand, L., Nedstrand, E., et al. (2007). Effects of acupuncture, applied relaxation, estrogens and placebo on hot flushes in post menopausal women: An analysis of two prospective, parallel, randomized studies. *Climacteric, 10*(1), 38–45.

VIII. Post-Treatment Care

Over the past 30 years, the number of cancer survivors has increased from 3 million persons to 10 million persons, including 270,000 childhood cancer survivors (American Cancer Society, 2008; Dickerman, 2007; Oeffinger & McCabe, 2006). Early diagnosis and advances in cancer treatment have increased the five-year relative survival rate for all cancers from 50% in the 1970s to 66% during 1996–2003 (American Cancer Society). Childhood cancers are now routinely cured; 80% of children and adolescents survive a cancer diagnosis (American Cancer Society; Dickerman). However, long-term cancer survivors are at risk for adverse effects from their life-saving treatment. Recent research suggests that more than 60% of survivors of childhood cancers have one or more treatment- or disease-related long-term effect(s) (Oeffinger et al., 2006). Less is known about the special health needs and long-term effects of cancer treatment for survivors of adult cancers. As more than 60% of cancer survivors are older than age 60, research efforts are under way to better understand the long-term effects of cancer treatment for adult cancers (Hewitt, Greenfield, & Stovall, 2005). Nurses have an important role in the continuing care of survivors, including monitoring, assessing, and treating children and adult survivors for the effects of treatment that emerge long after the completion of therapy. Nurses are vital in teaching survivors about leading a healthy lifestyle, thus minimizing the potential effects of cancer treatment.

A. General principles
1. Cancer survivors require follow-up care annually for life (American Cancer Society, 2008; COG, 2006; Hewitt et al., 2005; Oeffinger & McCabe, 2006). Early follow-up care may be more frequent and emphasizes surveillance and detection of disease recurrence. Long-term follow-up care transitions to a focus on identifying and anticipating chronic or late effects of the disease or treatment as well as surveillance for disease recurrence. A comprehensive treatment plan includes patient education, health promotion, and interventions to minimize or treat long-term effects (Aslett, Levitt, Richardson, & Gibson, 2007).
2. Essential components of survivorship care (Hewitt et al., 2005)
   a) Prevention of recurrent and new cancers and of other late effects
   b) Surveillance for cancer recurrence, metastasis, or second cancers
   c) Assessment of medical and psychosocial late effects
   d) Intervention for consequences of cancer and its treatment, including medical problems such as lymphedema and sexual dysfunction; symptoms including pain and fatigue; psychosocial distress experienced by cancer survivors and their caregivers; and concerns related to employment, insurance, and disability
   e) Coordination between specialists and primary care providers to ensure that all of the survivor's health needs are met
3. Information about "late effects" is an emerging body of knowledge that is expanding as the number of survivors and duration of survival increase. Surveys of cancer survivors overwhelmingly indicate the need for quality health information, as there is a perceived disparity between what they feel they have been told and what they would like to be told about their disease and its sequelae (Aslett et al., 2007).
4. Chronic or late effects may be exacerbated by numerous factors.
   a) Type of chemotherapy
   b) Duration of treatment
   c) Dose
      (1) Increasing cumulative dose and duration of therapy increases the risk of alkylating agent–induced leukemia (van Leeuwen & Travis, 2001).
      (2) An increase in the cumulative dose of an alkylating agent is associated with an increased risk of multiple health conditions (Oeffinger et al., 2006).
   d) Radiation: An increase in the cumulative dose of an alkylating agent in combination with any type of irradiation is associated with an increased relative risk (Oeffinger et al., 2006).
   e) Age
      (1) Developing organs in younger patients may be especially vulnerable to the effects of medication and radiation. Older patients who experience adverse effects from their disease or its treatment may be unable to compensate for lost function.
      (2) Childhood cancer survivors who received the diagnosis at an older age were significantly more likely to have one or more chronic health conditions as a sequela of their disease or its treatment (Oeffinger et al., 2006).
      (3) The cumulative incidence of a chronic health condition in childhood cancer survivors is more than 70% within 30 years of the cancer diagnosis, and more than 40% of these conditions will be severe, disabling, or fatal (Oeffinger et al., 2006).

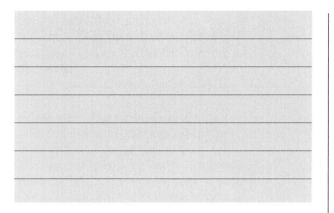

f) Gender: Female childhood cancer survivors were more likely than male survivors to have one or more chronic health conditions (Oeffinger et al., 2006).

g) Exposure to one of five specific combinations is associated with a risk of having a severe health condition that is at least 10 times the expected risk (Oeffinger et al., 2006).

   (1) Chest irradiation plus bleomycin

   (2) Chest irradiation plus an anthracycline

   (3) Chest irradiation plus abdominal or pelvic irradiation

   (4) Anthracycline plus an alkylating agent

   (5) Abdominal or pelvic irradiation plus an alkylating agent

5. Early recognition of problems and appropriate interventions may minimize long-term problems (Aziz & Rowland, 2003).

B. Types of effects
  1. Nonmalignant physical effects: See Table 36.
    a) Cardiac: Cardiomyopathy, subclinical left ventricular dysfunction, valvular disease, pericardial disease, and arrhythmias

      (1) The risk of developing anthracycline-associated cardiotoxicity increases with the total cumulative dose of doxorubicin: 1%–5% up to 550 mg/m^2; 30% at 600 mg/m^2; and 50% at ≥ 1g/m^2 (Carver et al., 2007).

      (2) Approximately 60% of children treated for childhood cancers receive an anthracycline; subsequently, there is a 0%–16% risk of heart failure and 0%–57% risk of subclinical cardiomyopathy (Dickerman, 2007).

      (3) Cardiac toxicity may have a latency period of 25 years, and the risk increases with time (Carver et al., 2007).

      (4) Cisplatin is associated with an increased risk of cardiovascular risk factors such as obesity, lipid abnormalities (decreased low high-density lipoprotein and elevated low-density lipoprotein), and hypertension (Carver et al., 2007).

    b) Pulmonary: Pulmonary fibrosis, restrictive-obstructive lung disease, and delayed interstitial pneumonia

    c) Renal: Nephropathy

    d) Musculoskeletal: Osteopenia, osteoporosis, avascular necrosis

    e) Endocrine: Hypothyroidism, growth hormone deficiency, gonadal failure. Hypothyroidism was seen in 25%–50% of Hodgkin disease survivors at 25 years (Dickerman, 2007).

    f) CNS: Cognitive deficits, neuropathy, leukoencephalopathy, cataracts, sensorineural, high-frequency hearing loss

  2. Psychosocial (COG, 2006)
    a) Psychosocial disorders: Social withdrawal, educational problems

    b) Mental health disorders: Depression, anxiety, post-traumatic stress

    c) Political and vocational issues: Employment, access to health care and insurance and educational assistance

C. Secondary malignancies (see Table 37)
  1. Definition: A secondary malignancy is a new cancer that is distinct from the original malignancy and does not represent metastatic disease from the primary tumor (Allan & Travis, 2005).

  2. Two major types of secondary malignancies
    a) Treatment-related AML/MDS generally presenting within five years of chemotherapy with alkylating agents or topoisomerase inhibitors. Two types of treatment-related leukemia (van Leeuwen & Travis, 2001)

      (1) "Classic" alkylating agent–induced AML

        (a) Risk begins 1–2 years after therapy, peaks at 5–10 years, then begins to decline.

        (b) More than half present as MDS, which typically progresses to AML within a year.

        (c) Development is associated with chromosome 5 and 7 aberrations.

      (2) Topoisomerase II inhibitor–induced acute leukemia

        (a) Risk begins shortly after therapy and peaks at two to three years.

Table 36. Late Effects Associated With Cancer Treatments

Organ System	Risk Factors	Potential Late Effects	Evaluation/Interventions
CNS—cognitive	Cytarabine (high-dose, IV or IT) MTX (high-dose, IV or IT) Cranial irradiation TBI CNS leukemia/lymphoma Relapsed leukemia/lymphoma treated with CNS-directed therapy Combination therapy with more than one neurotoxic IV or IT chemotherapy or with radiation involving the CNS Highest risk: • Age < 3 years old • Female • Premorbid or family history of learning or cognitive deficits • Radiation dose ≥ 24 Gy • Single-fraction TBI (10 Gy)	Neurocognitive dysfunction: • Executive function deficit (planning and organization) • Attention deficit • Impaired memory • Impaired processing speed • Impaired visual-motor integration • Learning deficits • Diminished IQ • Behavioral changes • Clinical leukoencephalopathy • Spasticity • Ataxia • Dysarthria • Dysphagia • Hemiparesis • Seizures • Progressive dementia	Assess cognitive, motor, and sensory neurologic function annually. Assess educational and/or vocational progress annually. Perform comprehensive neurologic examination annually. Obtain MRI of brain as indicated. Refer for formal neuropsychological evaluation at baseline and as clinically indicated. Refer patients with neurocognitive deficits to school liaison (psychologist, social worker, or school counselor) for educational assistance. Refer for vocational assistance as indicated. Refer to or consult with neurologist as indicated.
CNS—peripheral neuropathy	Vincristine Vinblastine Cisplatin Carboplatin Taxanes Highest risk: Cisplatin ≥ 300 mg/m^2	Peripheral neuropathy: • Tingling and numbness • Foot drop • Paresthesias • Areflexia • Weakness • Raynaud phenomenon	Assess for peripheral neuropathy or vasospasms of hands, feet, nose, lips, cheeks, or earlobes related to stress or cold temperatures. Perform neurologic examination annually. Treat neuropathic pain as appropriate. Encourage patients to protect the affected area from exposure to extreme temperature. Consider vasodilating medications for patients with severe, frequent vasospasm. Arrange for physical/occupational therapy as indicated. Provide a referral to pain team (for neuropathic pain management).
Ophthalmology	Busulfan Steroids Cranial, orbital, or eye radiation TBI	Cataracts Keratoconjunctivitis Retinopathy	Assess for visual changes annually. Recommend an annual ophthalmoscopic examination. Consult ophthalmologist as indicated.

(Continued on next page)

Table 36. Late Effects Associated With Cancer Treatments *(Continued)*

Organ System	Risk Factors	Potential Late Effects	Evaluation/Interventions
Ears/hearing	Carboplatin (in myeloablative doses) Cisplatin Highest risk: • CNS malignancy • Age < 4 years old • Combined with cranial/ear irradiation or ototoxic medications • Cisplatin ≥ 360 mg/m² • High-dose cisplatin (e.g., 40 mg/m² per day for 5 days per course) • Cisplatin administered after cranial/ear irradiation • Ear irradiation ≥ 30 Gy • Carboplatin conditioning for HCT	Sensorineural high-frequency hearing loss Tinnitus Vertigo	Assess for hearing difficulties, tinnitus, and vertigo annually. Perform otoscopic examination annually. Perform baseline audiogram, then annually if hearing loss is detected or as clinically indicated. If patient received ear irradiation, obtain audiogram annually for five years and then every five years. Recommend preferential seating in school, amplification, and hearing aids as indicated. Patients with hearing loss may require speech therapy. Refer to or consult with an otolaryngologist, an audiologist, and/or a neurologist as indicated.
Dental	Any patient who has not developed permanent dentition at the time of cancer therapy Any radiation treatment involving the oral cavity or salivary glands Highest risk: age < 5 years old	Dental abnormalities Tooth/root agenesis Root thinning/shortening Enamel dysplasia	Perform oral examination annually. Recommend dental examination and hygiene every six months. Promote regular fluoride applications. Obtain baseline panorex radiograph prior to dental procedures to evaluate root development.
Cardiovascular	Anthracyclines Cyclophosphamide Targeted agents, particularly trastuzumab Highest risk: • Anthracyclines combined with radiation involving the heart or other cardiotoxic cancer therapy • Female • Black/African race • Age < 5 years old • Comorbid cardiac medical conditions • Doxorubicin > 300 mg/m² • Chest irradiation ≥ 30 Gy	Cardiomyopathy Subclinical cardiomyopathy Valvular damage Arrythmias Coronary artery disease Pericardial damage	Assess cardiac history annually, including SOB, DOE, orthopnea, chest pain, and palpitations. Perform cardiac examination annually. Obtain ECG at baseline and as clinically indicated. Obtain echocardiogram or MUGA scan at baseline and as clinically indicated. Additional cardiac evaluation is indicated prior to or during pregnancy. Refer to a cardiologist as indicated. Consider cardiac medications for clinical or subclinical cardiac disease. Provide patient education regarding prevention of cardiac disease, including maintenance of appropriate weight and blood pressure, regular aerobic exercise, and a heart-healthy diet. Provide anticipatory guidance for symptoms of cardiac dysfunction and the side effects of cardiac medications.
	Carboplatin Cisplatin	Dyslipidemia	Obtain fasting lipid profile at baseline, then as indicated for preventive screening based on age and other risk factors. Consider treatment with statins for patients with dyslipidemia. Provide patient education regarding lipid-lowering strategies such as diet, exercise, and weight loss.

(Continued on next page)

Table 36. Late Effects Associated With Cancer Treatments *(Continued)*

Organ System	Risk Factors	Potential Late Effects	Evaluation/Interventions
Cardiovascular *(cont.)*	Cranial irradiation ≥ 40 Gy	Cerebrovascular dysfunction Stroke	Assess neurologic history annually, including hemiparesis, hemiplegia, weakness, or aphasia. Perform neurologic examination annually. Obtain brain MRI with angiography as indicated. Consult a neurologist or neurosurgeon as indicated. Refer to physical/occupational therapy as indicated.
Endocrine	Radiation to neuroendocrine axis Highest risk: Radiation ≥ 18 Gy	Growth hormone deficiency Metabolic syndrome	Assess nutritional status annually. Perform physical examination every six months until growth is completed and then annually, including height, weight, blood pressure, and BMI. Perform Tanner staging every six months until sexually mature. Obtain thyroid function tests. Obtain fasting blood glucose, serum insulin, and lipid profile every two years in overweight patients, every five years in normal weight patients, and as clinically indicated. Obtain x-ray for bone age in patients with delayed growth. Consult endocrinologist as indicated. Provide patient education regarding health promotion behaviors including maintenance of ideal body weight, exercise, and diet.
Pulmonary	Bleomycin Busulfan BCNU CCNU Highest risk: • BCNU ≥ 600 mg/m² • Busulfan ≥ 500 mg total dose • Bleomycin ≥ 400 units total dose • Combined with chest irradiation or TBI • Chlorambucil • Mitomycin • MTX • Cytarabine • Vinca alkaloids • Alkylating agents • Combination of radiation and radiation-sensitizing chemotherapy • Risk increased with younger age	Pulmonary fibrosis Interstitial pneumonitis Restrictive-obstructive lung disease	Assess pulmonary history annually, including cough, SOB, DOE, and wheezing. Perform pulmonary examination annually. Obtain a chest x-ray at baseline, then as clinically indicated. Perform PFTs, including diffusion capacity at baseline, then as clinically indicated and prior to anesthesia. Perform a CT scan if there is a significantly abnormal PFT result, chest x-ray, and/or clinical symptoms. Prescribe pneumococcal vaccine. Prescribe influenza virus vaccines annually. Refer patient to a pulmonologist as needed. Provide education regarding healthy behaviors, avoidance or cessation of smoking, and maintaining physical conditioning. Treat the patient's symptoms with corticosteroids, bronchodilators, expectorants, antibiotics, and oxygen as needed. Provide anticipatory guidance for those who have received bleomycin regarding the risk of pulmonary failure with high levels of oxygen (such as with general anesthesia or scuba diving).

(Continued on next page)

Table 36. Late Effects Associated With Cancer Treatments (Continued)

Organ System	Risk Factors	Potential Late Effects	Evaluation/Interventions
GI	Doxorubicin Dactinomycin MTX 6-MP RT Abdominal surgery	Fibrosis, strictures, obstruction Enteritis Adhesions Ulcers	Obtain height and weight annually. Obtain stool guaiac on an annual basis, and perform annual rectal examination after the age of 40 years. Obtain a CBC with MCV annually. Obtain blood chemistries annually. Provide anticipatory guidance regarding dietary modification as needed. Refer to or consult a gastroenterologist as needed. Dilate the fibrotic or obstructed area. Obtain radiographic studies as indicated. Educate the patient regarding medication administration and side effects as needed. Educate the patient regarding a high-fiber diet.
Hepatic	BCNU Dactinomycin MTX 6-MP Thioguanine	Abnormal liver function tests Hepatic fibrosis Cirrhosis Veno-occlusive disease	Perform annual physical examination including evaluation of sclera icterus, jaundice, ascites, hepatomegaly, and splenomegaly. Obtain LFTs at baseline and as clinically indicated. Obtain PT to assess synthetic function and hepatitis screen in patients with abnormal LFTs. Screen for viral hepatitis in patients with persistently abnormal liver function or any patient transfused prior to 1993. Recommend hepatitis A and B immunization for patients lacking immunity. Refer to or consult a gastroenterologist as needed. Educate patient about healthy behaviors, as well as avoiding alcohol or other hepatotoxic drugs. Educate patient regarding medication administration and side effects as indicated.
GU	Cyclophosphamide Ifosfamide Pelvic surgery combined with pelvic irradiation Decreased incidence with mesna use Highest risk: • Cyclophosphamide ≥ 3 g/m² • Pelvic irradiation dose ≥ 30 Gy	Hemorrhagic cystitis Bladder fibrosis Dysfunctional voiding Vesicoureteral reflux Hydronephrosis	Assess GU history annually, including hematuria, urinary urgency, frequency, urinary incontinence, dysuria, nocturia, and abnormal urinary stream. Obtain urinalysis annually. Counsel patient to report dysuria or hematuria. Obtain urine culture, spot urine calcium/creatinine ratio, and ultrasound of kidneys and bladder for patients with microscopic hematuria. Refer to nephrology or urology for culture-negative microscopic hematuria AND abnormal ultrasound and/or abnormal calcium/creatinine ratio. Refer to urology for culture-negative macroscopic hematuria.

(Continued on next page)

Table 36. Late Effects Associated With Cancer Treatments *(Continued)*

Organ System	Risk Factors	Potential Late Effects	Evaluation/Interventions
GU *(cont.)*	Cisplatin Ifosfamide Nephrectomy In combination with other nephrotoxic medications (e.g., aminoglycosides, immunosuppressants, etc.) Comorbid conditions: diabetes mellitus, hypertension Highest risk: • Age < 5 years old • Ifosfamide ≥ 60 g/m^2 • Renal irradiation dose ≥ 15 Gy • Cisplatin dose ≥ 200 mg/m^2	Glomerular dysfunction Tubular dysfunction Renal insufficiency	Perform an annual examination including blood pressure, height, and weight. Obtain BUN, SCr, and electrolytes at baseline and as clinically indicated. Obtain a urinalysis annually. Consult a nephrologist or urologist as indicated for patients with hypertension, proteinuria, or progressive renal insufficiency. Patients may require low-protein, low-salt dietary modifications. Patients may require medication for hypertension as indicated. Educate patients regarding kidney health after a nephrectomy, recommend that patients avoid contact sports and maintain hydration, and encourage patients to wear a Medic Alert® bracelet.
Reproductive—testes	Alkylating agents (busulfan, BCNU, chlorambucil, cyclophosphamide, ifosfamide, CCNU, mechlorethamine, melphalan, procarbazine, thiotepa) Carboplatin Cisplatin DTIC Temozolomide Surgery (orchiectomy or peritoneal node dissection) RT to abdomen/pelvis, testes, brain (neuroendocrine axis) Thyroid dysfunction Hormonal therapy Highest risk: • MOPP ≥ 3 cycles • Busulfan ≥ 600 mg/m^2 • Cyclophosphamide ≥ 7.5 g/m^2 • Any alkylating chemotherapy combined with testicular irradiation, pelvic irradiation, or TBI • Age (pubertal males have the highest risk for toxicity, but prepubertal status does not protect from gonadal injury)	Gonadal dysfunction Delayed/arrested puberty Hypogonadism Oligospermia, azoospermia Ejaculatory or other dysfunction Infertility	Assess pubertal history. Assess sexual function. Assess medication use affecting sexual function. Assess Tanner stage annually. Assess testicular volume by Prader orchidometry annually until sexually mature. Obtain LH, FSH, and testosterone levels at age 14 and when clinically indicated for signs of delayed puberty or testosterone deficiency. Obtain thyroxine and TSH levels. Refer to or consult an endocrinologist when necessary. Perform semen analysis as needed. Perform bone densitometry evaluation for osteopenia in hypogonadal patients or patients on hormone cancer therapy. Consider hormone replacement therapy for hypogonadal patients who do not have a history of hormone-sensitive cancer. Consult a reproductive endocrinologist reproductive endocrinology consultation for infertility. Provide anticipatory guidance regarding symptoms of testosterone deficiency or germ cell damage. Provide fertility counseling. Educate the patient regarding performing testicular self-examination. Provide education regarding hormone replacement therapy and side effects, if indicated. Educate patients regarding prevention of osteoporosis and atherosclerosis.

(Continued on next page)

Table 36. Late Effects Associated With Cancer Treatments *(Continued)*

Organ System	Risk Factors	Potential Late Effects	Evaluation/Interventions
Reproductive—ovaries	Alkylating agents (busulfan, BCNU, chlorambucil, cyclophosphamide, ifosfamide, CCNU, mechlorethamine, melphalan, procarbazine, thiotepa) Carboplatin Cisplatin DTIC Temozolomide Hormonal therapy Surgery (oophorectomy) Radiation to abdomen/pelvis, lumbosacral spine, brain (neuroendocrine axis) Highest risk: • MOPP > 3 cycles • Busulfan > 600 mg/m² • Cyclophosphamide > 7.5 g/m² • Alkylators combined with pelvic irradiation or TBI Gonadal function in females is preserved at higher cumulative doses than males.	Gonadal dysfunction Delayed/arrested puberty Oligomenorrhea Amenorrhea Premature menopause Infertility	Assess pubertal history. Assess menstrual/pregnancy history. Assess sexual function. Assess medication use affecting sexual function. Assess Tanner stage annually until sexually mature. Obtain LH, FSH, and estradiol levels at age 13 and when clinically indicated for delayed pubertal development, irregular menses, amenorrhea, or premature menopause. Obtain thyroxine and TSH levels. Perform bone densitometry evaluation for osteopenia in hypogonadal patients and patients on hormonal cancer therapy. Consider hormone replacement therapy for hypogonadal patients who do not have a history of hormone-sensitive cancer. Refer to or consult an endocrinologist when indicated. Refer to a reproductive endocrinologist for infertility evaluation. Provide anticipatory guidance regarding the symptoms of estrogen deficiency and early menopause. Provide fertility counseling and education regarding alternate strategies for parenting. Provide education regarding hormone replacement therapy and prevention of osteoporosis and atherosclerosis. Counsel women at risk for early menopause regarding fertility options. Counsel regarding contraception.

(Continued on next page)

Table 36. Late Effects Associated With Cancer Treatments *(Continued)*

Organ System	Risk Factors	Potential Late Effects	Evaluation/Interventions
Musculoskeletal	Steroids MTX Hormonal therapy Cranial radiation HCT recipients TBI Comorbid conditions: growth hormone deficiency, hypogonadism/delayed puberty, hyperthyroidism Lifestyle factors: inadequate intake of calcium/vitamin D, lack of weight-bearing exercise, smoking, alcohol use Highest risk: • Older age • MTX ≥ 40 g/m² • Prolonged corticosteroid therapy • Combination of corticosteroids and radiation to the bone Vinca alkaloids Amputation	Osteopenia Osteoporosis Avascular necrosis Muscle weakness Functional changes	Assess musculoskeletal history annually, including joint pain, swelling, mobility, and range of motion. Perform musculoskeletal examination annually. Obtain bone densitometry evaluation at baseline and as clinically indicated. Obtain MRI if symptoms of osteonecrosis are present. Consult an orthopedic surgeon if avascular necrosis presents on imaging. Perform physical therapy evaluation as indicated. Consider calcium and vitamin D supplementation. Consider use of bisphosphonates for patients with osteoporosis or high risk of fractures. Refer to endocrinologist as indicated. Make a careful comparison and measurement of irradiated and unirradiated areas. Obtain and plot on growth chart the patient's height, weight, and sitting height measurements annually. Perform radiographic studies of the irradiated area (baseline, yearly during rapid growth, and if normal, then every five years). Refer to or consult an orthopedist as clinically indicated. Encourage a routine physical exercise program for both range of motion and strengthening. Educate the patient about the importance of weight control and exercise. Provide anticipatory guidance regarding realistic expectations about potential growth and function of the affected area, and educate regarding osteoporosis prevention with calcium and vitamin D. Treat exacerbating or predisposing conditions (e.g., hypogonadism).

BCNU—carmustine; BMI—body mass index; BUN—blood urea nitrogen; CBC—complete blood count; CCNU—lomustine; CNS—central nervous system; CT—computed tomography; DOE—dyspnea on exertion; DTIC—dacarbazine; ECG—electrocardiogram; FSH—follicle-stimulating hormone; GI—gastrointestinal; GU—genitourinary; Gy—gray; HCT—hematopoietic cell transplantation; IQ—intelligence quotient; IT—intrathecal; IV—intravenous; LFT—liver function test; LH—luteinizing hormone; MCV—mean corpuscular volume; mg/m²—milligrams per meter squared; MOPP—mechlorethamine, vincristine, procarbazine, prednisone; MTX—methotrexate; MUGA—multigated acquisition; PFT—pulmonary function tests; PT—prothrombin time; RT—radiation therapy; MP—mercaptopurine; SCr—serum creatinine; SOB—shortness of breath; TBI—total body irradiation; TSH—thyroid-stimulating hormone

Note. Portions of this material have been adapted from the Children's Oncology Group *Long-Term Follow-Up Guidelines,* Version 2.0. Used with permission. Also based on information from Carver et al., 2007; Dickerman, 2007.

Table 37. Secondary Malignancies Related to Chemotherapy

Secondary Malignancy	Primary Malignancy Factors	Occurrence	Risk Factors
Leukemia	Breast cancer	Cumulative incidence less than 0.5% at 8–10 years	Alkylating agents (Curtis et al., 2006; Park et al., 2005)
	HD	Peaks 5–10 years after treatment: 0.07%–10% risk RR: 37.5	Risk of leukemia is higher (10% versus 0.7%) with MOPP than ABVD. (van Leeuwen et al., 2000; van Leeuwen & Travis, 2001)
	SCLC	RR: 6.57	Alkylating agents (Curtis et al., 2006)
	NSCLC	RR: 1.47	Alkylating agents (Curtis et al., 2006)
	MM	17% at 50 months	Alkylating agents
	NHL	Overall RR: 8.8 Occurs within 15 years Male: RR: 5.65 Female: RR: 19.89	CHOP (RR: 14.2) ACBVP Carmustine Procarbazine Mechlorethamine (RR: 13.0) Chlorambucil > 1,300 mg (RR: 6.5) (Andre et al., 2004; Curtis et al., 2006; Tward et al., 2007)
	Ovarian cancer	Up to 10 years after therapy	Alkylating agents, including cyclophosphamide, and melphalan Platinum-containing regimens (Curtis et al., 2006)
	Testicular cancer	RR:1.6–6.7 Median time to occurrence: 4.5 years	Etoposide (The risk appears to be increasing since PEB chemotherapy became standard in the 1990s.) (Richiardi et al., 2007; van den Belt-Dusebout et al., 2007)
NHL	HD	Within 5 years of treatment, then risk remains constant or increases over lifetime 25-year cumulative risk: 3.5% RR: 21.5	Risk factors are unclear but may be related to immunosuppression associated with the primary cancer (HD) or with combined chemoradiation treatment. (van Leeuwen et al., 2000; van Leeuwen & Travis, 2001)
Endometrial	Breast cancer	Associated with 35% increased risk	Tamoxifen (Curtis et al., 2006)
Bladder	NHL	Cyclophosphamide: 20–49 g, RR: 6.0 > 50 g, RR: 14.5	Cyclophosphamide > 20 g Radiation (Curtis et al., 2006; Tward et al., 2007)
	Testicular cancer	Median time to occurrence: 20 years RR: 3.9	RT including the iliac lymph nodes (This risk will likely decrease because from the mid-1980s RT has been directed to the para-aortic lymph nodes only.) No study noted increased risk of bladder cancer after chemotherapy alone; however, because PEB is carcinogenic to humans, and platinum is excreted in urine up to 20 years after treatment with PEB chemotherapy, prolonged platinum exposure may play a role in bladder cancer development. (van den Belt-Dusebout et al., 2007)
Brain	ALL	Risk is 17-fold after 5 years.	Cranial irradiation at doses of 18–24 Gy (Curtis et al., 2006)

(Continued on next page)

Table 37. Secondary Malignancies Related to Chemotherapy *(Continued)*

Secondary Malignancy	Primary Malignancy Factors	Occurrence	Risk Factors
Breast	HD	Peak incidence is 10–20 years after treatment ends. 25-year cumulative risk: 16% RR: 5.2	Mantle irradiation at age 40 or younger; risk increases with younger age. No excess risk of breast cancer observed in patients treated > 40 years old Patients treated with salvage chemotherapy had a lower risk of breast cancer than patients treated with initial RT or initial chemotherapy and RT, possibly due to chemotherapy-induced ovarian suppression. (Allan & Travis, 2005; Curtis et al., 2006; van Leeuwen et al., 2000; van Leeuwen & Travis, 2001)
Lung	HD	RR: 7.0 Chemotherapy-associated lung cancer occurs 1–4 years after therapy up to 15 years. Radiation-associated lung cancer occurs 5–9 years after therapy and for more than 20 years.	Thoracic irradiation Risk increases with dose of radiation. Smoking significantly increases risk (60% of lung cancers in HD survivors occur in patients who smoke). Alkylating agents (Allan & Travis, 2005; Curtis et al., 2006; Travis et al., 2002; van Leeuwen et al., 2000; van Leeuwen & Travis, 2001)
	NHL	RR: 1.6–2.45	Male gender Smoking Alkylating agents (Andre et al., 2004; Curtis et al., 2006; Tward et al., 2007)
Thyroid	HD	RR: 15.2	RT (Curtis et al., 2006; van Leeuwen et al., 2000)
Gastrointestinal	HD	RR: 8.4	RT (Dores et al., 2002; van Leeuwen et al., 2000)
	Testicular	RR: 1.27–2.1	RT (Richiardi et al., 2007; van den Belt-Dusebout et al., 2007)
Sarcoma	Breast cancer	RR: 3–6 Latency: 5–10 years	RT (Curtis et al., 2006)
	HD	RR: 12.1 Peak: 10–20 years	RT (Dores et al., 2002; van Leeuwen et al., 2000)
	Hereditary retino-blastoma	RR: 43 Up to 25 years after treatment	RT (Curtis et al., 2006)
	Soft-tissue tumors, neuroblastoma, Ewing sarcoma	Mean latency more than 15 years	RT and alkylating agents (Curtis et al., 2006)
Melanoma	HD	1–4 years after treatment RR: 5.5	May be related to immunosuppression associated with HD (van Leeuwen et al., 2000; van Leeuwen & Travis, 2001)
Head and neck	HD	RR: 9.8 (van Leeuwen et al., 2000)	–
Urogenital	Cervical cancer	10 to > 40 years after treatment	RT (Chaturvedi et al., 2007)
	HD	RR: 3.5 (van Leeuwen et al., 2000)	–

RR (observed cases/expected cases) compares the incidence rate to the baseline incidence rate of that cancer in the general reference population to determine increased (> 1.0) or decreased (< 1.0) risk (Curtis et al., 2006).

ABVD—doxorubicin, bleomycin, vinblastine, dacarbazine; ACBVP—doxorubicin, cyclophosphamide, bleomycin, vindesine, prednisone; ALL—acute lymphocytic leukemia; CHOP—cyclophosphamide, doxorubicin, vincristine, prednisone; Gy—gray; HD—Hodgkin disease; MM—multiple myeloma; MOPP—mechlorethamine, vincristine, procarbazine, prednisone; NHL—non-Hodgkin lymphoma; NSCLC—non-small cell lung cancer; PEB—cisplatin, etoposide, bleomycin; RR—relative risk; RT—radiation therapy; SCLC—small cell lung cancer

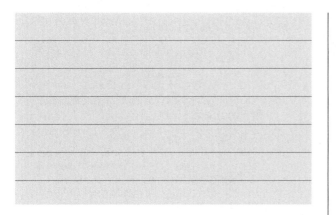

(b) It is not associated with preceding MDS.

(c) Development is associated with chromosomal translocations 11q23, 21q22, and 3q23.

b) Solid tumors, such as sarcomas, breast, lung, skin, and thyroid, generally present 10–20 years after treatment with radiation and alkylating agents.

3. Incidence

a) Cancer survivors have a 14% greater risk of developing another malignancy than the general population with 25 years of follow-up (Curtis et al., 2006).

b) The 25-year cumulative risk of secondary malignancy among survivors of childhood malignancies is 3.5%. Childhood cancer survivors have an eight-fold risk of secondary malignancy during the first 10 years after diagnosis; the risk declines to less than four-fold in 20-year survivors (Curtis et al., 2006).

c) Secondary malignancies are the leading cause of death in people who have survived more than 15 years following childhood cancer (Lawless, Puja, Green, & Mahoney, 2007) as well as in Hodgkin disease survivors (Aleman et al., 2003; Travis et al., 2006).

d) Radiation-induced leukemia and alkylating agent–induced leukemia occur within a few years of treatment, with a peak at 5–10 years, and incidence slowly declines thereafter (van Leeuwen & Travis, 2001).

e) Radiation-induced solid tumors generally are observed at least 5–10 years after treatment (van Leeuwen & Travis, 2001).

4. Patient-related risk factors

a) Age

(1) Younger age at cancer diagnosis increases the risk of developing a secondary malignancy. The risk of developing a subsequent cancer is 6-fold in childhood cancer survivors, 2–3-fold in patients diagnosed at ages 18–39, and 1.2–1.6-fold in patients diagnosed at ages 40–59 (Curtis et al., 2006).

(2) Adolescents appear to be at higher risk than younger patients (Barnard & Woods, 2005; Beaty et al., 1995; Oeffinger et al., 2006).

b) Gender: Overall, females have a slightly higher risk of secondary malignancies than males (Barnard & Woods, 2005; Beaty et al., 1995; Curtis et al., 2006).

c) Exposures (Curtis et al., 2006)

(1) Tobacco and alcohol exposure increase the risk of developing a secondary malignancy to approximately 35% (Curtis et al., 2006).

(2) Caloric excess, a diet low in fruits and vegetables, obesity, and physical inactivity likely contribute to the risk of secondary malignancies involving the upper aerodigestive tract, colon cancer, breast cancer, and cancers of the female reproductive organs (Curtis et al., 2006).

(3) Infections such as HPV, HIV, human herpes virus-8, Epstein-Barr virus, hepatitis B and C, and *Helicobacter pylori* may increase the risk of secondary malignancies.

d) Immunodeficiency increases the risk of secondary malignancies. Immune dysregulation may be associated with primary cancers such as leukemia and lymphoma, or with immunosuppressive treatment.

e) Genetic predisposition: Patients with genetic phenotypes that contributed to the development of their original cancer are at increased risk for a secondary cancer. Examples of genetic phenotypes that increase the susceptibility to a primary or secondary cancer include Fanconi anemia, Cowden disease, *BRCA1*- and/or *BRCA2*-related breast and/or ovarian cancer, and Li Fraumeni syndrome (Travis et al., 2006).

5. Therapy-related risk factors

a) Chemotherapy

(1) Chemotherapy is associated with an increased risk of treatment-related leukemia. There are inconsistent results reported with regard to the influence of radiation on the risk of leukemia in patients treated with chemotherapy (Abrahamsen et al., 2002; van Leeuwen & Travis, 2001).

(2) Combination chemotherapy with drugs possessing different mechanisms of ac-

tion may act synergistically to increase the risk of treatment-related leukemia (van Leeuwen & Travis, 2001).

   (3) Agents with known leukemogenic potential (COG, 2006)

      (a) Alkylating agents

         i) Busulfan

         ii) Carmustine

         iii) Chlorambucil

         iv) Cyclophosphamide

         v) Ifosfamide

         vi) Lomustine

         vii) Mechlorethamine

         viii) Melphalan

         ix) Procarbazine

         x) Thiotepa

      (b) Heavy metals

         i) Cisplatin

         ii) Carboplatin

      (c) Topoisomerase II inhibitors

         i) Epipodophyllotoxins (etoposide, teniposide)

         ii) Anthracyclines

      (d) Nonclassical alkylators

         i) Dacarbazine

         ii) Temozolomide

b) Radiation is associated with a risk of solid tumors that develop within or near the radiation fields and have a latency period of 5–10 years (Abrahamsen et al., 2002; van Leeuwen & Travis, 2001). Increased doses of radiation and alkylating agents are associated with increased risk of secondary malignancies (Allan & Travis, 2005).

6. Risk of secondary malignancy in patients with selected primary cancers

a) Hodgkin disease

   (1) The risk of developing a secondary cancer after treatment for Hodgkin disease is 28% at 25 years, and the overall relative risk is 7.0 (van Leeuwen et al., 2000).

   (2) Patients are at increased risk for AML, NHL, sarcomas, thyroid cancer, liver cancer, melanoma, lung cancer, breast cancer, stomach cancer, colon cancer, cervical cancer, and mouth/pharynx cancer (Curtis et al., 2006; Dores et al., 2002; van Leeuwen et al., 2000).

   (3) The risk of a secondary cancer increases greatly with younger age at the time of treatment, especially for adolescents treated at 15–20 years old (Aleman et al., 2003; Beaty et al., 1995; van Leeuwen et al., 2000).

   (4) Secondary malignancies are the leading cause of death in survivors of Hodgkin disease (Aleman et al., 2003; Travis et al., 2006).

   (5) The median time of increased risk for treatment-related leukemia is 5–10 years after treatment, while the risk of a secondary solid tumor persists more than 25 years (Abrahamsen et al., 2002; Aleman et al., 2003; Dores et al., 2002; van Leeuwen et al., 2000).

   (6) Patients ages 21–30 years at the time of treatment had the greatest risk of secondary AML/MDS, and the risk was greatest 5–10 years after treatment (Aleman et al., 2003).

   (7) There is an increased risk of breast cancer in patients younger than 40 years who were previously irradiated for Hodgkin disease, but not in patients older than 40 years at the time of therapy (van Leeuwen & Travis, 2001).

   (8) Chemotherapy does not appear to increase the risk of solid tumors when given as part of the initial therapy. However, salvage chemotherapy in relapsed patients appears to increase the risk of secondary solid tumors (other than breast cancer) from radiation. The risk of breast cancer is decreased in patients treated with salvage chemotherapy for relapsed disease compared with those treated initially with radiation or chemotherapy and radiation, possibly because of chemotherapy-induced ovarian suppression (Aleman et al., 2003; van Leeuwen et al., 2000).

b) NHL

   (1) The increased relative risk of a secondary cancer in NHL survivors is 1.14–1.47 over the general population

(Tward, Glenn, Pulsipher, Barnette, & Gaffney, 2007).

(2) Patients are at increased risk for AML, sarcomas, bladder cancer, cancers of the head and neck, melanoma, lung cancer, GI cancer, bladder cancer, kidney cancer, Hodgkin disease, and thyroid cancer (Tward et al., 2007).

(3) Chemotherapy increases the risk of AML, lung cancer, and bladder cancer (Tward et al., 2007).

(4) Radiation therapy increases the risk of sarcomas, breast cancer, and mesothelioma (Tward et al., 2007).

(5) Survivors of NHL have an overall significantly decreased risk of breast cancer, prostate cancer, and myeloma (Tward et al., 2007).

(6) The risk of a secondary cancer is greatest for survivors treated at a younger age, especially age < 25 years (Tward et al., 2007; Tward, Wendland, Shrieve, Szabo, & Gaffney, 2006).

c) Testicular cancer

(1) Testicular cancer survivors have a 1.7-fold increased risk for secondary malignancies compared to the general population (Richiardi et al., 2007; van den Belt-Dusebout et al., 2007).

(2) They have an increased risk of cancers of organs located in irradiated sites such as the stomach, gallbladder and bile ducts, pancreas, bladder, kidney, and thyroid; and soft-tissue sarcoma; nonmelanoma skin cancer; and chemotherapy-induced AML (Richiardi et al., 2007; van den Belt-Dusebout et al., 2007).

(3) Chemotherapy increases the risk of radiation-associated secondary malignancies (van den Belt-Dusebout et al., 2007).

(4) The risk of secondary malignancies increases with younger age at time of treatment (van den Belt-Dusebout et al., 2007).

(5) The median time to occurrence of secondary malignancy is 20 years (van den Belt-Dusebout et al., 2007).

d) Cervical cancer (Chaturvedi et al., 2007)

(1) Cervical cancer survivors have an increased risk for HPV-related cancers (of the pharynx, genital sites, and rectum/anus) and smoking-related cancers (of the pharynx, trachea/bronchus/lung, pancreas, and urinary bladder).

(2) Patients with cervical cancer treated with radiotherapy, but not those who did not receive radiotherapy, were at increased risk for all secondary cancers and cancers at heavily irradiated sites (colon, rectum/anus, urinary bladder, ovary, and genital sites) beyond 40 years of follow-up compared with women in the general population (Curtis et al., 2006).

(3) The 40-year cumulative risk of any secondary cancer was 22% among women diagnosed with cervical cancer before age 50 and 16% for those diagnosed after age 50.

e) Breast cancer: Breast cancer survivors are at increased risk for cancers of the salivary gland, esophagus, stomach, colon, breast, uterine corpus, ovary, and thyroid; sarcoma; melanoma; and AML (Curtis et al., 2006).

f) Pediatric malignancies

(1) The primary cause of death in five-year childhood cancer survivors is relapse of their malignancy (Barnard & Woods, 2005).

(2) Childhood cancer survivors are diagnosed with a secondary malignancy at a median age of 27 years, with a median elapsed time of 15 years to develop cancer in the genitourinary system (35%), head and neck area (32%), GI tract (23%), and other sites (10%) (Bassal et al., 2006).

(3) Risk of a secondary malignancy is significantly elevated following all childhood diagnoses except CNS neoplasms and is highest following neuroblastoma and soft-tissue sarcoma. In particular, survivors of neuroblastoma have a 329-fold increased risk of renal cell carcinomas; survivors of Hodgkin disease have a 4.5-fold increased risk

of GI carcinomas; and survivors of soft-tissue sarcoma, neuroblastoma, and leukemia have a significantly elevated risk of head and neck carcinoma (Bassal et al., 2006).

(4) The risk of treatment-related AML/MDS is 7.92, with a median time to diagnosis of six years (Barnard & Woods, 2005).

(5) Childhood soft-tissue sarcoma survivors are at an increased risk for AML, cutaneous melanoma, female breast cancer, sarcomas of the bone and soft tissue, and cancers of the oral cavity (Cohen, Curtis, Inskip, & Fraumeni, 2005).

(6) Childhood acute lymphocytic leukemia survivors have a five-fold risk of developing a secondary cancer at five years, particularly cancers of the brain, thyroid, buccal cavity (especially salivary gland), and bone and AML. The risk is greatest (17-fold) for survivors of brain cancers (Curtis et al., 2006).

g) HSCT recipients

(1) HSCT recipients are at risk for secondary solid tumors, treatment-related leukemia/MDS, and post-transplant lymphoproliferative disorders (Baker et al., 2003; Forrest et al., 2003).

(2) The risk of a post-transplant malignancy increases with younger age at time of transplant, especially for those younger than 10 years (Baker et al., 2003; Bhatia et al., 2001).

(3) The relative risk of thyroid carcinoma is 3.26 overall, with a significantly increased risk associated with age < 10 years, radiation, female gender, and chronic GVHD (Cohen et al., 2007).

7. Pathophysiology

a) Chemotherapy and radiotherapy cause DNA damage, which is the mechanism that leads to cell death. However, if nonlethal DNA damage occurs, then DNA repair is critical to prevent the development of a secondary cancer (Allan & Travis, 2005).

(1) Alkylating agents transfer an alkyl group to DNA, causing DNA mismatch and inhibition of DNA replication and transcription. A DNA mismatch repair mechanism is responsible for repairing this cell damage; otherwise, apoptosis occurs. If cells survive with dysfunctional DNA mismatch repair or genomic instability, this may lead

to malignancy (Allan & Travis, 2005; Tward et al., 2007).

(2) Topoisomerase inhibitors cause double-stranded DNA breaks, which lead to apoptosis. If the cell survives, these DNA breaks may cause chromosomal translocations of the mixed lineage leukemia gene or other crucial transforming genes that can lead to leukemia (Allan & Travis, 2005; Tward et al., 2007).

(3) Radiotherapy may induce DNA mutations that result in chromosomal aberrations or other genetic instability that, over time, may lead to malignancy (Tward et al., 2007).

b) Chemotherapy and radiotherapy interact with other factors such as tobacco use, genetic makeup, hormonal status, and immune function, which may contribute to the risk of developing a secondary cancer (Allan & Travis, 2005).

D. Collaborative management

1. Comprehensive survivorship care (COG, 2006; Hewitt et al., 2005; Oeffinger & McCabe, 2006): Patients completing primary treatment should be provided with a comprehensive care summary and follow-up plan that is clearly and effectively explained. This "Survivorship Care Plan" should be written by the principal provider(s) who coordinated oncology treatment. The care plan should summarize critical information needed for the survivor's long-term care.

a) Summary of cancer treatment

(1) Date of diagnosis

(2) Survivor's age at diagnosis

(3) Names of all chemotherapy agents and doses received

(4) All radiation field(s) and total radiation dose (in Gy) to each field (For chest,

thoracic spine, and upper abdominal radiation, include age at first dose.)
(5) Names of all relevant surgical procedures
(6) Names of all other therapeutic modalities
(7) Complications related to cancer treatment
   b) Potential long-term effects of cancer treatment
   c) Specific information about the timing and content of recommended follow-up
   d) Recommendations regarding preventive practices and how to maintain health and well-being
   e) Information on legal protections regarding employment and access to health insurance
   f) The availability of psychosocial services in the community
2. Models of survivorship care (Oeffinger & McCabe, 2006)
   a) Consultative model: Primary oncology team refers survivor for a one-time visit in long-term follow-up clinic where a comprehensive survivorship care plan is developed.
   b) Nurse practitioner (NP)-led survivor clinic: Survivors are transitioned to the care of the survivor NP who shares care of the survivor with the primary care physician. The NP and primary care physician communicate regularly, and the NP provides details of the patient's cancer history and patient-specific recommendations for follow-up care.
   c) Specialty multidisciplinary clinic: Modeled after pediatric long-term follow-up clinics, these clinics employ a team consisting of physicians, oncology NPs, social workers, psychologists, administrators, and a network of consulting physicians trained in the care of cancer survivors. NPs play a central role in the coordination and delivery of care.

E. Preventive screening recommendations
   1. Irradiated skin and soft tissues should be thoroughly evaluated and reassessed for the life of the patient.
   2. Survivors should follow adult cancer screening recommendations. This is especially important for childhood cancer survivors who have an additional risk for developing adult cancers prematurely.
   3. Women who have been treated with mantle-field irradiation should perform breast self-examination on a monthly basis at the time of puberty, and medical breast examination should be performed annually. Annual mammograms should begin eight years after irradiation (van Leeuwen & Travis, 2001).
   4. Patients should be counseled regarding smoking cessation (Curtis et al., 2006).
   5. Discuss weight management and exercise regimens with all cancer survivors.

F. Patient and family education
   1. Provide information about the treatment and potential late effects related to disease and treatment received.
   2. Explain the risks of secondary malignancy, the typical time to onset, signs and symptoms of secondary cancers, and the importance of follow-up visits.

G. Professional education
   1. Educate primary care professionals who may be working with survivors after the survivors are no longer followed by an oncologist. A survivorship plan that includes potential long-term effects of treatment and recommended follow-up is helpful for primary providers who may be unfamiliar with cancer and its treatments.
   2. Ensure that healthcare providers have the same information about secondary malignancies as do the patients and that they are aware of recommended follow-up.

H. Nursing assessment (see Table 36)
   1. Obtain history.
      a) Chemotherapy, surgery, and radiation received
      b) Toxicities experienced during therapy
      c) Physical and psychosocial systems
      d) Preexisting diseases that may exacerbate effects or contribute to synergistic effects of long-term effects or secondary malignancies
   2. Perform physical examination.

3. Review results of laboratory tests including CBC, blood chemistry panel, and urinalysis.
4. Review results of imaging studies as indicated (e.g., chest x-ray, bone densitometry).
5. Review results of pulmonary function tests and ECG as indicated.

References

Abrahamsen, A.F., Andersen, A., Nome, O., Jacobsen, A.B., Holte, H., Abrahamsen, J.F., et al. (2002). Long-term risk of second malignancy after treatment of Hodgkin's disease: The influence of treatment, age and follow-up time. *Annals of Oncology, 13*(11), 1786–1791.

Aleman, B.M.P., van den Belt-Dusebout, A.W., Klokman, W.J., van't Veer, M.B., Bartelink, H., & van Leeuwen, F.E. (2003). Long-term cause-specific mortality of patients treated for Hodgkin's disease. *Journal of Clinical Oncology, 21*(18), 3431–3439.

Allan, J.M., & Travis, L.B. (2005). Mechanisms of therapy-related carcinogenesis. *Nature Reviews. Cancer, 5*(12), 943–955.

American Cancer Society. (2008). *Cancer facts and figures, 2008.* Atlanta, GA: Author.

Andre, M., Mounier, N., Leleu, X., Sonet, A., Brice, P., Henry-Amar, M., et al. (2004). Second cancers and late toxicities after treatment of aggressive non-Hodgkin lymphoma with the ACVBP regimen: A GELA cohort study on 2837 patients. *Blood, 103*(4), 1222–1228.

Aslett, H., Levitt, G., Richardson, A., & Gibson, F. (2007). A review of long-term follow-up for survivors of childhood cancer. *European Journal of Cancer, 43*(12), 1781–1790.

Aziz, N.M., & Rowland, J.H. (2003). Trends and advances in cancer survivorship research: Challenge and opportunity. *Seminars in Radiation Oncology, 13*(3), 248–266.

Baker, K.S., DeFor, T.E., Burns, L.J., Ramsay, N.K.C., Neglia, J.P., & Robison, L.L. (2003). New malignancies after blood or marrow stem-cell transplantation in children and adults: Incidence and risk factors. *Journal of Clinical Oncology, 21*(7), 1352–1358.

Barnard, D.R., & Woods, W.G. (2005). Treatment-related myelodysplastic syndrome/acute myeloid leukemia in survivors of childhood cancer—An update. *Leukemia and Lymphoma, 46*(5), 651–663.

Bassal, M., Mertens, A.C., Taylor, L., Neglia, J.P., Greffe, B.S., Hammond, S., et al. (2006). Risk of selected subsequent carcinomas in survivors of childhood cancer: A report from the childhood cancer survivor study. *Journal of Clinical Oncology, 24*(3), 476–483.

Beaty, O., III, Hudson, M.M., Greenwald, C., Luo, X., Fang, L., Wilimas, J.A., et al. (1995). Subsequent malignancies in children and adolescents after treatment for Hodgkin's disease. *Journal of Clinical Oncology, 13*(3), 603–609.

Bhatia, S., Louie, A.D., Bhatia, R., O'Donnell, M.R., Fung, H., Kashyap, A., et al. (2001). Solid cancers after bone marrow transplantation. *Journal of Clinical Oncology, 19*(2), 464–471.

Carver, J.R., Shapiro, C.L., Ng, A., Jacobs, L., Schwartz, C., Virgo, K.S., et al. (2007). American Society of Clinical Oncology clinical evidence review on the ongoing care of adult cancer survivors: Cardiac and pulmonary late effects. *Journal of Clinical Oncology, 25*(25), 3991–4008.

Chaturvedi, A.K., Engels, E.A., Gilbert, E.S., Chen, B.E., Storm, H., Lynch, C.F., et al. (2007). Second cancers among 104,760 survivors of cervical cancer: Evaluation of long-term risk. *Journal of the National Cancer Institute, 99*(21), 1634–1643.

Children's Oncology Group. (2006). *Long-term follow-up guidelines for survivors of childhood, adolescent and young adult cancers.* Version 2.0-March 2006. Retrieved January 15, 2008, from http://www.survivorshipguidelines.org/pdf/LTFUGuidelines.pdf

Cohen, A., Rovelli, A., Merlo, D.F., van Lint, M.T., Lanino, E., Bresters, D., et al. (2007). Risk for secondary thyroid carcinoma after hematopoietic stem-cell transplantation: An EBMT Late Effects Working Party study. *Journal of Clinical Oncology, 25*(17), 2449–2454.

Cohen, R.J., Curtis, R.E., Inskip, P.D., & Fraumeni, J.F. (2005). The risk of developing second cancers among survivors of childhood soft tissue sarcoma. *Cancer, 103*(11), 2391–2396.

Curtis, R.E., Freedman, D.M., Ron, E., Ries, L.A.G., Hacker, D.G., Edwards, B.K., et al. (Eds.). (2006). *New malignancies among cancer survivors: SEER cancer registries, 1973–2000* (NIH Pub. No. 05-5302). Bethesda, MD: National Cancer Institute.

Dickerman, J.D. (2007). The late effects of childhood cancer therapy. *Pediatrics, 119*(3), 554–568.

Dores, G.M., Metayer, C., Curtis, R.E., Lynch, C.F., Clarke, E.A., Glimelius, B., et al. (2002). Second malignant neoplasms among long-term survivors of Hodgkin's disease: A population-based evaluation over 25 years. *Journal of Clinical Oncology, 20*(16), 3484–3494.

Forrest, D.L., Nevill, T.J., Naiman, S.C., Le, A., Brockington, D.A., Barnett, M.J., et al. (2003). Second malignancy following high-dose therapy and autologous stem cell transplantation: Incidence and risk factor analysis. *Bone Marrow Transplantation, 32*(9), 915–923.

Hewitt, M., Greenfield, S., & Stovall, E. (Eds.). (2005). *From cancer patient to cancer survivor: Lost in transition.* Washington, DC: National Academies Press. Retrieved January 15, 2008, from http://www.nap.edu/catalog.php?record_id=11468

Lawless, S.C.W., Puja, V., Green, D.M., & Mahoney, M.C. (2007). Mortality experiences among 15+ year survivors of childhood and adolescent cancers. *Pediatric Blood and Cancer, 48*(3), 333–338.

Oeffinger, K.C., & McCabe, M.S. (2006). Models for delivering survivorship care. *Journal of Clinical Oncology, 24*(32), 5117–5124.

Oeffinger, K.C., Mertens, A.C., Sklar, C.A., Kawashima, T., Hudson, M.M., Meadows, A.T., et al. (2006). Chronic health conditions in adult survivors of childhood cancer. *New England Journal of Medicine, 355*(15), 1572–1582.

Park, M.J., Park, Y.H., Ahn, H.J., Choi, W., Paik, K.H., Kim, J.M., et al. (2005). Secondary hematological malignancies after breast cancer chemotherapy. *Leukemia and Lymphoma, 46*(8), 1183–1188.

Richiardi, L., Scélo, G., Boffetta, P., Hemminki, K., Pukkala, E., Olsen, J.H., et al. (2007). Second malignancies among survivors of germ-cell testicular cancer: A pooled analysis between 13 cancer registries. *International Journal of Cancer, 120*(3), 623–631.

Travis, L.B., Gospodarowicz, M., Curtis, R.E., Clarke, E.A., Andersson, M., Glimelius, B., et al. (2002). Lung cancer following chemotherapy and radiotherapy for Hodgkin's disease. *Journal of the National Cancer Institute, 94*(3), 182–192.

Travis, L.B., Rabkin, C.S., Brown, L.M., Allan, J.M., Alter, B.P., Ambrosone, C.B., et al. (2006). Cancer survivorship—Genetic susceptibility and second primary cancers: Research strategies and recommendations. *Journal of the National Cancer Institute, 98*(1), 15–25.

Tward, J., Glenn, M., Pulsipher, M., Barnette, P., & Gaffney, D. (2007). Incidence, risk factors, and pathogenesis of second malignancies in patients with non-Hodgkin lymphoma. *Leukemia and Lymphoma, 48*(8), 1482–1495.

Tward, J.D., Wendland, M.M., Shrieve, D.C., Szabo, A., & Gaffney, D.K. (2006). The risk of secondary malignancies over 30 years after the treatment of non-Hodgkin lymphoma. *Cancer, 107*(1), 108–115.

van den Belt-Dusebout, A.W., de Wit, R., Gietema, J.A., Horenblas, S., Louwman, M.W.J., Ribot, J.G., et al. (2007). Treatment-specific risks of second malignancies and cardiovascular disease in 5-year survivors of testicular cancer. *Journal of Clinical Oncology, 25*(28), 4370–4378.

van Leeuwen, F.E., Klokman, W.J., van't Veer, M.B., Hagenbeek, A., Krol, A.D.G., Vetter, U.A.O., et al. (2000). Long-term risk of second malignancy in survivors of Hodgkin's disease treated during adolescence or young adulthood. *Journal of Clinical Oncology, 18*(3), 487–497.

van Leeuwen, F.E., & Travis, L.B. (2001). Second cancers. In V.T. DeVita Jr., S. Hellman, & S.A. Rosenberg (Eds.), *Cancer: Principles and practice of oncology* (6th ed., pp. 2939–2964). Philadelphia: Lippincott Williams & Wilkins.

IX. Nursing Education and Management

A. The clinical practicum
1. Course description: The clinical practicum allows the nurse to apply the knowledge gained in the didactic component to direct patient care situations. Emphasis is placed on the clinical skills that a nurse must demonstrate prior to being considered competent to administer chemotherapy and biotherapy (see Appendices 5 and 6).
2. Course objectives: At the completion of the clinical practicum, the nurse will be able to
   a) Demonstrate proficiency regarding the safe preparation, storage, transport, handling, spill management, administration, and disposal of chemotherapy drugs and equipment.
   b) Identify appropriate physical and laboratory assessments for specific chemotherapy agents.
   c) Demonstrate skill in venipuncture, including vein selection and sterile technique.
   d) Demonstrate skill in the care and use of various VADs.
   e) Identify patient and family education needs in relation to specific chemotherapy agents.
   f) Identify acute local or systemic reactions as a result of extravasation or anaphylaxis in association with specific chemotherapy drugs, and appropriate interventions.
   g) Demonstrate proficiency in the safe administration of chemotherapy and disposal of chemotherapy wastes and equipment.
   h) Verbalize knowledge of institutional policies and procedures regarding chemotherapy administration.
   i) Document pertinent information in the medical record.
3. Clinical activities
   a) The nurse should be supervised by a qualified preceptor to ensure safe practice.
   b) The preceptor and the nurse should establish specific objectives at the beginning of the clinical practicum. Ideally, the nurse and the preceptor should select a specific population of patients, and the nurse should assume responsibility for planning the care for these patients with supervision by the preceptor.
   c) The length of time spent in the supervised clinical practicum should be individualized depending on the nurse's ability and skill in meeting the specific objectives and institutional standards.
   d) After the nurse becomes proficient and independent in administering nonvesicants,

progression to vesicant administration can occur.
   e) The nurse should verbalize to the preceptor potential adverse reactions, side effects, toxicities, and measures to prevent and/or manage these reactions.
   f) Various clinical settings can be used for the nurse to demonstrate knowledge of chemotherapy administration. It may not be realistic for all settings or agencies to provide onsite chemotherapy education and training. Alternative methods should be used, such as
      (1) Contracting with major institutions to credential nurses for specific needs (e.g., vesicant, nonvesicant, IV push, short infusion, continuous infusion)
      (2) Creating a simulated lab to substitute for the clinical component when patients are not available.
4. Evaluation: An evaluation tool based on the practicum course objectives should be used to determine
   a) The nurse's knowledge of chemotherapy drugs and the associated nursing implications
   b) The nurse's knowledge of the necessary technical skills required for the administration of chemotherapy agents (e.g., venipuncture, VAD access and management, indwelling catheter management)
   c) The nurse's knowledge of patient and family education, which should be initiated based on the chemotherapy administered
   d) The nurse's knowledge of steps to be taken in the event of an untoward response following chemotherapy administration (e.g., anaphylaxis, hypersensitivity reaction, extravasation).
5. Following successful completion of the clinical practicum, the nurse should complete a skills inventory to demonstrate his or her ability to perform the four criteria described herein. This can be done in a simulated setting (e.g., skills lab) or as a precepted experience in the clinical setting. It is recommended that the learner administer at least three chemotherapy agents under the supervision of trained personnel. Two should be administered by IV push—the first should be a nonvesicant agent, the second should be a vesicant agent.
6. Annual education and competency evaluation is recommended. Educational content should, at a minimum, emphasize any new information available. Methods for evaluation may include but are not limited to clinical observation, quality improvement studies, chart audits, compe-

tency checklist, attendance at an educational program, literature review, and testing.

B. Policy and procedure
1. Policies help to promote standardization of practice within an institution. They provide an operational framework for organizational goals and objectives and may be required by regulatory and/or accrediting agencies. Procedures commonly outline the steps needed to accomplish a task (Scott & Harris, 2005).
2. Once a policy is implemented, it is imperative that it is enforced and followed by staff. Individuals can be held liable if patient harm results from a policy not being followed; institutions are liable if a policy is not followed by their staff. Consider staff in units outside of hematology/oncology. Are nurses administering hazardous drugs in obstetrics/gynecology or rheumatology? How is this addressed in your policy?
3. Interdisciplinary staff involvement is recommended when creating an antineoplastic policy and procedure. Input from pharmacy, medicine, nursing, and other departments will result in a more comprehensive policy.
4. Topics that may be included in an antineoplastic policy are drug administration, safety checks, disposal, home care, medical surveillance for staff, mixing, medication orders (e.g., who can write them, rounding volumes, format), PPE, linen handling, spill management, staff exposure to hazardous drugs, staff education, extravasation, documentation, storage, and transportation.
5. To maintain safety, it is important to accurately identify the patient prior to antineoplastic administration. Unique patient identifiers to be used are frequently standardized by the institution and may include the individual's name; date of birth; medical record number; account, visit, or admission number; photograph; and social security number. Many institutions will incorporate this data on a wristband that may be read or scanned electronically. Caution should be used when verifying patient identification with an identifier that can be easily changed, such as bed or chair number or a phone number.

C. Issues in antineoplastic administration affect nursing practice and patient safety. How these topics are addressed on an institutional level may vary. Some of the more recent issues are identified below.
1. *Vincristine:* The inadvertent administration of vincristine into the subarachnoid space (IT administration) has resulted in a number of tragic deaths around the world. Recent publications from JCAHO (2005) and WHO (2007) have prompted institutions to reevaluate their preparation and delivery of vincristine and of IT medications in general (Institute for Safe Medication Practices, 2006). A multidisciplinary review of the process of drug preparation and administration is advised. Several recommendations have been made to safeguard patients from receiving vincristine intrathecally.
   a) Both JCAHO and WHO recommended that vincristine and other vinca alkaloids be diluted and administered via a minibag. Opponents to this approach have cited the risk of extravasation, as many institutions have policies against the administration of vesicant chemotherapy by minibag into a peripheral IV line. Some centers in which these drugs are now administered by minibag require infusion through a CVC. Please see recommendations for administration of short IV infusions in the "Administration" portion of this text (page 101).
   b) Vincristine **must** be clearly labeled. WHO (2007) recommends "FOR INTRAVENOUS USE ONLY – FATAL IF GIVEN BY OTHER ROUTES." JCAHO (2005) recommends "FATAL IF GIVEN INTRATHECALLY. FOR IV USE ONLY. DO NOT REMOVE COVERING UNTIL MOMENT OF INJECTION," with each syringe inside an overwrap carrying the same label warning.
   c) Special procedures should be followed for the administration of IT medications: IT medications should be prepared in the pharmacy as closely as possible to the time of administration (JCAHO, 2005). Unique packaging and delivery to a separate location can further help to prevent errors.

d) Prior to the administration of all antineoplastic medications, it is recommended that the drug, dose, and route be independently verified by at least two qualified healthcare professionals.

2. *Antineoplastic medications administered outside the oncology areas:* It is the position of ONS that all RNs who administer and/or care for patients receiving chemotherapy should receive specialized education, including a didactic component and a practicum. See the ONS position on "The Education of the RN Who Administers and Cares for the Individual Receiving Chemotherapy and Biotherapy" in Appendix 7. This position applies to antineoplastic drugs regardless of route, indication, or setting.

a) All nurses should be knowledgeable about the drugs they administer; the mode of action, side effects, and toxicity; dosage range, rate, and route of excretion; potential responses; and interactions with other medications and foods.

b) Institutional policy should address the antineoplastic medication educational plan for nurses working within their facility. Some staff may require drug- or disease-specific education, whereas others will require comprehensive education for all antineoplastic medications.

3. *IC document:* With the exception of clinical trials, where IC is required for participation, each institution determines its own practice related to how and if a patient must provide written IC before receiving antineoplastic medications. **Note: It is good nursing practice to receive the patient's verbal affirmation that he or she would like to receive treatment before beginning the administration of chemotherapy at every treatment visit.** It is important to maintain consistency between policy and practice throughout the institution. Several approaches have been used and are noted below.

a) The general hospital "consent to treat" serves as the signed permission to provide antineoplastic medications.

b) A consent form designed specifically for the administration of antineoplastic medications is signed and part of the medical record.

c) Some centers use a general procedure consent form for antineoplastic medications.

d) A specific form is not signed, but consent is documented within the medical record.

D. Documentation
1. Consent document (see Appendix 8)
2. Flow sheets (see Appendices 1 and 2)
3. Extravasation flow sheet (see Appendix 9)
4. Competency checklist (see Appendices 5 and 6)

References

Institute for Safe Medication Practices. (2006, February 23). *IV vincristine survey shows safety improvements needed.* Retrieved July 6, 2008, from http://www.ismp.org/Newsletters/acutecare/articles/20060223.asp

Joint Commission on Accreditation of Healthcare Organizations. (2005, July 14). *Preventing vincristine administration errors. Sentinel Event Alert, Issue 34.* Retrieved July 6, 2008, from http://www.jointcommission.org/SentinelEvents/SentinelEventAlert/sea_34.htm

Scott, M.L., & Harris, J.Y. (2005). Organizational design and structure. In M.M. Gullatte (Ed.), *Nursing management: Principles and practice* (pp. 77–91). Pittsburgh, PA: Oncology Nursing Society.

World Health Organization. (2007, July 18). *Information exchange system alert no. 115, QSM/MC/IEA.115.* Retrieved July 6, 2008, from http://www.who.int/medicines/publications/drugalerts/Alert_115_vincristine.pdf

Appendix 1. Nursing Flow Sheet[a]

Name _____ Age _____ Diagnosis _____

Allergies _____

Medical problems _____

Date					
RN signature					
Type of visit					
VAD					
VAD flush					
Comments					
Vesicant location 1–5 R/L					
Reactions					
Mucositis 0–3					
Infection					
Rx					
Resolved					
Alopecia 0–3					
Bleeding Y/N					
Comments					
Diarrhea # episodes/24 hours					
Rx					
Constipation # BM/d/wk					
Normal/abnormal (N/ABNL)					
Rx					
Bladder symptoms 0–5					
Rx					
Relief Y/N					
Pain Y/N					
Sites					
Intensity 0–10					
Characteristics					
Analgesics					
Relief 0–10					
Relief adequate Y/N					
Comments					

[a]As used at Yale-New Haven Hospital, New Haven, CT

(Continued on next page)

Appendix 1. Nursing Flow Sheet[a] *(Continued)*

Date					
Insomnia Y/N					
Rx					
Rx effective Y/N					
Fatigue 0–10					
Nausea severity 0–3					
Vomiting # episodes/24 hours					
Duration					
Antiemetic relief					
Comments					
Appetite 0–4					
Diet 1–5					
Supplements, amount/24 hours					
Altered taste Y/N					
Other					
Cough Y/N					
Productive Y/N					
Rx					
Relief 1,2					
SOB 0–3					
O_2 specify					
Sexual difficulties 0–3					
Mobility 1–4					
Motor weakness 0–3					
Neuropathy 0–3					
Comments					
Anxiety 0–3					
Coping effectiveness Y/N					
Rx					
Counseling Y/N					
Homecare agency (specify)					
VNA/hospice					
HHA/homemaker					
Social services					
Patient education 1–7					
Education materials					
Other					

(Continued on next page)

Appendix 1. Nursing Flow Sheet[a] *(Continued)*

Nursing Flow Sheet Key

Date	
RN Signature	
Type of visit	P = Phone C = Clinic
VAD	P = Port H = Hickman
VAD flush	Check, specify heparin amount.
Comments	Note difficulty drawing blood, etc.
Vesicant location	1–5, see diagram R = right/L = left

Antecubital Space

2	Ventral Proximal Forearm		Dorsal Proximal Forearm	4
1	Ventral Distal Forearm		Dorsal Distal Forearm	3
			Dorsum of Hand	5

Reactions	Describe discomfort, burning, urticaria localized, follows vein path, entire extremity, phlebitis, extravasation (requires note), necrosis
Mucositis	0 = Absent 1 = Soreness 2 = Ulcerations, can eat 3 = Ulcerations, can't eat
Infection	Specify candida, herpes, bacteria, other.
Rx	Medication
Resolved	Check
Alopecia	0 = None 1 = Thinning 2 = 50% loss 3 = Complete hair loss
Bleeding	Y = Yes N = No
Comments	Specify sites
Diarrhea episodes	#/24 hours
Rx	Medication
Relief	Y = Yes N = No
Constipation	# BM/day/week
Normal/Abnormal	Above pattern normal for patient or not
Rx	Medication
Relief	Y = Yes N = No
Bladder symptoms	0 = None 1 = Dysuria 2 = Frequency 3 = Hematuria 4 = Incontinence 5 = Oliguria
Rx	Medication
Relief	Y = Yes N = No
Pain	Y = Yes N = No
Sites	
Intensity	0 = No pain–10 = worst pain imaginable
Characteristics	C = Constant I = Intermittent
Analgesics	Medication, schedule
Relief	0 = No relief–10 = Complete relief
Relief adequate	Y = Yes N = No

(Continued on next page)

Appendix 1. Nursing Flow Sheet[a] *(Continued)*

Nursing Flow Sheet Key	
Insomnia	Y = Yes N = No
Rx	Medication
Rx effective	Y = Yes N = No
Fatigue	0 = Quite rested–10 = Completely exhausted
Nausea severity	0 = None 1 = Mild 2 = Moderate 3 = Severe
Vomiting episodes	# vomiting episodes/24 hrs.
Duration	# hrs. after chemo vomiting started/stopped (e.g.,+3/+18)
Antiemetic relief	1 = Adequate 2 = Inadequate
Comments	
Appetite	0 = None 1 = 25% normal 2 = 50% normal 3 = 75% normal 4 = 100%
Diet	1 = Solids 2 = Liquids 3 = Soft 4 = 1,2 + Supplements 5 = Supplements
Supplements	Specify type and amount/24 hrs.
Altered taste	Y = Yes N = No
Comments	
Cough	Y = Yes N = No
Productive	Y = Yes N = No
Rx	Medication
Relief	1 = Adequate 2 = Inadequate
SOB	0 = None 1 = Mild 2 = Moderate 3 = Severe
O_2	Specify liter flow.
Sexual difficulties	0 = None 1 = Mild dysfunction 2 = Moderate dysfunction 3 = Severe limitations
Mobility	1 = Ambulatory 2 = Ambulatory with assist 3 = Wheel chair 4 = Bedridden
Motor weakness	0 = None 1 = Mild 2 = Moderate 3 = Severe
Neuropathy	0 = None 1 = Paresthesias, numbness/tingling feet and/or fingers 2 = Slapping gait, ataxia 3 = Visual, auditory disturbances
Comments	Location, etiology of muscle weakness, etc.
Anxiety	0 = None 1 = Mild 2 = Moderate 3 = Severe
Coping effectiveness	Y = Yes N = No
Rx	Medication
Counseling	Y = Yes N = No
Homecare agency	Specify name of agency, date initiated and discharged.
VNA/hospice	Check
HHA/homemaker	Check, note hrs./day or week
Social services	Check
Patient education	1 = Chemo side effects 2 = Symptom management 3 = Emergency 4 = Homecare resources 5 = Community 6 = Coping 7 = Specify
Education materials	Pamphlets or brochures given, videos used, etc.
Other	Other (e.g., complaints, problems, appliances [ostomies, trach, etc.])

Note. From "A Nursing Flow Sheet for Documentation of Ambulatory Oncology," by J.M. Moore and M.T. Knobf, 1991, *Oncology Nursing Forum,18*(5), pp. 933–939. Copyright 1991 by Oncology Nursing Society. Reprinted with permission.

Appendix 2. Chemotherapy Flow Sheet[a]

Rx: Antitumor Drugs and Dose (Meds, Rt, etc.)	Date							
	Day on study							
	Course							
	Dose							
	Transfusion							
Symptoms	Performance							
	Pain							
	Food intake							
	Vomiting							
	Diarrhea/constipation							
	Bleeding							
	Mucosa							
	Respiratory							
	Urinary							
	CNS							
	Weight							
Physical Findings	Temperature/respiration							
	Blood pressure/pulse							
	Skin/mouth							
	Breast/nodes							
	Chest							
	Heart							
	Abdomen							
	Liver/spleen							
	Neurologic							
	Rectal							
	Status							
Tumor Measurement	1.							
	2.							
	3.							
	4.							
Laboratory	WBC							
	Neutrophils							
	Lymphocytes							
	Monocytes							
	Hgb HCT							
	Retics							
	Platelets							
	BUN CREAT							
	Uric AC CA++							
	SGOT LDH							
	ALKP'TASE							
	BILI T/D							
	CEA							
	Radiology							
	Initials							

[a] As used at Beth Israel Deaconess Hospital in Boston, MA

Study _____ MR# _____

DX _____

Page _____ of Study _____

Continued remarks on reverse

Age _____

Height _____

M^2 _____

Weight (lb/kg) _____

(Continued on next page)

Appendix 2. Chemotherapy Flow Sheet[a] *(Continued)*

Administration	Date						
	IV site						
	Needle type and size						
	Adverse reaction						
	Treatment schedule: drug and adminstration method						
Patient Teaching	Instructions per institutional instruction sheet for:						
	1. Nausea/vomiting						
	2. Myelosuppression						
	3. Mouth						
	Self-care measures per institutional standards						
	Acknowledgment of initial teaching (patient signature)						
Nursing Observations/Assessments/Management							
	Nurse:						
	I = Initial teaching R = Reviewed W = Written materials P = See progress note N/A = Not applicable S = Side effects verbalized or reported						
Key	RN			RN		RN		RN
	RN			RN		RN		RN

Note. From "Flowsheet Documentation of Chemotherapy Administration and Patient Teaching," by M. Lynch and L. Yanes, 1991, *Oncology Nursing Forum, 18*(4), pp. 777–783. Copyright 1991 by the Oncology Nursing Society. Adapted with permission.

Appendix 3. Safe Management of Chemotherapy in the Home

You are receiving chemotherapy to treat your cancer. You must take special precautions to prevent the chemotherapy from coming into accidental contact with others. This document teaches you and your family how to avoid exposure to chemotherapy and how to handle the waste from the chemotherapy in your home.

Chemotherapy Drugs Are Hazardous
Chemotherapy drugs are hazardous. Equipment or items that come into contact with the medicines (such as syringes, needles) are considered contaminated. Regardless of how you take the medications, chemotherapy remains in your body for many hours and sometimes days after your treatment. Your body eliminates the chemotherapy in urine and stool. Traces of chemotherapy also may be present in vomit.

Disposal of Hazardous Drugs
Materials contaminated with chemotherapy must be disposed of in specially marked containers. You will be given a hard plastic container labeled "Chemotherapy Waste" or a similar warning. Place equipment and gloves that have been in contact with chemotherapy into this container after use. If the waste is too large to fit in the plastic container, place it in a separate plastic bag and seal it tightly with rubber bands. Place sharp objects in the hard plastic container. The company supplying your medicines and equipment will tell you who will remove the waste containers.

Body Wastes
You may use the toilet (septic tank or sewer) as usual. Flush twice with the lid closed for 48 hours after receiving chemotherapy. Wash your hands well with soap and water afterward, and wash your skin if urine or stool gets on it. Pregnant women should avoid direct contact with chemotherapy or contaminated waste.

Laundry
Wash your clothing or linen normally unless they become soiled with chemotherapy. If that happens, put on gloves and handle the laundry carefully to avoid getting drug on your hands. Immediately place the contaminated items in the washer and wash as usual. Do not wash other items with chemotherapy-soiled items. If you do not have a washer, place soiled items in a plastic bag until they can be washed.

Skin Care
Chemotherapy spilled on skin may cause irritation. If this happens, thoroughly wash the area with soap and water, then dry. If redness lasts more than one hour or if irritation occurs, call your doctor. To prevent chemotherapy from being absorbed through the skin, wear gloves when working with chemotherapy, equipment, or waste.

Eye Care
If any chemotherapy splashes into your eyes, flush them with water for 10–15 minutes and notify your doctor.

Questions and Answers
Is it safe for family members to have contact with me during my chemotherapy?
Yes. Eating together, enjoying favorite activities, hugging, and kissing are all safe.

Is it safe for my family to use the same toilet as I do?
Yes. As long as any chemotherapy waste is cleaned from the toilet, sharing is safe.

What should I do if I do not have control of my bladder or bowels?
Use a disposable, plastic-backed pad, diaper, or sheet to absorb urine or stool. Change immediately when soiled, and wash skin with soap and water. If you have an ostomy, your caregiver should wear gloves when emptying or changing the bags. Discard disposable ostomy supplies in the chemotherapy waste container.

What if I use a bedpan, urinal, or commode?
Your caregiver should wear gloves when emptying body wastes. Rinse the container with water after each use, and wash it with soap and water at least once a day.

What if I vomit?
Your caregiver should wear gloves when emptying the basin. Rinse the container with water after each use, and wash it with soap and water at least once a day.

Is it safe to be sexually active during my treatment?
Ask your doctor or your nurse this question. It is possible that traces of chemotherapy may be present in vaginal fluid and semen for up to 48 hours after treatment. Special precautions may be necessary.

How should I store chemotherapy at home?
Store chemotherapy and equipment in a safe place, out of reach of children and pets. Do not store chemotherapy in the bathroom, as high humidity may damage the drugs. Check medicine labels to see if your chemotherapy should be kept in the refrigerator or away from light. Be sure all medicines are completely labeled.

(Continued on next page)

Appendix 3. Safe Management of Chemotherapy in the Home *(Continued)*

Is it safe to dispose of chemotherapy in the trash?
No. Chemotherapy waste is hazardous and should be handled separately. If you are receiving IV chemotherapy at home, you should have a special waste container for the chemotherapy and equipment. This includes used syringes, needles, tubing, bags, cassettes, and vials. This container should be hard plastic and labeled "Hazardous Waste" or "Chemotherapy."

Can I travel with my chemotherapy?
Yes. Usually, traveling is no problem. However, because some chemotherapy requires special storage (such as refrigeration), you may need to make special arrangements. Check with your nurse, doctor, or medicine supplier for further instructions. Regardless of your means of travel (airplane, car, or other), always seal your chemotherapy drugs in a plastic bag.

What should I do if I spill some chemotherapy?
You will have a spill kit if you are receiving IV chemotherapy at home. In the event of a chemotherapy spill, open the spill kit and put on two pairs of gloves, the mask, gown, and goggles. Absorb the spill with the disposable sponge. Clean the area with soap and water. Dispose of all the materials—including gloves, mask, gown, and goggles—in the chemotherapy waste container.

Note. Based on information from International Agency for Research on Cancer. (2007). *Overall evaluations of carcinogenicity to humans.* Retrieved November 8, 2007, from http://monographs.iarc.fr/ENG/Classification/crthall.php

Appendix 4. Extravasation

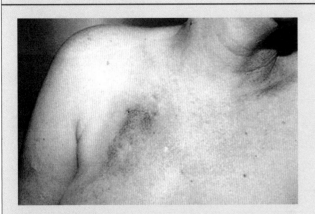

Photo 1. Erythema of site of port extravasation of doxorubicin (February 14)

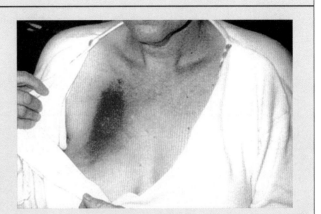

Photo 2. Skin necrosis begins (February 28).

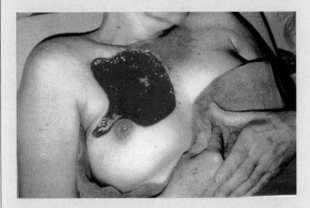

Photo 3. Area of extravasation following debridement (March 18)

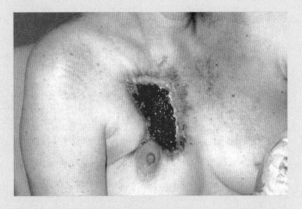

Photo 4. Outer areas of debrided area are granulating (June 5).

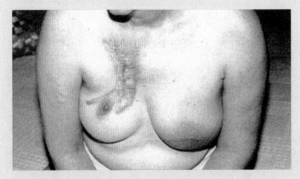

Photo 5. Ten months following extravasation, the area has healed and scars have formed (December 10).

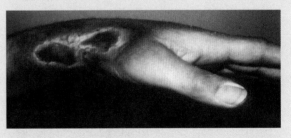

Photo 6. Severe Tissue Necrosis Secondary to Vesicant Extravasation

Note. Photos 1–5 from "Chemotherapy Extravasation From Implanted Ports," by L. Schulmeister and D. Camp-Sorrell, 2000, *Oncology Nursing Forum, 27*(3), p. 534. Copyright 2000 by Oncology Nursing Society. Reprinted with permission. Photo 6 courtesy of Rita Wickham, RN, PhD, AOCN®. Used with permission.

Appendix 5. Clinical Practicum Evaluation: Part I

Cancer Chemotherapy Administration Competency Record

Name _____

Chemotherapy-competent RN evaluators must validate competency on three occasions. Administer at least one vesicant under supervision.

RN Evaluators	Date	Drugs Administered

PRIOR TO ADMINISTRATION		Initials	
1. Coordinates time of administration with pharmacy and others as needed.			
2. Verifies that consent for treatment is signed.			
3. Checks that laboratory values are within acceptable parameters and reports results to MD/NP as needed.			
4. Verifies that original order is transcribed correctly.			
5. Recalculates BSA and drug doses.			
6. Checks chemotherapy order for drug, dose, schedule, and route.			
7. Verifies that patient education, premedication, prehydration, and other preparations are completed.			
ADMINISTRATION			
1. Compares original order to delivered drug (checks with pharmacist or RN).			
2. Verifies patient identification.			
3. Applies gloves and gown and uses safe-handling precautions.			
4. Verifies adequacy of venous access and appropriate IV-site selection.			
5. Checks IV patency and flushes line with 5–10 cc NS.			
6. Demonstrates safe administration:			
• Pushes through side arm, or at hub closest to patient; checks patency every 3–5 cc (or less if working with pediatric patients).			
• Ensures appropriate rate of administration.			
• Flushes between drugs.			
7. Demonstrates appropriate monitoring/observation for specific acute drug effects.			
8. Verbalizes appropriate action in the event of extravasation.			
9. Verbalizes appropriate action in the event of hypersensitivity reaction.			
AFTER ADMINISTRATION			
1. Flushes line with at least 5–10 cc NS.			
2. Appropriately removes device or flushes/maintains VAD.			
3. Disposes of chemotherapy waste according to procedure.			
4. Documents medications, education, and patient response.			
5. Communicates post-treatment considerations to patient, family members, and appropriate personnel.			

Appendix 6. Clinical Practicum Evaluation: Part II

Check the appropriate column to indicate whether the nurse performs the listed activities at a satisfactory level. If the nurse has not had the opportunity to carry out a particular activity, check the N/A (not applicable) column. Under Comments, provide examples of how the nurse met each objective or performed each activity.

	Yes	No	N/A
1. Participates in interdisciplinary care planning with physicians, nurses, and other healthcare professionals (e.g., home care or dietary workers). Comments:			
2. Anticipates complications of chemotherapy and takes action to prevent or minimize the complications. Comments:			
3. Involves the patient and family in care planning and attempts to establish interventions specific to the individual needs of the patient. Comments:			
4. Instructs the patient about hair and scalp care and takes measures to minimize hair loss and preserve body image. Comments:			
5. Reviews laboratory indices and gives a myelosuppressed patient correct information about conserving energy and taking precautions against infection and bleeding. Comments:			
6. Identifies patients at risk for stomatitis and instructs them about oral hygiene and preventive measures. Comments:			
7. Demonstrates knowledge of the use of drug therapy, relaxation, and diversional therapies in the prevention and management of nausea and vomiting. Comments:			
8. Instructs the patient about the prevention and management of gastrointestinal complications (e.g., constipation, diarrhea). Comments:			
9. Identifies and takes nursing action to prevent or manage potential or actual allergic reactions. Comments:			
10. Takes appropriate precautions in the preparation, handling, and disposal of chemotherapy. Comments:			
11. Demonstrates knowledge and skill in the assessment, management, and follow-up care of extravasation. Comments:			
12. Demonstrates skill in assessing the patient's need for a venous access device and knows the factors to be considered in selecting one type of device over another for a particular patient. Comments:			
13. Demonstrates knowledge of research trials by participating in data collection, drug administration, patient education, and follow-up. Comments:			

Appendix 7. Oncology Nursing Society Position on the Education of the RN Who Administers and Cares for the Individual Receiving Chemotherapy and Biotherapy

Specialized education and preparation of the RN who administers chemotherapy and biotherapy can ensure a safe level of care for the individual receiving these agents. Educational standards for oncology nurses are outlined in the *Standards of Oncology Nursing Education: Generalist and Advanced Practice Levels* (Oncology Nursing Society [ONS], 2003). Educational programs on chemotherapy and biotherapy offered by ONS include the Chemotherapy and Biotherapy Course, Cancer Chemotherapy and Biotherapy Renewal Course, Chemotherapy and Biotherapy Update, and Chemotherapy and Biotherapy Trainer Course (ONS, 2007). In addition, ONS provides up-to-date resources pertaining to new treatments using a variety of ongoing educational approaches. Guidelines and recommendations for oncology nurses providing chemotherapy and biotherapy are described in the *Core Curriculum for Oncology Nursing* (Itano & Taoka, 2005) and *Chemotherapy and Biotherapy Guidelines and Recommendations for Practice* (Polovich, White, & Kelleher, 2005). These publications describe the basic clinical content necessary to provide didactic information regarding the safe and competent administration of cytotoxic and biologic drugs. Successful completion of didactic learning must be followed by the successful completion of a clinical practicum under the auspices of an RN's institution or supporting agency.

It Is the Position of ONS That
- All curricula and syllabi developed for RNs administering chemotherapy and biotherapy include current and evidence-based content regarding
  - Principles of cancer chemotherapy and biotherapy
  - Types and classifications of chemotherapy and biotherapy
  - Pharmacology of cytotoxic and immunologic agents in cancer care
  - Chemotherapy and biotherapy indications in cancer care
  - Chemotherapy and radiotherapy protectants
  - Principles of safe preparation, storage, labeling, and disposal of chemotherapeutic and biologic agents
  - Proper use of personal protective equipment
  - Administration procedures, including administration schedule, dose, and route, as well as correct patient documentation
  - Monitoring patients receiving chemotherapy and biotherapy
  - Patient education on chemotherapy and biotherapy side effects and related symptom management
  - Post-treatment care and late and long-term effects, including psychosocial aspects of survivorship.

References
Itano, J.K., & Taoka, K.N. (Eds.). (2005). *Core curriculum for oncology nursing* (4th ed.). St. Louis, MO: Elsevier Saunders.

Oncology Nursing Society. (2003). *Standards of oncology nursing education: Generalist and advanced practice levels* (3rd ed.). Pittsburgh, PA: Author.

Oncology Nursing Society. (2007). *Treatment: Chemotherapy and biotherapy.* Retrieved May 25, 2007, from http://www.ons.org/ceCentral/treatment/chemo/index.shtml

Polovich, M., White, J.M., & Kelleher, L.O. (Eds.). (2005). *Chemotherapy and biotherapy guidelines and recommendations for practice* (2nd ed.). Pittsburgh, PA: Oncology Nursing Society.

Approved by the ONS Board of Directors 1992; revised 7/97, 6/99, 11/02, 7/05, 10/07.

Appendix 8. Consent Document

Consent for Treatment

Patient Name:_____ Date: _____

Diagnosis: _____

Medications: _____

Possible side effects may include any of the following or a combination of the following:

Allergic-like reactions	Skin and nail darkening	Risk of infection
Anemia	Skin ulceration at injection site	Menopausal symptoms
Fatigue	Skin rash	Menstrual irregularities
Constipation	Light sensitivity	Sterility
Diarrhea	Numbness or tingling	Dizziness
Loss of appetite	Hearing loss	Forgetfulness
Mouth sores	Heart damage	Secondary malignancy
Nausea or vomiting	Kidney damage	Muscle aching or weakness
Weight gain or loss	Low platelet count causing bleeding	
Liver damage	Low white blood cell count	
Hair loss		

Unexpected side effects may occur in addition to those noted above. Chemotherapy can be harmful to an unborn child. It is important to tell the doctor if I think I may be pregnant. It is important for both men and women who are being treated with chemotherapy and who are sexually active and fertile and who have a fertile partner to use a reliable form of birth control (birth control pills, a reliable barrier method, or a hormonal implant as recommended by your physician). **In rare instances, cancer treatment can cause life-threatening complications and death.**

_____ **(Patient Initials) A nurse has provided and reviewed with me written information on the drugs I will receive. I HAVE HAD THE CHANCE TO ASK ANY QUESTIONS ABOUT THE ABOVE DRUGS AND AM SATISFIED WITH THE INFORMATION PROVIDED.**

My doctor and nurse have explained my treatment plan in detail. My doctor has also discussed with me other methods of treating this disease and the risks and benefits of treatment. There is no guarantee that this treatment will give me the same results that other patients have received. If I change my mind and decide to stop treatment at any time, my doctor will continue to provide for my care in the future.

I have read the above information and understand the possible risks and benefits of the recommended treatment plan. I agree to accept the treatment and authorize Dr. _____ and his/her designated nurse to carry out the treatment plan.

Patient signature: _____ Date: _____

I have explained the expected response, side effects, and possibility of risks of the listed drugs to the above named patient.

Physician signature: _____

Nurse signature: _____

Appendix 9. Extravasation Flow Sheet

Chemotherapy Drug Extravasation Record

Patient: _____ Date of infiltration: _____ Time: _____ Today's date: _____

Drug: _____ Dilution (mg/ml): _____ Amount infiltrated _____

Vascular access	Infusion method	Pretreatment assessment
____ Peripheral IV Location:_____ ____ PICC ____ Implanted port Needle size and length:_____ ____ Tunneled catheter ____ Other	____ Side-arm infusion with IV running freely ____ Direct IV push ____ Minibag infusion ____ Continuous infusion Infusion pump used? ☐ Yes ☐ No	Location: _____ Type and size of needle/catheter: _____ _____ Description and quality of blood return: _____ _____ Comments: _____ ** Attach timed and dated photograph of site**

Description
Include topical cooling/heating applied, treatments, antidotes used, measurements of site, edema, and/or redness. Assess extremity for range of motion and discomfort with movement.

S: (Patient's symptoms) _____

O: (Observations – attach photo)_____

A: (Assessment) _____

P: (Treatment) _____

Physician notified: _____ Instructions: _____

Comments: _____

Consultations:

____ Plastic Surgery   Date: _____
____ Physical Therapy Date: _____
____ Other: _____

Follow-up:

Include return appointments, patient instructions on skin assessment, temperature monitoring, and reporting of pain.

Notes: _____

Signature: _____ Date: _____

Index

The letter f *after a page number indicates that relevant content appears in a figure; the letter* t, *in a table.*
NOTE: Most treatment medications are listed by their generic names. For brand-name equivalents, please see table on pages xii–xiii.

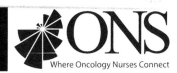
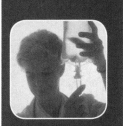

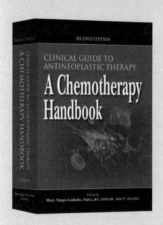
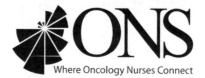